J. Tung

Presented to: _____

From: _____

NUTRITION
DURING
INFANCY

EDITORS

REGINALD C. TSANG, M.D.
Professor of Pediatrics, and Obstetrics and Gynecology
The David G. & Priscilla R. Gamble Professor of Neonatology
Director, Perinatal Research Institute
University of Cincinnati Medical Center
Children's Hospital Medical Center
Cincinnati, Ohio

BUFORD L. NICHOLS, M.D.
Professor of Pediatrics and Physiology
Head, Section of Nutrition and Gastroenterology
Department of Pediatrics
Scientific Director, Children's Nutrition Research Center
Baylor College of Medicine
Houston, Texas

HANLEY & BELFUS, INC. / Philadelphia
The C.V. Mosby Company / St. Louis • Toronto • London

Publisher: HANLEY & BELFUS, INC.
210 S. 13th Street
Philadelphia, PA 19107

North American and worldwide sales and distribution:
THE C.V. MOSBY COMPANY
11830 Westline Industrial Drive
St. Louis, MO 63146

In Canada: THE C.V. MOSBY COMPANY
5240 Finch Avenue East
Unit 1
Scarborough, Ontario M1S 4P2

The front cover illustration is a drawing by Pablo Picasso, 1904, Mother and Child and Four Studies of Her Right Hand (detail), black crayon on tan wove paper, 338 x 267 mm (1965.318 recto). Courtesy of The Harvard University Art Museums (Fogg Art Museum). Bequest of Meta and Paul J. Sachs.

NUTRITION DURING INFANCY   ISBN 0-932883-09-5

Last digit is the print number: 9 8 7 6 5 4

CONTENTS

CONTENTS

CONTRIBUTORS

William F. Balistreri, M.D.
Dorothy M. M. Kersten Professor of Pediatrics; Director, Division of Pediatric Gastroenterology and Nutrition; Children's Hospital Medical Center, University of Cincinnati College of Medicine, Cincinnati, Ohio

Sandra J. Bartholmey, Ph.D.
Nutrition Specialist, Gerber Products Company, Fremont, Michigan

Helen K. Berry
Director of Metabolic Disease Center/Basic Science Research, Children's Hospital Foundation, Cincinnati, Ohio

Nancy F. Butte, Ph.D.
Research Assistant Professor, Department of Pediatrics, Baylor College of Medicine, Houston, Texas

Clare E. Casey, Ph.D.
MacRobert Lecturer in Human Nutrition, Department of Medicine & Therapeutics, University of Aberdeen, Aberdeen, Scotland

David A. Cook, Ph.D.
Vice President, Food, Nutrition and Development, Mead Johnson Nutritional Group, Evansville, Indiana

Angel Cordano, M.D., M.P.H.
Director, Pediatric Nutrition, Mead Johnson Nutritional Group, Evansville, Indiana

Peter R. Dallman, M.D.
Professor of Pediatrics, University of California, San Francisco, San Francisco, California

Cutberto Garza, M.D., Ph.D.
Professor, Department of Pediatrics, Baylor College of Medicine, Texas Children's Hospital, Houston, Texas

Frank R. Greer, M.D.
Associate Professor of Pediatrics, University of Wisconsin—Madison, Madison, Wisconsin

Steven J. Gross, M.D.
Associate Professor of Pediatrics, State University of New York Health Science Center, Syracuse, New York

Margit Hamosh, Ph.D.
Professor of Pediatrics; Chief, Developmental Biology and Nutrition, Georgetown University Medical Center, Washington, District of Columbia

James W. Hansen, M.D., Ph.D.
Director, Pediatric Research, Mead Johnson Nutritional Group, Evansville, Indiana

Malcolm A. Holliday, M.D.
Professor of Pediatrics, University of California, San Francisco, California

Judy M. Hopkinson, Ph.D.
Research Instructor, Department of Pediatrics, Baylor College of Medicine, Houston, Texas

Leonard I. Kleinman, M.D.
Professor of Pediatrics; Director of Newborn Services, School of Medicine, State University of New York at Stony Brook, Stony Brook, New York

Winston W.K. Koo, M.B.B.S., FRACP
Assistant Professor of Pediatrics, University of Alberta; Staff Neonatologist, University of Alberta Hospital, Edmonton, Alberta, Canada

Abner H. Levkoff, M.D.
Professor of Pediatrics/Neonatology, Medical University of South Carolina, Charleston, South Carolina

Carlos H. Lifschitz, M.D.
Assistant Professor of Pediatrics, Baylor College of Medicine, Houston, Texas

John M. Lorenz, M.D.
Assistant Professor of Pediatrics, School of Medicine, State University of New York at Stony Brook, Stony Brook, New York

Stanley G. Miguel, Ph.D.
Nutrition Scientist, Liaison, Mead Johnson Nutritional Group, Evansville, Indiana

Kathleen J. Motil, M.D., Ph.D.
Assistant Professor of Pediatrics, Baylor College of Medicine, Houston, Texas

Buford L. Nichols, M.D.
Professor of Pediatrics and Director, Children's
Nutrition Research Center, Baylor College of
Medicine and Texas Children's Hospital,
Houston, Texas

William B. Pittard, III, M.D.
Associate Professor of Pediatrics/Neonatol-
ogy; Director of Neonatology, Medical University of South Carolina, Charleston, South
Carolina

George A. Purvis, Ph.D.
Vice President, Research and Development,
Gerber Products Company, Fremont, Michigan

Richard J. Schanler, M.D.
Assistant Professor of Pediatrics, Baylor College of Medicine and Texas Children's Hospital, Houston, Texas

Terri A. Slagle, M.D.
Fellow in Neonatology, State University of
New York Health Science Center, Syracuse,
New York

Bonny L. Specker, Ph.D.
Assistant Professor of Pediatrics and Biosta-
tistics/Epidemiology, University of Cincinnati
College of Medicine, Cincinnati, Ohio

John W. Suttie, Ph.D.
Professor of Biochemistry, University of
Wisconsin—Madison, Madison, Wisconsin

Reginald C. Tsang, M.D.
Professor of Pediatrics, and Obstetrics and
Gynecology; The David G. & Priscilla R. Gam-
ble Professor of Neonatology; Director, Divi-
sion of Neonatology; and Director, Perinatal
Research Institute, University of Cincinnati
School of Medicine and Children's Hospital
Medical Center, Cincinnati, Ohio

Philip A. Walravens, M.D.
Associate Clinical Professor of Pediatrics, Uni-
versity of Colorado Health Sciences Center,
Denver, Colorado

John C. Waterlow, M.D., Sc.D., FRCP, FRS
Emeritus Professor of Human Nutrition, Lon-
don School of Hygiene & Tropical Medicine,
University of London, London, England

Richard D. Zachman, Ph.D., M.D.
Professor of Pediatrics and Affiliate Professor
of Nutritional Sciences, University of Wisconsin Perinatal Center, Madison, Wisconsin

PREFACE

The art of nutrition dates back to antiquity; the science of nutrition has existed only for a few centuries. This book is an attempt to combine both the art and science of nutrition. The authors have taken on the challenge of communicating with nutritionists, nurses, pediatricians, and residents by producing a nutrition book that is informative, readable, entertaining, and, at times, provocative.

The book is a truly cooperative venture; authors were given opportunities to critique all manuscripts at a two-day intense session of "brainstorming."

Rather than traditional introductory remarks (which few persons read), we have chosen to introduce the book with a series of drawings by Dr. Wilhelm Camerer. Dr. Camerer's drawings illustrate the beginning of pediatric nutrition as a scientific discipline one hundred years ago. Born in 1842, Camerer unquestionably was one of the pioneers in scientific pediatric nutrition. Based on the data he gathered while conducting metabolic balance studies on his own five children, he published, in 1896, an important treatise on "Metabolism and Energy Requirements of Childhood From Birth to Maturation." It is reported that he carried out the chemical analyses in the kitchen of his home. He spent many years studying the composition of human milk and charting the growth of 283 infants during their first year of life.

This collection of drawings was first presented at a meeting of the German Academy of Pediatrics in Stuttgart, in September 1906.

REGINALD C. TSANG, M.D., Cincinnati, Ohio
BUFORD L. NICHOLS, M.D., Houston, Texas

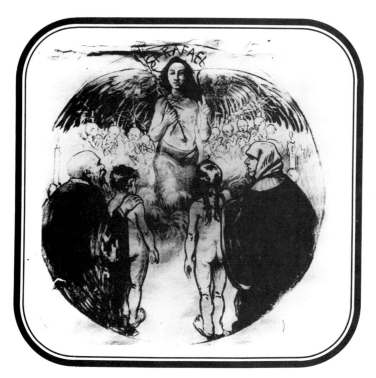

In this picture, Camerer, a Swabian knight, points out the high infant mortality that existed at the time of the birth of pediatric nutrition.

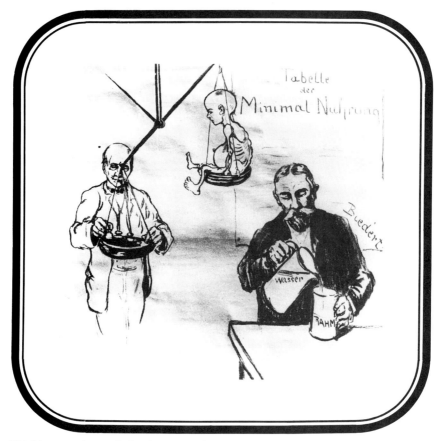

Weighing a malnourished infant. Note the infant's distended abdomen. Biedert, an early pediatrician, is mixing a formula composed of water and cream.

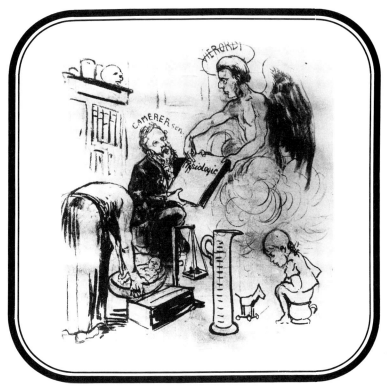

In this self-portrait, Camerer is pictured learning human physiology from Professor C. Vierordt at the Physiological Institute of the University of Tübingen in 1866. Camerer's wife is also depicted here, weighing one of their five children, while one of the other children collects samples for balance studies.

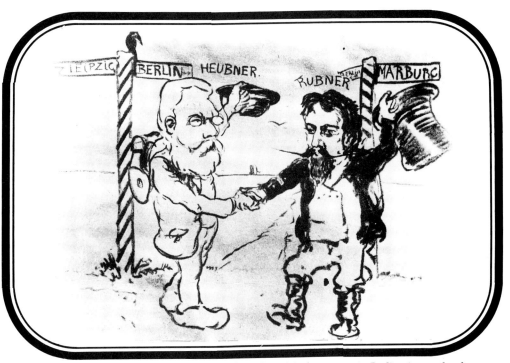

Otto Heubner from Leipzig and Max Rubner from Marburg meet in Berlin. As new faculty members associated with the Charity Hospital in Berlin, they collaborated on a report that contained information on the first quantitative investigations of infant energy metabolism, in 1898 and 1899.

In the next three sketches, Camerer introduces the three schools of German pediatrics: first, the school founded in Leipzig by Wunderlich, represented by Heubner; second, the school that was founded in Prague by Ritter von Rittershain, as personified by Keller; and third, the Munich school founded by Hauner and identified by Moro and Hamburger.

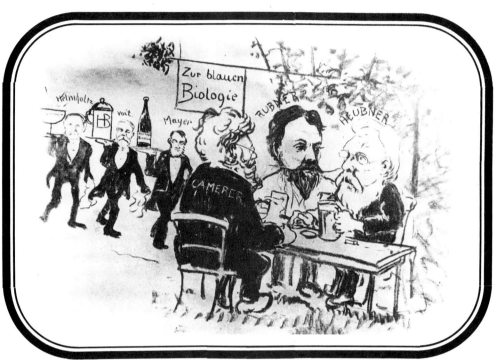

Camerer, Rubner, and Heubner meet at the biology tavern where they are waited on by the great geniuses of physiology, nutrition, and biochemistry: Helmholtz, Voit, and Mayer. This sketch represents the intellectual birth of scientific pediatric nutrition. Many early United States scientists trained under these scientific leaders.

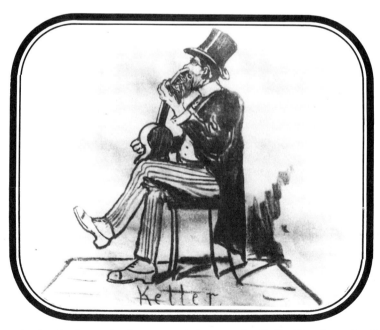

Keller trained at Breslau under Czerny, and also moved to Berlin. The picture implies that he lacks an adequate understanding of and interest in nutritional metabolism.

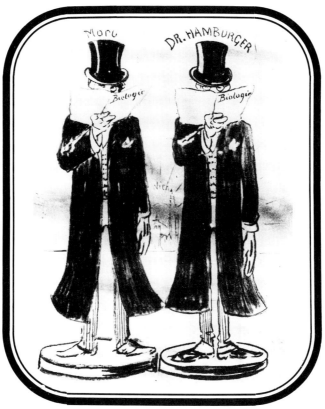

Camerer introduces two additional pediatricians, both from Munich: Moro and Hamburger. In this sketch, both are studying biology.

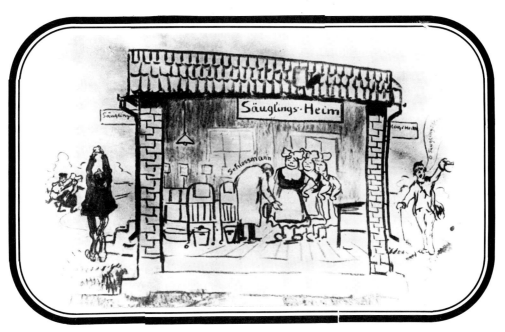

The Infants' Home. The doctor on the right is singing about the joys of working in the infants' ward, while Dr. Arthur Schlossmann of Düsseldorf (center) is shown welcoming three wet nurses. He anticipates a liter of milk from each. To the left, Dr. Schlossmann is greatly dismayed when one of the wet nurses leaves with her sweetheart. This scenario depicts the uncertainty over the supply of donated human milk, which leads to the next phase of pediatric nutrition.

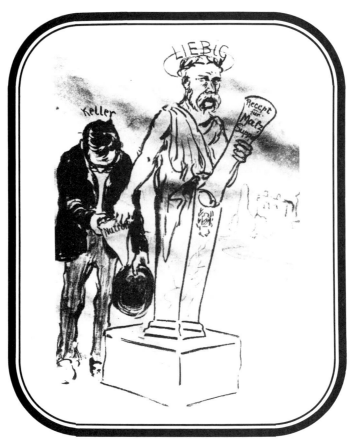

Justus von Liebig, the venerated founder of the science of nutrition, is immortalized here in a statue complete with a halo about his head. In his left hand is the recipe for maltsoup, a partially hydrolyzed starch used in the first stage of beer-making and recommended as a food for infants in 1866. Many heralded this publication as the founding of scientific artificial infant-feeding. Liebig was a scientific grandchild of Lavoisier, and the first to study the composition of human milk. In this picture, Keller contributes a pinch of sodium bicarbonate to the maltsoup, which improved its acceptability to infants.

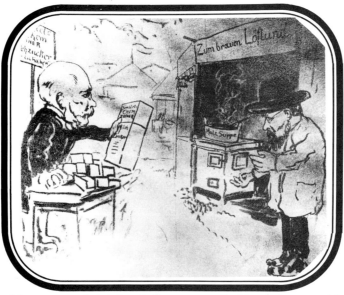

Two pediatricians promote their infant-feeding concepts. Soxhlet, the inventor of the method for terminal sterilization of infant formulas, promotes lactose and sucrose. Loflund is promoting various maltsoup preparations.

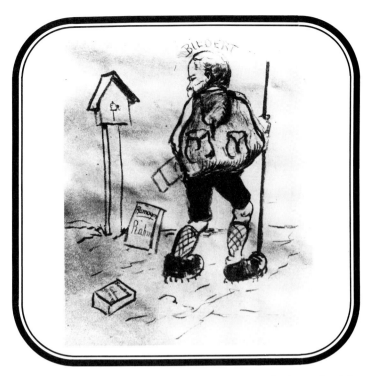

Biedert, who had studied with Leibig, is reintroduced. He was the first pediatrician to promote the theory that cow's milk casein was less digestible than human milk protein. In this picture, he derides the emphasis on carbohydrate and promotes an infant formula made with cream.

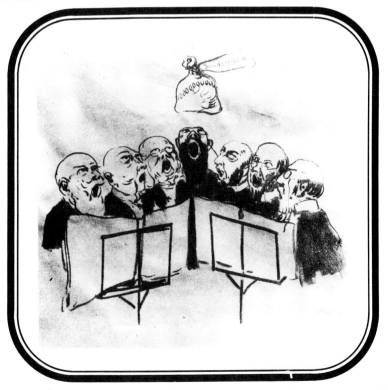

The industrialists are introduced. They discuss the uncertain qualities of mother's milk, and they rely on the unknown professor "Willig" to provide a testimonial that their formulas have miraculous powers. The Board of Directors sings the praise of formulas for their economic value, gazing at the purse of money that dangles over their heads.

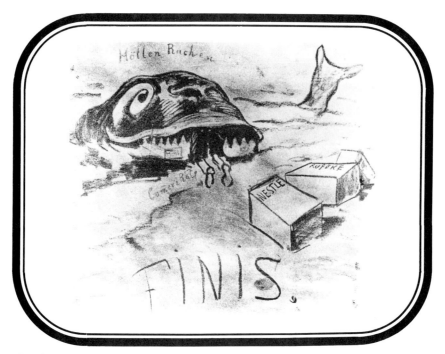

The whale of commercialism swallows the pediatrician. The Society of Pediatrics sings the epilogue extoling honesty and honor in their profession.

ACKNOWLEDGEMENTS

The editors are grateful to Mr. Stanley Coffman and his team of artists at the University of Cincinnati College of Medicine for providing most of the artistic renditions which make this text particularly interesting. Many thanks are due to Linda Belfus, publisher, for her personal interest and involvement in the design and production of this book. Mrs. Lyn Price was most helpful in editing the text and in improving the style of presentation. Mrs. Shirley Sizemore efficiently coordinated the review process for the book. We especially thank the Mead Johnson/Bristol Myers Company for a generous grant to host a stimulating authors' meeting where each manuscript was reviewed, critiqued and revised to meet the demands of interest, facts, and practical application for a wide variety of readership.

Basic Concepts in the Determination of Nutritional Requirements of Normal Infants

J. C. WATERLOW, M.D., Sc.D., F.R.S.

With a section on the requirements of low birthweight babies by O.G. Brooke, MD

"There is no diet so nourishing or so stimulating as to eat one's own words."

Attributed to SIR WINSTON CHURCHILL

"The anxious question is whether our arguments have begun right rather than whether they have had the good fortune to end right."

A. S. EDDINGTON, *The Nature of the Physical World*

"We must view with profound respect the infinite capacity of the human mind to resist the introduction of useful knowledge."

THOMAS R. LOUNSBURY, American philologist, 1838–1915

INTRODUCTION

It may be asked: "Why do we have to make detailed calculations of infants' needs? For thousands of years babies have been fed at the breast, weaned onto traditional mixtures of various kinds and then moved on to the family pot. Is it not enough simply to ensure that a baby gets enough food to fulfill its appetite and that the food is uncontaminated and clean?" However, three things have happened since the beginning of this century: (1) the decline in breastfeeding in industrialized countries, with more and more women having full-time jobs away from the home—a decline that is now beginning to be reversed; (2) the realization that in the Third World the traditional system does not necessarily work; and (3) our much greater capacity to preserve the lives of pre-term and very-low-birth-weight infants, who then have to be fed. All these trends lead to the same question: how much food does a baby need and what must its composition be to ensure good health and growth?

At the outset we have to distinguish between requirements and recommended daily allowances (RDAs). **The requirement is a physiological concept; the RDA is a generalization based on the physiological conclusions and represents an application of them to populations.** The RDA must therefore take account of the variablility between individuals. There is also the question, much stressed by Sukhatme,[1] of variation within an individual, from day to day or week to week, in intake, output or growth. The effect of this is to diminish the confidence with which we can draw conclusions from physiological measurements made over a short period.

Since the definition of RDAs needs a multidisciplinary approach, bringing together scientists and policy-makers, it has always been seen as one for committees rather than individuals. Since the end of World War II many national and international committees have made recommendations on energy and protein requirements, but unfortunately none so far has contained the ideal mixture of disciplines. In principle, the most authoritative recommendations should be those of the international agencies, because they are supposed to be of worldwide application, and in the composition of the committees the agencies are able to draw on experienced people from all over the world. In practice, however, things do not always work out in this way. Because in this chapter I shall draw heavily on the latest report of the Food and Agriculture Organization, the World Health Organization and the United Nations University,[2] it may be useful to say something from my own experience about the inevitable limitations of the international process.

The democratic approach to scientific truth is a contradiction in terms—the truth may most often be with the majority, but it is not always. The dissenters should be listened to carefully.

N. S. SCRIMSHAW[41]

In the first place, the UN system requries that a committee of no more than about 20 people should be reasonably representative of all parts of the world. This very requirement makes it difficult to ensure that collectively the committee has adequate expertise in all aspects of a complex subject. Second, if the expertise in a particular area is spread rather thin, the views of one or two members may become unduly dominant. Third, and most important, the international committees only meet once for some two weeks and then disperse, whereas national committtees are often able to convene many times. In the course of drafting an international report, gaps, difficulties and disagreements inevitably become apparent that can be resolved only by long and tedious correspondence. As a consequence, the reports are often long and delayed and may be superseded by later work.

Nevertheless, I am inclined to think that these drawbacks are more than outweighed by one great advantage. Precisely because the international committees are rather heterogeneous, with members drawn from different backgrounds and disciplines, there is a great deal of cross-fertilization of ideas and concepts. Each successive international committee has had a different approach from its predecessor and has generated new ideas for the future. This process is exemplified by the successive UN reports dealing with protein requirements.[3,4] Anyone who has the stamina to read them in succession will get a good picture of the progression of ideas over 20 years. I will add an example from my own experience (1963):

Waterlow (UK):   In my view the requirements of all men should be equal.
Masek (Czechoslovakia):   I am not so sure.

At the time I was astonished by Professor Masek's remark. Now I realize that he was right. The concept of a perfectly healthy person in a perfectly healthy environment is an unhelpful idealization.

If one asks "requirements for what purpose?" the standard answer is "to maintain health and satisfactory function," which in children includes growth. However, in the real world there is surely a range of states compatible with reasonable health and satisfactory function, rather than a single undefinable optimum. Consider the question of body weight. Requirements for both energy and protein are based on weight. It is always assumed in official

recommendation that the purpose is to maintain the status quo: that the body weight is as it should be. In fact, of course, there are large sections of the world in which a great many people weigh more than is good for them, and other areas in which many people perhaps weigh too little. We cannot, however, legislate for every situation. We can but say, as the 1985 report[2] does: if a person of given age, sex, weight and level of physical activity wishes to maintain existing body weight, here is an estimate of the average amounts of energy and protein that will be needed. If a different body weight is considered desirable, then an estimate can be made of the amounts needed to maintain that new body weight. We have to get away from the static concept of a reference man or woman. Thus a Western young man, weighing 70 kg, height 175 cm, body mass index (BMI) 22.8, with a total daily energy expenditure of $1.7 \times BMR$, would on average have an energy requirement of just under 3000 kcal/day. If he reduces his intake to 2600 kcal/day, at the same level of activity the body weight should in theory level off at 55.5 kg (BMI 18). His protein requirement would also be expected to fall by 20%. Who is to say that one state is better or worse than the other? Exactly the same considerations apply to children growing at different rates within the wide range of what may be considered normal.

When it comes to translating these concepts of average requirements for a particular type of person to recommended allowances for a group of similar people, an important difference emerges between energy and protein. **If body weights are to remain unchanged, the intake of energy per kg must be neither too great nor too small.** Hence the RDA is taken as equal to the *average* requirement. Admittedly people are not machines; within any group of apparently similar people living similar lives there is a wide variation in intake at constant body weight, presumably due to differences in metabolic efficiency. In setting the RDA for energy as equal to the average requirement, the theory is that those members of the group who need less will in fact eat less, and those who need more will eat more. This proposition seems so implausible that some workers have rejected as useless the concept of an RDA for energy. Nevertheless, it seems to work up to a point, when rations have to be provided for particular groups or even a whole population, as in Britain in World War II.

For protein the situation is different. As with energy, similar people differ in their requirements, with a coefficient of variation of 10–15%. However, there is no firm evidence of any harmful effect of eating rather more protein than the physiological requirement (sometimes called the minimum requirement). Unwanted nitrogen is simply excreted. **Therefore the RDA of a group for protein has been set as the average requirement + 2 SD, the so-called safe level, in order to cover the needs of virtually all members of the group.**

Although this approach seems logical for adults or older children, it breaks down for breastfed babies. Consider a group of exclusively breastfed infants growing normally. For each one the intake presumably meets his requirement. From these intakes we can calculate an average requirement for the group. It makes no sense to say that, in order to meet the requirements of all members of the group, an allowance should be recommended that in most cases is greater than the actual intake.

RDAs thus have no meaning for the infant while he or she is exclusively breastfed. What, then, are we to do on weaning? Are we to accept a sudden transition to some higher level of recommmended allowance? That would seem to be a very artificial approach, and therefore in this chapter I have confined myself to discussing average requirements. It is then left to the doctor, nurse or mother to exercise judgment and to decide in each case whether the baby needs more or less than the average. The only situation I can envisage in which the RDA for protein might be useful in this age group is if supplies are being calculated for feeding children in an orphanage or refugee camp.

PHYSIOLOGY OF THE INFANT'S ENERGY AND PROTEIN REQUIREMENTS

For both energy and protein, the infant's requirement is made up of two parts—for growth and for maintenance. The energy supply also has to meet a third need, that for physical activity (Fig. 1).

Growth

"Satisfactory" growth has traditionally and rightly been regarded as the main criterion that a baby is healthy and that its nutrient needs are being met. Therefore some discussion is necessary of the growth standards that form the basis of the charts widely used in clinics.

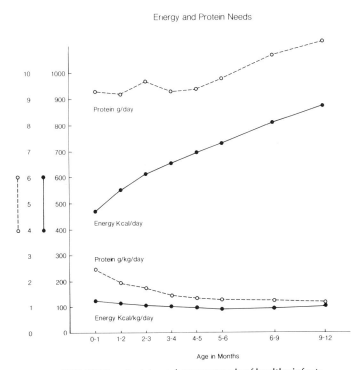

FIGURE 1. Protein and energy needs of healthy infants.

At the outset, as discussed in detail elsewhere,[5] it is necessary to distinguish between a *reference* and a *standard*. **A reference is simply a set of data used for normalizing measurements of weight and height so that they can be grouped, manipulated statistically and compared with other sets of measurements.** In principle the reference implies no value judgments and tells us nothing about optimal or satisfactory growth. For the time being, the World Health Organization (WHO) has chosen the data-base of the National Center for Health Statistics, NCHS (Department of Health, Education and Welfare)[6] as an international reference, mainly for technical reasons, because it is derived from a large sample and provides centiles and standard deviations, not only of weight and height for age, but also, for the first time, of weight for height.[7,8]

In contrast to the term "reference," in most languages "standard" does imply a value judgment. There has been a great deal of controversy about whether the NCHS reference, based on North American data, constitutes an appropriate standard for all ethnic groups in all countries. There is little doubt that there are genetic differences in height between individual children in any population, and perhaps there are small differences also between ethnic groups. However, Martorell in particular has argued convincingly that environmental factors (nutrition and infection) play a far greater part in the very large differences that we see within and between populations.[9]

I myself believe, in agreement with the WHO, that the NCHS reference does constitute an appropriate standard of expected growth in healthy children, if it is used sensibly. The following is an example of the kind of problem that is arising. A number of workers in developed countries have shown that in exclusively breastfed children, weight and height begin to fall away from the NCHS median at 4–6 months, to reach about the 25th centile. Whitehead and Paul[10,11] have argued that since the reference is derived largely from bottle-fed infants, many of whom may be too fat, if we accept breastfeeding as the optimum, the reference is inappropriately high. However, I doubt if the point is of much practical importance: no one need be concerned if an individual child grows along the 25th rather than the 50th NCHS centile. When it comes to populations, what matters is not so much the position of the mean or median but the dispersion, i.e., the proportion of children above the 95th reference centile if we are concerned about obesity, and below the 5th centile if we are concerned about malnutrition.

Growth velocity is a more sensitive indicator than attained weight or height. After all, in relation to requirements, what matters is whether the child is able to gain at an adequate rate. Observed gains can be compared with the increments of the reference population, but unfortunately we do not have enough information on the standard deviations and centiles of weight and height velocity to allow definition of a range for "adequate" gain. The classical velocity standards are those of Tanner and coworkers,[12] but the 3-monthly intervals at which their measurements were made in the first year of life are too long for assessing the adequacy of growth in infancy. The same applies to the more recent data of Karlberg et al. in Sweden.[13] There is a real difficulty here. As every pediatrician knows, a child does not grow at exactly the same rate every day and every week. The shorter the interval between two measurements, the greater the variability. Fomon's results show that the weight gain of normal infants over periods of 2–4 weeks has a coefficient of variation of 30–35%.[14] It therefore becomes very difficult to assess a lower limit for acceptable gain over such short periods.

Growth in length is as important a nutritional criterion as gain in weight. Healy and coworkers,[15] using longitudinal data from Sudan, have looked at month-to-month variations in height gain and have devised screening criteria to pinpoint the child whose growth faltering may be regarded as pathological, needing intervention. This approach could certainly be extended to weight gain.

The variability of growth, both within and between subjects, has a profound effect on the assessment of infants' needs and on framing recommended allowances. In the following sections I can but concentrate on the determination of *average* requirements. However, variability not only produces statistical problems in the application of average figures to an individual or a group; it is also of great interest in its own right. We need to know much more about the biological basis of the variations that are found even in apparently healthy children. Do they represent subclinical deviations from health? If so, is the main effect on appetite and intake, or on metabolic efficiency? It is noteworthy that in Fomon's series the coefficient of variation (CV) of energy intake (kcal/kg/day) was much less than that of weight gain, suggesting that the main fluctuations are in the efficiency of energy utilization.

Maintenance

The maintenance requirement (MR) for both energy and protein is the amount needed to maintain a steady state, with zero growth. A requirement for energy is obvious, since all the processes of life consume energy. In the words of Kleiber:

> Life involves much more than chemical potential, work and heat. Nutrition . . . is concerned with more than the supply of energy, yet energy transfer remains an important aspect of physiology in general and of nutrition in particular.
>
> M. KLEIBER, *The Fire of Life*

The problem is to quantitate this need. For energy the MR is larger than the basal or resting metabolic rate (RMR), because the latter by definition is measured in the fasting state, whereas the maintenance requirement must allow for the effects of food and for a minimal level of physical activity.

It is not so obvious why there should be a maintenance requirement for protein or nitrogen. That body proteins are turning over has been suggested as long as 170 years ago. In the words of Magendie (1817, cited by Munro[16]):

> It is extremely probable that all parts of the body of man experience an intestine movement, which has the double effect of expelling the molecules that can or ought no longer to compose the organs and replacing them by new molecules. This internal, intimate motion constitutes nutrition.
>
> MAGENDIE

We now know that 90 or even 95% of the nitrogen release by protein breakdown can be recycled to protein synthesis.[17] Why not 100%? The North American bear hibernates for 6 months, produces a fetus, yet does not eat or pass urine or feces and therefore loses no nitrogen.[18] In man, however, for reasons that we do not understand, there is a minimum obligatory nitrogen loss, mainly in the urine, that cannot be avoided (for details, see ref. 2).

For both energy and protein, the maintenance requirement is usually determined by interpolation from a plot of weight gain or nitrogen retention against intake at several levels above and below the maintenance level. The criticisms that may be raised against the balance method, at least in relation to protein requirements, are discussed in reference 2.

Physical Activity

In the infant physical activity accounts for only a small part of total energy expenditure until the second 6 months of life. Nevertheless, it is very important, since exploratory activity is essential for the child's behavioral and psychological development. Unfortunately, this component of energy expenditure is very difficult to measure in a baby. Time and motion studies have been made, but I do not know of any quantitative data in the literature for children below 6 months.[19,20]

Measurement of Intake

It is rather illogical to say, as has often been done: my requirement is what I actually eat. Nevertheless, when physiological information is not available we have to fall back on the observed intakes of healthy children growing normally. They are also a useful check on theoretical calculations. At least a baby's intake is less likely than that of an adult to be increased above its true needs by physiologically irrelevant social factors.

ESTIMATED REQUIREMENTS

NORMAL TERM INFANTS

Energy

We have enough information to make an informed guess of an infant's energy expenditure, which can then be compared with observed intakes. The components that have to be considered are: the basal or resting metabolic rate, which is by far the most important; physical activity; the thermic effect of food; the energy content of new tissue and the energy cost of depositing it; and finally, the energy losses in urine and feces (Fig. 2). There are various ways of making the calculation, according to how we combine the different components, but in the end they will give the same answer. The following calculations provide examples for children aged 3 months and 6 months, which span the critical period of weaning. All values are per kg body weight per 24 hours.

Basal or Resting Metabolic Rate. The information in the literature summarized by Schofield et al.[21] is quite consistent, that in an infant measured asleep 4–6 hours after the last feed, the BMR, extrapolated to 24 hours, may be taken as 48–55 kcal/kg. It does not seem

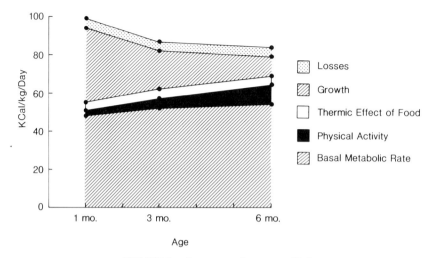

FIGURE 2.   Energy requirements of infants.

that the BMR is affected by the rate of growth, since according to the data collected by Schofield et al.,[21] the rate per kg remains virtually constant from birth to 3 years, during which time the rate of growth is changing a great deal. The evidence is consistent with the idea that growth does not occur in the basal state, but rather happens in bursts after meals.[22] Thus in adding the cost of growth to the BMR we are not counting the same thing twice.

Physical Activity.   At 3 months the average infant can only wriggle its limbs and move about; at 6 months it will be sitting and creeping. It is convenient to follow the FAO/WHO/UNU report[2] and express the costs of activity as multiples of the BMR. As a guess, since there is no hard information, and by analogy with adults, we might take the cost of activity at 3 months as + 0.2 BMR for 12 hours out of 24, and at 6 months as + 0.4 BMR for 12 hours in the day.

Thermic Effect of Food.   Again by analogy with adults, the thermic effect of food in the nongrowing state could be taken as 5% of the energy intake, or 4–5 kcal/kg/day. In actual measurements it is not possible to separate this effect from the energy cost of tissue deposition. Brooke and Ashworth[23] found that in infants 6–24 months of age recovering from malnutrition there was a linear relation between the amount of postprandial thermogenesis and the rate of weight gain, suggesting that a large part of the extra heat produced after a meal represented the energy cost of protein and fat synthesis. By taking a figure obtained in nongrowing adults we are again

avoiding the possibility of counting the same effect twice.

The Energy Cost of Growth.   As allowed for in this calculation, the energy cost of growth is the sum of the energy content (enthalpy) of the tissue laid down and the energy cost of synthesizing it. The value that has generally been used for tissue of normal composition is 5 kcal/gm of weight gain (for a full discussion see references 2, 24, 25). The infant at 3 months will be gaining weight at the rate of about 5 gm/kg/day, and at 6 months at the rate of about 3 gm/kg/day.

Losses.   If the amount and composition of the diet are known, the losses in feces and urine can be estimated from the difference between the enthalpy of fat and protein and their corresponding Atwater* factors. A reasonable estimate for losses might be 5 kcal/kg/day.

Thermoregulation.   Young infants have a different thermoneutral range than older children. Low-birthweight babies in particular may be exposed at times to too low a temperature and it is customary to make an allowance for cold stress. For normal weight infants under normal conditions such an allowance seems generally not to be considered necessary.

These calculations, which are necessarily approximations, are summarized in Table 1.

---

* The enthalpy is the heat of combustion: in round figures, 4.0, 5.7 and 9.4 kcal/gm for carbohydrate, protein and fat. The Atwater factors represent the available energy—4, 4, 9 kcal/gm respectively—after allowance has been made for losses in feces and urine. The appropriate values for these factors will vary with the nature of the diet, e.g., its fiber content. For a discussion see reference 2.

TABLE 1. Factorial Estimates of Energy Requirements of Infants (All Values as kcal/kg/day)

	AGE, MONTHS		
	1	3	6
BMR[1]	48	52	54
Physical activity[2]			
Rate of expenditure, × BMR (0.1, 0.2, 0.4)			
Energy cost	2.4	5.2	10.8
Thermic effect of food[3]	5	4.5	4.5
Growth[4]			
Rate, gm/kg/day	7.7	4.2	2.1
Energy cost	38.5	21	10.5
Losses[3]	5	4.5	4.5
TOTAL	99	87	84

[1]From Schofield et al.[21]
[2]Estimates—see text; it is assumed that the child is physically active, at the stated rate, for 12 hours out of 24, and basal for the other 12 hours.
[3]Taken as 5% of intake.
[4]Daily increments from NCHS median, boys. Cost taken as 5 kcal/gm gain.

The second most important component of expenditure after the BMR is the energy cost of growth. **This requirement is very sensitive to the fat content of the tissue laid down, because of the high energy content of fat.** Studies on somewhat older children recovering from malnutrition show considerable variations not only in rates of weight gain but also in the composition of the tissue laid down, and hence its energy cost.[26]

If we remove the energy cost of growth (Table 1) at 3–6 months, the remaining expenditure of 66–74 kcal/kg/day is 1.3–1.4 × BMR. This is rather lower than the estimate of 82 kcal/kg/day for the maintenance requirement derived by Spady et al.[27] from measurements of total energy expenditure extrapolated to zero weight gain but is in keeping with current estimates of maintenance requirements for adults.[2]

Observed Energy Intakes. In the 1973 FAO/WHO report[3] the energy requirements of infants were taken from the values determined by Fomon and coworkers[14] for the intakes of healthy babies receiving breast milk or formula ad libitum by bottle (Table 2). At the more recent UN meeting (1981) it was recognized that Fomon's results were based on rather small and highly selected groups. Therefore a survey was made of the literature on intakes of healthy infants in developed countries (Fig. 3).[2,28] For the intakes to be measured accurately they had to be obtained in bottle-fed children. These results also are given in Table 2. They show a very interesting phenomenon:

TABLE 2. Estimated Energy Requirements of Infants Based on Observed Intakes (kcal/kg/day)

Age, months	FAO/WHO (1973)[3]	FAO/WHO/UNU (1985)[2]
0–3	120	116
3–6	115	99
6–9	110	95
9–12	105	101

a decline in average intake between 3 and 9 months, with a rise again at 9 to 12 months. It seems reasonable to suppose that the falling-off represents the decreasing requirement for growth and the later rise an increased level of physical activity.

These observed intakes are on the whole lower than those of Fomon. Recent studies of the intakes of healthy breastfed infants give results that are lower still (Fig. 4). For example, Butte[29] has recorded an average intake as low as 70 kcal/kg/day at 3 months, although she obtains the usual value for BMR. It seems from Table 1 that such an intake would only be compatible with normal weight gain if the tissue laid down contained virtually no fat. The energy cost would then be about 2 kcal/gm gain. It is in fact often said that breastfed babies are leaner than bottle-fed ones.

The importance of these calculations, approximate though they are, is to help us to give the best advice to mothers on how long to continue exclusive breastfeeding before introducing supplements. If the physiological estimates

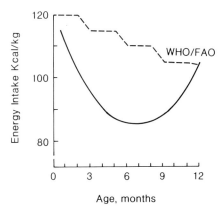

FIGURE 3. Energy intake per kilogram of body weight in the first year of life compared to the WHO/FAO (1973) recommendation. (From Whitehead RG, et al. A critical analysis of measured food energy intakes during infancy and early childhood in comparison with current international recommendations. J Hum Nutr 1981; 35:339-348, with permission.)

Breast Milk Intakes

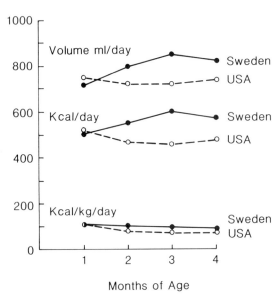

FIGURE 4. Breast milk intakes of healthy infants in Sweden and the U.S.A. (Sweden: from WHO Collaborative Breastfeeding Study;[74] and U.S.A.: from Butte et al.[29])

at 3 and 6 months (Table 1) , which are lower than those of either Fomon or Whitehead, are compared with average values for the energy supply from breast milk in healthy women, we get the results shown in Table 3. On the basis of the usual figure for the energy cost of weight gain (5 kcal/gm), one would expect that from 3–4 months the energy intakes of more and more babies would become inadequate if they are fed on breast milk alone. On the other had, if we take the minimum value for the cost of weight gain (2 kcal/gm), most infants would thrive on breast milk alone up to nearly 6 months. Therefore the usual advice, and indeed traditional practices, appear to be correct, that **in most cases exclusive breastfeeding should be adequate for 4–6 months.**

It is impossible to be more precise than this because of the many sources of variability: differences in body weight, rate of weight gain, physical activity, milk volume and energy content of breast milk. If each of these factors has a coefficient of variation of about 15%, the overall CV would be 33%. In the case of an individual child one can allow for these variations by following its progress on a weight chart. For populations the theoretical estimates of variability need to be supplemented by field observations. What is necessary is to

follow a sufficiently large cohort of exclusively breastfed children until they begin to falter according to some agreed upon criterion. Preliminary results from a study of this kind in the Sudan indicate that the mean time to faltering of exclusively breast fed babies was about 4 months, faltering being defined as a gain of less than −1 SD of the reference for 4 consecutive weeks.[3] There was, however, a wide range of variability, with 25% faltering by 8 weeks.

Protein

The question of the protein requirements of infants is normally less urgent than that of energy requirements, because if babies are fed on breast milk, cow milk formula or any reputable formula, as far as current knowledge goes, they will receive enough protein once their energy needs are met. However, problems may arise in developing countries if infants are not breastfed or are partially breastfed and given paps made of foods that are poor in protein, such as rice or starchy roots. There may also be concern about meeting protein needs to allow catch-up growth after repeated infections, or to provide for rapid enough growth in very-low-birth-weight infants.

It should be noted at the outset that in the physiological approach all values are in terms of nitrogen (N), which is then converted to protein by the usual factor 6.25 (sometimes 6.38 in the case of milk). These requirements are therefore nitrogen requirements and to call them protein requirements has led to misunderstanding (see below).

According to the classic "factorial" approach, the total requirement is the sum of the N needed for maintenance, obtained by N

TABLE 3.   Breast Milk Intakes of Healthy Infants

	Age, months			
	1	2	3	4
Volume, ml or gm				
Sweden[1]	719	795	848	822
U.S.A.[2]	751	725	723	740
Energy, kcal/day				
Sweden	503	556	594	575
U.S.A.	520	468	458	477
Energy, kcal/kg/day				
Sweden	114	105	98	87
U.S.A.	110	83	74	71

[1]From WHO Collaborative Breastfeeding Study.[74]
[2]From Butte et al.[29]

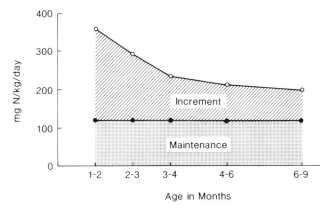

FIGURE 5.　Nitrogen requirements of infants.

balance, and the N deposited in the process of growth (Fig. 5). So much has been written about the balance method that very little need be said about it here. Balances can only be done over short periods, so they cannot take account of periodic changes in the efficiency of utilization or of possible long-term adaptations. For practical and indeed ethical reasons there is no information, to my knowledge, on children below 6 months other than neonates, so we have to rely on results from older children. However, if we compare one-year-olds with adults, the maintenance requirement seems to vary little with age. The results, admittedly scanty, summarized in the 1985 FAO/WHO/UNU report,[2] provide two useful pieces of information: first, they give an indication of the maintenance requirement for zero growth, for which the value proposed is 120 mg of N or 0.75 gm of protein/kg/day; second, they provide an estimate of the efficiency of utilization, which is taken as 70%. Both these values relate to milk, human or cow, as the source of protein. The latter figure (70%) is needed to calculate the requirement for growth, which is the product of the efficiency times the rate of protein accretion.

Here, however, we run into a difficulty. One cannot calculate the N increment simply from the expected weight gain multiplied by a fixed factor for the N content of the tissue gained, because apart from variations in fat gained, the N concentration in the lean body mass increases rapidly during the first year—the process known as maturation. Estimates of N increments at different ages have been very variable (see reference 3). The most recent estimates by Fomon et al.,[31] derived from measurements of body water, are probably the most

reliable. These values are given in Table 4, which shows the factorial calculation of N requirements up to 6 months.

I was responsible for most of the section of the 1985 UN report dealing with the protein requirements of infants. It seemed to me that this simple calculation omits one important factor. The "daily requirement," as the words are generally used, is meant to cover the needs over a period. However, as I have repeatedly emphasized, infants do not gain weight at the same rate from one week to another, and probably not at the same rate from day to day. Therefore any N which, for one reason or another, is not utilized for growth on one day must be made up for by an extra amount on the next day. If this argument is correct, the

TABLE 4.　Factorial Calculation of Nitrogen Requirement of Infants (mg/N/kg/day)

	Age, months				
	1-2	2-3	3-4	4-6	6-9
N increment[1]	112	80	55	43	37
N increment × 1.5[2]	168	120	81	64	56
N increment corrected for efficiency[3]	240	171	116	92	80
Maintenance[4]	120	120	120	120	120
TOTAL	360	291	236	212	200
From breast milk[6]	303	273	234	196	—
"Protein" gm/kg/day[5]					
factorial	2.25	1.82	1.47	1.32	1.25
from breast milk[7]	1.93	1.74	1.49	1.25	—

[1]From Fomon et al.[31]
[2]See text.
[3]Efficiency taken as 70%.
[4]From FAO/WHO/UNU.[2]
[5]"Protein" = total N × 6.25.
[6]Source as for 4, but value for 4-6 months from Butte et al.[29]
[7]Protein taken as N × 6.38.

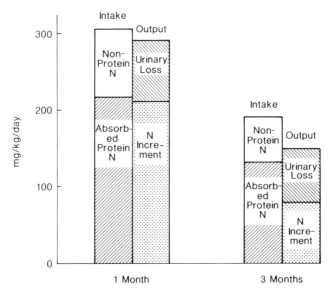

FIGURE 6.   Nitrogen intake from human milk versus nitrogen requirement. Non-protein N taken as 30% of total N.

amounts needed theoretically to cover the daily N increment should be increased—but by how much? We have no evidence on which to answer this question and therefore an empirical adjustment was made, of adding 50 percent to the theoretical daily increment. The rationale was that this maneuver brought the factorial estimate at the critical age of 3–4 months into close agreement with the average observed N intake from breast milk (Fig. 6). **This means that for N requirements, as for the requirements of many other nutrients, we are really using breast milk as the standard.**

Some people might conclude that the physiological or factorial approach is therefore a purely academic exercise. That would not be justified, because we have to have some method of estimating the N or protein requirements of infants during and after the weaning period, and these estimates must harmonize with data derived from breastfed infants before weaning. A sudden break, upward or downward, would not make physiological sense. This consideration leads on to the question of observed intakes.

Observed Intakes. In the earlier FAO/WHO reports of 1965[4] and 1973[3] no attempt was made to use the factorial method for computing protein requirements of infants below 6 months because the uncertainties were considered to be too great. Therefore in the first months of life the estimates were based on the data of Fomon and coworkers on the intakes

of babies fed human milk or formula ad libitum by bottle.[14] Because of the increased emphasis on breastfeeding, it is clearly more appropriate to determine N requirements from the average intakes of children who are fed at the breast. Representative values for milk from healthy mothers are shown in Table 4.

These values are given in terms of nitrogen rather than protein, because in recent years a certain confusion has arisen in the literature. Hambraeus et al.[32] and Räihä and coworkers[33] have reemphasized the fact, known indeed for many decades,[34] that in human milk about 30% of the N is non-protein nitrogen (NPN), of which about half is urea-N. Therefore, these authors conclude, the protein requirements of infants have been overestimated. It has certainly been a misleading practice of nutritionists to multiply the total N content of milk by 6.3 and call it the *protein* content. The inaccuracy, of course, is much smaller for cow milk, which contains less NPN, than for human milk. Nevertheless, in my opinion the conclusion that has been drawn by these workers is not realistic.

It may be useful to restate the question in terms of nitrogen, the "unit of currency" in balance studies. The question becomes: With normal milk intakes can the nitrogen contained in the true protein of human milk by itself satisfy the needs for growth and maintenance? We can calculate from available information (Table 5) that in a one-month-old baby the milk protein would supply just about

TABLE 5.   Comparison of Nitrogen Intake from Breast Milk with Nitrogen Requirement (mg/kg/day)

	Age, months	
	1	*3*
Intake		
Protein N	256	157
Absorbed protein N[1]	217	133
NPN	89	58
TOTAL	306	191
Output		
Weight gain, gm/kg/day	10.6	4.0
N increment[2]	212	80
Urinary loss	70	70
TOTAL	282	150

Data from Butte et al.[29] except where indicated.
[1]Absorption taken as 85%.
[2]N increment taken as 20 mg/gm weight gain.
At both 1 and 3 months the total N output into tissue protein + urine is greater than the absorbed protein N intake, even when no allowance is made for inefficiency of utilization.

enough N to provide for normal growth; however, the efficiency of utilization would have to be virtually 100% with no allowances for fluctuations in efficiency. The NPN associated with this amount of protein would barely cover the obligatory N losses in the urine. At 3 months protein N alone would not be enough to cover even the most conservative estimate of total N requirement.

Although there seems to be general agreement that on an isonitrogenous basis the N of cow milk is utilized as efficiently as that of human milk (see, for example, reference 35), the position with cow milk, if fed at the same level of protein, would be worse than with human milk, because the protein would be associated with less NPN. This brings us to the question of the availability of the NPN.

Hambraeus[32] has rightly said: "nutritionists need to discuss not only breast milk protein but also peptides, free amino acids and non-amino acid nitrogen." Since infants can be maintained parenterally on amino acid mixtures, it is reasonable to suppose that the free amino acids, peptides and probably the amino-sugars are utilized. About half the NPN consists of urea, and infants, like adults, can metabolize urea to some extent.[36] Since milk proteins contain a larger proportion of essential amino acids to total N than is found in tissue proteins, some "dilution" of milk protein with non-essential N is possible without impairing their capacity to form tissue protein, as demonstrated by Snyderman and Holt nearly 30 years ago.[37] For this reason it seems probable that N derived from hydrolysis of urea can

make a contribution to net protein synthesis.

The suggestion by Järvenpää and others[38] that protein requirements may have been set too high has been discussed at some length because it has important practical implications that could be dangerous, particularly in Third World countries. The question whether protein intakes greater than the requirement may be harmful is considered briefly in the section later in this chapter on Deficiency States.

Protein Quality.   Human milk is used as the gold standard for the pattern of essential amino acids needed by the infant.[2] Although cow milk proteins have a slighly different pattern, this does not seem to be of practical importance. Formulas based on soya, such as are used for treating children with cow milk intolerance, may need supplementation with methionine. The cereal paps, made for example of maize, that are fed to young children in developing countries, are likely to contain protein of low quality; this needs to be allowed for in calculating their requirement. **Partial breastfeeding, continued to the end of the first year or longer, is probably the most practical means of improving the quality of the protein intake.**

There is another aspect of protein quality that has come to the fore in recent years. We have to consider not only the chemical but also the biological properties of the infant's food. The most important difference between human and cow milk is the much higher concentration in the former of immunologically active proteins. The claim that all the secretory immunoglobulin (sIgA) in milk was excreted unchanged in the stools[39] aroused concern from the nutritional point of view, since if this were so it would be difficult for N requirements to be met. According to Butte et al.[40] at one month of age, the sum of the daily intake of lactoferrin + sIgA is about 400 mg/kg out of a total protein intake of 1600 mg/kg. If these proteins were excreted intact, it would be impossible to achieve the usual value of about 85% for the absorption of N from human milk. However, recent work from the same group[41] indicates that only about 10% of the sIgA and 3% of the lactoferrin ingested are excreted unchanged in the stools.

SPECIAL CASES: THE UNDERPRIVILEGED BABY AND THE LOW-BIRTHWEIGHT BABY

The discussion so far has been concerned with the needs of normal infants in a favorable environment. There are two other groups that need special attention: children in poor developing countries and very-low-birthweight babies. We can apply to both these groups the principles that have been set out, with some modification.

The Third World

The baby born in a deprived environment immediately has to face two handicaps. First, the evidence available so far suggests that poorly nourished mothers are often unable to produce the quantities of milk shown in Table 3. For example, in India, according to studies many years ago by Gopalan,[42] the volume of breast milk was about 500 ml/day from birth right up to 2 years of age. Similar results have been recorded from Mexico.[43] Clearly, these amounts, if correct, will not allow satisfactory growth to continue for very long on breast milk alone.

It is possible, however, that the classical test-feeding method systematically underestimates intakes when babies are being fed on demand, often many times in the night. It remains to be seen whether the new heavy water method[44] will produce an upward revision of the figures for breast milk output in Third World countries.

Second, from birth the infant is exposed to a high level of gastrointestinal and respiratory infection, and breastfeeding by no means provides complete protection. Even among children who survive the neonatal period there is a high mortality rate during the next few months.[45] Children may easily have diarrhea for 1–2 days out of every 10. The shortfall in intake arising from anorexia, together with actual catabolic losses, has to be made good by increased intakes of energy and protein at times when the infant is well. It is impossible to compute the magnitude of these extra requirements because conditions vary so much. **Probably the best guide is that the baby should be fed to appetite. In any situation where there is catch-up growth there is a relatively greater increase in the requirement for protein than for energy.**

The Low-birthweight Baby

The special needs of premature and very-low-birthweight infants are discusssed in more detail elsewhere in this book, but there are certain general aspects that need to be considered here.

First, it is important to distinguish between those low-birthweight infants who are mature but undergrown and those whose main problem is immaturity, since their energy and protein needs will be different. Mature small-for-gestation infants will have few of the metabolic difficulties that make protein quality and quantity critical in the very immature; neither will they have so much difficulty in nutrient absorption. On the other hand their requirements for catch-up growth will be very high, they are vulnerable to hypoglycemia, and they will have high thermoregulatory energy requirements.

Second, the requirements for growth in *all* low-birthweight infants will be greater than in normal mature neonates and older babies, since their weight gain is relatively greater. **The rate of weight gain of the infant between 28 and 35 weeks of gestation is, at about 15 gm/kg/day, greater than at any other time in the human lifespan and rivals that of infants recovering from severe protein-energy malnutrition.**

Finally, it is not possible in the low-birthweight infant to use observed intakes as a guide to energy and protein requirements, since appetite and feeding behavior are not sufficiently developed. Thus reliance has to be placed entirely on measurement, both of growth and of metabolic performance, and on calculations based on factorial determinations.

We now outline some specific differences in the energy and protein requirements of low-birthweight (LBW) infants in comparison with older babies.

Energy Requirements. Basal or resting metabolic rate is the most important component of energy expenditure in LBW infants as it is in all very young children. However it is very difficult to determine what is "basal" in such infants, and they cannot be fasted for long enough to be sure that the resting metabolism does not contain an important contribution from the energy cost of growth. There is evidence[46] that both resting and postprandial metabolic rate rise as energy intake increases, implying an increased contribution from synthesis, which is perhaps more continuous in these infants than in older ones. Resting metabolism is also extremely variable in preterm infants, depending on their weight and postnatal age, mean values in various studies ranging from 36 to 51 kcal/kg/day.[47-51] What evidence there is suggests that resting metabolism in LBW infants tends to be low in very immature infants in the early neonatal period, high in infants who are growing on high energy intakes, and has greater variability than in mature infants.

The component of energy expenditure due to physical activity in LBW infants is certainly lower than in full term neonates and older babies. Although short-term measurements have shown that activity may increase energy expenditure by two- to three-fold in preterm infants, such babies are inactive for much of the time. It is probable that activity accounts for about 7-8 kcal/kg/day, or about 6% of total energy expenditure.[52]

Some studies have shown that the energy cost of growth appears to be lower in preterm infants than has been found in older babies and in infants recovering from malnutrition.[53,54] However it seems likely that the values obtained in the published studies reflect the energy intakes of the infants in the studies, and hence the amount of fat being deposited during the period of study. The values of the energy cost of growth in the three recent studies that have specifically examined this issue show a trend to increase with increasing energy intake:

Source	Energy intake (kcal/kg/day)	Energy cost of growth (kcal/g)
Gudinchet et al., 1982[54]	130	3.0
Reichman et al., 1982[53]	149	4.9
Brooke et al., 1979[55]	181	5.7

It seems clear from several recent studies that fat deposition in preterm infants varies greatly depending on the composition of the feed and the energy intake, formula-fed infants laying down much more fat than infants fed on breast milk.[46,56]

The requirement for energy to meet the demands of thermoregulation is invariably greater in LBW infants than in larger babies, and is not negligible even in optimal nursing conditions. Infants nursed just below thermoneutrality increase their energy expenditure by 7-8 kcal/kg/day[57] and it has been suggested that a daily value of 10 kcal/kg should be allowed to cover incidental cold stress in the LBW infant.[58]

Finally, energy losses due to malabsorption, particularly of fat, are very important in preterm infants, since they are one of the few aspects of energy balance in these infants which something can be done about. **Fat malabsorption may, on occasions, account for as much as 40–50% of the dietary intake in otherwise apparently healthy infants,[55]** and is much influenced by the quality of fat in the feed.

Protein Requirements. The protein requirements of LBW infants are dominated on the one hand by the need to ensure an adequate protein intake during a period of very rapid growth, and on the other hand (and this is mainly of relevance to *preterm* infants) by the importance of avoiding such a high intake that immature pathways of intermediary metabolism are overwhelmed and potentially dangerous concentrations of toxic amino acids occur. Metabolic intolerance to high protein intakes in preterm infants is well described,[59] and results in acidosis, failure to thrive, hyperammonemia, and specific toxic states such as hypertyrosinemia. It seems unlikely from the published literature that such problems will occur if the daily protein intake is kept below 4 gm/kg, but there is little information about maximum tolerated intakes in infants under 1000 gm weight and 28 weeks of gestation, whose survival is increasingly commonplace.

In the attempt to avoid the problems of excessive protein intake, and also perhaps to minimize the risk of sensitization to cow milk and other animal proteins, there is a strong lobby which recommends the exclusive use of human milk in feeding LBW infants. However, if mature banked human milk is used the protein concentration may be very low (sometimes as low as 1.0 gm/100 ml) and there are serious doubts about its nutritional adequacy.[60,61] Such milk will provide only 2.0 gm/kg/day of protein when fed at maximum recommended volume intake and this is well below the requirement determined by factorial analysis.[62] Slow growth, particularly of the head, has been described in preterm infants fed in this way.[63] The milk of preterm mothers has a higher nitrogen content[64] but it is very variable and on occasions may even contain uncomfortably high protein concentrations.[61] The message seems to be that the feeding of such extremely vulnerable infants is too important to be hit-or-miss and, at least in developed countries, a well-designed formula of known protein content is preferable to human milk of unknown protein content, a very different recommendation from that generally made for full-term infants.

Conclusion

Requirements for energy and protein have been discussed separately, but this separation is artificial, since energy balance has a profound effect on N balance (see reference 2). Moreover, the relative requirements for maintenance and for growth are not the same for energy and for nitrogen. It can be seen from Tables 1 and 4 that at 3 months, for example, growth accounts for about 24% of the energy requirement but about 60% of the N requirement. The more rapid the growth the greater the disproportion, so that when catch-up growth is needed after an illness or in the preterm infant, not only is more food required per kg of body weight, but also a relative increase in the protein content of the food. Some attempt was made in the 1985 UN report[2] to calculate the extra amounts that might be needed for catch-up, but many assumptions have to be made and the calculations can only be regarded as examples.

For a LBW infant a protein intake of 3.5 gm/kg/day and an energy intake of 180 kcal/kg/day gives a protein-energy ratio of 0.078, compared with about 0.06 for a normal infant at 3 months (Tables 2 and 4).

The increased requirement for protein in these situations does not imply a return to the concept of high protein foods that was popular in the 1970s, but it does emphasize once again the importance in developing countries of continuing some breastfeeding long after supplementary foods have been introduced.[65]

DEFICIENCY STATES

Deficiencies of protein and energy usually occur together and are grouped under the general title "protein-energy malnutrition (PEM)." Table 6 provides a clinical classification, the so-called Wellcome classification,[66] of PEM into four groups (Fig. 7). This table was proposed by a meeting of workers from many parts of the world, held in Jamaica, to try to find agreed definitions for the various forms of PEM. Marasmus is easily defined; the main clinical features are gross wasting of fat and muscle, suggesting that the cause is simply a deficiency of food. Many specific features have been described in the kwashiorkor syndrome—edema, fatty liver, skin lesions, discoloration of the hair, etc. The Wellcome group agreed that the key characteristic, essential for the diagnosis, is edema. **It would be more precise,**

therefore, to refer to kwashiorkor as edematous malnutrition in childhood.

A general discussion of the characteristics and etiology of these different forms of infantile malnutrition is given in reference 67. **According to classical teaching, a specific deficiency of protein is the major factor in producing the edematous form of PEM.** The physiological, clinical and epidemiological evidence for this view has been summarized by Waterlow.[68] In the brief, the argument is: (1) a diet specifically low in protein compared with energy produces hypoalbuminemia; (2) hypoalbuminemia predisposes to edema formation, although other factors, particularly potassium deficiency, may be implicated; and (3) edematous malnutrition occurs particularly in those parts of the world where the staple is low in protein and develops at a time when the children are completely weaned from the breast.

However, there is a contrary opinion that regards this story as an oversimplification. Golden[70] has produced interesting evidence to suggest that many features of the kwashiorkor syndrome result from the damaging effect of free radicals. The argument is not yet resolved.

Since this book is concerned with infants below one year of age, it should be noted that marasmus may occur in quite young infants, for example at 3 months if breastfeeding fails and there is no adequate alternative. Kwashiorkor, however, is less often seen in the first year of life, its peak prevalence being in the second and third years.

It has often been pointed out that kwashiorkor and marasmus represent only the tip of the iceberg. The group described in Table 6 as "undernutrition," i.e., a moderate deficit in weight for age, is many times more common. In recent years it has become customary to divide deficit in weight for age into two components, low weight for height (wasting) and low height for age (stunting).[5,7] Wasting and stunting are frequently found together in the same child; nevertheless, they are physiologi-

TABLE 6. The Wellcome Classification of Severe PEM[63]

Weight (% of standard)	Edema –	Edema +
80–60	Undernutrition	Kwashiorkor
<60	Marasmus	Marasmic kwashiorkor

Allowances per kg bodyweight per day for Total Parenteral Nutrition in Infants and Children (Sufficient for Growth in All but Severe Stress Conditions)

Age (years)	0–1	1–6	6–12	12–18
Water (ml)	120–150	90–120	60–90	30–60
Energy (MJ)	0.38–0.50	0.31–0.38	0.25–0.31	0.13–0.25
Energy (kcal)	90–120	75–90	60–75	30–60
Glucose (g)	12–20	6.0–12.0	3.0–6.0	2.0–4.0
Fat (g)	2.5–4.0	2.0–3.0	2.0–3.0	2.0–2.5
Amino acids (g)	2.0–3.0	1.5–2.5	1.3–2.0	1.0–1.3
Sodium (mmol)	1.0–2.5	1.0–2.0	1.0–2.0	1.0–1.5
Potassium (mmol)	2.0–2.5	1.0–2.0	0.9–2.0	0.7–1.2
Calcium (mmol)	0.5–1.0	0.3–0.7	0.2–0.7	0.11–0.20
Magnesium (mmol)	0.15–0.40	0.08–0.20	0.06–0.20	0.04–0.08
Phosphorus (mmol)	0.4–0.8	0.20–0.50	0.18–0.50	0.15–0.25
Iron (μmol)	2.0–3.0	1.5–2.5	1.5–2.5	1.0–1.5
Copper (μmol)	0.2–0.4	0.1–0.3	0.1–0.3	0.07–0.12
Zinc (μmol)	0.5–0.7	0.4–0.5	0.4–0.5	0.2–0.4
Manganese (μmol)	0.8–1.0	0.7–0.9	0.7–0.9	0.6–0.8
Chlorine (mmol)	1.8–4.3	1.5–2.5	1.5–2.5	1.3–2.3
Iodine (μmol)	0.03–0.05	0.02–0.04	0.02–0.04	0.015–0.03
Vitamins (water soluble)				
Thiamine (mg)	0.05	—	—	0.02–0.04
Riboflavine (mg)	0.10	—	—	0.03–0.05
Nicotinamide (mg)	1.00	—	—	0.20–0.50
Pyridoxine (mg)	0.10	—	—	0.03–0.05
Folic acid (μg)	20.00	—	—	3.00–6.00
Cyanocobalamin (μg)	0.20	—	—	0.03–0.10
Pantothenic acid (mg)	1.00	—	—	0.20–0.50
Biotin (μg)	30.00	—	—	5.00–10.00
Ascorbic acid (mg)	3.00	—	—	0.50–1.00
Vitamins (fat soluble)				
Retinol (μg)	100.00	—	—	10.00–25.00
Cholecalciferol (μg)	2.50	—	—	0.04–1.00
Phytylmenaquinone (μg)	50.00	—	—	2.00–10.00
α-Tocopherol (mg)	3.00	—	—	1.50–2.00

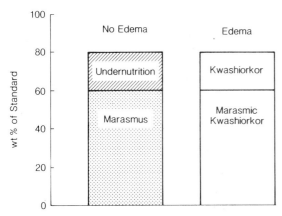

FIGURE 7. Wellcome classification of severe protein-energy malnutrition.

cally different states and there is no statistical relation between them.[69] One may speculate that wasting and stunting also have different causes. It seems obvious that wasting results from an inadequate energy intake. The wasted child usually does not have specific signs of other deficiencies. However, since the diet probably has been low in many nutrients as well as energy, there are likely to be latent deficiencies. If the diet during rehabilitation does not provide all the factors necessary for growth, specific nutrients may become limiting and latent deficiencies become manifest. This

has been described for potassium, magnesium, zinc, vitamin D and folic acid.

We do not yet understand the cause of stunting in linear growth, which in Third World countries is much commoner than wasting. It has been suggested that it may result from a specific deficiency of protein or of factors associated with protein in foods, such as zinc or calcium.[5,70,71] This, of course, is a completely different situation from the dwarfism due to growth hormone deficiency in industrialized countries.

TOXICITY

Energy

In infants, as in people of any age, excess energy intake leads to overweight and obesity. In the past it was recognized that bottle-fed infants tended to be heavier than breastfed babies, perhaps because of the use of unsuitable formulas such as sweetened condensed milk. There has been much concern that obesity in infancy may predispose to obesity in later life. However, it seems that although some fat children were indeed fat in infancy, most fat babies do not in fact develop into fat children.[72,73] The opposite sequence could in fact be proposed: that inadequate energy intake in infancy permanently programs the

TABLE 7. Daily Average Requirement of Infants for Energy and Protein[1]

Age, months	Median weight, kg[2]	Energy requirement[3]		Protein requirements[4]	
		kcal/kg	kcal/day	gm/kg	gm/day
Boys					
0-1	3.8	124	470	2.46	9.3
1-2	4.75	116	550	1.93	9.2
2-3	5.6	109	610	1.74	9.7
3-4	6.35	103	655	1.47	9.3
4-5	7.0	99	695	1.34	9.4
5-6	7.55	96.5	730	1.30	9.8
6-9	8.55	95	810	1.25	10.7
9-12	9.7	101	970	1.15	11.2
Girls					
0-1	3.6	124	445	2.39	8.6
1-2	4.35	116	505	1.93	8.4
2-3	5.05	109	545.	1.78	9.0
3-4	5.7	103	590	1.53	8.7
4-5	6.35	99	630	1.34	8.5
5-6	6.95	96.5	670	1.30	9.0
6-9	7.95	95	750	1.25	9.9
9-12	9.05	101	905	1.15	10.4

[1]It is recognized that these figures are unrealistically detailed, but they provide the basis for more approximate practical calculations. *Note that these values are average requirements and not safe levels.*
[2]50th centile. NCHS reference.
[3]From reference 2, Table 21.
[4]Intake of breastfed infants up to 3 months (reference 2, Table 29); from 3 months, calculated requirements (reference 2, Table 32).

child to economize energy and so predisposes to obesity later on. This subject needs further investigation.

Although I have no statistical support for this suggestion, I have been impressed by (1) how many adults that I have attempted to treat for obesity reported having been miserable puny babies, as a result of failure of breastfeeding, chronic gastroenteritis, pyloric stenosis, etc; and (2) the great frequency of obesity in adult women, such as the Jamaican or Ghanaian market women, in countries where infantile marasmus is common.

An immediate disadvantage of a baby being overweight is that it will limit its physical activity at a time when its musculature is still poorly developed.

Protein

There are no clearly documented effects of excess protein intake. Järvenpää et al.[38] have expressed concern that plasma concentrations of amino acids and urea are higher on intakes of 1.5 than on 1.2 gm/kg/day of protein, but are cautious about concluding that the higher levels are harmful. If they are, then the protein requirement of infants must be very finely balanced between too little and too much. Presumably any deleterious effects of a high protein intake will be greater in younger infants in whom renal function is not fully developed.

Protein in a meal is generally considered to have a greater thermic effect (specific dynamic action) than carbohydrate or fat. Perhaps this explains reports in the literature of infants in very hot countries such as Arabia dying of heat stroke after feeds high in protein.

Allergy to proteins such as those of cow milk is discussed in a subsequent chapter. It is probable that such effects depend more on the composition of the proteins than on their amounts.

CASE REPORT

Baby AB, a Jamaican male aged 10 months, was brought to the hospital by his mother because "him swell up" one week ago. He was breastfed for only 3 months because his mother had to work. The baby was then fed sweetened corn meal porridge and "tea." He had a poor appetite for 3 months and diarrhea for 2 weeks.

Examination: apathetic baby. Pitting edema of legs and feet. Liver edge 5 cm below costal margin. No mucosal or skin lesions. Hair sparse and slightly discolored. Some loss of skin turgor over trunk. Temperature, 36.5°. Chest and ears clear. Weight, 5.2 kg. Length, 66 cm. 55% weight for age; 90% height for age; 70% weight for

height. Urine: only 40 ml in first 24 hours; no albumin or blood. Blood: serum albumin 25 gm/L; K 3.2 mmol/L, Na 128 mmol/L. Hemoglobin, 7gm/dl. Liver function tests normal. Stools: liquid, acid, no worms or pathogenic organisms.

Diagnosis: Marasmic kwashiorkor.

Treatment: In view of the persisting diarrhea and the need to avoid dehydration, for first two days therapy consisted of continuous intragastric infusion of hypotonic saline (1/5 normal) + 5% dextrose with added K and Mg (see references 75 and 76). After 2 days, one-quarter strength formula by mouth every 2 hours.

Over next 4 days, strength and volume of feeds increased and frequency decreased, until by 7 days the baby was getting its maintenance requirements of energy and protein (about 80 kcal and 0.7 gm/kg/day of protein).

By day 10 stools reduced to 3 per day, appetite was improving, and there was no change in weight. Pitting edema was still present. From day 10 the energy and protein content of the feed was increased to provide 2.5 gm of protein and 150 kcal/kg/day in 6 feeds given every 3 hours. Over the next 4 days there was an abrupt loss of weight with disappearance of edema.

From then on the baby gained weight rapidly. He was fed ad libitum and achieved an average intake of 3 gm of protein and 170 kcal/kg/day. By the sixth week he had achieved the expected weight for height. A mixed diet (in addition to milk, cereals, crushed vegetables, minced meat, and eggs) was then introduced and he was discharged 10 days later.

Other treatment: A broad-spectrum antibiotic was administered to prevent undetected infection. Note that the undernourished baby cannot produce a pyrexia or adequate leukocytosis. From 2 days, folic acid 1 mg daily was provided. Note that many such infants have a "latent" folic acid deficiency. The rehabilitation diet is made up of skim milk powder, sucrose and arachis or coconut oil to provide about 1300 kcal and 32 gm of protein per liter. At 6 kg the infant would be given per day 5 feeds of 160 ml. This would provide approximately 170 kcal and 4.25 gm gm/kg/day of protein. Figure 8 shows that this would be enough to allow for weight gain at the rate of 15 gm/kg/day, assuming that 5 kcal are needed for each gram of gain. With this intake energy is likely to be limiting rather than protein. Full details of treatment are given in references 75 and 76.

Questions and Answers

Q. What responses of the infant would result in slower advances in strength or volume of feed?

A. The commonest cause is poor appetite. It is dangerous, and may even cause death, to try to achieve too high an intake during the first 1–2 weeks. The child's appetite is a good guide. The motto should always be: "festina lente" (Latin for "make haste slowly"). Some children may have prolonged anorexia for psychological reasons, particularly deprived children from orphanages or broken homes. These children need careful coaxing—what Cicely Williams calls TLC (tender loving care).

The second main cause of a poor response is persistent diarrhea. In some cases, not very common in our experience, there is an acquired lactose intolerance that responds well to a lactose-free formula. Note that if this is a formula based on soya, additional zinc may be neces-

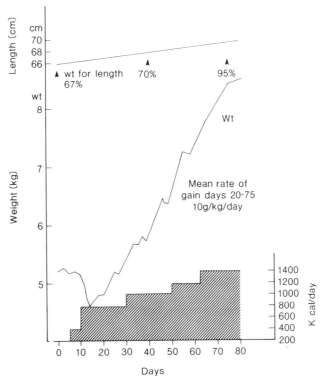

FIGURE 8.   Weight gain of malnourished infant on high
energy intake.

sary.* In other cases there is persistent colonization of the
small bowel. We have found metronidazole to be very
helpful.

Q. Is recurrence common? What advice should be given
to the parents to prevent recurrence?
A. Our practice has been not to discharge children until
they have regained their expected weight for height,
although they are usually still somewhat stunted and
therefore below expected weight for age. In our experience recurrence is rare with this regimen except in
children admitted with severe malnutrition below the age
of 6 months.

However, to regain expected weight for height means
keeping the children in hospital for 2-3 months, with the
disadvantages of expense and possibly psychological
damage. Providing plenty of toys and actually playing with
the children is very important. The question is
now being studied whether earlier discharge, before the
children are fully rehabilitated, carries an increased risk of
relapse.

The advice to the parent is the usual kind of thing: the
importance of hygiene, oral fluids if there are bouts of
diarrhea, and amounts and types of food appropriate for
the child's age.

---

*Golden MHN, Golden, BE. Effect of zinc supplementation on the
dietary intake, rate of weight gain and energy cost of tissue
deposition in children recovering from severe malnutritiion. Am J
Clin Nurs 1981; 34: 900-908.

REFERENCES

1. Sukhatme PV, Margen S. Autoregulatory homeostatic nature
   of energy balance. Am J Clin Nutr 1982; 35:355-365.
2. World Health Organization Energy and Protein Requirements. Report of a Joint FAC/WHO/UNU Meeting. Tech
   Rep Ser No. 724. WHO, Geneva, 1985.
3. Food and Agriculture Organization. Energy and protein requirements. Report of a Joint FAO/WHO Ad Hoc Expert
   Committee. FAO Nutrition Meetings Rep Ser 52, 1973.
4. World Health Organization: Protein Requirements. Report of
   a Joint FAO/WHO Expert Group. WHO Tech Rep Ser No.
   301. WHO, Geneva, 1965.
5. Waterlow JC. Current issues in nutritional assessment by
   anthropometry. In Brozek J, Schurch B (eds): Malnutrition
   and Behavior: Critical Assessment of Key Issues. Lausanne,
   Nestle Foundation, 1984; 77-90.
6. Hamill PVV, Drizd TA, Johnson CL, et al. Physical growth:
   National Center for Health Statistics percentiles. Am J Clin
   Nutr 1979;32:607-629.
7. Waterlow JC, Buzina R, Keller W, et al. The presentation and
   use of height and weight data for comparing the nutritional
   status of groups of children under the age of 10 years. Bull
   WHO 1977;55:489-498.
8. World Health Organization. Measuring Change in Nutritional
   Status. WHO, Geneva, 1983.
9. Martorell R. Child growth retardation: a discussion of its
   causes and of its relationship to health. In Blaxter KL,
   Waterlow JC (eds): Nutritional Adaptation in Man. London,
   Libbey, 1985;13-30.
10. Whitehead RG, Paul AA. Growth charts and the assessment of
    infant feeding practices in the Western world and in
    developing countries. Early Hum Dev 1984; 9:187-207.
11. Salmenperä L, Perheentupe J, Siimes MA. Exclusively breast
    fed healthy infants grow slower than reference infants.
    Pediatr Res 1985;19:307-312.

12. Tanner JM, Whitehouse RH, Takaishi W. Standards from birth to maturity for height, weight, height velocity and weight velocity . British children, 1963, part II. Arch Dis Child 1966;41:613-635.

13. Karlberg P, Taranger J, Engstrom, I, et al. Physical growth from birth to 16 years and longitudinal outcome of the study during the same age period. Acta Paediatr Scand 1976;Suppl. 176:7-77.

14. Fomon SJ. Infant Nutrition 2nd ed. Philadelphia, W.B. Saunders Co., 1974; 118-151.

15. Healy, MJR, Yang Min, Tanner JM, Zumrawi FY. Short term increments in weight and length in growth monitoring in infancy. In Guesry P Goyens P, Waterlow JC (eds): Nestle Nutrition Workshop, 1987.

16. Munro HN. Historical Introduction: the origi and growth of our present concepts of protein metabolism. In Munro HN, Allison JB (eds): Mammalian Protein Metabolism. New York Academic Press, 1964; 7.

17. Waterlow JC. Observations on the mechanism of adaptation to low protein intakes. Lancet 1968;2:1092-1097.

18. Nelson RA. Protein and fat metabolism in hibernating bears. Fed Proc 1980;39:2955-2958.

19. Torun B. Physiological measurements of physical activity among children under free-living conditions. In Pollitt E, Amande P. (eds): Current Topics in Nutrition and Disease, Vol.11. New York, Liss, 1984;159-184.

20. Chavez A, Martinez C. Behavioral measurements of activity in children and their relation to food intake in a poor community. In Pollitt E, P Amande P (eds): Current Topics in Nutrition and Disease, Vol. 11. New York, Liss, 1984; 303-322.

21. Schofield WN, Schofield C, James WPT. Basal metabolic rate - review and prediction, together with an annotated bibliography of source material. Hum Nutr Clin Nutr 1985; 39C, Suppl. 1:5-41.

22. Ashworth A. Metabolic rates during recovery from protein-calorie malnutrition the need for a new concept of specific dynamic action. Nature 1969;223:407-409.

23. Brooke OG, Ashworth A. The influence of malnutrition on the post-prandial metabolic rate and respiratory quotients. Br J Nutr 1972;27:407-415.

24. Forbes GB, Kreipe RE, Lipinski B. Body composition and the energy cost of weight gain. Hum Nutr Clin Nutr 1982; 36C:485-487.

25. Millward DJ, Garlick PJ, Reeds PJ. The energy cost of growth. Proc Nutr Soc 1976;35:339-349.

26. Reeds PJ, Jackson AA, Picou D, Poulter N Muscle mass and composition in malnourished infants and children and changes seen after recovery. Pediatr Res 1978;12:613.

27. Spady DW, Payne PR, Picou D, Waterlow JC. Energy balance during recovery from malnutrition. Am J Clin Nutr 1976; 29:1073-1088.

28. Whitehead RG, Paul AA, Cole TJ. A critical analysis of measured food energy intakes during infancy and early childhood in comparison with current international recommendations. J Hum Nutr 1981;35:339-348.

29. Butte NF, Garza C, O'Brien Smith E, Nichols BL. Human milk intake and growth in exclusively breast-fed infants. J Pediatr 1984;104:187-195.

30. Zumrawi FW, Dimond H, Waterlow JC. Growth faltering in infants in the Sudan. Hum Nutr Clin Nutr 1987;41C:387-396.

31. Fomon SJ, Haschke F, Ziegler EE, Nelson SE. Body composition of reference children from brith to age 10 years. Am J Clin Nutr 1982;35:1169-1175.

32. Hambraeus L, Fransson GB, Lonnerdal B. Nutritional availability of breast milk protein. Lancet 1984; 2:167-168.

33. Järvenpää AL, Räiha NCR, Rassin DK, Gaull GE. Milk protein quantity and quality in the term infant. I. Metabolic responses and effects on growth. Pediatrics 1982;70:214-220.

34. Macy IG. Composition of human colostrum and milk. Am J Dis Child 1949; 79:589-603.

35. Waterlow JC, Wills VG, Gyorgy P. Balance studies in malnourished Jamaican infants. I Comparison of absorption and retention of nitrogen and phosphorus from human milk and a cow's milk mixture. Br J Nutr 1960;14:199-205.

36. Picou D, Phillips M. Urea metabolism in malnourished and recovered children receiving a high or low protein diet. Am J Clin Nutr 1972;25:1261-1266.

37. Snyderman SE, Holt LE Jr, Dancis J, et al. Unessential nitrogen: a limiting factor for human growth. J Nutr 1962;78:57-72.

38. Järvenpää AL, Rassin DK, Räihä NCR, Gaull GE. Milk protein quanitity and quality in the term infant. II. Effects on acidic and neutral amino acids. Pediatrics 1982;70:221-223.

39. McClelland DBL, McGrath J, Samson RR. Antimicrobial factors in human milk. Studies of concentration and transfer in human milk. Studies of transfer to the infant during the early stages of loctation. Acta Paediatr Scand 1978;67, Suppl.271: 1-20.

40. Butte NF, Goldblum RM, Fehl LM, et al. Daily ingestion of immunologic components in human milk during the first four months of life. Acta Paediatr Scand 1984;73:296-301.

41. Schnaler RJ, Goldblum RM, Garza C, Goldman AS. Enhanced fecal excretion of selected immune factors in very low birthweight infants fed fortified human milk. Pediatr Res in press.

42. Gopalan C. Effect of nutrition on pregnancy and lactation. Bull WHO 1962;26:203-211.

43. Chavez A, Martinez C. Effects of maternal undernutrition and dietary supplementation on milk production. In Aebi H, Whitehead RG (eds): Maternal Nutrition during Pregnancy and Lactation. Bern, Huber, 1980;274-286.

44. Coward WA, Cole TJ, Sawyer MB, Prentice AM. Breast milk intake measurement in mixed-fed infants by administration of deuterium oxide to their mothers. Hum Nutr Clin Nutr 1982;36C:141-148.

45. Ashworth A, Waterlow JC. Infant mortality in developing countries. Arch Dis Child 1982;57:882-884.

46. Brooke OG. Energy expenditure in the fetus and neonate: sources of variablity. Acta Paediatr Scand 1985; Suppl 319:128-134.

47. Mestyan J, Fekete M, Bata G, Jarai I. The basal metabolic rate of premature infants. Biol Neonate 1964; 1:11-25.

48. Scopes JW Ahmed I. Minimum rates of oxygen consumption in sick premature newborn infants. Arch Dis Child 1966;41:407-412.

49. Hill JR Robinson DC. Oxygen consumption in normally-grown small-for-dates and large-for-dates newborn infants. J Physiol 1968;199:683-693.

50. Brooke OG, Alvear J. Postprandial metabolism in infants of low birthweight. Hum Nutr Clin Nutr 1982;36C:167-175.

51. Abdulrazzak YM, Brooke OG. Respiratory metabolism in preterm infants: the measurement of oxygen consumption during prolonged periods. Pediatr Res 1984; 18:928-319.

52. Committee on Nutrition of the Preterm Infant, European Society of Paediatric Gastroenterology and Nutrition. Nutrition and feeding of preterm infants. Acta Paediatr Scand in press.

53. Reichman B, Chessex P, Putet G, et al. Partition of energy metabolism and energy cost of growth in the very-low-birthweight infant. Pediatrics 1982;69:446-451.

54. Gudinchet F. Schutz Y, Micheli J-L, et al. Metabolic cost of growth in very low-birth-weight infants. Pediatr Res 1982:16:1025-1030.

55. Brooke OG, Alvear J, Arnold M. Energy retention, energy expenditure and growth in healthy immature infants. Pediatr Res 1979;13:215-220.

56. Brooke OG Energy needs in infancy. In Fomon SJ, Heird WC (eds): Energy and Protein Needs during Infancy. Orlando, Florida, Academic Press, 1986;3-18.

57. Glass L, Silverman W Sinclair JC. Effect of the thermal environment on cold resistance and growth of small infants after the first week of life. Pediatrics 1968;41:1033-1046.

58. Sinclair JC (ed). Temperature Regulation and Energy Metabolism in the Newborn. New York, Grune and Stratton, 1978.

59. Raiha NCR, Heinonen K, Rassin DK, Gaull GE, Milk protein quality and quantity in low-birth-weight infants: 1. Metabolic responses and effects on growth. Pediatrics 1976;57:659-174.

60. Brooke OG. Nutrition in the preterm infant. Lancet 1983; 1:514-515.

61. Lucas A, Hudson GJ. Preterm milk as a source of protein for low birthweight infants. Arch Dis Child 1984;59:831-836.

62. Ziegler EE. Protein requirements of preterm infants. In Fomon SJ, Heird WC (eds): Energy and Protein Needs during Infancy. Orlando, Florida, Academic Press, 1986.

63. Davies DP. Adequacy of expressed breast milk for early growth of preterm infants. Arch Dis Child 1977;52:296-299.
64. Lemons JA, Moye L, Hall D, Simmons M. Differences in the composition of preterm and term human milk during early lactation. Pediatr Res 1982;16:113-117.
65. Jelliffe DB, Jelliffe EF. The volume and composition of human milk in poorly nourished communities. Am J Clin Nutr 1978;31:492-515.
66. Wellcome Trust Working Party. Classification of infantile malnutrition. Lancet 1970;2:302-303.
67. Alleyne GAO, Hay RW, Picou DI, et al. Protein-Energy Malnutrition. London, Arnold, 1977.
68. Waterlow JC. Kwashiorkor revisited: the pathogenesis of oedema in kwashiorkor and its significance. Trans R Soc Trop Med Hyg 1984;78:436-441.
69. Keller W. choice of indicators of nutritional status. In Schürch B (ed): Evaluation of Nutrition Education in Third World Communities. Bern, Huber, 1983;101-114.
70. Golden M. The consequences of protein deficiency in man and its relationship to the features of kwashiorkor. Blaxter KL, Waterlow JC (eds): Nutritional Adaptation in Man. London, Libbey, 1985; 169-188.
71. Waterlow JC. Observations on the assessment of protein-energy malnutrition with special reference to stunting. Courier 1978;28:455-458.
72. Garrow JS. The outlook for the obese baby. Ann Nestlé 1981;1-13.
73. Poskitt EME, Cole TJ. Do fat babies stay fat? Br Med J 1977; 1: 7-9.
74. World Health Organization. The Quantity and Quality of Breast Milk. Report on the WHO Collaborative Study on Breast-feeding. WHO, Geneva, 1985.
75. Waterlow JC, Golden MHN, Patrick J. Protein-energy malnutrition: treatment. In Dickerson JWT, Lee MA (eds): Nutrition in the Clinical Management of Disease. London, Arnold, 1980;49-71.
76. World Health Organization. The Treatment and Management of Severe Protein Malnutrition. WHO, Geneva, 1981.

2

Physiology of Lactation

CUTBERTO GARZA, M.D., Ph.D.
JUDY HOPKINSON, Ph.D.

ABSTRACT

The production of sufficient human milk to nourish an infant adequately is the goal of the successful management of lactation. Mechanisms for milk synthesis and secretion will not develop optimally if the mammary gland is not appropriately stimulated. This stimulation is dependent upon a normally functioning maternal physiology and effective physical stimulation of the nipple and areola in a favorable environment. Although it is unusual for the hormonal changes needed to support lactation not to proceed normally immediately after parturition, failure to consider normal lactation physiology after the immediate postpartum period is common. When physiologic principles are not applied, the cytologic structures and the hormonal milieu for milk synthesis are not maintained. The consequence is lactation failure, a preventable condition in most cases.

INTRODUCTION

Current guidelines for infant feeding published by the American Academy of Pediatrics[1] state that infants should be breastfed for 4 to 6 months. The most common reason given by women who wean their infants before the recommended time is an insufficient milk supply.[2] Lactation failure does occur but it should be a relatively uncommon condition.[3] Previous suggestions that the mother's capacity to provide sufficient energy and protein is outgrown by the 3- to 4-month-old infant[4] have been challenged by intake and growth data of normal populations. Recent data have documented that ad libitum intakes of normally growing, exclusively breastfed infants [5,6] and of infants fed human milk and solid food[7,8] are significantly below (approximately 20 to 30%) previous estimates of energy requirements.

Lactation failure is preventable in almost all cases if sound physiological principles are applied during the initiation, establishment, and maintenance periods of lactation. Although information on human lactation physiology remains incomplete, sufficient knowledge from human and animal studies is available to develop useful guidelines for the successful management of lactation.

BREAST ANATOMY

The most prominent external features of the breast are the nipple and areola (Fig. 1). The nipple varies greatly in size among women. It contains the openings of 10 to 15 lactiferous ducts through which milk is either ejected or expressed. The nipple is surrounded by the areola, a circular area of melanin-pigmented cells (melanophores) that darken early in the first pregnancy. The areola also varies in size. The nipple and subareolar area contain smooth muscle fibers arranged concentrically and radially. These smooth muscles contract the areola and compress the base of the nipple. This involuntary action likely helps empty lactiferous ducts underlying the nipple and areola.

The areola contains many small tubercles, most prominent in the lactating woman, which overlie sebaceous glands whose secretion appears to provide protection to the skin against vigorous sucking. The skin overlying the breast is innervated by the supraclavicular and intercostal nerves.[9] The nipple and areola are richly innervated and supplied with a dense array of sensory end organs that may be of special importance to the successful initiation and establishment of lactation. The nipple and areola appear to be innervated solely by the interior branch of the fourth intercostal nerve.[10]

The breast consists of adipose and glandular tissue. Each breast contains 15 to 20 lobes of glandular tissue; each lobe in turn contains many lobules. The basic secretory unit of the breast is the alveolus or acinus. Multiple acini make up each lobule. Each acinus consists of secretory cells surrounded by contractile myoepithelial cells. Acini empty into small ducts which channel milk from the acinar lumen to lactiferous sinuses or ampullae located beneath the nipple. *True acini do not develop until the first pregnancy.* At puberty, the epithelial ducts

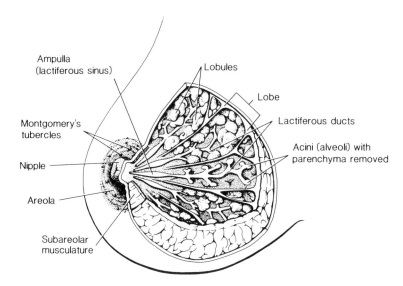

Ampulla
(lactiferous sinus)

Lobules

Lobe

Montgomery's
tubercles

Lactiferous ducts

Acini (alveoli) with
parenchyma removed

Nipple

Areola

Subareolar
musculature

FIGURE 1. *Anatomy of the breast.* Key anatomical features of special importance during lactation are illustrated as well as the basic secretary units (alveoli) of the mammary gland and the ducts leading from the alveoli to the ampulla. (From Townsend CM. Clinical Symposia. Issue 2, vol. 32, 1980, p. 4, with permission.)

develop and adipose tissue increases markedly in response to endocrine signals from the hypothalamus, anterior pituitary, and, in later puberty, the ovaries. Estrogen is especially important in the initial maturation of the ductal system and in the periodic and transient increases in the vascularity of the gland and the proliferation of supporting connective tissue which occur during each menstrual cycle. Vascular dilatation and engorgement are also noted during the progesterone-dominant phase of menses. Other hormones, such as insulin and thyroxin, play permissive roles in these processes. These changes are even more pronounced during pregnancy when glandular proliferation is most evident. The reader is referred to standard gynecological texts for a detailed discussion of the endocrine stimuli that characterize the menstrual cycle.[11]

INITIATION OF LACTATION

Endocrine Stimuli

Three approaches have been used to study the physiology of lactation initiation. Each approach has concentrated on the endocrine aspects of the process. First, tissue culture experiments have identified the endocrine stimuli necessary to initiate lactation and those that enhance milk synthesis.[12] These studies have identified a need for insulin and adrenocortical steroids for acinar proliferation. Prolactin is necessary for lactogenesis (synthesis of milk), although other hormones (such as growth hor-

mone and placental lactogen) can induce milk synthesis under tissue culture conditions.

Second, exogenous hormones have been administered to intact animals and to animals with various excised endocrine glands. These studies have supported results of tissue culture experiments. The role of prolactin has been particularly well described in these experiments. Prolactin administration under appropriate conditions will result in the biochemical and anatomical changes required for milk production in parous animals.[13] These responses can be inhibited if bromocriptine, a prolactin-inhibiting drug, is administered to normal animals in the early postpartum period.[14]

In contrast to the action of prolactin, progesterone has been demonstrated to inhibit the initiation of lactation. Bilateral oophorectomy or removal of the corpus luteum from pregnant animals will initiate lactation.[15] The simultaneous administration of progesterone with either procedure blocks the initiation of milk synthesis. These types of experiments have identified the two basic components of lactation initiation: a prolactin-induced initiation and a progesterone-modulated inhibition of initiation.[16]

Third, these components of lactation initiation also have been demonstrated by hormonal measurements obtained in humans throughout pregnancy, parturition, and lactation. Prolactin levels increase progressively as pregnancy advances. Progesterone and estrogen levels also rise throughout pregnancy. If urinary excretion is used as an index of total production, progesterone levels appear to increase linearly after approximately 20 weeks of gestation.[17] Estrogen levels also increase steadily after approximately 20 weeks of gestation. Serum estrogen increases gradually 3 to 5 weeks before parturition and then markedly approximately 2 weeks before delivery.

At parturition prolactin levels surge. With the expulsion of the placenta, progesterone and estrogen levels fall. Elevated baseline levels of prolactin observed during the immediate postpartum period decline steadily in the subsequent 3 to 4 weeks if lactation is not maintained.[18] If lactation continues, elevated prolactin levels may be observed for as long as 2 years.[19] When the infant nurses, prolactin levels increase in bursts above elevated baseline levels. Although baseline prolactin levels have not been correlated with the degree of milk production, the magnitude of the increase during suckling has been related to absolute milk volumes.[20] Basal prolactin levels in late lactation are much lower than those observed in the early postpartum period. This observation suggests that prolactin is more critical for the initiation than it is for the maintenance of milk production.

Animal studies show that the administration of small doses of estrogen may lead to increased milk production, whereas large doses tend to suppress lactation. The timing of estrogen administration, however, is important; the administration of small doses of estrogen to sheep in early lactation was associated with an increase in the fat content of milk but no increase in milk volume; in late lactation, estrogen administration was associated with an increase in milk production. In humans, long-acting preparations of estradiol or testosterone have been administered immediately after delivery to suppress lactation. The mechanism of action of this response is not clear; prolactin levels are not suppressed by the administration of either steroid.[22,23] Those preparations may interfere with prolactin's lactogenic effects.

The mechanisms by which prolactin and supporting hormones induce milk production are not known. Prolactin appears to induce the proliferation of its own receptors by increasing the number of secretory cells and the number of receptors per cell.[16] Proliferation of prolactin receptors has been documented at parturition, a response that is thought to be necessary for successful lactogenesis. Estrogen also increases the number of prolactin receptors; progesterone suppresses this estrogenic response.

Two mechanisms have been proposed to explain the initiation of events that lead to milk synthesis after prolactin binds to its receptor: the "second messenger" mechanism common to steroid hormones and the cellular internalization of a prolactin fragment leading to specific genomic responses by the secretory cells.

As lactation is initiated, the secretory cells produce colostrum. This secretion has a higher protein and lower fat and lactose content than does mature milk. **Colostrum is especially rich in immunoglobulins, mostly sIgA, and a variety of immunologically competent mononuclear cells.** Colostrum is produced over the first 3 to 5 days of lactation. This secretion is followed by so-called "transitional milk." Mature milk usually is produced by two weeks after parturition. None of these periods is fixed. The marked changes in composition that characterize the transition from colostrum to mature milk are followed by less rapid compositional alterations. A relatively stable composition is observed after approximately 12 weeks.[24]

The control of prolactin secretion during lactation is not well understood. Generally, prolactin secretion occurs in bursts in response to suckling. Afferent nerve fibers from the nipple and areola carry signals through the spinothalamic tract to the anterior pituitary via the hypothalamus. Prolactin secretion may be under the tonic inhibition of dopamine and there is evidence that the serotonergic system may activate its secretion.[25] Thyrotropin releasing factor also stimulates its secretion. The possibility of a specific prolactin releasing factor has been reported and is not ruled out.

Synthesis and Secretion of Milk Protein

The basic biochemical mechanisms responsible for the synthesis of milk proteins, lipids, and carbohydrates are well understood. Major gaps, however, exist in the understanding of mechanisms that regulate their production. Milk proteins are synthesized mostly from free amino acids taken up from the blood stream by acinar secretory cells (Fig. 2). Amino acid uptake is a function of the arterial concentration of amino acids, the rate of mammary blood flow, and the efficiency of the extraction process across the basal membrane of the secretory cell.[26] After amino acid uptake, protein synthesis follows the usual pathways of DNA transcription and mRNA directed translation.

Many human milk proteins are modified by the addition of phosphate or carbohydrate groups. These modifications result in a distinct heterogeneity of individual proteins. The significance of this heterogeneity is difficult to assess but is likely to be more important from a functional than from a nutritional standpoint.

A central role in the secretion of milk proteins has been proposed for the endoreticulum (ER) and other cellular membranes.[27] Secretory proteins appear to move from the ER to the Golgi bodies with portions of the ER membrane. Vesicles containing modified proteins bud off from the Golgi bodies and move toward the apical portion of the cell. Secretory vesicles from the Golgi bodies fuse with the plasma membrane of the secretory cell and empty into the acinar lumen. Membrane transfers occur throughout these successive movements. Extensive reviews are available of the relationships among the primary structure of a protein, the structure and membranes of

secretory cells, and the synthesis and secretion of proteins.[28,29]

Not all proteins, however, are synthesized de novo in the mammary gland. Some are transferred from blood or extracellular fluid to milk through the secretory cell. The transfer mechanisms are not well understood. The protein most studied is IgA. Most milk secretory IgA (sIgA) is thought to originate in local plasma cells.[30] IgA produced by these cells is transported across the acinar cells to milk, but some IgA may be transferred from blood. The secretory piece is added to IgA during its transfer through the secretory cell. If the transfer of whole proteins from blood to milk occurs, a possible model for protein uptake may be found in the highly selective pinocytotic transfer of antibodies described in the neonatal rat.[31]

The appearance of a wide spectrum of specific antibodies in human milk has been of particular interest. The principal im-

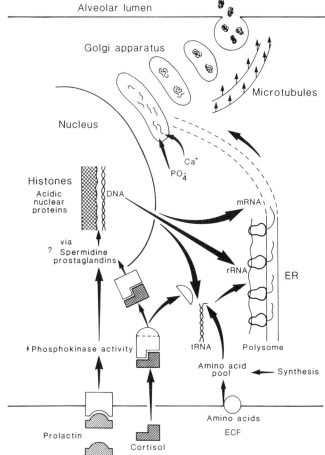

FIGURE 2. A schematic representation of factors involved in milk protein synthesis and secretion. Gene derepression by the action of prolactin (membrane receptor) and cortisol (mobile receptor) is believed to be mediated by spermidine and/or prostaglandins. Proteins synthesized on the endoplasmic reticulum (ER) are conveyed to the Golgi apparatus, where they enter associations with other proteins (e.g., caseins aggregate in micelles). Golgi vesicle migration is thought to involve microtubules, while release from the cell is predominantly by reverse pinocytosis (From Mepham TB. Synthesis and secretion of milk proteins. In Peaker M (ed.). Comparative Aspects of Lactation. New York, Academic Press, 1977, p. 63, with permission.)

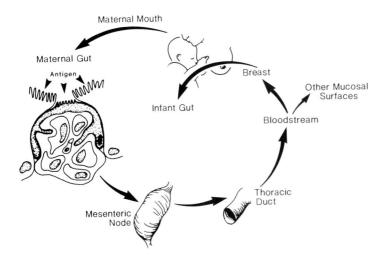

FIGURE 3. *Enteromammary Pathway.* Cells in gut-associated lymphoid tissue are sensitized to antigens in the maternal intestinal tract and migrate via the thoracic duct to the systemic circulation. During lactation these cells populate the mammary gland and secrete IgA. IgA is transported into the mammary gland's secretory cell. The secretory piece is attached to the IgA and sIgA is secreted in milk. (From Kleinman RE Walker WA. The enteromammary immune system. Dig Dis Sci 1979;24: 880, with permission.)

munoglobulin found in human milk is sIgA. **The specificity of human milk sIgA is dependent upon the mother's antigenic exposure.** Mechanisms responsible for the appearance of these antibodies are understood partially. Plasma cells are transported from the gastrointestinal and bronchotracheal-associated lymphatic tissues to multiple mucosal surfaces including the mammary gland, where they produce IgA for secretion in milk (Fig. 3).[32] The particular hormonal milieu that induces lactogenesis appears necessary for these cells to be directed to the mammary gland.[30]

The ability of the mother to secrete antibodies directed against specific antigens in her environment imparts to human milk an environmental specificity with significant protective potential.[33] There is limited understanding of the dynamics and properties of this response, which appears to be very complex. From accumulated evidence, the sIgA response in human milk following maternal mucosal exposure to diverse antigens is not uniform. It is not known if the requirements necessary for a signficant positive sIgA response in milk reside exclusively in the antigen or in the manner in which the antigen is presented to and processed by the immunologic system.

The complexities of the sIgA response are evident from recent work of Hanson and coworkers.[34-36] Oral immunization with live poliovirus vaccine of lactating women previously exposed naturally to the virus did not result in an expected enhancement of specific sIgA antibodies against polio in milk but did result in a reduction in titer.[34] Simultaneous

cholera vaccination further decreased the response to the polio vaccine.[35] In related experiments, subcutaneous immunization against cholera resulted in a significant rise in sIgA titer in the milk of 70% of Pakistani women tested but in none of the Swedish women used as a comparison group.[36] The Swedish group did not respond following a booster dose of 14 days after the initial immunization. These results suggest that the capacity of parenterally administered cholera vaccine to stimulate the production and secretion of sIgA in milk differs between naturally sensitized and nonsensitized women.

The stage of lactation [37] and the length of gestation[38] influence the total content and relative amounts of specific proteins in human milk. However, the physiologic mechanisms that regulate these changes have not been identified nor has the role of the mother's nutritional state been defined well. The total protein concentration of human milk does not appear to differ between populations at distinct levels of nutritional risk,[39] but difficulties are encountered in the interpretation of published data because protein often has been estimated from measurements of total milk nitrogen rather than from measurements of protein nitrogen. In contrast to field studies of diverse populations, evaluations of well-nourished women in controlled metabolic centers[40] have demonstrated that **acute increases in dietary protein (from 8 to 20% of total energy) are associated with increases in total protein** concentration (approximately 8%) in milk and in 24-hour milk protein output (21%). The duration of these responses has not been evaluated.

FIGURE 4. Diet and breast milk fat.

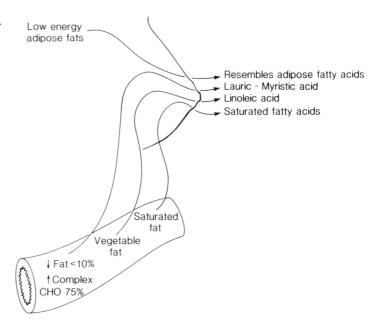

Low energy adipose fats

Resembles adipose fatty acids
Lauric - Myristic acid
Linoleic acid
Saturated fatty acids

Saturated fat

Vegetable fat

↓ Fat <10%
↑ Complex CHO 75%

Synthesis and Secretion of Milk Fat

Human milk lipids usually are classified as triglycerides, free fatty acids, sterols, or phospholipids. This discussion will focus on triglycerides and free fatty acids. The origin of milk triglycerides and free fatty acids is dependent upon the composition and energy level of the mother's diet. Under most dietary conditions, except possibly extreme undernutrition, mature milk contains approximately 3.5 gm/dl of total fat. The composition of the fat, however, is markedly dependent on the diet (Fig. 4).[41,42] Women who consume diets that are high in complex carbohydrates (75% of total energy), low in fat (approximately 10% or less), and supply energy at or in excess of requirement produce milks with relatively high levels of lauric and myristic acids. These medium-chain fatty acids are synthesized de novo by the mammary gland. **Women with high content of vegetable fat in the diet produce milk with relatively high concentrations of linoleic acid.** Those with very high intakes of saturated fat produce milk with a fat composition that reflects their diets. When women consume diets that do not meet their energy needs, milk fat composition resembles the fat composition of their adipose tissue.

Most fats in milk are transported in blood to the mammary gland as triglycerides in chylomicrons or very low density lipoproteins (VLDL).[43] Lipoprotein lipase (LPL) on the luminal surfaces of mammary gland capillaries catalyzes the hydrolysis of triglycerides in the chylomicrons and VLDL and makes available fatty acids and partial glycerides to the mammary gland. Most free fatty acids (FFA) released by LPL hydrolysis are carried away by the blood stream; partial glycerides are taken up by the capillary endothelium where they undergo further hydrolysis and are transported across the capillary wall into the interstitial space between the capillary and the mammary gland's secretory cells. FFA and partial glycerides are transported into the secretory cell from the interstitial space.

LPL activity is controlled partially by prolactin. The level of this hormone increases after parturition and rises further with suckling. Prolactin stimulates LPL activity in the mammary gland, but inhibits it in adipose tissue. Therefore fat uptake by the mammary gland is facilitated.

De novo synthesis of fat by the mammary gland follows the usual pathways catalyzed by the enzyme complex, fatty acid synthase, resulting in condensation of successive malonyl-Co A units derived from acetyl-Co A and bicarbonate, with one important exception.[44] In most tissues, thioesterase I terminates the growth of acyl chains on the fatty acid synthase complex when fats reach 16 carbon units. In the mammary gland, thioesterase II modifies the usual product specificity by catalyzing the hydrolysis of the thioester linkages of medium-

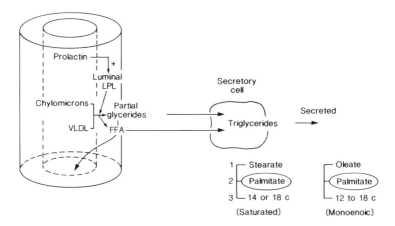

FIGURE 5.

chain moieties attached to the fatty acid synthase complex. **Most of the medium-chain fats, therefore, are the products of in situ lipid synthesis;** the longer chain fats are transported to the mammary gland and are of immediate dietary or adipose tissue origin.

Fatty acids synthesized in situ or transferred from blood chylomicrons or VLDL are esterified to form triglycerides in the secretory cell (Fig 5). Fatty acids of specific chain length and saturation are not distributed randomly between positions 1 and 2 of the glycerol moiety.[45] The fully saturated triglycerides usually contain stearate and palmitate in positions 1 and 2 respectively; position 3 is esterified by fatty acids of 14 or 18 carbon chain length. Monoenoic triglycerides consist of 1-oleate, 2-palmitate, and position 3 is filled with fatty acids of 12 to 18 carbon chain lengths. The selective placement of palmitate in the 2 position and stearate and oleate in the 1 and 3 positions is notable in human milk. Preliminary stable isotope-tracer studies of the transfer of dietary lipids into human milk by Hachey and coworkers support the selective conservation of palmitate 2-monoglycerides across the blood into the acinar lumen.

The process by which fat is secreted into the acinar lumen is partially analogous to protein secretion. Small fat droplets without any apparent membrane form in the basal portion of the secretory cell. As these droplets progress toward the apex of the secretory cell, they are surrounded peripherally by vesicles produced by the Golgi bodies. Fat droplets fuse with the vesicles originating in the Golgi bodies and with the plasmalemma of the secretory cell. Fat is thereafter extruded from the cell packaged as globules surrounded by a membrane that originates from the plasmalemma of the secretory cell and the Golgi bodies.

Synthesis and Secretion of Milk Carbohydrate

Lactose contents rise rapidly during the initiation of lactation and reach a fairly stable level at approximately 7 gm/dl in mature milk.[3] Small amounts of glucose, oligosaccharides and glycoproteins are found also in milk (Fig. 6). Oligosaccharides and glycoproteins may be of functional importance to the infant in the modulation of the infant's colonic flora[47] and in protecting the infant against infection.[48] Oligosaccharides in human milk resemble receptors found on the surface of retropharyngeal cells which bind bacteria. The milk oligosaccharides may bind potential pathogens by mimicking the receptors on retropharyngeal cells and thereby protect the infant. The regulation of oligosaccharide content in human milk is not understood.

Lactose is the most tightly regulated component of human milk. The interindividual coefficient of variablity is less than 3.5% in women consuming the usual Western type of diet.[12] Normal milk has an osmolar concentration very close to that of blood, and lactose accounts for 60 to 70% of the total osmolar concentration of milk. **From its major role as an osmotic agent and its tightly controlled concentration it is suggested that lactose is a major regulator of milk volume.**[49] Lactose concentrations appear to be maintained even under severe nutritional stress. Lactating rats fed 75% of their usual ad libitum diet, for ex-

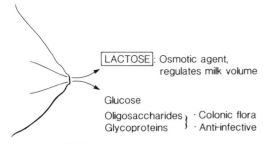

FIGURE 6.   Milk carbohydrates.

ample, demonstrate a marked reduction in the quantity of milk produced but none in the concentration of lactose in the milk that is secreted.[50]

The pathway for lactose synthesis is described in most standard textbooks of biochemistry.[51] The basic substrate is glucose, which is epimerized to galactose (Fig. 7). Lactose synthesis is accomplished by lactose synthetase, an enzyme complex that consists of galactosyltransferase and (alpha)-lactalbumin. Galactosyltransferase interacts with (alpha)-lactalbumin to specify the transfer of galactose to glucose to form the galactose-glucose disaccharide, lactose. Progesterone has an inhibitory effect on the biosynthesis of lactose and, more specifically, on the production of (alpha)-lactalbumin;[52] prolactin promotes the production of (alpha)-lactalbumin. Animal studies demonstrate that by the latter half of pregnancy, mammary gland galactosyltransferase activity reaches near maximal values, whereas levels of (alpha)-lactalbumin remain low and do not increase to maximal values until after parturition.[53] Based on these and other similar data it is suggested that the ratio of prolactin to progesterone is an important factor in the control of (alpha)-lactalbumin synthesis. As this ratio increases, the stimulatory effect of prolactin on the synthesis of (alpha)-lactalbumin is expected to increase.

The potential role of lactose as a determinant of milk volume has led to studies of glucose utilization by the mammary gland. Perfusion of the mammary gland with a glucose-poor medium results in the secretion of a protein- and fat-rich fluid that bears little resemblance to milk.[54] In cows, a linear relationship is observed between plasma glucose concentrations and milk volume at plasma glucose concentrations below 55 mg/dl.[55] Kuhn et al.[56] also have reported that lactose synthesis increases linearly in incubated rat mammary acini in media with concentrations of glucose up to 270 mg/dl. Although the importance of glucose appears to be evident from these types of studies, specific mechanisms responsible for the regulation of lactose synthesis have not been identified.[56] Many of the difficulties in identifying specific regulatory mechanisms have centered on the problems of measuring substrate concentrations in the Golgi lumen where lactose synthesis occurs.

Cardiovascular Adaptations

There are few studies in humans which evaluate cardiovascular status during lactation. The best animal studies published are those of Hanwell and Linzell.[52,58] These investigators report a heightened flow of blood to the mammary gland and to organs of the alimentary system. Cardiac output remains above pregnancy levels when lactation follows pregnancy. In rats, the high cardiac output results in an increased blood flow to all organs in early lactation; in later stages a greater proportion of the cardiac output is directed to the mammary gland and alimentary organs. Whether these changes occur in the human is not known with confidence.

The mechanisms which support these cardiovascular changes also are not well described. Hanwell and Linzell[59] demonstrated that increased cardiac output in rats appears to be dependent upon the suckling stimulus and not necessarily on milk removal. From earlier experiments by these investigators[60] it was suggested that this response may be linked to prolactin or growth hormone since administration of either hormone maintained mammary blood flow and high cardiac outputs. Chemical signals also may induce the dilatation or constriction of blood vessels in the mammary gland and thereby modulate local blood flow.[61] Changes in the blood flow of the mammary glands also may be modulated by milk in the breast, which compresses blood vessels.

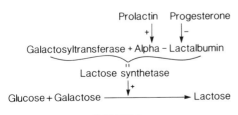

FIGURE 7.

ESTABLISHMENT AND MAINTENANCE OF LACTATION

A steady and adequate milk production is believed to be dependent upon adequate maternal nutrient stores and intake. So entrenched is this viewpoint that many health professionals believe that there is a direct association between maternal nutrition and lactation performance, i.e., as nutritional status is upgraded, lactational performance improves. Field studies do not always conform with this view. Recent studies of well-nourished, upper-middle-income women in North America[12,62] and in women at signficant nutritional risk in the Gambia[63] indicate that both groups produce milk of similar volumes and composition. **Lactating women, therefore, are able to produce normal quantities of milk of normal quality under widely varying environmental and nutritional conditions.** Furthermore, studies that assess the impact of supplemented diets on groups of women at nutritional risk are inconclusive; they neither support nor refute the relative independence of general lactation performance and diet. In reaching this conclusion, however, it is important to point out the limitations of this general observation. Under conditions of extreme deprivation, milk volume and composition are affected adversely,[64] and in less extreme conditions, maintenance of normal volumes likely leads to a deterioration of maternal nutrient status.

Endocrine Stimuli

The physiologic principles that normally regulate the establishment and maintenance of lactation are that (1) milk is produced on demand, and (2) involution of the mammary gland is initiated rapidly if milk is not removed from the breast. Adequate release of prolactin and oxytocin is essential for the establishment and maintenance of lactation. As reviewed in the previous section, high baseline serum prolactin concentrations and significant increases above baseline during each nursing episode are noted more commonly in early than in later stages (> approximately 4 months) of milk production. Elevated prolactin concentrations maintain casein and lactose synthesis by unidentified mechanisms.[65]

Oxytocin is the mediator of the "letdown" or "milk-flow" reflex. Oxytocin release is directly responsible for the contraction of myoepithelial cells that surround the acini of the mammary gland. Current views maintain that the contraction of myoepithelial cells promotes the secretion of milk fat and causes milk stored in the distal ducts and acinar lumen to move into the larger ducts and lactiferous sinuses.[66] This action occurs repeatedly during a nursing episode. The practical

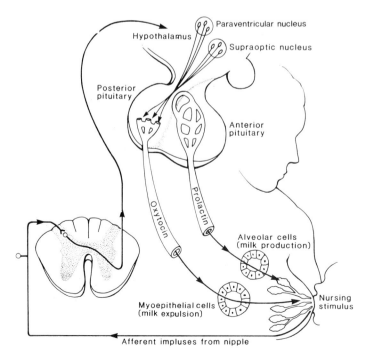

FIGURE 8. *Neuroendocrine influences on lactation.* Prolactin and oxytocin are released from the anterior and posterior pituitary, respectively. Their release is initiated by suckling. The afferent stimulus is carried via the spinothalamic tract to the hypothalamus and from the hypothalamus to the pituitary. (From Goldfarb J, Tibbetts E. Breast Feeding Handbook. Hillside NJ, Enslow Publishers, 1980;34, with permission.)

outcome of this reflex is that milk fat content early in a feeding may be as low as approximately 1 gm/dl. If the feeding progresses normally, the fat content may rise to 8 gm/dl or higher as the breast is emptied.[67]

Signals for oxytocin release are carried via the spinothalamic tracts to the posterior pituitary via the hypothalamus (Fig. 8). Oxytocin release usually is stimulated by suckling (tactile stimuli); however, auditory, visual, or olfactory stimuli also may induce its release. Excitement of the sympathetic nervous system appears to inhibit the let-down reflex by directly inhibiting the contraction of myoepthelial cells or by decreasing the blood concentrations of oxytocin which reach the breast.[68] Mammary blood vessels appear to be very sensitive to the vasoconstrictive action of adrenaline and noradrenaline.[69] Failure of milk production during highly stressful periods is likely partially due to these responses.

The mechanism by which frequent removal of milk from the breast promotes an increased synthesis of milk is not well described. The response may depend, in part, on the heightened release of prolactin which likely accompanies frequent milk expression. Experiments in ruminants have demonstrated that blood flow to the mammary gland rises with increases in the frequency of milk expression.[70] The increase in blood flow is associated with a higher rate of nutrient delivery to the secretory cells and a higher exposure to hormonal stimuli. How these processes lead to an increased proliferation and activity of secretory cells is not known. Failure to remove milk results in stasis. Milk stasis is associated with early changes of mammary gland involution characterized by a progressive atrophy of the anatomical structures that support milk production and a slowing of the biochemical processes which maintain milk synthesis.[71]

Maternal Nutrient Utilization During Lactation

The mean milk output during the first four postpartum months is approximately 750 ml/day.[12] Changes in milk volume after this period appear to be highly variable and to depend upon whether the child is exclusively breastfed or is fed a combination of human milk and other foods. If protein and energy substrates are used with 100% efficiency for milk production, the cost of lactation to the mother in terms of protein and calories is approximately 7.4 gm of protein and 500 kcal/day; if the efficiency is 80%, the cost is 9 gm of protein and 625 kcal/day. Women who gain 11 to 12.5 kg of body weight during pregnancy should have stored 2 to 4 kg of adipose tissue. These energy stores provide 200 to 300 kcal/day for three months to meet the additional energy needs of lactation.

Factors that influence the use of protein, calories, and other nutrients for the production of milk rather than for the maintenance of maternal tissues have been investigated, but not extensively.[63,72] As in other normal physiologic processes, endocrine signals are expected to participate in the control of the balance between tissue mobilization for milk production and metabolite uptake by the mammary gland and other tissues. Animal studies have shown that the dietary intake during the preceding pregnancy plays an important physiologic role in the resulting balance between these processes.

Studies in the sow have demonstrated that milk production, assessed by litter weight gain, is not hampered by dietary deprivation during pregnancy if adequate or surplus nutrients are given during the subsequent lactation.[73] If, however, an inadequate diet is consumed during lactation, previous dietary treatments have an interactive effect with lactation performance. Little information, however, is available which assesses mechanisms that account for differing rates and degrees of mobilization of maternal tissues under distinct maternal physiologic states.

Recent data from human studies have begun to provide this type of information. Lipolysis and lipoprotein lipase (LPL) activity have been studied in biopsies of femoral and abdominal adipose tissue depots of healthy nonpregnant women and during pregnancy and lactation.[74] Basal lipolytic rates were not significantly different between sites in nonpregnant women but were signficantly higher in the femoral depot than in other adipose sites of lactating women. The lipolytic effect following noradrenaline administration was similar in both regions in lactating women but was significantly less in femoral fat than in abdominal fat of nonpregnant women and during early pregnancy.

LPL activity in abdominal adipose tissue remained the same in all three physiologic states. This enzyme hydrolyzes serum triglycerides; liberated fatty acids are transported into the tissues. LPL activity was higher in the femoral region of pregnant and nonpregnant

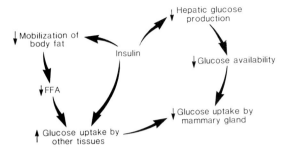

FIGURE 9. *Insulin, glucose, and free fatty acid interrelationships.* Influence of insulin on lipolysis and subsequent effects on glucose availability are represented schematically. (From Garza C Butte NF The effect of maternal nutrition on lactational performance. In Kretchmer N (ed): Frontiers in Clinical Nutrition. Rockville, MD, Aspen Press, 1985;22, with permission.)

women than in lactating women. From this array of findings it is suggested that in both nonpregnant and pregnant women, lipid assimilation is favored in femoral stores over the abdominal depot. During lactation, the femoral region undergoes unique adaptations. Its LPL activity falls and the response to lipolytic stimuli increases. Lipid mobilization therefore is favored by this tissue during lactation.

Under defined physiologic states, specific adipose tissue sites appear to be specialized in their function as energy sources. Previous longitudinal studies of the body composition of lactating women over the first four postpartum months also detected a nonuniform mobilization of adipose tissue stores.[72] Subscapular skinfold thickness was noted to decrease at a greater rate than that of the triceps or suprailiac regions. Analogous responses in other adipose tissue sites or other types of tissue have not been examined.

Endocrine controls during the periods of lactational maintenance have been evaluated primarily in animals.[55,75,76] Studies suggest that animals with high yields of milk tend to maintain lower serum insulin concentrations than do those with low yields. The link between insulin and milk production may be the relative availability of glucose (Fig. 9). Relatively low serum concentrations of insulin should be associated with high glucose output by the liver, decreases in uptake of glucose by competing tissues, and higher rates of lipolysis. Higher serum concentrations of free fatty acids from lipolysis would decrease glucose oxidation by tissues able to metabolize either fat or glucose. The net result would be a higher availability of glucose for milk production.

Augmented serum concentrations of growth hormone have been noted in animals with high milk yields. Increased growth hormone levels complement the expected effects of relatively low serum insulin concentrations; gluconeogenesis, glycogenolysis, and lipolysis would be promoted under conditions of relatively increased growth hormone production. Modulation of nutrient use for milk production similar to that described for a relatively low insulin output state is possible under conditions of increased growth hormone. In animals treated with growth hormone or saline, total glucose utilization is similar, but animals treated with growth hormone channel a greater proportion of available glucose to milk production. Uncritical extrapolation of these findings to human physiology is not warranted by these limited observations, but they do provide insights into potential regulatory mechanisms that are accessible to experimental evaluation.

REFERENCES

1. American Academy of Pediatrics and American College of Obstetricians and Gynecologists. Guidelines for Perinatal Care. Washington, AAP and ACOG, 1983;172.
2. Sjolin S, Hofvander Y, Hillervik C. Factors related to early termination of breast feeding. A retrospective study in Sweden. Acta Paediatr Scand 1977;66:505-511.
3. Lawrence R. Successful breastfeeding. Am J Dis Child 1981;135:595-596.
4. Waterlow JC, Thomson AM. Observations on the adequacy of breastfeeding. Lancet 1979;2:238-242.
5. Butte NF, Garza C, Smith EO, Nichols BL. Human milk intake and growth performance of exclusively breast-fed infants. J Pediatr 1984;104:187-195.
6. Dewey KG, Lonnerdal B. Milk and nutrient intake of breastfed infants from 1 to 6 months: relation to growth and fatness. J Pediatr Gastroenterol Nutr 1983;2:497-506.
7. Stuff J, Garza C, Boutte C, et al. Sources of variation in milk and caloric intakes in breast-fed infants: implications for lactation study design and interpretation. Am J Clin Nutr 1986;43:361-366.
8. Stuff JE, Garza C, Boutte C, Nichols BL. Caloric intakes of older breast-fed infants: human milk and solid food. Am J Clin Nutr 1986; 43:418.
9. Lockhart RD, Hamilton GF, Fyff FW. Anatomy of the Human Body, 2nd ed. Philadelphia, J.B. Lippincott Co. 1969; 6-9.
10. Farina MA, Newby BG, Alani H. Innervation of the nipple-areola complex. Plastic Reconstruct Surg 1980;66:497-501.
11. Green TH Jr: Gynecology: Essentials of Clinical Practice, 2nd ed. Boston, Little, Brown, 1971.
12. Tucker Allen H. General endocrinological control. In Larson BL, Smith VR (eds): Lactation, Vol. I, New York, Academic Press, 1974;277-326.
13. Lyons WR. Hormonal synergism in mammary growth. Proc Roy Soc (Lond) Sec B, 1958;149:303-325.
14. Martin RH, Glass MR, Chapman C, et al. Suppressions by bromocriptine of the lactalbumin peak associated with human lactogenesis. Clin Endocrinol, 1981;14:363-366.

15. Kuhn JN. Progesterone withdrawal as the lactogenic trigger in the rat. J Endocrinol 1969;44:39-54.
16. Schams D. Hormonal control of lactation. In Elliott K, Fitzsimons DW (eds): Breastfeeding and the Mother. New York, Elsevier, 1976;53-83.
17. Oakey RE. Estrogen and progesterone production in human pregnancy. In James ML (ed): The Endcrinology of Pregnancy and Parturition. New York, Academic Press, 1983;193-229.
18. Tyson JE, Hwang P, Guyda H, Friesen HG. Studies of prolactin secretion in human pregnancy. Am J Obstet Gynecol 1972;113:14-20.
19. Delvoye PM, Demaegd U, Nyampeta U, Robyn C. Serum prolactin, gonadotropin and estradiol in menstruating and amenorrheic mothers during two years of lactation. Am J Obstet Gynecol 1978;130:635-639.
20. Aono T, Takenori S, Tsuneo S, Kurachi K. The initiation of human lactation and prolactin response to suckling. J Clin Endocrinol Metab 1977;44:1101-1106.
21. Fulkerson WJ, McDowell GH. Effect of estrogen administered in early or late lactation on the yield and composition of milk in sheep. J Endocrinol 1974;63:175-180.
22. Tyson JE, Huth J, Smith S, Thomas P. Prolactin induced alterations in human milk. Abstr Clin Res 1973;21:64.
23. Weinstein D, Ben-David M, Polishuk WZ. Serum prolactin and the suppression of lactation. Br J Obstet Gynaecol 1976;83:679-682.
24. Dewey KG, Finley DA, Lonnerdal B. Breast milk volume and composition during late lactation. J Pediatr Gastroenterol Nutr 1984; 3:713-720.
25. MacLeod RM and Lehmeyer LE. Regulation of the synthesis and release of prolactin. In Wolstenholme GEW, Knight J (eds): Lactogenic Hormones. Edinburgh, Churchill Livingstone, 1972;53-83.
26. Mepham TB. Amino acid utilization by lactating mammary gland. J Dairy Sci 1982;65:287-298.
27. Keenan TW, Frnake WW, Mather IH, Morre DJ. Endomembrane composition and function in milk formation. In Larson BL (ed): Lactation: A Comprehensive Treatise, Vol. IV. New York, Academic Press, 1974;405-436.
28. Saacke RG, Heald CW. Cytological aspects of milk formation and secretion. In Larson BL, and Smith VR (eds): A Comprehensive Treatise, Vol. II. New York, Academic Press, 1974;147-189.
29. Kelly RB. Pathways of protein secretions in eukaryotes. Science, 1985;230:25-31.
30. Weisz-Carrington P, Roux ME, McWilliams M, et al. Hormonal induction of the secretory immune system in the mammary gland. Proc Natl Acad Sci 1978;75:2928-2932.
31. Rodewald R. Intestinal transport of antibodies in the newborn rat. J Cell Biol 1973;58:189-211.
32. Kleinman RE, Walker WA. The enteromammary immune system. An important concept in breast milk host defense. Dig Dis Sci 1979;24:876-882.
33. Goldman AS, Smith CW. Host resistance factors in human milk. J Pediatr 1973;82:1082-1090.
34. Svennerholm AM, Hanson LA, Holmgren J, et al. Milk antibodies to live and killed polio vaccines in Pakistani and Swedish women. J Infect Dis 1981;143:707-711.
35. Hanson LA, Ahlstedt S, Andersson B, et al. Ann NY Acad Sci 1983; 409:1-21.
36. Svenerholm AM, Hanson LA, Holmgren J, et al. Different secretory IgA antibody response to cholera vaccination in Swedish and Pakistani women. Infect Immunol 1980;30:427-430.
37. Goldman AS, Garza C, Nichols BL, Goldman RM. Immunologic factors in human milk during the first year of lactation. J Pediatr 1982;100:563-567.
38. Goldman AS, Garza C, Nichols BL, et al. Effects of prematurity on the immunologic system in human milk. J Pediatr 1983;101:901-905.
39. Garza C, Butte NF. The effect of maternal nutrition on lactational performance In Kretchmer N (ed): Frontiers in Clinical Nutrition. Rockville MD, Aspen, 1985;15-36.
40. Forsum E, Lonnerdal B. Effect of protein intake on protein and nitrogen composition of breast milk. Am J Clin Nutr 1980;1809-1813.
41. Insull W, Hirsch J, James T, Ahrens EH Jr. The fatty acids of human milk. II. Alterations produced by manipulation of caloric balance and exchange of dietary fats. J Clin Invest 1959;38:443-450.
42. Read WWC, Lutz PG, Tashjian A. Human milk lipids. III. Short-term effects of dietary carbohydrates and fat. Am J Clin Nutr 1965;17:180-181.
43. Gleockler DH, Ferreri LF, Flaim E. Lipoprotein patterns in normal lactating Holstein cows bled at various times. Effects of milking. Proc Soc Exp Biol Med 1980;165:165:118-122.
44. Smith S. Mechanism of chain length determination in biosynthesis of milk fatty acids. J Dairy Sci 1980;63:337-352.
45. Breckenbridge WC, Marai L, Kuksis A. Triglyceride structure of human milk fat. Can J Biochem 1969;47:761-769.
46. Wooding FBP. The mechanism of secretion of the milk fat globule. J Cell Sci 1971;9:805-821.
47. Gyorgy P. The uniqueness of human milk: biochemical aspects. Am J Clin Nutr 1971;24:970-995.
48. Svanborg EC, Andersson B, Hagberg L, et al. Receptor analogues and anti-pili antibodies as inhibitors of bacterial attachment in vivo and in vitro. Ann NY Acad Sci 1983;409:580-592.
49. Peaker M. Lactation: some cardiovascular and metabolic consequences, and the mechanisms of lactose and iron secretion into milk. In Elliot K, Fitzsimons DW (eds): Breastfeeding and the Mother. New York, Elsevier, 1976; 87-102.
50. Wilde CJ, Kuhn NJ. Lactose synthesis in the rat and the effects of litter size and malnutrition. Biochem J 1979;182:287-294.
51. Lehninger AL. Principles of Biochemistry. New York, Worth Publishers, 1982.
52. Turkington RW, Brew K, Vanaman TC, Hill RL. The hormonal control of lactose synthesis in the developing mouse mammary gland. J Biol Chem 1968;243:3382-3387.
53. Turkington RW, Hill RL. Lactose synthesis: progesterone inhibition of the induction of (alpha)-lactalbumin. Science 1969;163:1458-1460.
54. Linzell JL, Peaker M. Mechanisms of milk secretion. Physiol Rev 1971;51:564-597.
55. Kronfeld DS. Major metabolic determinations of milk volume, mammary efficiency, and spontaneous ketosis in dairy cows. J Dairy Sci 1982;65:2204-2212.
56. Kuhn NJ, Carrick DT, Wilde CJ. Lactose synthesis: The possibilities of regulation. J Dairy Sci 1980;63:328-336.
57. Chatwin AL, Linzell JC, Setchell BP. Cardiovascular changes during lactation in the rat. J Endocrinol 1969;44:247-254.
58. Hanwell A, Linzell JL. The time course of cardiovascular changes in lactation in the rat. J Physiol 1973;233:93-109.
59. Hanwell A, Linzell JL. The effect of engorgement with milk and of suckling on mammary blood flow in the rat. J Physiol 1973;233:111-125.
60. Hanwell A, Linzell JL. Elevation of cardiac output in the rat by prolactin and growth hormone. J Endocrinol 1972;53:57A-58A.
61. Dhondt G, Houvenaghel A, Peeters G, Verschooten K. Influence of vasoactive hormones on blood flow through the mammary artery in lactating cows. Arch Int Pharmacodyn. 1973;204:89-104.
62. Dewey KG, Lonnerdal B. Milk and nutrient intake of breast-fed infants from 1 to 6 months: relation to growth and fatness. J Pediatr Gastroenterol Nutr 1983:2:497-506.
63. Prentice AM, Lunn PG, Watkinson M. Dietary supplementation of lactating women. II. Effect of maternal health, nutritional status and biochemistry. Hum Nutr Clin Nutr 1983;372:65-74.
64. Burger GCE, Drummond JC, Sandstead HR (eds). Malnutrition and Starvation in Western Netherlands The Hague, The Netherlands, The Hague General Printing Office, 1948;93.
65. Kohmoto K, Sakai S. Prolactin receptors in the mammary gland. In Yokoyama A, Mizuno, H Nagasawa H (eds): Physiology of Mammary Glands. Baltimore, University Press, 1978;231,248.

66. Tindal JS. Central pathway in oxytocin and prolactin release. In Yokoyama A, Mizuno H, Nagasawa H, (eds): Physiology of Mammary Glands. Baltimore, University Press, 1978; 305-322.

67. Watson MA, Alford ES, Dill CW, et al. Compositional changes during sequential sampling of human milk. Nutr Rep Int 1982;26:1105-1111.

68. Cross BA. Neurohormonal mechanisms in emotional inhibition of milk ejection. J Endocrinol 1955;12:29-37.

69. Linzell JL. Mammary blood flow and methods of identifying and measuring precursors of milk. In Larson BL, Smith UR (eds): Lactation, Vol I. New York, Academic Press, 1974;143-225.

70. Shinde Y. Role of milking in initiation and maintenance of lactation in the dairy animal. In Yokoyama A, Mizuno H, Nagasawa H (eds): Physiology of Mammary Glands. Baltimore, University Press, 1978;347-360.

71. Lascelles AK, Lee CS. Involution of the mammary gland. In Larson BL (ed): Lactation, Vol. IV. New York, Academic Press, 1978;115-181.

72. Butte NF, Garza C, Stuff JE, et al. Effect of maternal diet and body composition on lactational performance. Am J Clin Nutr 1984;39:296-306.

73. Mahan DC, Mangan LT. Evaluation of various protein sequences on the nutritional carry over from gestation to lactation with first litter sows. J Nutr 1975;105:1291-1298.

74. Rebuffe-Scrive M, Enk L, Crona N, et al. Fat cell metabolism in different regions in women. Effect of menstrual cycle, pregnancy, and lactation. J Clin Invest 1985;75:1973-1976.

75. Hart IL, Bines JA, Morant SV, Ridley JL. Endocrine control of energy metabolism in the cow: comparison of the levels of hormones (Pri, GH, Ins,Thy) and metabolites in the plasma of high-and low-yielding cattle at various stages of lactation. J Endocrinol 1978;77:333-345.

76. Bines JA, Hart IL. Metabolic limits to milk production, especially rates of growth hormone and insulin. J. Dairy Sci 1982;65:1375-1389.

3

Anatomic and Biochemical Ontogeny of the Gastrointestinal Tract and Liver

WILLIAM F. BALISTRERI, M.D.

"No subject has been treated more extensively, more eagerly, sometimes even more spitefully than that of infant feeding. The philosopher's stone has not been so anxiously sought for, nor been so often found in medical journals, books, and societies as the correct infant food and the appropriate treatment of cow's milk. . . . the digestive capabilities of the infants differ, just as those of adults, and nature therefore provides a variety of good breast-milks adapted to the individual idiosyncrasy of the special infant. With this fact impressed upon us, we can well see that in artificial feedings no routine mixture will, in all cases, prove successful. We are in need of a means by which we can prescribe exactly according to the idosyncrasy of the digestion we are dealing with." (Contributions to Pediatrics, vol III. WJ Robinson, ed. New York, The Critic and Guide Company, 1909.)

A. JACOBI

The only thing new in the world is the history you don't know.

HARRY S. TRUMAN

At the turn of this century Jacobi, in the work cited above, reflected upon studies by Korowin and Zweifel performed more than 20 years before which assessed the digestibility of starch in the saliva and pancreatic juice of young infants.

"Korowin made infusions of pancreas and of parotids, added starch, and the result was that the pancreatic infusion changed starch at a later period than did the infusion of the parotids. In his experiments, the pancreas did not change starch in the first month, only slightly in the second month, but noticeably in the third month. The infusion of the parotids, however, was efficient in the first few days of life, particularly in infants of large size and well developed." (Korowin: Centalbl f.d. med. Wissensch, 1873 XI, 261.)

A. JACOBI

INTRODUCTION

The magnitude and the number of obstacles that the newborn faces in maintaining nutrient balance are inversely related to gestational age. There is clearly a high "start-up" cost in establishing functional maturity of the digestive system. The gastrointestinal tract of the preterm infant and perhaps the term infant may not be ready to provide the vital functions of nutrient intake, processing, assimilation, metabolism and distribution to other organs. There is over a century of documentation of this concept. Current theories and the results of contemporary studies focusing on the development of the gastrointestinal tract and the tolerance to various foodstuffs are in many cases not novel. Our predecessors in pediatrics knew the limitations they had to overcome in planning an infant nutrition regimen. Current practice differs little—we are simply attempting to feed smaller and sicker babies in our newborn intensive care units. Feeding techniques must remain apace the technology. However, other than refinements in our understanding of regulatory processes, intermediary metabolism, and the needs of infants in special circumstances, basic tenants hold.

It was also noted that "the effect produced by the saliva was able to persist in the stomach, although the effect ceased within two hours." (Zweifel: Untersuch ii. d. Verdaungsapparat der Neugebaren, 1874). Nicory (Biochem J 1922;16:387) suggested that "any diastatic activity is inconsiderable until the increased secretion of saliva begins."

Jackson (Arch Pediatr 1923;40:324) noted that in children with esophageal atresia, if saliva was expectorated into a funnel connected with a gastrostomy tube, nutrition improved immediately, suggesting that saliva did play an important part in nutritive processes of children. In their classic 1927 textbook The Diseases of Infants and Children, Griffith and Mitchell viewed the contribution of salivary glands to digestion as not signficant since "much of the fluid runs out of the mouth."

The trophic effect of feeding on gastrointestinal motility, an area which today is a favorite

33

research topic, was evident to Eli Ives, M.D. of New Haven, Connecticut, who was a Professor of Materia Medica, Botany, and Diseases of Children at Yale in 1820. Among his observations, recently cited by Pearson,[1] was that:

"The meconium is the dark green substance resembling tar, but more mucilagenous, which is found in the bowels of infants at birth. This is ordinarily evacuated by the first milk of the mother (colostrum) which has a laxative quality. The infant may be put to the breast one or two hours from birth. This course will produce permanent contraction of the uterus stopping hemorrhages, and will prevent milk fever. The child loses its affinity to nurse if it is delayed two or three days. Sometimes molasses and water are given to evacuate, but it is not generally necessary. When the infant is first born it is well to wet its mouth with half a teaspoon of cold water. I give it nothing else until applied to the breast. The bowels are evacuated partly in consequence of their sympathy with the skin, which is excited by the air and other external impressions." (Lectures on the diseases of children. The first American academic course in pediatrics. The Medical Institution of Yale College, New Haven, CT, 1813–1852. Pearson, MA (ed), p. 48, 1986.)

ELI IVES

Ives also placed the common phenomenon that has been subsequently termed "gastroesophageal reflux" in proper perspective. He is quoted as saying, "After nursing the milk sometimes seems to regurgitate without the least effort. No serious evil will arise unless young, anxious mothers should give medicine and make the child sick." Over 100 years ago Gubaroff (Arch. f. Anat. u. Entweckelungsgeschechte, p. 395, 1886) suggested that the "pseudo-valvular opening at the gastric end of the esophagus is imperfectly developed in infancy." This was cited as accounting in part for the greater ease with which vomiting occurred at this time.

Other specific disturbances, such as the physiologic malabsorption of fat in infants, were common knowledge in the early 1900s. "Fat diarrhea" was seen as a frequent symptom in early life but was not viewed as dangerous. It was further noted that "mucous membranes, when moistened with bile, allow fat to penetrate more readily than when not so treated. When bile is prevented from reaching the intestine, for instance, in mild duodenal catarrh, with thickening of the mucous membrane, 60 or 80% of the ingested fat may be found in the feces, in place of the 4 or 5 or 10% which are met within the normal evacuation." (Muller, cited by Jacobi, Vol II, p. 251.) Tedious documentation of bile acid kinetics, performed

60-70 years later by other investigators, provided verification!

Investigation of the ontogeny of the "nutritive organs" should therefore provide us with few surprises. However, important aspects remain to be delineated such as precise definition of work capacities at various stages, developmental interrelationships and alternative (compensatory) pathways. Those areas that are not readily explained by intuitive reasoning may reflect an important teleologic principle. Koldovsky has suggested that **in early life low activity of one functional system may in fact present an advantage to a parallel process.**[2] There are several examples: (1) the transport capacity for two different substrates that compete for an uptake process may exhibit disparate emergence (e.g., essential amino acid uptake predominates over bile acid transport in newborn rats), (2) the relatively alkaline pH of the gastric contents of a newborn might allow lingual lipase and bile-salt–stimulated lipase to mediate lipolysis intragastrically as well as permit the establishment of bacterial flora, (3) the low activity of pepsin may also allow intragastric processes such as absorption of immunoglobulins from milk to occur, and (4) undigested ("malabsorbed") lactose may serve to promote bacterial colonization.

ONTOGENY OF GASTROINTESTINAL TRACT STRUCTURE AND FUNCTION

"The digestion and absorption of food is, like the respiration of air, a function which the infant has had no opportunity of practicing during its fetal career. The circulation of blood, the assimilation from the blood of food substances for growth, and the formation of urine, are activities which have been either assumed or attempted by the organism *in utero*. But the gastrointestinal tract has had only slight opportunities for utilizing its muscles and practically none at all for exercising its chemical and absorptive powers before birth. Moreover, the digestive tract must soon process a relatively large amount of raw material." (The Physiology of the Newborn Infant. Springfield, IL, Charles C Thomas, 1945.)

CLEMENT A. SMITH

The ability to consistently supply appropriate nutrients to infants is limited to varying degrees by immaturity of digestive organ function. This stricture occurs at a time of high metabolic demands—during maturation and differentiation of tissue and sustenance of organ growth.

Successful utilization of ingested nutrients involves the timely interaction of multiple intestinal, pancreatic, and hepatic events; (1)

sucking, swallowing and motility to ensure orderly delivery to and transit through digestive sectors; (2) secretion of digestive and trophic compounds; (3) membrane transport (or uptake) processes mediating nutrient absorption and transfer to metabolic sites; and (4) blood flow to provide critical organ oxygenation and compartmentation of nutrients. Obviously multiple enzymes must be recruited to catalyze many of these processes. Thus efficient function requires not only that the individual components be functional but that coordination and integration occur.

Our understanding of the studies of the ontogeny of the gastrointestinal tract is limited by the fact that many observations of organ function have been made in many different species as well as in humans and integrated concepts may not be readily available. Key information on cell proliferation and turnover in the gastrointestinal tract of the human fetus is, for obvious reasons, lacking. These issues have recently been discussed by Klein et al.[3]

The role of the intestine and liver in fetal nutrient transport and metabolism is of course limited, yet the newborn must abruptly make a transition from placental to intestinal nutrition. Gastrointestinal tract and hepatic function must permit the interrelated events of absorption and metabolism to sustain growth and development. It appears that the physiologic and biochemical "stage is set" during late gestation; therefore in the full-term infant the curtain need only be raised and the play can begin. Feeding and the release of regulatory peptides in response to nutrient input function as seminal events. Lagerkrantz and Slotkin recently characterized the perinatal mileau—during birth the fetus generates markedly elevated levels of "stress" hormones, such as adrenaline and noradrenaline.[4] This catecholamine surge is believed to be important in preparing the newborn to survive after in utero existence is terminated.[4,5] Paradoxically these hormones actually divert blood away from the intestines; however, this in itself may serve as a signal or stimulus. Mulvihill et al. have suggested that the swallowing of amniotic fluid by the fetus is essential in fetal gastrointestinal development.[6] The effect is mediated via the luminal trophic actions of peptides such as epidermal growth factor (EGF) and gastrin.

In the rat, the processes of digestion and absorption are considered to be "immature" in the first two weeks and undergo rapid changes by the third week so that adult-like activities

are reached by the fourth week. This temporal sequence parallels weaning, yet weaning is not the sole modulator; hormonal effects are a key. Generally, there is a narrow window of hormonal responsiveness.[7] Polyamines and ornithine decarboxylase (ODC) also may be factors responsible for developmental maturation or adaptive hyperplasia.[8]

Martin and Henning have shown that adrenal corticosteroids are potent determinants of the rate of developmental changes of intestinal hydrolases; these hormones, however, are not necessary for the enzymes to ultimately reach adult levels of activity.[9] It is possible that stress induces a precocious surge of corticosteroids which stimulates intestinal development. O'Loughlin et al. have shown that both systemic and oral administration of EGF is effective in regulating growth, cellular proliferation and postnatal maturation of the gastrointestinal tract.[10] Inositol phosphatase activity increases rapidly during the suckling period, suggesting a relationship to cell proliferation rate in the mucosa of the small intestine.[11]

Ingested nutrients entering the lumen and regulatory peptides or hormones released in response to consistent enteral feeding play a major role in adaptation to extrauterine life (Fig. 1). The mechanism by which food provides the strong stimulation to growth of gastrointestinal mucosa involves both direct and indirect effects mediated by hormones, secretory products, and nerves.[12,13] It has been determined that, in the animal model, qualitative and quantitative differences in diet composition, such as changing from liquid to a solid meal and from predominance of disaccharides to a diet consisting of complex polysaccharides, proteins, and lipids, require that enzymatic and transport systems be dynamic to adapt to the ingested diet. In addition, dietary composition in early life may have long-term consequences for nutrient transport mechanisms and adaptability; this has been termed critical period programming.[14] An understanding of these concepts may allow more efficient means of delivery of calories, especially to the low-birthweight infant.

ANATOMIC AND BIOCHEMICAL DIFFERENTIATION

The developing organism will undergo a series of species-specific sequential coordinated changes in morphology and metabolism, i.e., differentiation of epithelial cells and

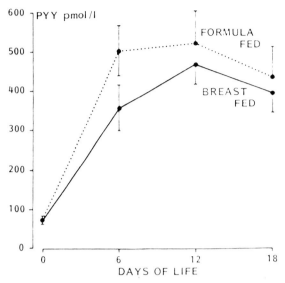

FIGURE 1.   PYY, a peptide that exerts potent effects on motility (reduces the rate of gastric emptying and slows the rate of intestinal transit, thereby increasing the efficiency of absorption), is a candidate hormone for modulation of adaptation of the neonatal gut to enteral nutrition. This graph depicts PYY concentrations in umbilical venous plasma (day 0) and in prefeed plasma from preterm infants receiving either human milk or milk formula at 6, 12, and 18 days of postnatal life (mean ± SE) and demonstrates the dramatic postnatal rise associated with feeding. (From Adrian et al. Pediatr Res 1986;20:1225, with permission).

hepatocytes and emergence of constituent enzymes.[15-19] This will result in the formation of organized arrangements of specialized cells in organs of the digestive tract. Anatomic differentiation precedes functional competency, the former occurring in the human at approximately the mid-portion of gestation, the latter following by 6-8 weeks.

ANATOMIC DIFFERENTIATION

Differentiation of the Liver

The hepatic anlage appears during the 4th week of gestation in the human fetus as a solitary diverticulum from the duodenum growing within the ventral mesentery to reach the septum transversum where it proliferates to form anastomosing cords (Fig. 2).[20-22] The cranial portion of this hepatic diverticulum differentiates into hepatic glandular tissue and bile ducts; the caudal portion becomes the gallbladder and cystic duct. Identifiable hepatic lobes are noted by the 6th week, and at the 9th week of gestation the liver achieves its

peak relative size, constituting approximately 10% of the total fetal weight.

During the various stages of development hepatic compositional changes occur. In early gestation (at approximately 7 weeks) the hepatic anlage contains significantly more hematopoietic cells than functioning hepatocytes. This reflects the subservient role of the liver as a source of extramedullary blood formation during fetal life and in the early postnatal period. Of interest, the hepatocytes that are present are small (approximately 20 μ vs. 30-35 μ at maturity) and contain a paucity of glycogen. At the end of gestation hepatocytes have assumed a larger proportion of the organ volume. The amount of deposited glycogen increases; hematopoietic cells decrease and are absent by the end of the first postnatal month.

The dynamics of human liver development were studied by Novometsky.[23] Using stereologic measurements to quantitate human fetal hepatic morphology, the authors noted a continuous increase in volume density (or percent) of hepatocytes during the increase in gestational age of the fetus. There was a parallel decrease of the sinusoidal network volume density. It is of interest to note that in intrauterine growth-retarded fetuses the rise of hepatocyte volume density was significantly lower in comparison with their physiologically developed counterparts. Using a quantitative electron microscopic technique, de la Iglesia et al. have shown less endoplasmic reticulum in livers of children under one year of age[24] when compared with adults, which correlates with experimental studies documenting low activities of microsomal-bound enzymes and a relative inability to metabolize xenobiotics.

Koga et al. have studied the development of the intrahepatic bile ducts of the human fetus.[25] Well-developed bile canaliculi, which appear as highly specialized loci of the liver cell membrane with microvilli and junctional complexes, were found before 6 weeks and large bile canaliculi bounded by 4 to 7 liver cells were noted. Subsequently bile canaliculi between 3 or 4 adjoining liver cells were present. This arrangement persisted for the duration of fetal life. The intrahepatic bile ducts develop around the portal vein as epithelial cell plates derived from the hepatic duct, and branches sprout from cell plates in several areas. Formation of intrahepatic bile ducts is completed by the 3rd month of gestation. The cystic duct and the gallbladder arise as a solid

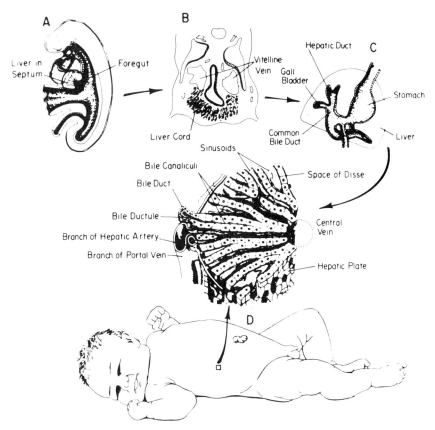

FIGURE 2. Schematic diagram of events occurring during hepatic embryogenesis. A, Ventral outgrowth of hepatic diverticulum from foregut endoderm occurs in the 3.5 week embryo. B, The enlarging hepatic diverticulum between the two vitelline veins buds off epithelial cords which become the liver parenchyma; the endothelium of capillaries—the sinusoids—align about this tissue (4 week embryo). C, Hemisection of embryo (7.5 weeks) demonstrating recanalization of the hepatic biliary tract. D, The hepatic lobule in the newborn infant. (From Andres JM, et al. J Pediatr 1977;90:686, 964, with permission).

epithelial cylinder from the hepatic diverticulum, becoming recanalized sequentially during the first 7-8 weeks.[20,21,26]

The hepatic blood flow component of liver embryogenesis arises from several sources—the hepatic artery, the portal vein, and the umbilical vein; the latter two form the portal sinus.[27,28] Portal venous blood supplies the right hepatic lobe while umbilical venous blood is distributed primarily to the left lobe. A small portion of the portal venous blood joins the umbilical venous flow to fill the ductus venosus. The latter functions to direct blood into the hepatic vein, bypassing the sinusoidal network. **Oxygen saturation in portal venous blood is low in comparison to that of the umbilical venous blood; therefore the right lobe of the liver is less well oxygenated.**[27,28] This may account for the observation that in the fetus the right lobe has greater hematopoietic activity. Because of these flow patterns to and through the liver, this organ has a significant influence on venous return to the heart and in the regulation of oxygen and in energy distribution to the fetus. Sinusoids develop as a permanent dense capillary network formed by the anastomosis between the portal vein and the inferior vena cava. Kupffer cells, which arise as large macrophages along the sinusoidal and epithelial lining, may play a significant role in host defense even in early life.

In the postnatal period, growth of the liver occurs in proportion to height, weight, and age.[29] There is, in addition, a change in the proportions of the liver. The liver accounts for up to 10% of the total fetal body volume, 5% of the body weight at birth, but only 2% of the adult human body weight. Alison has recently reviewed the regulation of hepatic growth in the postnatal period.[26]

Differentiation of the Gut

Small Intestine. In the human fetus the primitive gut can be defined as a tubular structure by the 4th week of gestation. At approximately the 5th-6th week of gestation the nascent intestine elongates rapidly, so as to outstrip the bounds imposed by the peritoneal cavity, and therefore forms a loop that protrudes along the yolk sac into the umbilical cord. At the 6th-8th week of embryogenesis the majority of the intestine remains within the umbilical cord; the developing intestine rotates around the axis of the superior mesenteric vessels in a counterclockwise fashion. The duodenum and splenic flexure of the colon are held in position by mesenteric bands and do not enter into the cord. The small intestine continues to elongate and at approximately the 10th week of gestation reenters the abdominal cavity led by the jejunum, which fills the left portion of the space. The right half of the abdominal cavity is filled by the ileum. The colon reenters and the cecum becomes fixed near the iliac crest, with the ascending and transverse colon lying in their respective adult positions. Abnormalities of this orderly process are associated with various types of nonrotation or malrotation.

A characteristic sequence of intestinal ontogenesis is differentiation and maturation progressing from the proximal to the distal portions of the digestive system. In the rat differentiation of small intestinal mucosa occurs late, i.e., during the last 5 days of a 22-day gestation period.[18,19,30] In contrast, in the human, the mucosa is gradually altered from an undifferentiated stratified epithelium, devoid of villi, to a mucosa with a villous structure and a simple columnar epithelium. Villi are present in the proximal small intestine by 9 weeks and are present in the entire small intestine by 14 weeks of gestation. Intestinal epithelial cell proliferation initially takes place along the entire length of the nascent villi; proliferative activity is confined to the crypts at the base of the villi after approximately the 12th week.

Cellular differentiation is apparent in the stomach by the development of gastric pits at the 7th-8th week of gestation and the appearance of parietal cells at 11 weeks and chief cells at 12 weeks; functional activity, i.e., acid secretion, then may occur. Microvilli, noted at 8-10 weeks, are initially short and irregularly spaced, with a partially developed glycocalyx. This is followed by chemoarchitectural differentiation or enzymatic specialization of brush border enzymes. The physiologic significance of the relatively early development of the human small intestine, compared to various animal models, is not known but presumably reflects both the dynamic demands as well as specific protective mechanisms.

The Developing Colon. Johnson observed in the early 1900s that the immature human colon has villi. (The development of the mucous membrane of the esophagus, stomach and small intestine in the human embryo. Am J Anat 10:521–561, 1910.) In the rat the configuration of the fetal colon is also similar to that of the small intestine, having well developed villous structures.[15,17,30] As a correlate, the functional capacity is also unique, i.e., transepithelial active transport of amino acids and glucose has been demonstrated to occur in the fetal colon.[31]

Potter and Burlingame[32] have clearly documented also that in early life, the rat colon is a distinct organ capable of the absorption of sodium in co-transport with glucose. This unique feature is lost in the process of gaining the transport characteristics of the adult during the first few weeks of life. The loss of glucose-dependent sodium transport capacity precedes the disappearance of the colonic villi.[32] Significant carbonic anhydrase activity is demonstrable in the neonatal rat colon, further suggesting the importance of this segment in transport function.[33] **It is conceivable that the fetal and possibly the neonatal colon serves a nutritive function,** perhaps as a salvage pathway to rescue both carbohydrate and nitrogen. This is discussed below. The colon is actively involved in maintaining salt and water homeostasis and may absorb other essential nutrients to partially compensate for the decreased absorption by the small intestine during development.[34-37]

A component of the anatomic adaptation must be the development of the mucosal barrier to prevent ingress of noxious products. Dietary antigens are ingested and, as the bacterial flora proliferates, toxins are produced. These products, if allowed to penetrate the epithelial barriers, may lead to allergic or inflammatory processes. Immunologic (cellular elements and immunoglobulins) and nonimmunologic (secretion, peristalsis, antibacterial substances such as bile acids, etc.) mechanisms have evolved in the mature gut to prevent uptake of macromolecules. The newborn gastrointestinal tract, however, does not present an impermeable barrier and the local defense mechanisms are ineffective. Prior to "closure," antigen uptake into the systemic circulation or transport of intact macromolecules may occur via pinocytosis.[19,38-40] The intestinal micro-villous membrane (MVM) obtained from new-born animals is more "fluid" and disorganized compared with adult animal membranes, due in part to a greater lipid-to-protein ratio in the MVM of newborns.[41,42] This may contribute to the permeability of the mucosal barrier to macromolecules. **Macromolecule absorption in early life may, however, serve a useful function, i.e., stimulation of specific immune responses, and antigenic recognition.**[43]

Quantitative and qualitative differences in glycosphingolipid composition exist between fetal and adult intestinal mucosa in several experimental animals.[44] The functional significance of this observation is unclear; however, glycosphingolipids are involved in multiple phenomena such as transmembrane transport, cell growth, cellular adhesion, and the binding of hormones, enzymes, and toxins by these cells.

Differentiation of the Pancreas

The morphologic development of the human exocrine pancreas proceeds in an orderly manner. Dorsal and ventral anlagen are detectable at the 5th week of gestation, and by the 7th week, the anlagen fuse to form the definitive pancreas. Exocrine (and endocrine) tissue is identifiable at 12-14 weeks.

Acinar cells and islets of Langerhans are first noted in the human fetus at the 3rd month of gestation. By the 5th month, well differentiated zymogen granules are noted in acinar cells.[17-19,45] Tryptic activity can be seen as early as the 16th week of gestation, with a marked rise occurring near the end of gestation. Of note is the fact that intestinal enterokinase activity, which initiates intraluminal proteolytic activity, is detected in fetuses from the 26th week of gestation. However, the activity is low at birth in comparison to adult levels (approximately 20%).

Adequate adult-like function of the pancreas requires an adequate number of cells, in an appropriate arrangement, along with a patent ductular network. There must be exportable enzymes present in stores which are responsive to appropriate neural and hormonal stimuli for secretion. Morphologically, the pancreatic tissue is mature by term. There are emerging data regarding the presence and functional capacity of pancreatic cell membrane and cytosolic receptors in early life.[46]

The ductular network is clearly patent prior to term. Basal enzyme and ion (Na^+ and HCO_3^-) secretion has been noted in preterm in-

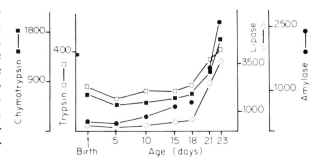

FIGURE 3.   Analysis of the total enzymatic activities of the pancreas in the rat from birth to weaning. Note the rises which occur prior to or at weaning (21 days of age). (From Corring T, et al. In World Review of Nutrition and Dietetics, vol 39, Basel, S. Karger, 1982;124-190, with permission.)

fants. During the early postnatal phase, the exocrine pancreas undergoes rapid changes in total content and in the rate of synthesis of exportable secretory proteins (Fig. 3). Pancreatic *proteases* are first detectable at 25-27 weeks of gestation. *Lipases* are present in fetal pancreatic tissue homogenates at 16-18 weeks of gestation; however, their concentration in duodenal fluid remains low in comparison to adult values. Data regarding the relative content of colipase and phospholipase are meager; however, there is a suggestion of low levels of activity. *Amylase* is first detectable in amniotic fluid at 16-18 weeks, but the concentration in fetal pancreatic tissue homogenates is nearly undetectable. There is little or no amylase present in duodenal fluid obtained from newborn infants. Any amylase activity present may be of salivary origin. Adult levels of amylase activity may not be reached until 6 months of age.

Preterm infants do not respond to mediators of secretion (gastrin, cholecystokinin (CCK), secretin, insulin, acetylcholine, etc.) in a manner that is quantitatively similar to that detected in the mature pancreas. Administration of pharmacologic doses of secretagogues does not elicit enzyme output in the infantile pancreas.[45,47-50]

FUNCTIONAL ALTERATIONS DURING DEVELOPMENT

"A good deal of the work which must be mentioned in this section (i.e. enzymes in ontogenesis) seems to have been inspired by the idea that, if one could get hold of the original egg-cell, no enzymes would be found to be present at all, and that they all arise, one after the other, in a kind of ontogenetic procession from an ovum completely innocent of any. This idea has only to be stated for its ab-surdity to be recognised, and it is far more probable that no living cell can exist without at least a protease, a lipase, and an amylase (and, of course, many oxidizing enzymes). In so far as the theory of recapitulation was lying behind the idea in question, the confusion was greater, for the presumably primitive bacteria are noted for the variety and catholicity of the enzyme reactions they can bring about. In any case, it seems likely that the embryonic body starts life with an assortment of fundamental en-zymes, or a collection of fundamentally necessary active surfaces, to which, as development goes on, certain others are added, and from which possibly some are sub-tracted. Apart from the identification of the basal en-zymes, therefore, there remains the task of determining the variations in activity of those which are present, and the more exact description of their kinetics, e.g., by chart-ing variations in specificity, optimum pH, and other properties." (Chemical Embryology, vol III. New York, The MacMillan Company, p. 1289, 1931.)

J. NEEDHAM

As mentioned above, apparent deficiencies in digestive organ function have been obser-ved repeatedly in normal, healthy newborn in-fants. This has led to extensive investigation of specific alterations such as the quantitative pattern of various enzymes during embryonic development. Despite marked inter-species differences, several general concepts can be stated. During late fetal or early postnatal development, the differentiation of tissue func-tion depends on de-novo synthesis of en-zymes, not on activation of enzymes already present in embryonic tissue.[51] Greengard, in documenting the quantitative pattern of en-zymatic differentiation in early life,[51] noted that the increase in activity or "emergence" oc-curred in certain clusters which correlate with the changing functional requirements of the developing organism (Figs. 4-6). **Substrate and hormonal flow across the placenta and dietary and hormonal input in the postnatal period modulate the development of these various enzymatic processes.** The lipid com-position of cell and organelle membranes changes rapidly in response to alterations in the composition of dietary lipids. The role of *genetic preprogramming* i.e., intrinsic timing mechanisms (the biologic clock), also is to be considered in understanding the ontogeny of enzyme activities. The emergence of enzymes in clusters suggest that these coordinated developmental changes have common control mechanisms. Lamers et al. have furthered these observations by noting that the develop-mental patterns of blood hormonal concen-trations (glucagon, insulin, throxine, etc.) are consistent with the observed developmental pattern of enzymic maturation of the gastroin-

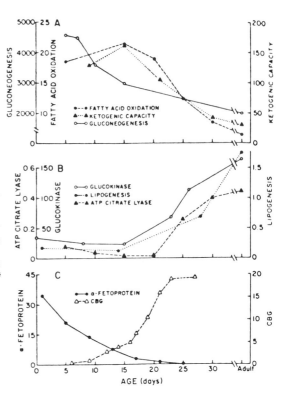

FIGURE 4.   Depiction of the concept of "emergence" of hepatic functional activity in clusters. A, Examples of liver functions that show high activity during suckling period: (1) gluconeogenesis (o——o) is shown by rate of incorporation of labeled amino acids into glycogen in liver slices; (2) fatty acid oxidation (•---•) is shown as percent conversion of palmitate into acid-soluble products by liver homogenates in the presence of carnitine and (3) ketogenic capacity (▲....▲) is shown by activity of mitochondrial acetoacetyl-CoA thiolase. B, Liver func-tions that show low activity during suckling period: (1) glucokinase activity (o——o); (2) lipogenesis (•....•) is shown as incorporation of acetate into fatty acids in liver slices; and (3) ATP citrate lyase activity (▲----▲). C, Developmental changes in secretory capacity of rat liver: (1) plasma concentrations of α-fetoprotein (•——•) are shown as estradiol-binding capacity; and (2) plasma con-centrations of corticosteroid-binding globulin (CBG, Δ----Δ) are shown as corticosterone-binding capacity. (From Henning SJ. Am J Physiol 1981;241:G204, with permis-sion).

testinal tract, which play a critical role in the adaptation to the extrauterine environment.[52]

Functional Development of the Liver

Hepatic Excretory Function.   Bile secre-tion begins at approximately the 12th ges-tational week. The relative composition of the major components of bile, i.e., bile acids,

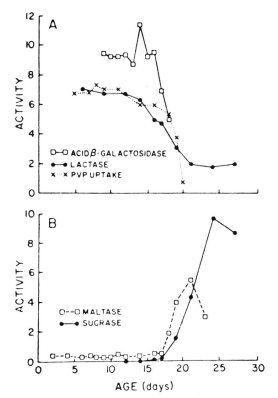

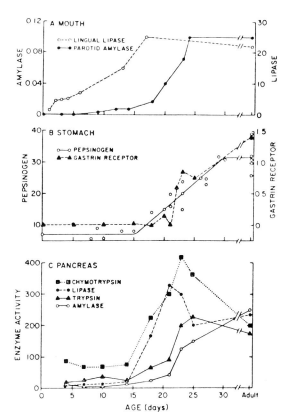

FIGURE 5.   Depiction of the concept of "emergence" of intestinal functional activity in clusters. *A*, Examples of intestinal functions that show high activity during suckling period: (1) lysosomal enzymes, as represented by acid β-galactosidase (□——□); (2) brush-border (neutral) lactase (●——●); and (3) pinocytotic capacity is represented by polyvinyl pyrrolidone (PVP) % uptake (x----x). *B*, Examples of intestinal enzymes that show increased activity at time of weaning: (1) maltase (□----□); and (2) sucrase (●——●). (From Henning SJ. Am J Physiol 1981;241:G203, with permission).

FIGURE 6.   *A*, Development of lingual lipase (o----o) and parotid amylase (●——●) in infant rats. Amylase values are mg/mg prot. Lipase values are U/gm body weight in posterior half of tongue. *B*, Changes in content of pepsinogen (o——o) and gastrin receptors (▲----▲) in gastric mucosa of rats of various ages. *C*, Changes in activities of pancreatic hydrolases in small intestine of neonatal and weanling rats. Lipase (●——●) and trypsin (▲——▲) are expressed as U/100 gm body weight; chymotrypsin (■....■) is given as 0.5 × U/100 gm body weight; and amylase (o——o) is given as 0.1 × U/100 body weight. (From Henning SJ. Am J Physiol 1981; 241:G202, with permission).

lecithin, cholesterol, and inorganic salts, varies throughout development. Bile obtained from the duodenum of infants contains less cholesterol and phospholipid than that of older children or adults.[53,54] Biliary excretion of other organic anions is also low, but matures rapidly.

Gallbladder and ductular bile water reabsorption, canalicular secretion and hormone-induced choleresis (i.e., induction of bile flow) are "deficient processes" in the newborn dog.[55-57] In addition to hepatic and intestinal events, a major factor governing the concentration of bile acids that reach the proximal gut lumen is gallbladder contractility.[55,56,58] Gallbladder motility has been addressed in a few studies. Denehy et al. showed that the newborn gallbladder develops a lower intraluminal pressure than the adult organ following stimulation due to decreased smooth muscle contractility.[58]

There are qualitative and quantitative differences in the fetal and newborn bile acid composition.[59,60] Fetal serum bile acid concentrations are maintained at a low level by transport across the placenta to the mother.[61] Newborn infants demonstrate low intraluminal concentrations of total bile acids as well as an absence of bacterially-derived secondary bile acids.[62] Any of the latter that are found are most likely of placental origin. There also may be atypical bile acids present in hepatic bile, reflecting the primitive nature of bile acid synthetic pathways[63,64] and quantitative differences in the activity of enzymes involved in bile acid metabolism. With maturation, the bile acid pool size increases and there is a major redistribution of the pool from the liver to the gut.[59,60,65]

Bongiovanni, in 1965, noted bile acids in human gallbladder bile at 14-16 weeks of gestation;[66] chenodeoxycholate was noted to be the predominant bile acid in human fetal bile with taurine conjugation being dominant.[66-69] There is some suggestion that low-birthweight infants born to mothers who had been treated with corticosteroids show earlier intrauterine maturation of bile acid synthetic and transport processes.[70,71] The type of feeding, e.g., formula versus breast milk, but not the availability of taurine for bile acid conjugation can influence kinetics and intraduodenal levels in the newborn (Fig. 7).[68,69,72]

The overall efficiency of hepatic excretory function and of intraluminal fat digestion is dependent upon effective bile formation.[73,74] **Biliary elimination of bile acids, which is the main determinant of bile flow in a mature animal, is critical for the biliary excretion of other endogenous and exogenous compounds.** The physiologic components of the enterohepatic circulation of bile acids are well defined and there appears to be an age-related impairment of many of the processes involved in the transport and metabolism of these compounds (Fig.8).[55,57,59,60] The net effect is that efficient bile flow does not ensue. This is manifested by an elevation in the serum concentration of the primary bile acids in early life (Table 1).[59,60,75] Impaired uptake of bile acids by hepatocytes is further suggested by the finding of an exaggerated postprandial rise in the serum bile acid levels seen in healthy newborns.[59,60,75] This has been directly confirmed by the documentation of reduced bile acid transport in experimental systems such as isolated rat hepatocytes or liver membrane vesicles (Figs. 9,10).[76-78]

Efficient enterohepatic circulation of bile acids depends, in part, on the appearance and the degree of developmental maturity of the putative bile acid carriers in the brush border membrane of enterocytes in the terminal ileum. In the adult, active uptake of conjugated bile acids by ileal cells is a saturable, Na^+-dependent transport system; however, in the developing animal, ileal reabsorption of bile acids is less efficient. Saturable, Na^+–bile acid-

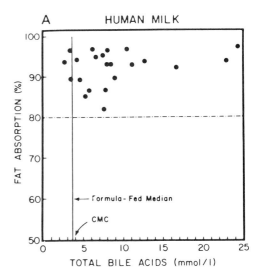

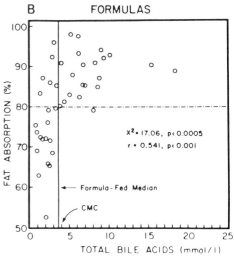

FIGURE 7.   Correlation of fat absorption (% of intake) with duodenal concentration of total bile acids in preterm infants fed either human milk (A) or formula (B). Human milk-fed median or formula-fed median = median concentration of bile acids in infants in either group. Note that correlation coefficient (r) in formula-fed infants (B) is for nontransformed (arithmetic) bile acid concentration; CMC = critical micellar concentration. (From Jarvenpaa A-L. Pediatrics 1983;72:686, with permission).

coupled transport is absent in rat ileum throughout the suckling period.[59,60,79] Maturation occurs near weaning predominantly through an increase in the number of functional bile acid carriers within the ileal brush border membrane.[79] **The emergence of active transport processes for bile acids is concurrent with the surge in plasma concentrations of endogenous corticosterone[80,81] and thyroxine,[82,83]** as well as alterations in the

FIGURE 8.   Bile acid transport and metabolism in immature versus mature (rat/human).

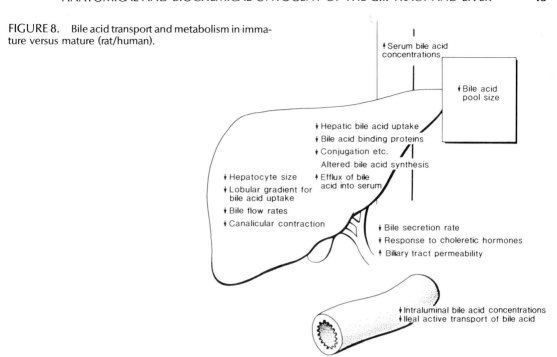

TABLE 1.   Anatomic and Physiologic Differences in Hepatic Excretory Function and Bile Acid Transport and Metabolism in Immature Versus Adult Organisms[59,60]

A. *Physiologic*
  1. ↑ Peripheral serum bile acid levels[75,154,157]
  2. ↓ Hepatic uptake of bile acids (isolated hepatocytes, membrane vesicles) and xenobiotics (indocyanine green (ICG), bromsulphthalein (BSP), bilirubin)[76-78,88,89,158,159]
  3. ↑ Efflux of bile acids from hepatocytes[60,158]
  4. ↓ Bile acid binding proteins (cytoplasmic)[158,160]
  5. ↓ Conjugation, ↓ sulfation, ↓ glucuronidation[152,161-163]

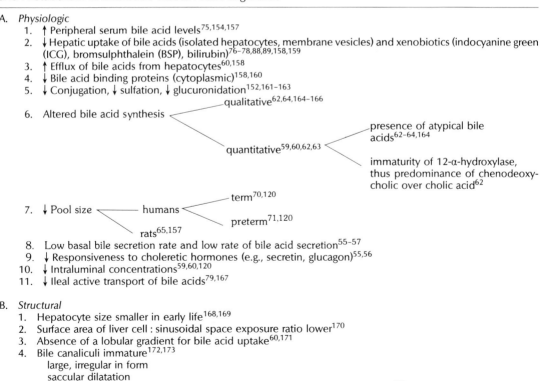

  6. Altered bile acid synthesis ——— qualitative[62,64,164-166]
      quantitative[59,60,62,63] —— presence of atypical bile acids[62-64,164]
      — immaturity of 12-α-hydroxylase, thus predominance of chenodeoxycholic over cholic acid[62]

  7. ↓ Pool size —— humans —— term[70,120]
      —— preterm[71,120]
      — rats[65,157]
  8. Low basal bile secretion rate and low rate of bile acid secretion[55-57]
  9. ↓ Responsiveness to choleretic hormones (e.g., secretin, glucagon)[55,56]
  10. ↓ Intraluminal concentrations[59,60,120]
  11. ↓ Ileal active transport of bile acids[79,167]

B. *Structural*
  1. Hepatocyte size smaller in early life[168,169]
  2. Surface area of liver cell : sinusoidal space exposure ratio lower[170]
  3. Absence of a lobular gradient for bile acid uptake[60,171]
  4. Bile canaliculi immature[172,173]
        large, irregular in form
        saccular dilatation
  5. ? Cytoskeletal dysfunction (↓ frequency and force of canalicular contraction)[174]
  6. ↑ Biliary tract permeability[58]

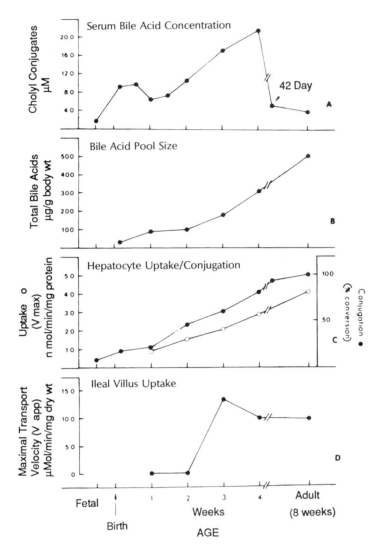

FIGURE 9. Diagrammatic representation of alterations that occur in various processes involved in bile acid metabolism during development of the rat. *A*, Pattern of the serum concentration of cholyl conjugates, the primary bile acid found in this species, at various developmental ages. *B*, Progressive increase in total bile acid pool size with age. *C*, Graphic depiction of the maturation of hepatic bile acid uptake (○) and conjugation (●) of bile acids with taurine. *D*, Variation in maximal ileal transport velocity with age. (From Balistreri WF, et al. J Pediatr Gastroenterol Nutr 1983;2:351, with permission).

microvillous membrane microenvironment.[84,85] Onset of active bile acid transport occurs in concert with expansion of the bile acid pool, which results from maturation of the events occurring in the liver, namely uptake, synthesis, and excretion as described above.[59,60,71]

Hepatic Metabolic Function. Hepatic metabolic function is also immature in the newborn; this is best reflected in bilirubin physiology and by the inefficiency of xenobiotic metabolism. "The degree of hyperbilirubinemia is a measure of the functional maturity of the infant at the time of birth."[86]

There is decreased activity of UDP-glucuronyl transferase, the rate-limiting enzyme in excretion of bilirubin.[87] Postnatal development of transferase activity occurs in prematurely born infants irrespective of gestational age, in contrast to a slow development in utero, indicating that **birth-related rather than age-related factors are of importance in the emergence of this enzyme.**[87-90] This is one of multiple functional "impairments" that are present to varying degrees in the newborn which result in a large mass of unconjugated bilirubin being delivered to an immature ex-

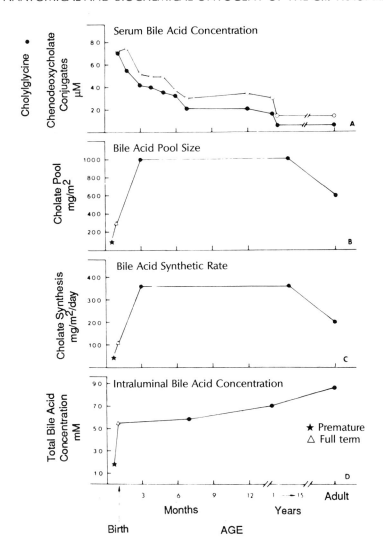

FIGURE 10. Graphic depiction of compiled data regarding developmental changes in various aspects of bile acid metabolism in humans. *A,* Progressive decline in the serum concentration of the primary bile acids, cholyglycine (●) and conjugated chenodeoxycholate(○), with age. *B and C,* Bile acid kinetics studied by isotopic dilution reflected in bile acid pool size and bile acid synthetic rate. *D,* Total bile concentration in duodenal samples. (From Balistreri WF, et al. J Pediatr Gastroenterol Nutr 1983;2:352, with permission.)

cretory system (Table 2, Fig. 11).[91] Similarly, numerous studies have demonstrated a transient period during which the newborn exhibits a decreased capacity to metabolize and detoxify various drugs.[92] For example, in preterm infants the half-life of elimination of theophylline is markedly prolonged compared with adults.[93] The inefficiency of drug metabolism in newborn infants is related to the low levels of activity of the hepatic cytochrome P450 monooxygenase system. The importance of this low capacity for biotransformation in early life was

dramatically demonstrated by the description of fatal cardiovascular collapse due to the toxic accumulation of chloramphenicol in newborn infants.[94]

Lipid Metabolism. A major source of energy in early life, in addition to glycogenolysis and gluconeogenesis, is fatty acid oxidation. In human newborns the restricted capacity for hepatic ketogenesis during the immediate perinatal period might limit the ability of the newborn to tolerate a period of fasting.[95] Ketone production from endogenous fatty

TABLE 2.   Alterations in Bilirubin Transport and Metabolism Responsible for Elevated Serum
Concentrations of Unconjugated Bilirubin in Early Life

1. Cessation of placental transport and maternal detoxification
2. Dynamic status of hepatic blood flow, bilirubin shunted away from the sinusoid
3. Bilirubin production rates high in neonates due to:
      large red-cell mass
      short red-cell life span
      inefficient erythropoiesis
      increased heme oxygenase activity
4. Less efficient albumin binding in newborn due to:
      lower serum albumin concentration
      decreased albumin binding capacity
      stress (e.g., sepsis, acidosis, hypoxia)
5. ↓ uptake and ↓ intracellular binding by hepatocytes (decreased Y protein)
6. Decreased conjugation (↓ activity of glucuronyl transferase)
7. Impaired bile secretion
8. Altered enterohepatic circulation of bilirubin
      ↓ bacterial flora, thus ↓ formation of urobilinogen
      hydrolysis of conjugated bilirubin to unconjugated bilirubin by way of **intestinal** β-glucuronidase with
          subsequent reabsorption
      human milk β-glucuronidase mediating deconjugation

Modified from Balistreri WF, Schubert WK. Liver disease in infancy and childhood. In Schiff L, Schiff E (eds): Diseases of the Liver. Philadelphia, J.B. Lippincott Co., 1982; 1265–1348.

acids provides the energy for hepatic gluco-neogenesis and also provides an alternative fuel for cerebral metabolism when the glucose supply is limited.

Although the ability of the newborn liver to oxidize fatty acids is underdeveloped at birth, there is a rapid maturation during the first few days of life. This is of particular significance since milk, which is the major source of calories in this period of life, presents a large fat load. On a high fat, low carbohydrate diet the newborn must generate active gluconeogenesis to maintain blood sugar concentrations. During the suckling period in the rat there is abundant fatty oxidation in view of the increasing postnatal activity of ketogenic enzymes. Hepatic ketone body production occurs at a high rate. These enzyme activities decline to adult activity toward the end of the suckling phase.[51,96]

Carbohydrate Metabolism.   The pattern of development of enzymes involved in hepatic carbohydrate metabolism is coordinated with dietary intake and the transition from suckling to weaning periods.[96] Since efficient regulation of glycogen synthesis, storage, and degradation develops near term, this may be a factor responsible for altered glucose homeostasis in those born before term. Despite efficient utilization of dietary galactose for conversion to

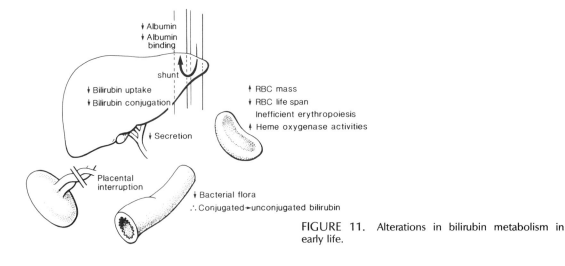

FIGURE 11.   Alterations in bilirubin metabolism in early life.

glucose, there still remains a dependence upon gluconeogenesis in early postnatal life. This is especially important if glycogen storage is limited. Gluconeogenic activity is not present in the fetal liver of certain species. **The capacity for synthesizing glucose from various precursors is acquired after birth** (Fig. 12). Gluconeogenesis may take place, however, in the small intestine of the developing rat.[97] The onset of gluconeogenesis occurs in concert with the appearance of cytosolic phosphoenolpyruvate carboxykinase.[98] The capacity for gluconeogenesis is then highest in early postnatal life with a subsequent decline toward adult levels.[96-98] Brennan and Aprille have shown rapid accumulation of adenine nucleotides in the liver mitochondria of newborn mammals, which is responsible for the activation of pyruvate carboxylation and gluconeogenesis in the immediate postnatal period.[99] In this study, tissue oxygenation and changes (namely a decrease) in the insulin-to-glucagon ratio appeared to be important stimuli for the change in the subcellular compartmentation of hepatic adenine nucleotides.

Protein Metabolism. Elegant studies performed by Dancis et al. in the early 1950s suggested that the **fetal liver is capable of synthesizing all plasma proteins except gammaglobulin,** and this may be the only plasma protein derived from the mother, since the placenta otherwise does not contribute significantly to the plasma proteins of the fetus.[100]

Specific decarboxylases that are rate-controlling in the biosynthesis of polyamines are much higher in fetal liver than in the mature organ.[101] The synthesis of physiologically important polyamines may be directly related to the metabolism of RNA and the modulation of rapid growth. The accumulation of polyamines during embryogenesis parallels phases of growth characterized by alterations in the content of nucleic acid and protein. The synthesis of albumin and secretory proteins in the developing liver parallels quantitative changes in the endoplasmic reticulum. Albumin synthesis occurs in a reciprocal relationship to α-fetoprotein, becoming active in the 3rd or 4th month of gestation, a phenomenon reflected in the disparate dynamics of the serum concentrations of these two proteins.

Biochemical immaturity of protein synthetic processes in the newborn may have a significant impact on nutritional management. In the absence of cystathionase, the transulfuration pathway, by which dietary methionine is converted to cysteine, is "inefficient" and the infant must be supplied with the latter nutrient. There may be a similar dietary requirement for taurine.[102] In view of the alterations in the capacity of the immature liver to metabolize certain amino acids, it has been postulated that calculation of an amino acid molar ratio may be a reliable and useful index of hepatocellular maturity of the newborn.[103]

Development of Intestinal Function

Motility and Secretion. In the human there is a cranial to caudal migration of neuroblasts which occurs during the 5th-12th weeks of gestation, and by the 24th week the distribution of ganglion cells is established. Swallowing has been noted to occur in the human fetus at the 16-17th week of intrauterine life.[18,19] The fetus is estimated to ingest approximately 2-7 ml of amniotic fluid every 24 hours. At the 20th week of gestation amniotic fluid is ingested at the rate of approximately 16-20 ml per day. The term infant swallows approximately 450 ml of amniotic fluid per day.[104,105]

There is poor coordination of esophageal motility in response to deglutition. Simultaneous nonperistaltic contractions occur along the entire length of the esophogus. Lower esophageal sphincter pressure is decreased in comparison to that of the adult and gastric

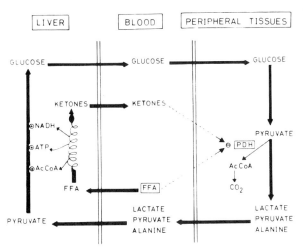

FIGURE 12. Interrelationships that suggest an essential role of hepatic fatty acid oxidation in maintaining active gluconeogenesis in the newborn. Feeding MCT may increase glucose production in fasting neonates by increasing the supply of gluconeogenic precursors (lactate, pyruvate, alanine) to the liver, activating hepatic gluconeogenesis. (From Girard J. Biol Neonate 1986;50:251, with permission).

emptying time is delayed; therefore there is an enhanced risk of gastroesophageal reflux. Motility accelerates during development; administered contrast material reaches the cecum of the 32-week infant in 9 hours, whereas in the term infant transit time is 4-7 hours.[17-19,106] The primitive nature of the muscular layers of the intestine, incoordination of peristaltic waves, increase in the number of anti-peristaltic waves, and decreased secretion of several hormones all contribute to the prolonged transit time. This may be beneficial, i.e., slower transit may facilitate absorption by maximizing the use of the existing transport processes due to longer exposure or contact. Absent or impaired rectal sphincteric reflexes have been noted in preterm infants and may at times resemble a functional obstruction. **It is rare to note the passage of meconium by a preterm infant in utero even when subjected to severe hypoxia** (Tab 3, Fig. 13). There is a decreased capacity for retention in the infantile colon, therefore diapers are required because of the frequent passage of stools that are of small volume yet have a high water content!

In the infant, the stomach capacity is to some degree volume-limited; therefore the caloric density of formulas may need to be high to meet the voracious energy requirements. Other key functions of the stomach, namely mixing and emptying, are slow to reach adult levels of efficiency. The muscular layer of the stomach is thin; therefore the churning activity is feeble. Gastric emptying or antral motility involves a complex series of interacting events: (1) the hydrostatic pressure of the bolus, (2) rhythmic gastric contractions, and (3) relaxation of the pylorus. There is an apparent but a poorly understood interplay of distention, position, and nature of the dietary constituents (i.e., osmolality, composition, pH) as well as the hormones released in response to feeding, such as gastrin or enterogastrone.[106] It has been suggested, however, that colostrum plays a role in stimulating maturation of many of these steps of gastric physiology. Gastrin, which clearly serves as a stimulus to gastric secretion in the adult, may also be trophic for cellular differentiation and "development" of gastric function, and may affect lower esophageal sphincter (LES) pressures. Tseng and Johnson have shown that thyroxine plays an indirect role in the functional development of chief and parietal cells in the stomach by increasing serum corticosterone concentration.[107]

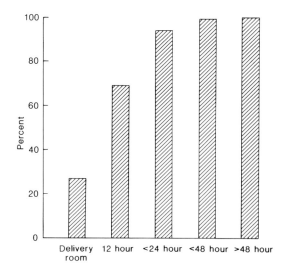

FIGURE 13.   The timing of first stool. (See Table 3 for details.)

TABLE 3.   Time of Passage of First Stool by 500 Full-term Infants*

	NO.	%	CUMULATIVE %
Delivery Room	136	27.2	27.2
12 hours	209	41.8	69.0
12-24 hours	125	25.0	94.0
24-48 hours	29	5.8	99.8
Over 48 hours	1†	0.2	100.0

*From Sherry SN, Kramer I. The time of passage of the first stool and first urine by the newborn infant. J Pediatr 1955; 46:158–159, with permission.
† Sixty-two hours.

During postnatal development in the rat, basal and stimulated gastric acid secretion is noted to increase rapidly early in life and to decrease as the animal matures. Basal acid output and maximal acid output are much higher in the rat during the post-weaning phase (i.e., 30 days) than in either the pre-weaning (15 days) period or in the mature rat.[108] Jacobs et al. have shown this phenomenon to be related to the fact that individual parietal cells of the 30-day-old rat secrete more H^+ than corresponding cells of 100-day-old rats under comparable conditions of stimulation.[109]

Human newborns have high serum gastrin concentrations, yet the basal acid secretion rate is low; exogenous gastrin is also an ineffective stimulant. This phenomenon occurs despite the presence of parietal cells, suggesting end-organ insensitivity to gastrin. The ab-

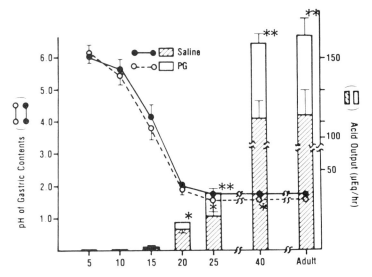

FIGURE 14.   Ontogeny of gastric mucosal gastrin receptor and response. pH of gastric contents and acid output in rats of various ages in response to saline or pentagastrin (250 μg/kg). Each point (pH) or bar (H$^+$ output) represents mean ± SE of 6 determinations. *$P < 0.05$. **$P > 0.01$. (From Takeuchi K, et al. Am J Physiol 1981; 240: G165, with permission).

sence of gastrin responsiveness in newborn rats is due to a lack of gastrin receptors (Fig. 14).[110]

Younoszai et al. studied water and electrolyte transport in the intestine of the developing rat and showed that, for a given osmotic load, the flux of solute and water into the lumen was inversely related to maturity.[111]

Digestive/Absorptive Function.   In general, the mechanisms involved in absorption of various nutrients include (1) intraluminal events, i.e., hydrolysis via specific enzyme activity; (2) membrane-related events—absorption, intrinsic enzymatic hydrolysis and transport; and (3) intracellular events such as endocytosis. Postnatal development of these essential gastrointestinal functions has been extensively studied and shown to be governed by the previously described interacting determinants—the genetic endowment, intrinsic timing mechanisms (biologic clock), dietary composition and other environmental influences—as well as by hormonal input, which serves as a regulatory or triggering mechanism.[112,113] It has even been suggested that iron content of the weaning diet may play a critical role in "terminal" maturation of the rat small intestine.[114] Each brush border membrane transport system seems to possess a distinctive developmental timetable that can be affected by these genetic, dietary, and hormonal factors.[115]

Intragastric digestion (mediated by lipase, amylase, etc.) has been an important recent discovery. The major contribution of enzymes originating proximal to the stomach is a concept that had not been previously appreciated. In fact, in the third edition of Smith's classic text, *Physiology of the Newborn*, published in 1959, the author states, "The conclusion seems justified that gastric digestion is not a factor of primary importance to nutrition at this time of life."

Lipid Digestion and Absorption.   The majority of the calories ingested by a newborn are triglycerides. The percentage of ingested fat appearing in the stool of an infant is greater than that found in older infants and children. This suggests that the processes mediating the intraluminal phases of fat digestion and absorption are ineffective. As discussed above, the enterohepatic circulation of bile acids, which play a critical role, matures sequentially to ensure acclimation of fat absorption after the termination of gestation. This serves as a prototype of the coordinated and interrelated events needed to ensure efficient digestion. The severity of the inefficiency of fat digestion is inversely related to the length of gestation.

It has been noted that lipid may be absorbed by pinocytosis from the gut of a 12-week old human fetus. However, efficient postnatal fat digestion and absorption are much more complex events. The transfer of insoluble triglycerides from the gut lumen to the aqueous environment is initiated by key intraluminal events: (1) emulsification of fat globules, (2) enzymatic hydrolysis of triglycerides via lipase with colipase, (3) solubilization of the lipolytic products by bile acids, and (4) transfer across the intestinal mucosa.[116,117] Intestinal mucosal events, such as lipid uptake, triglyceride synthesis and chylomicron formation, have not been well studied in the newborn period. Chylomicrons have been noted in the serum of newborn infants in the first few days of life. The mucosal phase of fat absorption or re-esterification therefore is seemingly well developed at birth.

However, there is low pancreatic enzyme lipase activity and a low intraduodenal bile acid concentration in the newborn.[59,118,119] Pancreatic lipase activity increases three-to-four-fold in the first week in preterm babies. Therefore **luminal events that require bile acids and lipase in order to function efficiently are rate-limiting overall in fat absorption**. There are sufficient animal data to document immaturity of many of the processes involved in the enterohepatic circulation of bile acids (see Table 1).[59,60,120]

Fat malabsorption in early life ("physiologic steatorrhea") is predominantly due to intraluminal bile acid deficiency, which leads to inadequate micelle formation and reduced solubilization of dietary triglycerides.[120,121] Infants will not achieve adult levels of efficiency of fat absorption until approximately 4-5 months of age.[122] Estimates of the coefficient of lipid absorption range from approximately 60-90% in preterm infants and from 70-95% in full-term infants.[122,123] These ranges in main part reflect the type and amount of fat ingested. Absorption of human milk fat is less dependent on bile acids than is absorption of cow milk fat.[122,123] Inefficient utilization of dietary fats is exaggerated by a predominant long-chain triglyceride diet.

In premature infants, the importance of intragastric lipolysis mediated by lingual lipase, non-nutritive sucking, or "humanization" of lipid formulations prepared for infant feeding to compensate for ineffective intraluminal lipid digestion and absorption remains to be determined. In enterally fed preterm infants, oral calcium supplementation may significantly alter the efficiency of lipid absorption.[124]

Carbohydrate Absorption. Carbohydrate digestion is primarily a mucosal cell surface event; starch digestion is initiated in the intestinal lumen by alpha-amylases.[125,126] Digestion of starch and glycogen begins in the mouth via action of salivary amylases. Amylase activity is detectable in salivary and pancreatic tissue by 22 weeks of gestation. However, the amylase content of duodenal juice is low in neonates.[126-128] The relative impact of salivary amylase on starch digestion therefore may be great; however, this enzyme is not active in the acidic gastric environment for prolonged periods.[129] Breast milk derived amylase may also in part compensate for low pancreatic amylase. Glucoamylase, an intestinal brush border enzyme that removes glucose from the non-reducing end of starch, may also serve as an alternative. The glucoamylase activity that is demonstrable at one month is similar to that found in the adult.[130] **This may be the rationale behind the apparent success of inclusion of glucose oligomers in infant formula.**

Disaccharidases or intestinal hydrolases demonstrate topographical specialization.[131-134] There is also longitudinal specialization of the small intestine with gradients evident during development.[131] These enzymes are localized to the microvillous membrane;[131-133] their appearance follows a clear developmental sequence that may represent an example of hormonal modulation of an intrinsic program of enzymatic expression in terms of time, degree, and functional competence (Figs. 15,16). In experimental studies in which organ development occurs in media devoid of hormones, this intrinsic program is still manifest.[2,133,134] The expression of programmed activity is seemingly also dependent upon direct contact with intraluminal nutrients and hepatobiliary and pancreatic secretions. There is a variation in sucrase activity with the amount of substrate ingested. Hormones present in breast milk may also play a role.

With the exception of lactase (β-glucosidase), the activity of disaccharidases (i.e. α-glucosidases) reaches adult tissue concentrations by the 28th week of gestation. The activity of lactase reaches term levels at approximately 36 weeks.[135,136] High lactase activity is found in the intestinal mucosa of rats at birth. Precocious appearance can be induced by steroids.[137] In the rat, after the suckling period, when there is little need for this hydrolase activity, the levels decline.[138] Breath hydrogen testing, as an index of carbohydrate absorption, suggests that most preterm infants

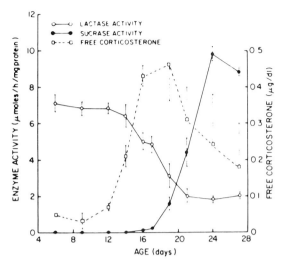

FIGURE 15. Developmental patterns for the activities of the enzymes lactase and sucrase in jejunal mucosa of the rat as compared with free corticosterone in plasma. Values are given as mean ± SEM. (From Henning SJ. Ann Rev Physiol 1985;47:236, with permission.)

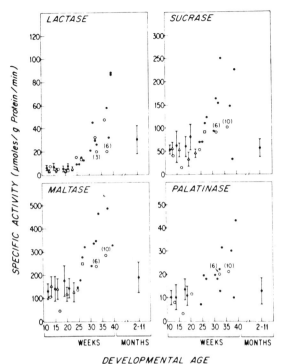

FIGURE 16. Development of disaccharidase activities in human fetal jejunum. (Data compiled by Grand, et al.) Numbers in parentheses refer to number of observations. (From Grand RJ. Gastroenterology 1976;70:803, with permission.)

will demonstrate lactose malabsorption;[34,36] however, growth rates and stool patterns are unremarkable in otherwise healthy preterm infants on lactose-containing formula.[135,139] **Malabsorbed lactose undergoes fermentation mediated by the colonic bacterial flora.** This results in production of volatile organic acids which are absorbed by the colon, which in early life is anatomically unique as described above. The "colonic salvage" pathway functions to rescue malabsorbed carbohydrates and may be quantitatively important for lactose absorption in the presence of low lactase activity. This phenomenon may minimize energy loss. The administration of broad-spectrum antibiotics may alter the colonic flora; similarly, diversion of the intestinal stream by surgery may place the preterm infant at a nutritional disadvantage.[35]

The rate-limiting step in carbohydrate absorption following hydrolase activity is intestinal glucose transport. Glucose (and amino acid) active transport can be mediated by the fetal small intestine; however, it is not clear what role this serves. Glucose absorption, however, is less efficient in the developing intestine than in the mature intestinal tract.[2,19,139,140]

Protein Absorption. Pepsin initiates protein digestion in the acid environment of the mature stomach. However, following a brief, brisk gastric acid output in the first 24 hours of life, acid secretion declines; therefore the pH of gastric contents is neutral to mildly alkaline in newborn infants. This is due to decreased basal or stimulated hydrochloric acid secretion and prolonged buffering by the ingested stomach contents.[108,109,141] The small amount of pepsin that is secreted is inactivated at alkaline pH and there is very little intragastric digestion of protein noted in infants less than 2 weeks of age.[142]

Protein hydrolysis must therefore occur primarily in the proximal small intestine and is dependent on pancreatic proteases and membrane or cytosolic peptidases. The activity of chymotrypsin and carboxypeptidase B is low in newborn infants, whereas **trypsin activity is relatively high; thus the limitations to protein absorption, despite low enterokinase activity, are minimal.**[143] Functional studies correlate with biochemical changes, i.e., newborns can digest and absorb sufficient quantities of dietary protein, and 85% of the dietary nitrogen intake may be absorbed by infants regardless of dietary composition, age, or relative maturity.[144] Newborn infants completely digest the quantity of protein found in cow milk formulas.

There is avid active transport of amino acids in the fetal gut.[145] Taurine, which is a sulfur-containing β-amino acid, is present in high concentrations in human milk. There is a low rate of endogenous synthesis of taurine; therefore this amino acid may be "conditionally essential" during development (i.e., essential during certain conditions). Of interest is the fact that there is no carrier system for β-amino acids in the adult rat jejunum. Moyer et al. have found a sodium-dependent carrier mechanism for taurine transport present in the brush border membrane of suckling rat jejunum.[146] The activity of this carrier decreases or disappears after weaning. This has led to the speculation that, in contrast to the adult, carrier-mediated intestinal transport of taurine is critical to the maintenance of taurine homeostasis during early life.

IMPLICATIONS OF IMMATURE GASTROINTESTINAL TRACT FUNCTION

The deliberations of this chapter were meant to provide sufficient data to illustrate that a major stimulus to development of gastrointestinal, and most likely hepatobiliary and pancreatic, function is the presence of intraluminal nutrients. Aynsley-Green has provided much data in human infants to suggest that postnatal surges in the rate of secretion of peptides is a key influence regulating the postnatal adaptation to enteral feedings.[147] Administration of intravenous glucose as the sole nutrient input to preterm infants for the first 3 days of life is associated with an *absence* of the normal postprandial surge in various gastrointestinal hormones.[147-151] This is in contrast to the dramatic surge in a number of gastrointestinal hormones noted in infants who are fed enterally (Figs. 17,18). Enteral feeding is clearly a triggering mechanism. Therefore, early consistent enteral nutrition or even "minimal enteral feeding" seems to offer a benefit to the infant.[147,151]

A practical demonstration of the beneficial effects of enteral feeding is regularly seen in babies who are deprived of this modality of nutrient input, i.e., those receiving exclusive parenteral nutrition. In these children, pan-

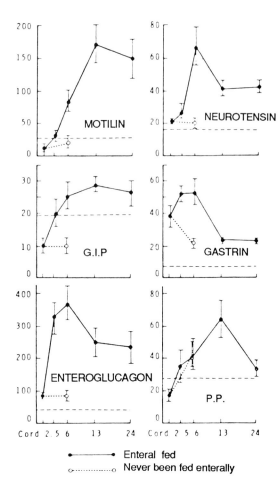

FIGURE 17.   Postnatal surges following enteral feeding in plasma concentrations of gut hormones (all values = pmol/L± SEM) in preterm infants measured at birth (cord blood) and at days 2.5, 6, 13 and 24. Plasma concentrations are also shown from a group of preterm infants who had received only intravenous fluids from birth on account of hyaline membrane disease. Broken lines show mean adult fasting values. (From Aynsley-Green A. Am J Clin Nutr 1985;41:406, with permission.)

creatic hyposecretion, intestinal mucosal atrophy, and the accumulation of biliary sludge reflecting decreased bile flow are all present. Each of these aberrations can be readily reversed with the initiation of feedings.

CASE REPORT

G.W., a 1500 gm infant, had persistent problems with gastric distention and guaiac-positive stools, which suggested necrotizing enterocolitis. He was therefore placed on total parenteral nutrition (TPN) and given no intake by mouth (NPO). After receiving TPN for a period of 2 weeks, the baby was noted to have a persistent increase in serum

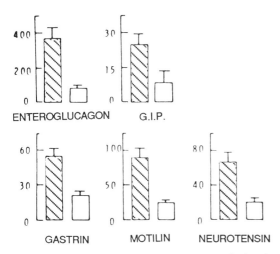

FIGURE 18.   Demonstration of the changes in the basal plasma concentration of various gut hormones (pmoles/L±SEM) measured on the sixth day of life in preterm infants who had been enterally fed since birth (N) compared with those who, because of respiratory distress, had been deprived of enteral feedings since birth and maintained on intravenous dextrose (□). (From Lucas A. In New Aspects of Clinical Nutrition. Karger, Basel, 1983;581-594, with permission.)

bile acid concentrations followed by a rise in the serum conjugated bilirubin level; these biochemical abnormalities were consistent with TPN-associated cholestasis. Ultrasonography revealed the presence of "sludge" in his gallbladder. Initial attempts at feeding in hopes of ameliorating the hepatobiliary dysfunction were unsuccessful. The baby had voluminous watery diarrhea that contained unabsorbed carbohydrate. Gradual tolerance to oral feedings was achieved by slowly increasing the volume of continuously infused elemental formula. The serum bile acid and bilirubin concentrations declined slowly, implying that the liver disease had resolved. After 4 weeks, "bolus" feedings were tolerated.

This case illustrates the problems encountered in trying to provide adequate calories to the low-birthweight infant. The infantile intestinal tract and hepatobiliary system present precarious physiologic balances, which can rapidly become pathophysiologic entities. Immaturity of hepatic excretory and metabolic function may result in the possibly toxic accumulation of drugs in plasma,[152] retention of endogenous compounds (bilirubin and bile acids) and possibly an increased susceptibility to cholestasis as seen in patients with gram-negative sepsis[153] or during total parenteral nutrition.[154,155]

The case also places the work of Aynsley-Green in perspective; his observations suggest that the method of administering feeds to preterm infants will determine the endocrine

milieu.[147,148,150] Major differences in these physiologic changes are present in infants who are bolus fed compared with continuously fed infants. In turn, infants made NPO have an ablation of important physiologic surges in regulatory peptides. "Milk could be given in small volumes as a therapeutic maneuver to induce gut development rather than for nutritional reasons."[147]

There are alternative pathways or enhanced specific compensatory processes which may ameliorate the impact of impaired gastrointestinal physiology in early life. For example, in the presence of low pancreatic lipase activity, extrapancreatic lipases may serve to ensure adequate fat digestion. Lingual lipase may mediate intragastric lipolysis and in part compensate for the relative pancreatic lipolytic "defect."[155,156] The ingestion of breast milk will deliver to the intestinal tract trophic factors such as epidermal growth factor and other hormones, as well as a bile salt stimulated lipase. These can complement the activity of lingual lipase and result in adequate hydrolysis of dietary triglycerides. In the presence of inefficient utilization of orally administered lipids, the critical need for bile acids may be reduced by the administration of formulas that include medium-chain triglycerides as a caloric source; the latter is well absorbed, even the face of reduced lipolysis and micelle solubilization.

The feeding of the low-birthweight infant remains an important area for future investigation. At present we must respect the limitations imposed by premature birth and take these factors into account when designing a feeding plan and when calculating nutrient requirements.

Questions and Answers

Q.   If one were to use milk to induce gut development, is there a difference between human milk and cow milk formulas?
A.   Possibly, due to EGF, hormones, etc. present in breast milk.

Q.   Are there "magic numbers" that one could use for serum bile acid or bilirubin concentrations that would imply serious liver dysfunction or require further workup to exclude primary liver disease?
A.   Bile acids in our laboratory are directly related to age; therefore we cannot evaluate without knowing the age. The level of bilirubin that is commonly used is bilirubin–direct (conjugated) > 2.0 mg/dl.

REFERENCES

1. Pearson HA. Lectures on the diseases of children by Eli Ives, M.D., of Yale and New Haven: America's first academic pediatrician (special article). Pediatrics 1986; 77:680.
2. Koldovsky O. Development of human gastrointestinal functions: interaction of changes in diet composition, hormonal maturation, and fetal genetic programming. J Am Coll Nutr 1984;3:131-138.
3. Klein RM. Models for the study of cell proliferation in the developing gastrointestinal tract. J Pediatr Gastroenterol Nutr 1986;5:513.
4. Lagerkrantz H Slotkin TA. The "stress" of being born. Scientific American April 1986;100.
5. Fisher DA. The unique endocrine milieu of the fetus. J Clin Invest 1986;78:603-611.
6. Mulvihill SJ, Stone MM, Fonkalsrud EW, Debas HT. Trophic effect of amniotic fluid on fetal gastrointestinal development. J Surg Res 1986;40:291-296.
7. Henning SJ, Leeper LL. Coordinate loss of glucocorticoid responsiveness by intestinal enzymes during postnatal development. Am J Physiol 1982;242:G89-G94.
8. Yang P, Baylin SB, Luk GD. Polyamines and intestinal growth: absolute requirement for ODC activity in adaptation during lactation. Am J Physiol 1984;247:G553-G557.
9. Martin GR, Henning SJ. Enzymic development of the small intestine: are glucocorticoids necessary? Am J Physiol 1984;246:G695-G699.
10. O'Loughlin EV, Chung M, Hollenberg M, et al. Effect of epidermal growth factor on ontogeny of the gastrointestinal tract. Am J Physiol 1985;249:G674-G678.
11. Rao RK, Ramakrishnan CV. Inositol phosphatase in developing rat duodenum, jejunum and ileum. Biol Neonate 1986;50:165-170.
12. Johnson LR. Regulation of gastrointestinal growth. In Johnson LR (ed): Physiology of Gastrointestinal Tract. New York, Raven Press, 1981;169-196.
13. Kedinger M, Simon PM, Raul F, et al. The effect of dexamethasone on the development of rat intestinal brush-border enzymes in organ culture. Develop Biol 1980;74:9-21.
14. Karasov WH, Solberg DH, Change SD, et al. Is intestinal transport of sugars and amino acids subject to critical-period programming? Am J Physiol 1985;249:G770-G785.
15. Corring T, Durand G, Henry Y. Some aspects of development and nutrition in the monogastric animal during postnatal life. In Bourne GH (ed): World Review of Nutrition and Dietetics, Vol 39. Basel, Karger, 1982;124-190.
16. Colony PC. Successive phases of human fetal intestinal development. In Kretchmer N, Minkowski A (eds): Nutritional Adaptation of the Gastrointestinal Tract of the Newborn. New York, Nestle, Vevey/Raven Press, 1983;3-28.
17. Kammeraad A. The development of the gastrointestinal tract of the rat: Histogenesis of the epithelium of the stomach, small intestine and pancreas. J Morphol 1942;70:323-351.
18. Lebenthal E, Lee PC. Structure and function of the gastrointestinal tract. Pediatrics Update, 1981;105.
19. Grand RJ, Watkins JB, Torti FM. Development of the human gastrointestinal tract (a review). Gastroenterology 1976; 70:790-810.
20. Arey LB. Developmental Anatomy, 2nd ed. Philadelphia, W.B. Saunders, 1965.
21. Hoar RM, Monie IW. Comparative development of specific organ systems. In Kimmel CA, Buelke-Sam J (eds): Developmental Toxicology. New York, Raven Press, 1981;13-33.
22. Andres JM, Mathis RK, Walker WA. Liver disease in infants. I. Developmental hepatology and mechanisms of liver dysfunction. J Pediatr 1977;90:686-697.
23. Novometsky F, Plank J, Levcik A. Developmental trends of liver parenchyma in the terminal period of gestation: a stereological approach. Exp Pathol 1982;21:187-192.

24. de la Iglesia FA, Sturgess JM, McGuire EJ, Feuer G. Quantitative microscopic evaluation of the endoplasmic reticulum in developing human liver. Am J Pathol 1976;82:61-70.
25. Koga A. Morphogenesis of intrahepatic bile ducts of the human fetus: light and electron microscopic study. Z Anat Entwickl-Gesch 1971;135:156-184.
26. Alison MR. Regulation of hepatic growth. In Physiological Reviews, vol 66. The American Physiological Society (Publishers), 1986;499-541.
27. Lind J. Changes in the liver circulation at birth. Ann NY Acad Sci 1963;111:110-120.
28. Rudolph AM. Hepatic and ductus venosus blood flows during fetal life. Hepatology 1983;3:254-258.
29. Coppoletta JM, Wolbach SB. Body length and organ weights of infants and children: a study of the body length and normal weights of the more important vital organs of the body between birth and 12 years of age. Am J Pathol 1933; 9:55.
30. Trier JS, Moxey PC. Morphogenesis of the small intestine during fetal development. In Ciba Foundation Symposium 70 (new series), Development of Mammalian Absorptive Processes. Amsterdam, Excepta Medica, 1979;3-20.
31. Potter GD, Schmidt KL, Lester R. Glucose absorption by in vitro perfused colon of the fetal rat. Am J Physiol 1983;245:G424-G430.
32. Potter GD, Burlingame SM. Glucose-coupled sodium absorption in the developing rat colon. Am J Physiol 1986;250:G221-G226.
33. Lacy ER, Colony PC. Localization of carbonic anhydrase. Gastroenterology 1985;89:138-150.
34. MacLean WC Jr, Fink BB, Schoeller DA, et al. Lactose assimilation by full-term infants: relation of ^{13}C) and H breath tests with fecal (^{13}C) excretion. Pediatr Res 1983; 17:629-633.
35. Bhatia J, Prihoda AR, Richardson CJ. Parenteral antibiotics and carbohydrate intolerance in term neonates. Am J Dis Child 1986;140:111-113.
36. MacLean WC Jr, Fink BB. Lactose malabsorption by premature infants: magnitude and clinical significance. J Pediatr 1980;97:383-388.
37. Moog F. The differentiation and redifferentiation of the intestinal epithelium and its brush border membrane. In Ciba Foundation Symposium 70 (new series), Development of Mammalian Absorptive Processes. Amsterdam, Excerpta Medica, 1979;31-44.
38. Moxey PC, Trier JS. Specialized cell types in the human fetal small intestine. Anat Rec 1978; 191:269-286.
39. Moxey PC, Trier JS. Structural features of the mucosa of human fetal intestine. Gastroenterology 1975;68:1002.
40. Moxey PC, Trier JS. Endocrine cells in the human fetal small intestine. Cell Tissue Res 1977;183:33-50.
41. Pang K-Y, Newman AP, Udall JN, Walker WA. Development of gastrointestinal mucosal barrier. VII. In utero maturation of microvillus surface by cortisone. Am J Physiol 1985; 249:G85-G91.
42. Pang K-Y, Bresson JL, Walker WA. Development of the gastrointestinal mucosal barrier. Evidence for structural differences in microvillus membranes from newborn and adult rabbits. Biochem Biophys Acta 1983;727:201-208.
43. Tomasi TB, Larson L, Challacombe S, McNabb PJ. Mucosal immunity: The origin and migration patterns of cells in the secretory system. J Allergy Clin Immunol 1980;65:12.
44. Dahiya R, Brasitus TA. Glycosphingolipid patterns of fetal and adult small intestinal mucosa in the sheep. Biochem Biophys Acta 1986;875:220-226.
45. Lebenthal E, Heitlinger LA. Perinatal development of the exocrine pancreas. In Tanner MA, Stocks RJ (eds): Neonatal Gastroenterology. Newcastle-Upon-Tyme, .Intercept 1984;179-192.
46. Pollack PF, Verbridge J, Thornburg W, et al. Isolated pancreatic acini from suckling and weanling rats: changes in amino acid incorporation and carbachol-stimulated amylase secretion with age. Biol Neonate 1986;49:344-350.
47. Lebenthal E, Lee PC. Development of functional response in human exocrine pancreas. Pediatrics 1980;66:556-560.
48. Spooner BS, Cohne HI, Faubion J. Development of mammalian embryonic pancreas: the relationship between

morphogenesis and cytodifferentiation. Develop Biol 1977;61:119-130.

49. Van Nest GA, MacDonald RJ, Rauran RK, Rutter RJ. Protein synthesized and secreted during rat pancreatic development. J Cell Biol 1980;86:784-794.

50. Werlin SL, Stefaniak J. Maturation of secretory function in rat pancreas. Pediatr Res 1982;16:123-125.

51. Greengard O. Enzymic differentiation of human liver: comparison with the rat model. Pediatr Res 1977;11:669-676.

52. Lamers WH Mooren PG, Griep H, et al. Hormones in perinatal rat and spiny mouse: relation to altricial and precocial timing of birth. Am J Physiol 1986;251:E78-E85.

53. Heubi JE, Soloway RD, Balistreri WF. Biliary lipid composition in healthy and diseased infants, children and young adults. Gastroenterology 1982;82:1295-1299.

54. von Bergmann J, von Bergmann K, Hadorn B, et al. Biliary lipid composition in early childhood. Clin Chim Acta 1975;64:241-246.

55. Tavoloni N. Bile secretion and its control in the newborn puppy. Pediatr Res 1986;20:203-208.

56. Tavoloni N, Jones MJT, Berk PD. Postnatal development of bile secretory physiology in the dog. J Pediatr Gastroenterol Nutr 1985;4:256-267.

57. Shaffer EA, Zahavi I, Gall DG. Postnatal development of hepatic bile formation in rabbit. Dig Dis Sci 1985;30:558-563.

58. Denehy CM, Ryan JR. Development of gallbladder contractility in the guinea pig. Pediatr Res 1986;20:214-217.

59. Balistreri WF, Heubi JE, Suchy FJ. Immaturity of the enterohepatic circulation in early life: factors predisposing to "physiologic" maldigestion and cholestasis. J Pediatr Gastroenterol Nutr 1983;2:346-354.

60. Balistreri WF, et al. Immaturity of the enterohepatic circulation of bile acids in early life: factors responsible for increased peripheral serum bile acid concentrations. In Proceedings of Falk Symposium No. 42, VIII International Bile Acid Meeting, Bern, Switzerland. MTP Press Limited, 1985;87-93.

61. Itoh S, Onishi S, Isobe K, et al. Foetal maternal relationships of bile acid pattern estimated by high-pressure liquid chromatography. Biochem J 1982;204:1411-1415.

62. Colombo C, Zuliani G, Rochi M, et al. Biliary bile acid composition of the human fetus in early gestation. Pediatr Res in press.

63. Street JM, Balistreri WF, Setchell KDR. Bile acid metabolism in the perinatal period—excretion of conventional and atypical bile acids in meconium. Gastroentrology 1986; 90:1773.

64. Back P and Walter K. Developmental pattern of bile acid metabolism as revealed by bile acid analysis of meconium. Gastroenterology 1980;78:671.

65. Little JM, Richey JE, Van Thiel DH, Lester R. Taurocholate pool size and distribution in the fetal rat. J Clin Invest 1979;63:1042-1049.

66. Bongiovanni AM. Bile acid content of gallbladder of infants, children and adults. J Clin Endocrinol Metab 1965;25: 678-685.

67. Sharp HL, Peller J, Carey JB, Krivit W. Primary and secondary bile acids in meconium. Pediatr Res 1971;5:274-279.

68. Jarvenpaa A-L. Feeding the low-birth-weight infant IV. Fat absorption as a function of diet and duodenal bile acids. Pediatrics 1983;72:684-689.

69. Jarvenpaa A-L, Rassin DK, Kuitunen P, et al. Feeding the low-birth weight infant. III. Diet influences bile acid metabolism. Pediatrics 1983;72:677-683.

70. Watkins JB, Ingall D, Szczepanik P, Klein PD, et al. Bile-salt metabolism in the newborn. N Engl J Med 1973;288:431-434.

71. Watkins JB, Szczepanik P, Gould JB et al. Bile salt metabolism in the human premature infant. Gastroenterology 1975;69:706-713.

72. Watkins JB, Jarvenpaa AL, Szczepanik-Van Leeuwen P, et al. Feeding the low-birth-weight infant. V. Effects of taurine, cholesterol and human milk on bile acid kinetics. Gastroenterology 1983;85:793-800.

73. Boyer JL. New concepts of the mechanisms of hepatocyte bile formation. Physiol Rev 1980;60:303-326.

74. Hofmann AF. The enterohepatic circulation of bile acids. Clin Gastroenterol 1977;6:3-24.

75. Suchy FJ, Balistreri WF, Heubi JE, et al. Physiologic cholestasis: elevation of the primary serum bile acid concentrations in normal infants. Gastroenterology 1981; 80:1037-1041.

76. Suchy FJ, Balistreri WF. Uptake of taurocholate by hepatocytes isolated from developing rats. Pediatr Res 1982; 16:282-285.

77. Suchy FJ, Couchene SM, Blitzer BL. Taurocholate transport by basolateral plasma membrane vesicles isolated from developing rat liver. Am J Physiol 1985;248:G648-G654.

78. Suchy FJ, Bucuvalas JC, Goodrich AL, et al. Taurocholate transport and Na^+ K^+ −ATPase activity in fetal and neonatal rat liver plasma membrane vesicles. Am J Physiol in press.

79. Moyer MS, Heubi JE, Goodrich AL, et al. Ontogeny of bile acid transport in brush border membrane vesicles from rat ileum. Gastroenterology 1986;90:1188-1196.

80. Allen C, Kendall JW. Maturation of the circadian rhythm of plasma corticosterone in the rat. Endocrinology 1967; 80:926-930.

81. Bartova A. Functioning of the hypothalamic-pituitary-adrenal system during postnatal development in rats. Gen Comp Endocrinol 1968;10:235-239.

82. Henning SJ. Biochemistry of intestinal development. Environ Health Perspect 1979;33:9-16.

83. Henning SJ. Permissive role of thyroxine in the ontogeny of jejunal sucrase. Endocrinology 1978;102:9-15.

84. Schwarz SM, Ling S, Hostetler B, et al. Lipid composition and membrane fluidity in the small intestne of the developing rabbit. Gastroenterology 1984;86:1544-1551.

85. Schwarz SM, Hostetler B, Ling S, et al. Intestinal membrane lipid composition and fluidity during development in the rat. Am J Physiol 1985;248:G200-G207.

86. Davidson LT, Merritt KK, Weach AA. Hyperbilirubinemia in newborn. Am J Dis Child 1941;61:958.

87. Kawade N, Onishi S. The prenatal and postnatal development of UDP-glucuronyltransferase activity towards bilirubin and the effect of premature birth on this activity in the human liver. Biochem J 1983;196:257-260.

88. Oppe TE, Gibbs IE. Sulfobromophthalein excretion in premature infants. Arch Dis Child 1959;34:125-130.

89. Yudkin S, Gellis SS. Liver function in newborn infants with special reference to the excreton of bromosulfophthalein. Arch Dis Child 1949;24:12-14.

90. Warner A. Drug use in the neonate: interrelationships of pharmacokinetics, toxicity, and biochemical maturity. Clin Chem 1986;32:721-727.

91. Balistreri WF, Schubert WK. Liber disease in infancy and childhood. In Schiff L, Schiff E (eds): Diseases of the Liver. Philadelphia, J.B. Lippincott Co. 1982;1265-1348.

92. Soyka LF, Redmond GP (eds): Drug Metabolism in the Immature Human. Raven Press, New York, 1981.

93. Brashear RE, Veng-Pedersen P, Rhodes ML, Smith CN. Theophylline elimination in the pregnant and fetal rabbit. J Lab Clin Med 1982;100:15-25.

94. Sutherland JM. Fatal cardiovascular collapse of infants receiving large amounts of chloramphenicol. Am J Dis Child 1959;97:761-767.

95. Stanley CA, Gonzales E, Baker L. Development of hepatic fatty acid oxidation and ketogenesis in the newborn guinea pig. Pediatr Res 1983;17:224-229.

96. Henning SJ. Postnatal development: coordination of feeding, digestion and metabolism. Am J Physiol 1981;241: G199-214.

97. Westbury K, Hahn P. Fructose-1,6-biphosphatase activity in the intestinal mucosa of developing rats. Am J Physiol 1984;9:G683-G686.

98. El Manoubi L, Callikan S, Duee P-H, et al. Development of gluconeogenesis in isolated hepatocytes from the rabbit. Am J Physiol 1983;244:E24-E30.

99. Brennan WA Jr, Aprille JR. Regulation of hepatic gluconeogenesis in newborn rabbit: Controlling factors in presuckling period. Am J Physiol 1985;249:E498-E505.

100. Dancis J, Braverman N, Lind J. Plasma protein synthesis in

the human fetus and placenta. J Clin Invest 1957;36: 398.

101. Janne J, Holtta E, Guha SK. Polyamines in mammalian liver during growth and development. In Popper H, Schaffner F (eds): Progress in Liver Diseases, vol V. New York, Grune and Stratton 1976;100-124.

102. Gaull GE. Taurine in human milk: growth modulator or conditionally essential amino acid? J Pediatr Gastroenterol Nutr 1983;2:S266-S271.

103. Glasgow JFT, Moore R. Plasma amino acid ratio as an index of hepatocellular maturity in the neonate. Biol Neonate 1983;44:146-152.

104. Abramovich DR. Fetal factors influencing amniotic fluid volume and composition of liquor amni. J Obstet Gynaecol Br Commonw 1970;77:865-877.

105. Pritchard JA. Fetal swallowing and amniotic fluid volume. Obstet Gynecol 1966;28:606-610.

106. Siegel M, Krantz B, Lebenthal E. Effect of fat and carbohydrate composition on the gastric emptying of isocaloric feedings in premature infants Gastroenterology 1985; 89:785-790.

107. Tseng C-C, Johnson LR. Role of thyroxine in functional gastric development. Am J. Physiol 1986;251:G111-G116.

108. Hyman PE, Clarke DD, Everett SL, et al. Gastric acid secretory function in preterm infants. J Pediatr 1985;106: 467-471.

109. Jacobs DM, Ackerman SH, Shindledecker RD. Ontogeny of gastric secretion in the rat. Ultrastructural changes in relation to secretory changes. Gastroenterology 1986;91: 667-672.

110. Takeuchi K, Peitsch W, Johnson LR. Mucosal gastrin receptor. V. Development in newborn rats. Am J Physiol 1981;240:G163-G169.

111. Younoszai MK, Sapario RS, Laughlin M. Maturation of jejunum and ileum in rats. Water and electrolyte transport during in vivo perfusion of hypertonic solutions. J Clin Invest 1978;62:271-281.

112. Lebenthal E, Lee PC, Heitlinger LA. Impact of development of the gastrointestinal tract on infant feeding. J Pediatr 1983;102:1-9.

113. Henning SJ. Ontogeny of enzymes in the small intestine. Ann Rev Physiol 1985;47:231-45.

114. Buts J-P, Delacroix DL, Dekeyser N, et al. Role of dietary iron in maturation of rat small intestine at weaning. Am J Physiol 1984;246:G725-G731.

115. Shehata AT, Lerner J, and Miller DS. Development of nutrient transport systems in chick jejunum. Am J Physiol 1984;246:G101-G107.

116. Weijers HA Drion EF, Van De Kamer JH. Analysis and interpretations of the fat-absorption coefficient. Acta Paediatr Scand 1960;49:615-521.

117. Watkins JB. Mechanisms of fat absorption and the development of gastrointestinal function. Pediatr Clin North Am 1975;22:721-730.

118. Zoppi G, Andreotti G, Pajno-Ferraro F, et al. Exocrine pancreas function in premature and full-term neonates. Pediatr Res 1972;6:880-886.

119. Signer E, Murphy GM, Edkins S, et al. Role of bile salts in fat malabsorption of premature infants. Arch Dis Child 1974; 49:174-180.

120. Heubi JE, Balistreri WF, Suchy FJ. Bile salt metabolism in the first year of life. J Lab Clin Med 1982;100:127-136.

121. Westergaard H, Dietschy JM. Delineation of dimensions and permeability characteristics of the two major diffusion barriers to passive mucosal uptake in rabbit intestine. J Clin Invest 1974;54:718-732.

122. Foman SJ, Ziegler EE, Thomas LM, et al. Excretion of fat by normal full-term infants fed various milks and formulas. Am J Clin Nutr 1970;23:1299-1313.

123. Barltrop D, Oppe TE. Absorption of fat and calcium by low birth weight infants from milk containing butter fat and olive oil. Arch Dis Child 1973;48:496.

124. Chappell JE, Clandinin MT, Kearney-Volpe C, et al. Fatty acid balance studies in premature infants fed human milk or formula: effect of calcium supplementation. J Pediatr 1986;108:439-447.

125. Freeman HJ, Quamme GA. Age-related changes in sodium dependent glucose transport in rat small intestine. Am J Physiol 1986;251:G208-G217.

126. Lebenthal E. Infant nutrition: metabolism and the digestive system. J Pediatr Gastroenterol Nutr 1983;2:S57-S338.

127. Kerzner B, Sloan HR, Haase G, et al. The jejunal absorption of glucose oligomers in the absence of pancreatic enzymes. Pediatr Res 1981;15:250-253.

128. Keene MFL; Hewer EE. Digestive enzymes of the human fetus. Lancet 1929;1:767.

129. Heitlinger LA, Ping CL, Dillon WP, Lebenthal E. Mammary amylase: possible alternate pathway of carbohydrate digestion in infancy. Pediatr Res 1983;17:15.

130. Lebenthal E, Lee PC. Glucoamylase and disaccharidase activities in normal subjects and in patients with mucosal injury of the small intestine. J Pediatr 1980;97:389.

131. Koldovsky O. Longitudinal specialization of the small intestine: developmental aspects. Gastroenterology 1983;85: 1436-1437.

132. Semenza G. Anchoring and biosynthesis of small-intestinal sucrase-isomaltase. In Kretchmer N, Minkowski A (eds): Nutritional Adaptation of the Gastrointestinal Tract of the Newborn. New York, Nestle, Vevey/Raven Press, 1983;290-42.

133. Black BL. Morphological development of the epithelium of the embryonic chick intestine in culture: influence of thyroxine and hydrocortisone. Am J Anat 1978;153:573-599.

134. Black BL, Moog F. Alkaline phosphatase and maltase activity in the embryonic chick intestine in culture: influence of thyroxine and hydrocortisone. Dev Biol 1978;66:232-249.

135. Lebenthal E, Antonowicz I, Shwachman H. Correlation of lactase activity lactose tolerance and milk consumption in different age groups. Am J Clin Nutr 28:595, 1975.

136. Welsh JD, Poley JR, Bhata M, Stevenson DE. Intestinal disaccharidases activities in relation to age, race and mucosal damage. Gastroenterology 75:847, 1978.

137. Doell R, Rosen G, Kretchmer N. Immunochemical studies of intestinal disaccharidases during normal and precocious development. Proc Natl Acad Sci USA 1965;54:1268-1273.

138. Jonas MM, Montgomery RK, Grand RJ. Intestinal lactase synthesis during postnatal development in the rat. Pediatr Res 19:956-962, 1985.

139. Koldovsky O Digestion and absorption. In Stave U (ed): Perinatal Physiology. New York, Plenum Publishing Corp. 1977;317-356.

140. Koldovsky O, Heringova A, Jirsova V, et al. Transport of glucose against a concentration gradient in everted sacs of jejunum and ileum of human fetus. Gastroenterology 1965;48:185.

141. Avery GB, Randolph JC, Weaver T. Gastric acidity in the first day of life. Pediatrics 1966;37:1005.

142. Harries JT Fraser AJ. The acidity of the gastric contents of premature babies during the first 14 days of life. Biol Neonate 1966;12:186.

143. Antonowicz I, Lebenthal E. Developmental pattern of small intestinal enterokinase and disaccharidase activities in the human fetus. Gastroenterology 1977;72:1299-1303.

144. Auricchio S, Stellato A, DeVizia B. Development of brush border peptidases in human and rat small intestine during fetal and neonatal life. Pediatr Res 1981;15:991.

145. Rubino A, and Guandalini S. Dipeptide transport in the mucosa of developing rabbits. In Elliott K, O'Connor M (eds): Peptide Transport and Hydrolysis. Ciba Foundation Symposium 50. Amsterdam, Elsevier, 1977;61-71.

146. Moyer MS, Goodrich AL, Suchy FJ: Ontogenesis of intestinal taurine transport: evidence for a carrier system in developing rat jejunum. Gastroenterology 1986;90:1558.

147. Aynsley-Green A. Metabolic and endocrine interrelations in the human fetus and neonate. Am J Clin Nutr 1985;41:399-417.

148. Aynsley-Green A, Adrian TE, Bloom SR. Feeding and the development of enteroinsular hormone release in the preterm infant: effects of continuous gastric infusion of human

milk compared with intermittent boluses. Acta Paediatr Scand 1982;71:379-383.

149. Lucas A. Endocrine aspects of enteral nutriton. In New Aspects of Clinical Nutrition. Basel, Karger, 1983;581-594.

150. Lucas A, Bloom SR, Aynsley-Green A. Metabolic and endocrine consequences of depriving preterm infants of enteral nutrition. Acta Paediatr Scand 1983;72:245-249.

151. Aynsley-Green A, Lucas A, Bloom SR. The effects of feeds of differing composition on enter-insular hormone secretion in the first hours of life in human neonates. Acta Paediatr Scand 1979;68:265-270.

152. Klinger W. Biotransformation of drugs and other xenobiotics during postnatal development. Pharmacol Ther 1982; 16:377-429.

153. Bernstein RB, Novy MJ, Piasecki GJ, et al. Bilirubin metabolism in the fetus. J Clin Invest 1969;48:1678-1688.

154. Sondheimer JM, et al. Cholestatic tendencies in premature infants on and off parenteral nutrition. Pediatrics 1978; 62:984.

155. Hamosh M. Lingual and breast milk lipases. In Barness LA (ed): Advances in Pediatrics vol 29. Chicago, Year Book Medical Publishers, 1982;31-67.

156. Liao TH, Hamosh P, Hamosh M. Gastric lipolysis in the developing rat: Ontogeny of the lipases active in the stomach. Biochem Biophys Acta 1983;754:1-9.

157. Belknap WM, Balistreri WF, Suchy FJ, et al. Physiologic cholestasis. II. Serum bile acids reflect the development of the enterohepatic circulation in rats. Hepatology 1981;1: 613-616.

158. Belknap WM, Zimmer-Nechemias L, Suchy FJ, et al. Bile acid efflux from suckling rat hepatocytes. Unpublished data.

159. Gartner LA, Lee KS, Lane D, et al. Development of bilirubin transport and metabolism in the newborn rhesus monkey. J Pediatr 1977;90:513-530.

160. Stolz A, Sugiyama Y, Kuhlenkamp J, et al. Cytosolic bile acid binding protein in rat liver: radioimmunoassay, molecular forms, developmental characteristics and organ distribution. Hepatology 1986;6:433-439.

161. Suchy FJ, Couchene SM, Balistreri WF. Ontogeny of hepatic bile acid conjugation in the rat. Pediatr Res 1985;19:97-

101.

162. Balistreri WF, Zimmer L, Suchy FJ, et al. Bile salt sulfotransferase: Alteration during maturation and non-inducibility during substrate ingestion. J Lipid Res 1984;25: 228-235.

163. Suchy FJ, Balistreri WF. Maturation of bile acid conjugation in hepatocytes from fetal and suckling rats. Gastroenterology 1980;78:1324.

164. Strandvik B, Witstrom SA. Tetrahdroxylated bile acids in healthy human newborns. Eur J Clin Invest 1982;12:301-305.

165. Subbiah TR, Hassan AS. Development of bile acid biogenesis and its significance in cholesterol homeostasis. Adv Lipid Res 1982;19:137-161.

166. Danielsson H, Rutter WJ. The metabolism of bile acids in the developing rat liver. Biochemistry 1968;7:346-351.

167. deBelle RC, Vaupshas V, Vitullo BB, et al. Intestinal absorption of bile salts: Immature development in the neonate. J Pediatr 1979;79:371-377.

168. Rohr HP, Wirz A, Henning LC, et al. Morphometric analysis of the rat liver cell in the perinatal period. Lab Invest 1971;24:128-139.

169. Daimon T, David H, Zglinicki TV, et al. Correlated ultrastructural and morphometric studies on the liver during perinatal development. Exp Pathol 1982;21:237-250.

170. Miller DH, Zanolli CS, Gumucio JJ. Quantitative morphology of the sinusoids of the hepatic acinus. Gastroenterology 1979;76:847.

171. Suchy FJ, et al. Absence of a hepatic lobular gradient for bile acid uptake in the suckling rat. Hepatology 1983;3:847.

172. DeWolf-Peeters C, et al. Electron microscopy and histochemistry of canalicular differentiation in fetal and neonatal rat liver. Tissue Cell 1976;4:379.

173. DeWolf-Peeters C, et al. Electron microscopy and morphometry of canalicular differentiation in fetal and neonatal rat liver. Exp Mol Pathol 1974;21:339.

174. Miyairi M, Watanabe S, Phillips MJ. Cell motility of fetal hepatocytes in short term culture. Pediatr Res 1985;19: 1225-1229.

4

Ontogeny of the Kidney

JOHN M. LORENZ, M.D.
LEONARD I. KLEINMAN, M.D.

"The kidneys advise and the heart comprehends."
TRACTATE SHABBAT, 33B (*Talmud*)

ABSTRACT

The kidney is the principal organ responsible for the fine adjustment of water and electrolyte excretion in relation to intake so that body fluid composition is maintained within limits compatible with optimal function. Although the functional capabilities of the perinatal kidney are limited relative to those of the adult kidney, still these capabilities are adequate even in the moderately premature infant to deal with water, electrolyte, and acid loads presented to the kidney as a result of breast milk or formula intake. However, the perinatal kidney is unable to compensate for deficits or excesses of water and electrolytes as efficiently as can the adult kidney. These deficits and excesses are most likely encountered by infants with complicating illnesses who require intravenous fluid, electrolyte, and caloric maintenance. The factors responsible for these limitations vary as a function of the stage of development of the kidney. Depending on the stage of development, the predominant factor initially may be lesser number of nephrons, subsequently may be histologic immaturity of nephrons, and finally may be lesser filtrative and reabsorptive surface areas per nephron. **A major factor responsible for the limited ability of the perinatal kidney to respond to water and electrolyte excesses is its low glomerular filtration rate (GFR).** However, the perinatal kidney requires a low GFR in order to assure a reasonable degree of glomerular-tubular balance.

INTRODUCTION

It has been said that "we are what we eat." From the perspective of body and electrolyte content, it would be more accurate to say that we are what we eat minus what we excrete. It is the kidney that is the principal organ responsible for the fine adjustment of water and electrolyte excretion in relation to intake so that the *milieu interior* of the body is maintained within limits compatible with optimal function. In the developing organism, this process is complicated by the continuing accretion and modification of body water and electrolytes as growth and differentiation occur. Fortunately,

even with limitations imposed by renal immaturity, the preterm newborn infant seems more capable of appropriately regulating water and electrolyte excretion than we as their caretakers sometimes are in appropriately regulating intake.

In the fetus, body water and electrolyte homeostasis is maintained largely by the placenta, so that renal maturation in utero is geared primarily to prepare the kidney for its extrauterine role. As a result, the functional capabilities of the fetal kidney are much greater than its normal functional requirements. Indeed, fetuses without functioning kidneys often manifest no body water or electrolyte abnormalities. Even with preterm birth, then, substantial anatomic and functional maturation has already occurred so that the kidney is prepared to assume its responsiblity for maintaining body water and electrolyte homeostasis. However, as we shall discuss in this chapter, the capabilities of the immature kidney in most cases fall short of those of the mature kidney and further maturation occurs in the postnatal period.

ANATOMIC MATURATION

The mammalian kidney develops through three successive but overlapping systems: the pronephros, the mesonephros, and the metanephros. Each of these three systems develops bilaterally in succession from the cervical to sacral regions of the embryo from the intermediate (i.e., between the somites and intraembryonic coelom) mesoderm. The first two systems have no functional activity in the human embryo and regress during development. The definitive mammalian kidney, the metanephros, develops from the union of the metanephric blastema with the cranial part of the ureteral bud. The metranephric blastema arises from the lower lumbar and sacral intermediate mesoderm. The nephroblastic cells of the metanephric blastema develop into the glomerulus, proximal convoluted tubule, loop of Henle, and distal convoluted tubule. The ureteral bud arises as an outgrowth of the mesonephric duct. It penetrates the metanephric blastema and eventually forms the collecting ducts, renal calyces and pelves, and ureters.

The metanephric kidney undergoes three basic phases of development, with a good deal of overlap among phases. The first phase is nephrogenesis, the development of new nephrons. The first nephrons to develop are those whose glomeruli will be located in the juxtamedulary region of the mature kidney. (See Figure 1 for anatomy of the kidney.) Glomerular filtration begins between the 9th and 12th weeks of gestation. At 22 weeks of gestation, only one-third of the eventual complement of nephrons is formed and all are juxtamedullary. Over the next 14 weeks nephrogenesis progresses toward the capsule. **Nephrogenesis is complete at 36 weeks' gestation,** so that the full-term newborn has as many nephrons as he will have during the rest of his life, while the prematurely born infant will continue to produce new nephrons for some time after birth.

The second phase of development is the histologic maturation of nephron segments. By the time that nephrogenesis ceases at 36 weeks, more recently formed nephrons will still manifest anatomic immaturity. This histologic immaturity disappears within several weeks. The final phase of renal development is that of increase in nephron size with no apparent change in histologic characteristics.

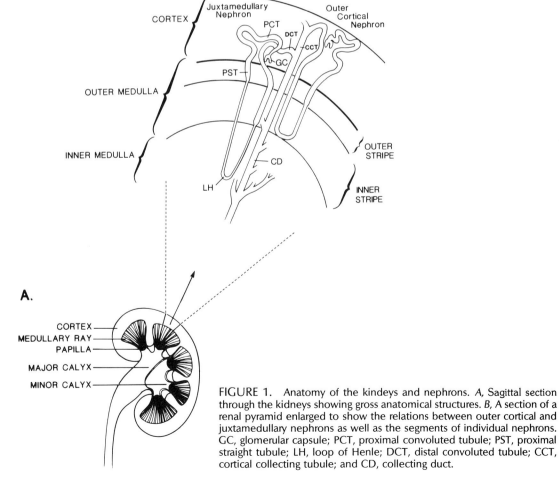

FIGURE 1. Anatomy of the kindeys and nephrons. A, Sagittal section through the kidneys showing gross anatomical structures. B, A section of a renal pyramid enlarged to show the relations between outer cortical and juxtamedullary nephrons as well as the segments of individual nephrons. GC, glomerular capsule; PCT, proximal convoluted tubule; PST, proximal straight tubule; LH, loop of Henle; DCT, distal convoluted tubule; CCT, cortical collecting tubule; and CD, collecting duct.

The developing kidney is a thoroughly heterogenous organ. As a consequence of the sequence of nephrogenesis, the microarchitecture of the cortex develops from the *inner* juxtamedullary region toward the peripheral region. Moreover, although growth of all nephron segments occurs as the infant matures, the rate of growth differs among segments within a nephron. Anatomically, there is *glomerular over tubular preponderance* in the perinatal kidney. At birth, the ratio of glomerular surface area to proximal tubule volume is approximately 27. The subsequent rate of growth of the proximal tubules is greater than that of the glomeruli. Thus the ratio of glomerular surface area to proximal tubule volume decreases to 8 at six months of age and then gradually approaches the adult level of 3 during late adolescence.[1]

Approximately 20% of the loops of Henle at birth are too short to reach into the medulla.[2] Even though total cortical thickness is increasing during this time as a consequence of glomerular and proximal tubular growth, the loops of Henle are growing at an even faster rate, so that by adulthood only 1-2% of all loops fail to reach into the medulla.

RENAL HEMODYNAMICS IN THE PERINATAL KIDNEY

In adult man, about 20-25% of the cardiac output goes to the kidneys, even though the kidneys constitute less than ½% of the total body weight. This large flow per unit organ weight, the largest of any organ in the body, is necessary because the kidney receives blood not merely for its nutrient and oxygen supply, as do all other organs, but also in order to alter the water and electrolyte content of the blood.

Results of various studies have all indicated that renal blood flow is *lower* in the perinatal animal than in the adult of the same species.[3-9] Moreover, the fraction of the cardiac output going to the kidney is usually lower in the perinatal animal than in the adult. In the fetus, of course, the largest part of the cardiac output goes to the placenta (about 40-50% of the combined right and left heart output). In the baboon fetus, for example, less than 5% of the combined cardiac output goes to the kidney, a fraction less than that going to the gastrointestinal tract.[10] The postnatal distribution of cardiac output varies with the species studied. In the rat, the kidneys receive 3.6% of the cardiac

output at birth and 16.6% at maturity.[11] In the monkey, there is no difference between the newborn and adult in the renal fraction of cardiac output.[5]

Renal blood flow (RBF) is continuously increasing with development but so is renal mass. In the fetal lamb, the increase in renal growth and renal blood flow occur at approximately the same rate, so that renal blood flow per unit kidney mass does not change.[12] However, after birth renal blood flow increases at a greater rate than kidney mass.

Blood flow to the kidney does not develop in a homogeneous pattern. Figure 2 reveals the maturational characteristics of blood flow to the inner and outer cortex of the newborn dog.[13] Blood flow to the *outer* cortical region increases continuously with age (corrected for renal mass in this region), whereas *inner* cortical flow changes little at first (again corrected for regional renal mass) and then increases with age.

Another way to evaluate the maturational pattern of intrarenal blood flow is to look at the relative flows to the two different regions, i.e., the developmental characteristics of the ratio of blood flow to the inner and outer cortex (Fig. 2). Early in life the ratio of inner to outer cortical blood flow is approximately one, and during the first 2 weeks the ratio declines (due primarily to the increase in outer cortical flow, Fig. 3) and then remains constant thereafter. Note that in the case of the neonatal dog the developmental change in relative intrarenal blood flow distribution occurs during the period of nephrogenesis and ceases at 2 weeks after birth when nephrogenesis is complete. This correlation of intrarenal blood flow distribution maturation to anatomical maturation does not hold for all animals studied, however.[14]

There is a complicated interplay of renal pressures and resistances during kidney maturation. Fortunately, this interplay provides blood to those nephrons that are *most mature* and presumably those that function best. As new nephrons mature, intrarenal vascular resistances are altered so that more blood can be distributed to these nephrons. This process results in a reasonable degree of *nephron-perfusion balance* throughout the renal maturational period.

Factors that control and regulate the intrarenal distribution of vascular resistance still need to be studied. There is enhanced activity of the renin-angiotensin system during the

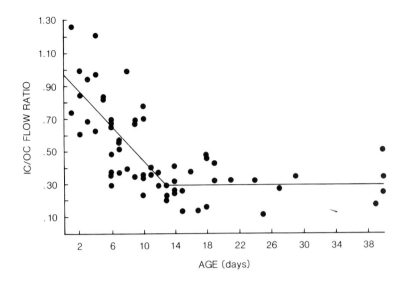

FIGURE 3. Maturation of intrarenal blood flow distribution in newborn dog. IC/OC, ratio of plasma flow of inner cortex (IC) to that of outer cortex (OC). Plasma flow to each region of the kidney is factored by dry mass of the region (From Kleinman LI, Reuter JH. J Physiol (London) 1973; 228:91, with permission.)

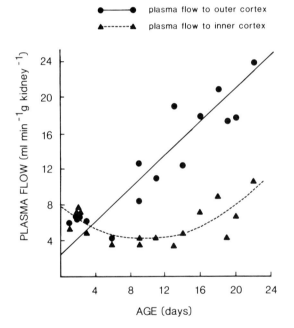

FIGURE 2. Maturation of plasma flow to outer cortex (circles and solid line) and inner cortex (triangles and dashed line) of kidney of newborn dogs. Flow to each region of the kidney is factored by dry mass of the region. (From Kleinman LI, Reuter JH. J Physiol (London) 1973; 228:91, with permission.)

perinatal period,[15-19] and this increased activity may contribute to the generally high renal vascular resistance usually found in the perinatal animal. Conceivably, a changing intrarenal pattern of the synthesis and release of renin during the perinatal period may account for the changing intrarenal distribution of vascular resistances. Alternatively, renal vascular response to catecholamine release, through either humoral or neural mechanisms, may be responsible for the changing pattern of renal hemodynamics in the perinatal animal. In the newborn dog for example, there is a greater renal vascular sensitivity to epinephrine than exists in the adult.[20] Finally, changes in other humoral agents known to affect renal hemodynamics, such as the prostaglandins, may contribute to the changing pattern of renal blood flow.

GLOMERULAR FILTRATION RATE IN THE PERINATAL ANIMAL

In the adult animal, approximately 20-25% of the plasma flowing through the kidney is filtered at the glomerulus. The kidney of an average-size man filters about 120 ml of water every minute.

Developmental changes in glomerular filtration (GFR) parallel those for renal blood flow (RBF) both in terms of intrarenal distribution and whole-kidney development. Thus glomerular filtration at a certain stage of development is lower in the outer than inner cortex but then increases at a greater rate in the outer than in the inner cortex.[21] With regard to the whole kidney, GFR increases as the animal matures, but as in the case of renal blood flow, the relative rates of increase for GFR and kidney mass depend on the stage of development.

Based on studies of different species it is possible to define three stages of GFR devel-

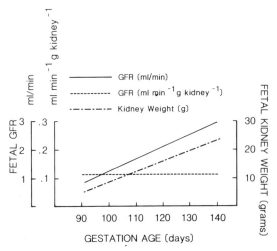

FIGURE 4. Maturation of glomerular filtration rate (GFR) in fetal lamb. GFR is expressed in units of ml/min (—) and units of ml min^{-1}g kidney^{-1} (----). Rate of kidney growth is also shown (—·—). (Based on data of Robillard et al.[12] From Kleinman LI. The Physiologist 1982; 25:104, with permission.)

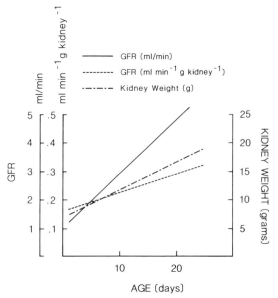

FIGURE 5. Maturation of glomerular filtration rate (GFR) in neonatal dog. GFR is expressed in units of ml/min (—) and units of ml min^{-1}g kidney^{-1} (----). Rate of kidney growth is also shown (—·—). (Based on data of Kleinman and Lubbe.[8] From Kleinman LI. The Physiologist 1982; 25:104 with permission.)

opment. These functional stages, however, do not necessarily correlate with the anatomical phases mentioned previously. It is important, nevertheless, to be aware of these different functional stages when comparing results from one species to another. The first stage, exemplified by the fetal lamb, is characterized by equivalent rates of increases of GFR and kidney mass, so that there is no change with age in GFR per gram of kidney (Fig. 4). The second stage, exemplified by the newborn dog (Fig. 5)—but also by the human infant during the first 4 months of life,[23] the neonatal lamb during the first 2 months,[24] the neonatal piglet during the first 2 months,[25] and the rat for the first 40-50 days of life[26]—is characterized by a greater rate of increase in GFR than in kidney growth. Thus, GFR per gram kidney weight is increasing during this period. In the final phase of development, glomerular filtration increases at the same rate as that of kidney mass.

Analysis of mechanisms of RBF and GFR development is made difficult by these three different stages of development which, as mentioned above, do not necessarily correlate with the three different phases of anatomical growth. Nevertheless, it may be possible to clarify some of these mechanisms based on a multitude of studies from various species at different stages of development. Table 1 summarizes the patterns of development of renal growth, RBF, GFR, and factors that might af-

fect RBF and GFR, such as arterial blood pressure, renal vascular resistance, glomerular capsular hydrostatic pressure (P_{gc}), individual glomerular plasma flow (GPF), and filtration coefficient (K_f) (Figs. 6, 7).

The two primary factors that affect renal blood flow are blood pressure and renal vascular resistance. In the early period in the fetal lamb there is only a slight increase in blood pressure and a marked *decrease* in renal vascular resistance with maturation,[14] so that the rise in total renal blood flow during this period is clearly due to the change in renal vascular resistance. However, the change in vascular resistance is parallel to the change in renal growth, so there is little or no change in renal vascular resistance per unit renal mass and little or no change in renal blood flow per gram kidney.

Blood pressure rises during the second developmental period (Table 1).[8] Although renal vascular resistance falls during this period in all species studied, there is controversy about the change in vascular resistance per unit renal mass. In the pig,[7] guinea pig,[21] and some studies in dogs[20] vascular resistance per gram kidney has been shown to fall with maturation; in other studies in dogs there is no change,[8] and in the rhesus monkey it actually

$$\text{GBF} \propto P_a \left(\frac{1}{R_a} + \frac{1}{R_e} \right)$$

$$\text{GFR} \propto K_f \left[\left(\bar{P}_c + \pi_{gc} \right) - \left(P_{gc} + \bar{\pi}_c \right) \right]$$

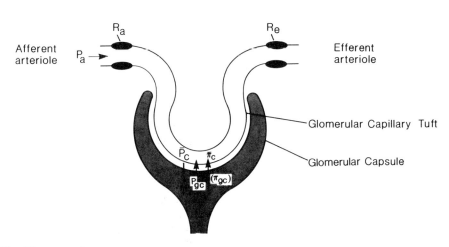

FIGURE 6.   Diagrammatic and mathematic representation of the factors that determine glomerular blood flow (GBF) and glomerular filtration rate (GFR). K_f, *filtration coefficient* (a function of glomerular capillary surface area and hydraulic conductivity); P_a, arterial blood pressure; P_{gc}, hydrostatic pressure in the glomerular capsule; $\bar{P}_c$, mean glomerular capillary hydrostatic pressure; R_a, *afferent* glomerular arteriolar resistance; R_e, *efferent* glomerular arteriolar resistance; π_{gc}, glomerular capsule oncotic pressure (negligible); $\bar{\pi}_c$, mean glomerular capillary oncotic pressure.

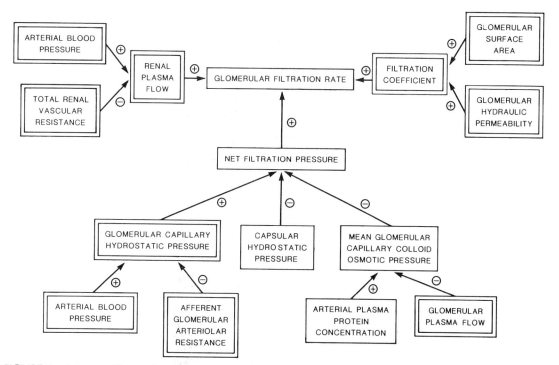

FIGURE 7.   Scheme of factors that affect the GFR. (+) Indicates that an increase in the causal factor will produce an increase in the resultant factor; (−) indicates that an increase in the causal factor will produce a decrease in the resultant factor; a double box indicates a factor that may contribute to low GFR in the perinatal kidney.

TABLE 1.   Developmental Periods of RBF and GFR Maturation

| | DEVELOPMENTAL PERIOD* | | |
	Early	Mid	Late
Animal model	Sheep fetus	Neonatal dog < 10 wks Neonatal guinea pig Newborn lamb < 2 mo Infant rat < 40 days Newborn infant < 4 mo	Young dog Young lamb Infant rat > 40 days Infant human
Kidney growth	Nephrogenesis Nephron maturation Nephron growth	Nephrogenesis (some species part of period) Nephron maturation Nephron growth	Nephron maturation (some species part of period) Nephron growth
Change in blood pressure	Slight increase	Large increase	Slight increase
RBF			
1. Total	Increase	Increase	Increase
2. Per kidney mass	Slight increase or no change	Increase	Slight increase or no change
3. Distribution	Toward outer cortex (slight)	Toward outer cortex	No change
RVR			
1. Total	Decrease	Decrease	Decrease
2. Per kidney mass	No change	Slight decrease or no change	Slight decrease or no change
Change in GFR			
1. Total	Increase	Increase	Increase
2. Per kidney mass	No change	Increase	No change
3. Single nephron	Slight increase or no change	Increase	Increase
P_{gc}	Slight increase or no change	Increase	Slight increase or no change
GPF	Slight increase or no change	Increase	Increase
K_f	Increase	Increase	Increase

*Developmental periods are arbitrary and vary from species to species. RBF, renal blood flow; GFR, glomerular filtration rate; RVR, renal vascular resistance; P_{gc}, glomerular capillary hydrostatic pressure; GPF, individual glomerular plasma flow; K_f, filtration coefficient.

rises slightly.[5] Thus the increase in renal blood flow per kidney mass during this period is probably related to the increase in blood pressure and perhaps (in certain species at least) to the fall in renal vascular resistance.

Factors determining the rate of glomerular filtration include glomerular plasma flow (GPF), plasma oncotic pressure ($\bar{\pi}_c$), glomerular capillary hydrostatic pressure ($\bar{P}_c$), glomerular capsular hydrostatic pressure (P_{gc}), and the glomerular filtration coefficient (K_f). Detailed discussion of the role of each of these factors in the maturaton of GFR is too complex for the present review. A summary, however, is presented in Table 1. There is a progressive maturational increase in the glomerular filtration coefficient (K_f) during the entire perinatal period. The increase in K_f is related largely to an increase in surface area of the glomerulus,[27] but also perhaps to an increase in hydraulic conductivity (pore size).[28] In the early period, since there is little change in GPF[14] and presumably therefore little change in single nephron GFR, the increase in total kidney GFR is probably due to the increasing number of nephrons. It is likely that during the second (mid) developmental period maturational increases in glomerular capillary hydrostatic pressure, $\bar{P}_c$, play an important role. The relative importance of the low K_f on the one hand or the low GPF on the other during this period is not known. In the third period of development (at least in the rat) there is evidence that the increase in nephron GFR is largely related to increases in glomerular plasma flow (GPF).[26]

TUBULAR TRANSPORT IN THE PERINATAL KIDNEY

The function of the kidney tubules is to alter the glomerular filtrate by transporting solutes and water across the tubular epithelium. Transport from the tubular lumen to interstitial fluid or peritubular capillaries is termed *reabsorption,* and transport from capillary to tubular lumen is called *secretion* (Fig. 8). Transport can be either passive (along an electrochemical gradient and requiring no metabolic energy) or active (against an electrochemical gradient and requiring metabolic energy).

Classically, renal tubular function has been evaluated by measuring rates of transport of various substances between tubular lumen and peritubular capillary. Transport rates of certain substances appear to be limited by a *transport maximum* (T_m); measurement of the T_m for these substances has been utilized as an index of tubular function. The T_m for glucose (T_{mG}), a substance that is transported from proximal renal tubule to peritubular capillary, and the T_m for PAH (T_{mPAH}), a substance that is transported from peritubular capillary to proximal renal tubule, have both been used as a measure of renal tubular function.

Absolute values for T_{mPAH} are low in newborn animals,[29] including human beings.[23,30] The low values for T_{mPAH} apply even when corrected for body weight or surface area, kidney weight, and more importantly, GFR. Glucose T_m is also lower in the neonate than in the adult when comparison is made on a body-weight or surface-area basis.[29,31] Early investigators found the ratio T_{mG}/GFR to be lower in the newborn infant than in the adult,[29] but more recent investigations have found the ratio to be the same in the adult and newborn infant.[32]

Perhaps one source of the difficulty in measuring the T_{mG}, or even the T_{mG}/GFR, which is more appropriate, is that proximal tubular glucose transport appears to be related to proximal tubular sodium reabsorption.[33] When a large fraction of the filtered sodium is reabsorbed, the T_{mG}/GFR is large and vice versa. Studies of the T_{mG}/GFR in newborn dogs initially indicated that tubular transport of glucose might be limited.[34] More recent studies, however, suggest that the low T_{mG}/GFR was due to the lower fractional sodium reabsorption in the proximal tubule that occurred in the newborn animal during glucose loading.[35] At any level of sodium reabsorption, the T_{mG}/GFR was the same for the newborn and adult.

The constancy of the T_{mG}/GFR ratio throughout maturation is a reflection of the balance of glomerular and tubular function of the whole kidney. The kidney, however, consists of a million nephrons, and it is as important for each of these individual nephrons to maintain glomerular tubular balance as it is for the kidney as a whole. Thus, if there exist certain nephrons with tubules of a low transport capability, it would be beneficial to have these tubules attached to glomeruli with low filtration rates; conversely, tubules that function well should be matched with glomeruli that filter well. Such a situation would result in functional glomerular-tubular balance, with a homogeneous population of nephrons with similar ratios of glomerular to tubular function. If the opposite situation occurs, i.e., poorly functioning glomeruli with well-functioning tubules (high T_m/GFR) or vice versa (low T_m/GFR), there would result functional *glomerular-tubular imbalance,* with a heterogen-

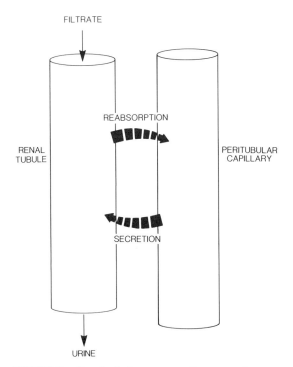

FIGURE 8. Renal tubular transport. Transport of water or solute from the tubular lumen to the peritubular capillary is referred to as *reabsorption.* Transport (active or passive) of water or solute from the peritubular capillary to the tubular lumen is referred to as *secretion.*

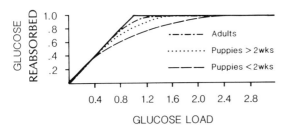

FIGURE 9.   Relationship between filtered glucose load and tubular reabsorption of glucose. The 45° solid-line segment is a hypothetical line representing complete reabsorption of glucose; the horizontal solid-line segment represents constant maximum glucose reabsorption when the load is greater than T_m. (Based on data from Baker and Kleinman.[35] From Kleinman LI. The kidney. In Stave U (ed): Perinatal Physiology. New York, Plenum Medical Book Co., 1978 with permission.)

eous population of nephrons with different ratios of glomerular to tubular function.

Functional analysis of homogeneity or heterogeneity of glomerular-tubular balance may be made by examining a titration curve of a substance such as glucose that has a transport maximum or overall T_{mG}/GFR (Fig. 9). As the filtered glucose load is progressively increased by raising plasma glucose, all the glucose in each nephron will be reabsorbed until the T_{mG}/GFR for that nephron is reached; additional reabsorption will then cease, and the excess filtered glucose will be excreted. If the T_{mg}/GFR were identical for each nephron (perfect nephron homogeneity), reabsorption would cease at the same glucose load for each nephron and for the kidney as a whole. This situation is represented by the solid line in Figure 9, which shows a continuing increase in total kidney glucose reabsorption equal to that of the filtered load (the line has a slope of 45°), and then a cessation of reabsorption when the transport maximum is reached (the line becomes horizontal).

If some nephrons have a lower T_{mG}/GFR than others, glucose reabsorption will cease in these tubules before it does in others, and there will be a deviation from the solid line. This deviation is referred to as "splay," and is shown in Figure 9 as the curved dashed lines connecting the two segments of the solid lines. The degree of splay is largely a function of the degree of nephron heterogeneity. As can be seen in Figure 9, there is a progressive decline in the degree of splay as the newborn dog matures. This physiologic nephron heterogeneity in the newborn animal is consistent with the anatomic nephron heterogeneity discussed previously.

Nephron heterogeneity not only produces splay in a glucose titration curve, but also *lowers the plasma threshold for glucose*, i.e., the plasma glucose concentration at which glucose first appears in the urine. As soon as glucose reabsorption ceases in the tubule, the excess glucose that is filtered will be excreted in the urine. Thus, as soon as the function in Figure 9 deviates from the 45° straight line, it represents the point at which glucose will appear in the urine.

This situation is made more apparent in Figure 10 in which urinary glucose excretion is plotted against plasma glucose. In the adult dog, no glucose appears in the urine until plasma glucose is well above 200 mg/dl. In puppies less than 2 weeks old, however, glu-

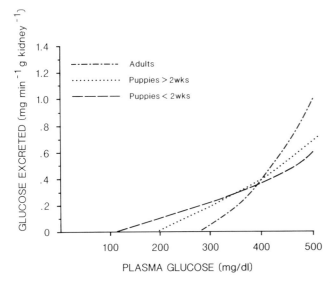

FIGURE 10.   Relationship between plasma glucose and glucose excreted in the urine. The plasma concentration at which glucose first appears in the urine is referred to as the plasma threshold for glucose. (Based on data from Baker and Kleinman.[35] From Kleinman LI. The kidney. In Stave U (ed): Perinatal Physiology. New York, Plenum Medical Book Co., 1978, with permission.)

cose is excreted when the plasma glucose is only 100 mg/dl. This degree of depression of the glucose threshold in the perinatal animal means that the immature kidney will excrete glucose at blood levels only slightly above the physiologic level for the adult. This probably accounts for the frequently observed clinical phenomenon of very premature infants with glucosuria at plasma concentrations of glucose below 100 mg/dl.

EXCRETION OF SODIUM BY THE PERINATAL KIDNEY

In the adult, under non-diuretic conditions, more than 99% of filtered sodium is reabsorbed by the tubules. Micropuncture studies reveal that about 70% of filtered sodium is reabsorbed in the proximal tubule; the rest is reabsorbed more distally, largely in the ascending limb of the loop of Henle (Fig. 11). Sodium reabsorption in the proximal tubule is due primarily to the active transport of sodium. In addition, the net proximal reabsorption of sodium is also a function of the reabsorption of glucose, bicarbonate and amino acids as well as physical forces of the peritubular environment such as colloid osmotic and hydrostatic pressures, the permeability characteristics of

the proximal nephron and the integrity of the intercellular tight junctions.

In the adult animal, under most circumstances, as the filtered load of sodium is increased, proximal tubular sodium reabsorption is proportionately increased, and as filtered sodium falls, proximal sodium reabsorption decreases. As a result, the fraction of filtered sodium reabsorbed proximally remains relatively constant, testifying to the existence of glomerular tubular balance for sodium reabsorption.

In the guinea pig and newborn dog the fractional reabsorption of water (and presumably sodium) at the end of the proximal tubule has been found to be relatively constant during maturation and similar to that for the adult.[21,37] In these animals the GFR increases as the animal matures; concomitantly, there is a proportional increase in proximal tubular sodium and water load and consequently in reabsorption. Similarly, in the newborn rat, as single-nephron GFR increases with maturation, proximal tubular sodium reabsorption increases proportionately.[38] Although these studies might suggest that the development of tubular sodium reabsorption simply involves a proportional increase in reabsorptive capacity with that of glomerular filtered load, other experiments studying the maturation of the renal response to sodium loading reveal that the

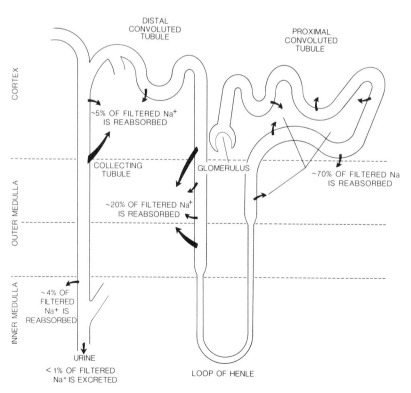

FIGURE 11. A schematic representation of segmental sodium reabsorption in the nephron under normovolemic conditions.

developmental pattern of tubular sodium reabsorption is somewhat more complex.

In normovolemic neonatal dogs when filtered sodium load is increased there is a proportionate increase in proximal tubule sodium reabsorption, so that fractional sodium reabsorption remains relatively constant.[39] However, during extracellular volume expansion when filtered sodium is increased, the increase in proximal tubule sodium reabsorption is not proportionate to the increase in filtered sodium, so that fractional sodium reabsorption decreases (derived from data in reference 40). Thus, there is good proximal tubule glomerular-tubular balance in the normovolemic neonatal dog but this balance is disrupted somewhat during volume expansion. In the volume-expanded adult animal, proximal tubule glomerular-tubular balance, although not perfect, is better preserved than in the newborn dog.

When the adult is given a large sodium load, there is an immediate expansion of the extracellular fluid space. This expansion stimulates the kidney to decrease tubular sodium reabsorption, resulting in increased excretion of sodium and a relatively rapid return of the extracellular fluid space to preload condition. When newborn infants and animals are given a sodium load, they experience a rise in serum sodium concentrations, abnormal increases in weight, and generalized edema.[40] **The poor renal response of the infant to a sodium load is due to its low GFR and its relatively high fractional tubular sodium reabsorption during the sodium loading. The ability to excrete the sodium load increases with age throughout the first year of life.** This maturational increase in sodium excretion is due both to the increase in filtered sodium (due to maturational increase in the GFR) and to an increase in fractional sodium excretion.[42]

Paradoxically, infants born prematurely before 36 weeks' gestation have a better sodium excretory response to sodium loading than do infants born later in gestation.[43] As the premature infant matures over the first few weeks of life, its ability to excrete the sodium load declines rather than improves. **Thus the developing kidney, in the human at least, seems to undergo a parabolic response to sodium loading—a slightly decreasing response with age early in development followed by an increasing response later in development.**

The newborn dog has been used as a model for studying maturation of renal function, since its renal response to sodium loading is similar to that of the newborn infant. Newborn dogs excrete only 5% of a sodium load administered intravenously after 2 hours, compared with 30% excretion of an equivalent load administered to adult dogs.[44] The major reason for the difference in response is that the adult dog excretes 6-8% of the filtered sodium compared with only 1-2% excreted by the puppy (under nonexpanded conditions both adult and newborn dogs excrete about 0.2% of the filtered load). There is a slight fall in the renal response during the second week of life and then a gradual increase as the animal matures (Fig. 12). Thus the maturational pattern in the neonatal dog corresponds to that of the preterm infant. Note that the maturational pattern of tubular response to saline expansion differs from that for intrarenal blood flow distribution (Fig. 3) and GFR (Fig. 5).

Elucidation of the mechanisms involved in maturation of sodium excretion during control and volume-expanded conditions can be obtained from results of experiments analyzing the tubular segmental locus of sodium reabsorption (Fig. 11). For the purpose of this discussion the kidney tubule is divided into two portions, proximal and distal. The proximal portion consists anatomically of the proximal convoluted tubule and the proximal straight

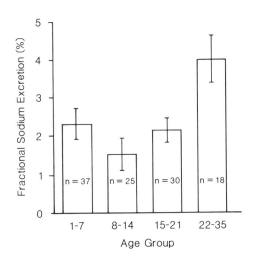

FIGURE 12. Maturation of fractional tubular sodium excretion in saline-expanded newborn dogs. (Based on data from various studies by one of the authors.[39,40,45] From Kleinman LI. The Physiologist 1982;25:104, with permission.)

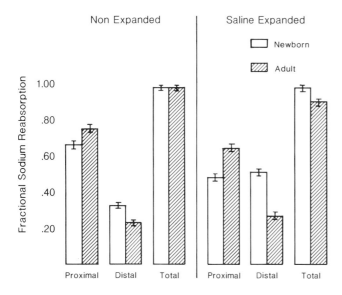

Non Expanded   Saline Expanded

☐ Newborn
▨ Adult

FIGURE 13. Fractional sodium reabsorption in proximal, distal, and total nephron during non-expanded and saline-expanded states in newborn and adult dogs. Means ± standard errors are depicted. During saline expansion, suppression of sodium reabsorption by the proximal nephron is more pronounced in the newborn than in the adult; however, distal sodium reabsorption is enhanced in the newborn but not in the adult. The net result is a higher fractional sodium reabsorption in the newborn than in the adult during saline expansion. (From Kleinman LI, Banks RO. Proc Soc Exp Biol Med 1983;173:231, with permission.)

tubule. The distal nephron consists of Henle's loop, the distal convoluted tubule, and collecting ducts.

Under nonexpanded conditions there are only small differences in the way the adult and newborn dog reabsorb filtered sodium (Fig. 13).[46] Approximately 70-75% of the filtered sodium is reabsorbed proximally while 20-25% is reabsorbed distally for a total reabsorption of greater than 99% of the filtered sodium. During saline expansion in the adult, proximal sodium reabsorption falls to about 60%, distal reabsorption changes little, and total reabsorption is about 92-94%, i.e., 6-8% of the filtered sodium is excreted. In the neonatal kidney, saline expansion results in a fall of proximal sodium reabsorption to less than 50%—a greater inhibition of sodium reabsorption than in the adult. However, the distal nephron reabsorbs more sodium than in the adult, so that in the end, a total of 98% of the filtered sodium is reabsorbed—greater than in the mature kidney. The major portion of this increased distal sodium reabsorption probably occurs in the loop of Henle.[46]

Of particular interest are the findings in the proximal nephron in the dog. Without saline expansion fractional sodium reabsorption is about the same in the adult and neonatal proximal tubule, but during saline expansion fractional sodium reabsorption is less in the neonatal proximal tubule. These findings may be explained in terms of mechanisms of proximal tubule sodium reabsorption that include active sodium reabsorption, passive sodium reab-

sorption, and some degree of "back leak" into the tubular lumen across the intercellular "tight" junction (Fig. 14). Back leak across the tight junction is enhanced during volume expansion. **There is ultrastructural evidence of a "less tight" intercellular junction in the immature kidney.**[47] In addition, microperfusion studies of proximal tubules of neonatal rabbits reveal increased leakiness compared with more mature tubules,[48] and distal blockade studies reveal the proximal nephron of the newborn dog to be more susceptible to an osmotic diuresis than the adult.[49] Moreover, when renal perfusion pressure is increased there is greater inhibition of proximal tubule sodium reabsorption in the neonatal than in the adult kidney.[40] These studies are consistent with the hypothesis that there is greater propensity for back leak in the neonatal proximal tubule.

Another possible explanation for the lower proximal tubule sodium reabsorption capacity during saline loading in the neonatal kidney is that the immature tubule may not be able to generate enough energy (weak sodium pump) to transport sodium against transtubular sodium gradients that are higher than baseline. Support for this hypothesis can be found in the study[38] in which the absolute rate of sodium transport was found to be less in the immature than in the mature proximal tubule of the rat, in the study that demonstrated that the proximal tubule of the newborn dog was unable to generate a transtubular sodium gradient as great as that of the adult,[49] and finally in the

TUBULAR
LUMEN

PROXIMAL TUBULE
CELLS

PERITUBULAR
CAPILLARY

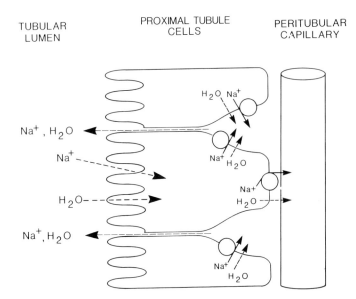

FIGURE 14. Diagrammatic representation of sodium transport in the proximal tubule. Solid arrows represent active transport and dashed arrows represent passive diffusion. Water reabsorption occurs iso-osmotically as a consequence of sodium reabsorption.

finding of lower Na-K-ATPase activity (believed to be responsible for the sodium pump) in
the immature than in the mature proximal
tubule of the rabbit kidney.[50]

Both the back leak and weak pump hypotheses explain the finding that under non-
expanded conditions, when there is minimal
back leak and strain on the sodium pump,
there is little or no difference in proximal
tubular sodium reabsorption between mature
and immature kidneys. However, during extracellular volume expansion, which would enhance back leak and stress the sodium pump,
proximal sodium reabsorption is less in the immature than in the mature kidney.

A model of the maturational response to
saline expansion is presented in Figures 15
and 16. In the proximal tubule (Fig. 15) sodium load is continuously increasing during
development due to the increase in GFR. Proximal tubule sodium reabsorption is also increasing (due both to an increase in active
transport capacity and to a decrease in back
leak). However, *sodium reabsorption is increasing at a greater rate than the sodium
load,* so that the proximal sodium reabsorption

PROXIMAL NEPHRON

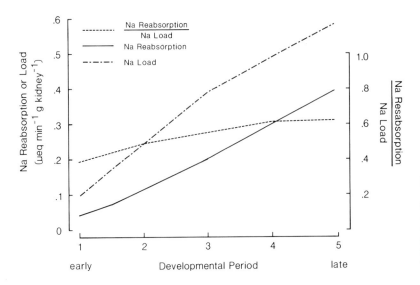

FIGURE 15. Maturational
pattern of *proximal* sodium
handling during saline expansion. Developmental periods
are arbitrary and do not necessarily correspond to those
described in Table 1. (From
Kleinman LI. The Physiologist
1982;25:104, with permission.)

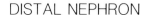

DISTAL NEPHRON

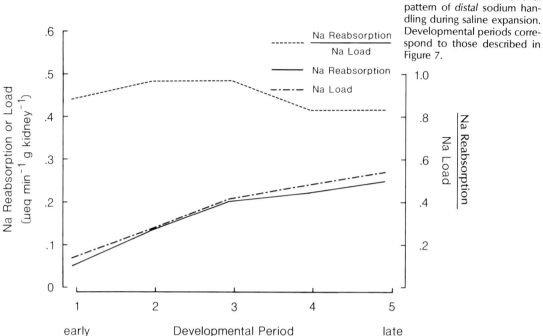

FIGURE 16. Maturational pattern of *distal* sodium handling during saline expansion. Developmental periods correspond to those described in Figure 7.

divided by filtered load (fractional sodium reabsorption in the proximal tubule) continues to increase throughout periods 1 to 4. If the developmental increase in fractional sodium reabsorption during volume expansion is due largely to diminishing back leak or strengthening sodium pump, then it would not be apparent during nonexpansion and it would explain the finding of similar proximal fractional sodium reabsorption in newborn and adult animals during nonexpansion.

In the distal nephron, sodium load (the amount of sodium not reabsorbed proximally) increases throughout the developmental period (Fig. 16) due to the increase in GFR, but it does not increase as much as the increase in load to the proximal tubule because of the maturational rise in proximal tubular sodium reabsorption. Distal sodium reabsorption increases continuously but at different rates than distal sodium loads. Thus from periods 1 to 2 the rate of increase of sodium reabsorption is greater than the rate of increase of distal sodium load, so that the ratio of sodium reabsorption to load (distal fractional sodium reabsorption) is increasing during this period. Since proximal fractional sodium reabsorption is also increasing (Fig. 15), overall fractional sodium reabsorption is increasing and fractional sodium excretion is decreasing during this period. This would correspond to the

developmental pattern in the preterm infant when overall fractional sodium excretion is decreasing.

During the next developmental period the rate of increase of distal sodium load equals that of distal sodium reabsorption, so there is no change in the ratio. From the developmental periods 3 to 4 the rate of increase in distal sodium reabsorption is less than that of the sodium load, so that the ratio decreases to the mature level. However, this ratio falls at a greater rate than proximal fractional sodium reabsorption is increasing, so that overall fractional reabsorption decreases. This period corresponds to the maturational decrease in overall fractional sodium reabsorption seen in most animals.

Support for this model in human infants is provided by clinical studies that have shown that water-loaded premature infants (less than 35 weeks' conceptual age) have lower proximal fractional sodium reabsorption, increased distal nephron fractional sodium reabsorption, and overall greater fractional sodium excretion than infants greater than 35 weeks' conceptual age.[51] Furthermore, this model of development of proximal and distal sodium reabsorption capacity described above provides an explanation for the parabolic change in renal response to saline expansion in the human neonate and still allows for a continuous matu-

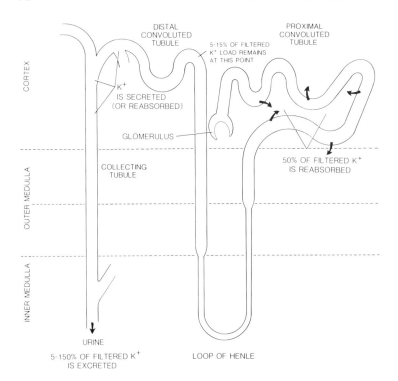

FIGURE 17. A simplified schematic representation of the renal processes involved in potassium excretion.

rational increase in reabsorptive capacity for both proximal and distal tubules.

EXCRETION OF POTASSIUM BY THE PERINATAL KIDNEY

Potassium is freely filterable at the glomerulus. There is substantial reabsorption of potassium in the proximal convoluted and straight tubules and in the thick ascending limb of the loop of Henle. Over a wide range of potassium intake approximately 50% of the filtered potassium load remains at the end of the proximal convoluted tubule and approximately 10% at the beginning of the distal tubule. As a result, a remarkably constant 5-15% of the filtered load is delivered to the early distal tubule, largely independent of intake. **Net potassium secretion occurs in the late distal tubule and cortical collecting tubule under most circumstances**.[52] It is these nephron segments that primarily regulate urinary potassium excretion under a variety of peritubular and luminal influences. A variable, relatively small amount of potassium reabsorption occurs along the length of the medullary collecting duct (Fig. 17).

Figure 18 is a schematic representation of the essential components of the cellular transport system for potassium in the late distal and cortical collecting tubules. The main elements of this system are (1) the peritubular

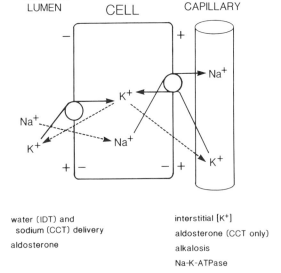

FIGURE 18. Cell schema of the essential components of potassium and sodium transport system in the late distal tubule (IDT). Solid arrows indicate active transport and dashed arrows indicate passive diffusion. Factors that increase net potassium flux across the basolateral membrane into the cell are listed at the lower right. Factors that increase net potassium flux across the luminal membrane into the tubular lumen are listed at the lower left. The situation in the cortical collecting tubule (CCT) is similar.

(basolateral) membrane sodium-potassium exchange pump, (2) relatively high intracellular potassium activity, (3) movement of potassium from cell to lumen across a permeable luminal membrane driven by a favorable concentration gradient and opposed by a small cell negative voltage, and (4) a potassium-accumulating pump in the luminal membrane.[52] The balance between the latter and the electrochemical potential difference for potassium ions across the luminal membrane determine the net secretory rate across the luminal membrane. Entry of sodium into tubular cells across the luminal membrane is necessary for cation exchange at the peritubular surface.

Factors that stimulate potassium secretion in the late distal and cortical collecting tubules, and thereby urinary potassium excretion, do so by increasing intracellular potassium activity or net potassium flux across the luminal membrane of cells in these segments (Fig. 18). Increases in extracellular potassium concentration,[54,55] pH,[56,57] aldosterone concentration,[54] and basolateral membrane Na-K-ATPase activity[58] increase uptake of potassium across the basolateral membrane and, as a result, increase intracellular potassium activity. Increases in sodium and water delivery increase the flux of potassium from cell to lumen across the apical membrane of cells in the late distal tubule and cortical collecting tubules.[59,60] Aldosterone increases luminal membrane permeability to sodium and potassium.[61] Decreases in these factors inhibit potassium secretion in these nephron segments.

Potassium is handled in a qualitatively similar manner by the immature kidney. With usual or high potassium intakes, more than 80% of the filtered load is reabsorbed in the proximal tubule and loop of Henle. **The bulk of urinary potassium excretion is the result of tubular secretion.**[62,63]

There is little information available concerning the relative ability of the newborn to respond to pertubations in potassium homeostasis. There is evidence that even preterm newborns can increase potassium secretion in response to appropriate stimuli.[64] Animal studies, however, indicate that the newborn cannot excrete excess potassium as readily as the adult.[63] This is the result of a limited secretory capacity of immature late distal and cortical collecting tubules. Possibilities that could contribute to the limited secretory capacity of the immature distal nephron include low Na-K-ATPase activity in late distal and cortical

collecting tubules,[50] lower responsiveness to aldosterone,[65] low water and sodium delivery as a result of low GFR[63] and low tubular surface area or low luminal membrane permeability to potassium (no data available).

EXCRETION AND CONSERVATION OF WATER IN THE PERINATAL KIDNEY

Although the concentration of solutes in human plasma is held fairly constant at about 300 mOsm/L, the concentration of solutes in the urine of an adult human varies from 50–1500 mOsm/L depending on the amount of water intake.

All mammalian fetuses studied excrete urine hypotonic to plasma. The fetal lamb at 81-93 days' gestation excretes urine that has a solute concentration of 239 mOsm/L, and the urine becomes progressively more dilute with gestation, so that at 130-142 days, urinary solute concentration has fallen to 166 mOsm/L.[66] Interestingly enough, while the urine is becoming more and more dilute, the urinary urea concentration is increasing.

The infant of a few days of age is not able to excrete a water load as well as can an adult. Infants given a water load of 3% of their body weight excreted only 10% of the load in the first 3 hours, whereas an adult excreted all of it during this time.[67] Infants of 6-18 days excreted 57% of a water load equal to 5% of body weight, compared with an adult who excreted 100% of an equivalent water load in that time.[68] The ability to respond to a water load improves rapidly during the first few weeks of life, reaching adult capabilities by 1 month of age.[67]

Newborn animals also have a limited renal response to water loading. Newborn dogs given a water load of 5% of their body weight excreted only 56% of the dose in 4 hours, compared with an 85% excretion of similar dose in the adult. In addition, maximum urine flow rate per unit body weight in the puppies was only 65% of that in adults.[69]

The ability to excrete a water load is a function of the amount of water presented to the diluting segment (ascending limb of the loop of Henle and early distal convoluted tubule) and the ability of this segment to dilute the urine (Fig. 19). The amount of water presented to the diluting segment is a function of the GFR and of proximal tubular water reabsorption.

Diluting ability, in turn, is a function of the ability of the ascending limb of the loop of Henle to transport sodium chloride against a

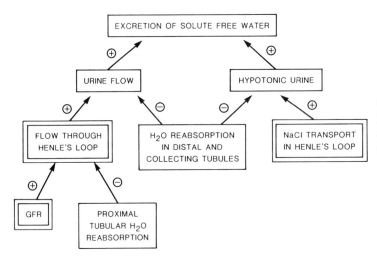

FIGURE 19. Scheme of factors that affect the excretion of solute free water. (+) Indicates that an increase in the causal factor will produce an increase in the resultant factor; (−) indicates that an increase in the causal factor will produce a decrease in the resultant factor; a double box indicates a factor found to contribute to the decreased ability of the perinatal kidney to respond to a water load.

concentration gradient and the ability of the distal convoluted tubule and the collecting duct to remain impermeable to water. Newborn infants can dilute their urine to the same degree as can adults (to 50 mOsm/L).[68,70] The reason for the poor response of the newborn animal to a water load is therefore likely to be the decreased load presented to the diluting segment; this decrease, in turn, is most likely due to the low GFR.

The newborn animal and infant are not as capable of responding to dehydration or hypertonic solute loading by excreting as con-

centrated a urine as the adult.[71-73] An adult man normally excretes a urine of about 800-1000 mOsm/L, and is able to increase the concentration of solutes to 1400 mOsm/L under conditions of dehydration. *A newborn infant usually excretes urine hypotonic to plasma, and can concentrate the urine to only 600-700 mOsm/L under conditions of water deprivation.*

The ability to produce a concentrated urine is a function of the ability to produce and maintain a solute concentration gradient in the interstitial fluid of the kidney from the inner

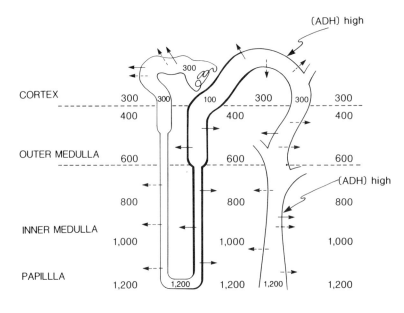

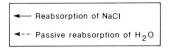

FIGURE 20. Schematic representation of the renal countercurrent system under conditions of antidiuresis. Nephron segments depicted with heavy lines indicate very low permeability to water. The permeability of the late distal tubule and collecting duct is ADH-dependent. In the presence of ADH, these nephron segments are permeable to water. The numbers refer to osmolality (mOsm/kg H_2O) of tubular or interstitial fluid. (From Valtin H. Renal Function: Mechanisms of Conserving Water and Solute Balance in Health, 2nd ed. Boston, Little, Brown and Co., 1983, with permission.)

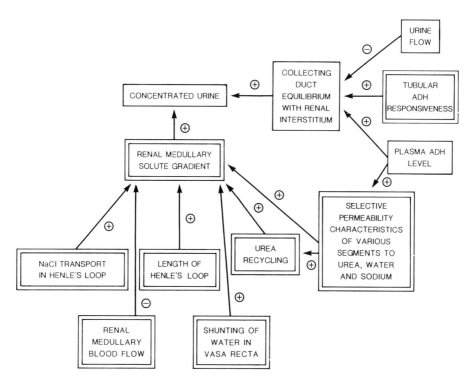

FIGURE 21. Scheme of factors that affect the ability of the kidney to concentrate the urine. (+) indicates that an increase in the causal factor will produce an increase in the resultant factor; (−) indicates that an increase in the causal factor will produce a decrease in the resultant factor; a double box indicates a factor that may contribute to the poor concentrating ability in the perinatal kidney.

medulla to the corticomedullary junction, and also of the ability of fluid within the collecting duct to equilibrate with the interstitial fluid of the medullary region (Figs. 20, 21). The ability to produce the renal medullary interstitial solute gradient is a function of: (1) the ability of the thick portion of the ascending limb of the loop of Henle to transport sodium chloride; (2) the length of the loops of Henle; (3) the selective permeability characteristics of the various segments of the loops of Henle to sodium, chloride, water, and urea; and (4) the amount of urea presented to the medullary portion of the kidney. The ability of the kidney to maintain the medullary solute gradient is a function of the blood flow to the renal medulla and the degree to which water in the medullary vasculature is shunted from descending to ascending limbs of the vasa recta. The vasa recta are postglomerular vascular loops that descend in bundles to various depths in the inner medulla in association with the ascending limbs of Henle and collecting ducts. The more water is shunted from descending to ascending limbs of the vasa recta, the less water reaches the deep medullary tissue to dissipate the solute gradient.

The ability of the collecting duct to equilibrate with the interstitial fluid of the renal medulla is a function of the amount of antidiuretic hormone (ADH) present, the ability of the collecting duct to respond to ADH, and the amount of urine flow in the collecting duct.

The major reason an immature animal cannot excrete urine as concentrated as that of an adult is that the kidneys of newborn animals have smaller medullary solute gradients than do those of adult animals.[75-77] There is an increase in the medullary sodium gradient and a much larger increase in the urea gradient as the animal matures. The major reasons for the changing medullary solute gradient in the developing kidney is the increase in active sodium chloride transport by the thick ascending limb of Henle's loop[78,79] and the changing anatomic pattern of the loops of Henle dipping into the deep portions of the medulla with maturation.[2,71,80] A recent computer-simulated study[78] indicated that maturation of these two factors could account not only for the maturational change in the sodium chloride gradient but also for the much larger change in the urea gradient.

Other reasons for the initially low urea gradient in the immature kidney may include the low renal excretion of urea (due primarily to the positive nitrogen balance in maturing animals) and the anatomic immaturity of the loop of Henle, which might retard cycling of the urea in the medulla.[71,77] **Infants on high-protein diets or urea supplements can concentrate their urine to a greater degree than can infants on low-protein diets,**[81,82] further emphasizing the importance of renal delivery of urea to the concentrating mechanisms in maturing animals. Newborn infants on high-protein or urea diets and newborn animals receiving urea loads, however, cannot increase the concentration of urinary nonurea solutes[77,81] as can adult animals.[83] Moreover, urea loads given to immature animals do not produce increases in the renal medullary solute gradient (for either urea or nonurea solutes) as they do in more mature animals.[77] These findings support the concept of the immaturity of the medullary urea-cycling mechanism.

Other factors that may contribute to the relatively small medullary solute gradient in the immature kidney include the relatively high fractional blood flow to the medullary region of the kidney of the developing animal,[84-86] which may increase the dissipation of the solute gradient, and the anatomical immaturity of the vasa recta, which may retard countercurrent water recycling.[77]

Earlier studies using insensitive bioassay suggested that serum ADH concentrations were lower in immature than in mature animals; however, more recent studies using radioimmunoassay techniques have demonstrated that fetal and neonatal animals are capable of attaining very high circulating levels of ADH.[87-89] There is some question, however, of the ability of the immature kidney to respond to ADH. Although the lower medullary solute gradient can account for the lower maximal concentrating ability with ADH in the immature than in the mature kidney, water conductivity and cyclic AMP response to ADH has been shown to increase with development.[78,79,90] On the other hand, there is evidence of adequate equilibration between collecting duct and medullary interstitium in neonatal dogs,[37] which would indicate that response to ADH is adequate.

Differences in urinary solute concentration between perinatal and adult animals largely reflect their different needs. Adult mammals usually excrete a concentrated urine, since there is need to conserve free water (water without solutes). They usually have a low intake of water and, in addition, they excrete free water through the skin and lungs. The fetus, of course, does not excrete free water through its skin or through its lungs. Ingestion of hypotonic amniotic fluid requires excretion of hypotonic urine; this the fetal kidneys are apparently well designed to do. The newborn animal subsists largely on a hypotonic liquid intake, and it too needs to excrete a dilute urine. As the newborn animal matures and as nitrogen excretion (in the form of urea) increases, the capacity to concentrate urine improves. During the period of low urea output, however, the kidneys are unable to maximally concentrate urine, and are consequently unable to conserve free water. **Under conditions of water deprivation or hypertonic solute loading, the neonatal animal is thus extremely prone to hypertonic dehydration.**

Furthermore, the limited concentrating ability of the newborn limits renal solute excretion and consequently limits the amount of solute able to be infused (including urea-generating protein) with any given volume of free water (Fig. 22). For example, in a neonate with a maximum concentrating ability of 400 mOsm/L and a renal solute load of 20 mOsm/kg/day, the infant will need to excrete at least 50 ml/kg/day of urine to prevent plasma hypertonicity. Thus, enough fluid must be infused to generate this amount of urine as well as water for insensible water losses. If fluid were infused

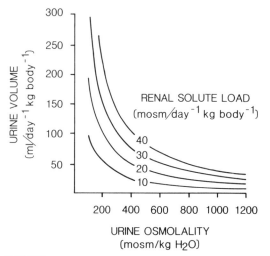

FIGURE 22.   Graphic representation of the relationships among urine volume, urine osmolality, and renal solute load.

at a rate that could generate only 25 ml/kg/day of urine, then only 10 mOsm/kg/day of solute could be excreted (Fig. 22). In an adult who is able to concentrate the urine to 1000 mOsm/L, only 20 ml/kg/day of urine need to be excreted to excrete 20 mOsm/kg/day of solute.

ACID EXCRETION BY THE PERINATAL KIDNEY

Normally, the average human adult produces approximately 13,000 mEq of acid (hydrogen ions) per day. Most of this acid is produced from tissue respiration in the form of carbon dioxide or carbonic acid. The nonrespiratory acid production, usually derived from metabolism of ingested food, amounts to only 30-100 mEq of hydrogen ions per day, depending, of course, on the diet and metabolic state of the individual. During steady state, all the acid produced is excreted. The respiratory acid is excreted by the lungs and the nonrespiratory acid by the kidneys.

The kidney assists in the maintenance of body acid-base homeostasis in two fundamental ways: (1) it regulates extracellular bicarbonate ion concentration and (2) it excretes the nonrespiratory acid produced by metabolism. Both of these mechanisms involve active secretion of hydrogen ions into the tubular lumen.

Under normal circumstances, all filtered bicarbonate is reabsorbed by the tubules, about 90% proximally and the rest in the distal convoluted tubule and collecting duct. Under certain circumstances, the load presented to the tubules may be too large, and bicarbonate will consequently be excreted in the urine.

There is general agreement that at least some, if not all, of the bicarbonate ions are reabsorbed as a consequence of the active secretion of hydrogen ions by the tubules. Bicarbonate reabsorption via the hydrogen secretory mechanism occurs in the following manner (Fig. 23). Within the tubular cell, CO_2 is converted to hydrogen and bicarbonate ions. This reaction is accelerated by the enzyme *carbonic anhydrase*. The hydrogen ion is actively pumped out of the cell into the tubular lumen in exchange for sodium. Once in the tubular lumen, the hydrogen ion combines with the bicarbonate to form CO_2, which then diffuses back into the cell. In the cell, the CO_2 is converted to hydrogen and bicarbonate ions. The bicarbonate ion diffuses into the peritubular blood, and the hydrogen ion is resecreted into the tubular lumen. The net effect, therefore, is the reabsorption of bicarbonate.

In the proximal tubule, along the brush border, there is carbonic anhydrase, so that the production of CO_2 from the hydrogen and bicarbonate ions is accelerated in the tubular lumen. This acceleration permits a rapid lowering of the hydrogen ion concentration in the tubular lumen toward its equilibrium concentration. Consequently, the pH of proximal tubular fluid is lowered only slightly (to approximately 7.0), and the active transport of hydrogen ions from cell to lumen occurs against only a small concentration gradient, resulting in more efficient hydrogen ion secretion and

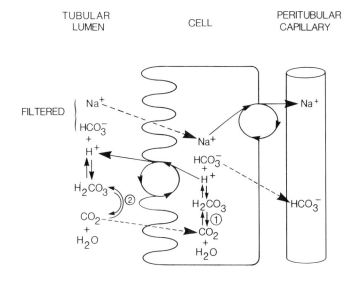

TUBULAR LUMEN   CELL   PERITUBULAR CAPILLARY

FIGURE 23. Diagrammatic representation of bicarbonate reabsorption and hydrogen secretion in the renal tubule. Solid arrows indicate active transport and dashed arrows indicate passive diffusion. Note that the net effect of this process is the transport of sodium and bicarbonate from tubular lumen to peritubular capillary. In the proximal and distal tubules, intracellular carbonic anhydrase increases reaction rate 1 in the proximal tubule; intraluminal brush border carbonic anhydrase increases reaction rate 2. In the absence of intraluminal carbonic anhydrase, the dehydration of carbonic acid is slowed, and the intraluminal hydrogen ion concentration increases.

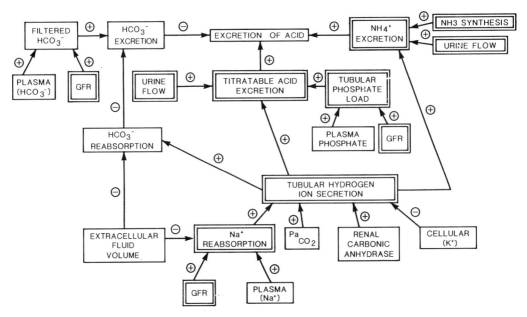

FIGURE 24. Scheme of factors that affect bicarbonate reabsorption and the excretion of acid. (+) Indicates that an increase in the causal factor will produce an increase in the resultant factor; (−) indicates that an increase in the causal factor will produce a decrease in the resultant factor; a double box indicates a factor that mat contribute to the decreased ability of the perinatal kidney to respond to an acid load. Renal carbonic anhydrase is low in the perinatal kidney, but the significance of this lower enzyme activity with respect to the decreased hydrogen ion secretion in the perinatal kidney is questionable.

bicarbonate reabsorption. There is no evidence of intraluminal carbonic anhydrase in the distal hydrogen secreting sites, although there is ample activity of this enzyme within the cells at this locus.

Bicarbonate reabsorption can be influenced by the following factors (Fig. 24): (1) GFR—increases in GFR result in increases in bicarbonate reabsorption; (2) arterial P_{CO_2}—increases in P_{aCO_2} result in increases in bicarbonate reabsorption; (3) body potassium—decreases in body potassium result in increases in bicarbonate reabsorption; (4) activity of renal carbonic anhydrase—substantial decreases in carbonic anhydrase activity decrease bicarbonate reabsorption; (5) extracellular fluid volume—increases in extracellular fluid volume decrease bicarbonate reabsorption; and (6) sodium reabsorption—increases in sodium reabsorption result in increases in bicarbonate reabsorption.

Acid is excreted by the kidney as free hydrogen ions and hydrogen bound to certain buffers in the urine. There are two classes of urinary buffers: (1) those filtered by the glomerulus, the most important being phosphate,

and (2) the buffer produced by the tubular cells, ammonia. The amount of acid excreted as free hydrogen ion plus the hydrogen bound to the filtered buffers is known as the *titratable acid*, since it is measured by titrating the urine back to a pH of 7.4. *Net renal acid excretion* is the acid excreted as urinary titratable acid plus urinary ammonium minus urinary bicarbonate excretion.

The maximum amount of acid that can be excreted by the kidney is limited by the maximum gradient for hydrogen ions that can be maintained between the tubular lumen and the tubular cell and the amount of buffer present in the urine. In adult man, the maximum urine : blood free hydrogen ion gradient is about 1000:1, which means that the kidney of man can lower its urinary pH to about 4.4. If the kidney had to excrete all its hydrogen ions in the free ionic form, then the normal kidney would be able to excrete less than 1% of the body's normal nonrespiratory acid production. Therefore, practically all the hydrogen excreted by the kidney must be buffered.

The basic cellular mechanisms involved in acid excretion are essentially the same as those for bicarbonate reabsorption (Fig. 25). Hydrogen ions are actively secreted into the tubular lumen. Those ions not utilized for

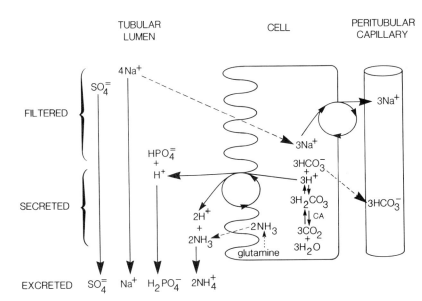

FIGURE 25. Diagrammatic representation of the formation of titratable acidity (in this case as $H_2PO_4^-$) and ammonium in the renal tubule. The excretion of $SO_4^=$ with $2NH_4^=$ is shown here to indicate how filtered Na_2SO_4 (which is derived from buffering of H_2SO_4 in the body) is handled.

bicarbonate reabsorption are then buffered by one of the two classes of buffers. The amount of hydrogen ions excreted is therefore related to the amount of bicarbonate remaining in the tubules. At the end of the proximal tubule, approximately 10% of the filtered bicarbonate remains unreabsorbed, and the pH of the tubular fluid is about 7.0. The free hydrogen ions in this segment are buffered by the filtered buffer with a relatively high pK, phosphate, and the renal buffer ammonia.

In the distal acid-secreting sites, the remainder of the bicarbonate ions are usually reabsorbed, and the urine is acidified to a degree dependent on the excess of free hydrogen ions secreted up to the production of a urine with a minimum pH of 4.4. The hydrogen ions here are buffered primarily by ammonia and the filtered buffers with a low pK such as creatinine and beta-hydroxybutyrate. Under conditions of high bicarbonate filtered loads or decreased tubular reabsorption of bicarbonate or both, less acid will be excreted. Indeed, if there is significant excretion of bicarbonate, then the pH of the urine will rise to values above that of blood, and there will be a net excretion of base, not acid. **Under conditions of decreased renal phosphate load or decreased synthesis of ammonia, net acid excretion will be impaired.**

The fetus is capable of acidifying its urine. In the fetal pig, the pH of the allantoic fluid (consisting primarily of urine) decreases progressively from 7.0 at 22 days' gestation to 5.8 at 90 days'. Titratable acidity and ammonia con-

centration of this fluid both increase progressively during this period.[91] The human infant is born with a bladder filled with a urine at a pH of about 6.3.[92] Although the fetus is clearly capable of excreting an acid urine, its renal acidifying capacity, estimated by measuring response to acid loading, is not as efficient as that of the adult.

When fetal lambs were infused with small to moderate amounts of hydrochloric acid, there was little change in urine pH and total acid excretion.[93] With infusion of larger amounts of hydrochloric acid, there was a greater fall in urine pH (to about 5.8) and a significant increase in urinary titratable acidity and ammonia concentration, but not to the same degree as obtained in adults.[93,94] Similar results were obtained from a study in which lactic acid was infused over a 90-min period into in situ fetal lambs.[95] Blood pH fell to 7.13 during the infusion, but urinary pH fell no lower than 6.25, and net acid excretion by the kidney over a 3-hour period following initiation of the acid infusion amounted to only a small fraction of the acid load. Although much of the infused acid must have been excreted by extrarenal mechanisms (the rise in extracellular pH and buffer base during the recovery period could not be accounted for by renal excretion of acid), the small amount of renal acid excretion accompanied by depression of extracellular pH during the acid infusion indicates that a relative inefficiency of one or more of the mechanisms of renal acid secretion exists in the fetus.

The newborn animal and infant are also unable to adequately excrete an imposed acid load.[93,96-103] In the human neonate, the more prematurely born infants respond less well than do more mature infants to acid loading.[101,103] The ability to excrete acid in the newborn human improves rapidly over the first few weeks of life. **By one month of age, the infant can excrete as much hydrogen ion on acid loading as can the older child.**[104] Low total acid excretion in the face of an acid load in the newborn is the result of low titratable acid excretion, low ammonia excretion, and in some species a relatively high minimum urinary pH.

Factors that affect the renal excretion of acid are schematized in Figure 24, and the following discussion will be presented from the perspective of the relevance of these factors to perinatal acid excretion. The relatively poor ability of the perinatal kidney to excrete an imposed acid load could be due to the inadequate excretion of urinary buffers and/or to limited ability of its tubules to secrete hydrogen ions against a large concentration gradient (i.e., generate a low urinary pH). **There is good evidence that the relatively poor ability of the perinatal kidney to respond to acid loading is related to inadequate excretion of urinary buffers.** The amount of filtered buffers presented to the tubules depends on the glomerular filtration rate, which is low in the perinatal kidney. In addition, the amount of phosphate presented to the tubules is also related to the amount of phosphate ingested. In the human infant before feeding commences, only 10-25% of the acid is excreted as titratable acid.[92] In babies fed cow milk, a diet containing large amounts of phosphate, total acid excretion is high and 60% of the urinary acid is titratable acid. In breastfed babies, both total acid excretion and the proportion of acid excreted as titratable acid are lower.[91] Total acid excretion is lower in these babies because the lower protein content of human milk decreases the metabolic production of acid, and the lower phosphate content of this milk decreases the titratable acid excretion.

When one-week-old infants were given an acid load of ammonium or calcium chloride, they were not able to excrete as much titratable acid or ammonia as were adults. Babies loaded with phosphate before the acid load demonstrated a marked increase in urinary titratable acidity and excreted 2.5 times as much acid in 8 hours as did infants not receiving phosphate.[98,100] That low phosphate excretion is not the complete explanation for the poor

response of the newborn infant to acid loading can be deduced from the finding that adults excreted twice as much as acid as did the phosphate-loaded infants.

Inadequate excretion of ammonium also plays an important role in the inability of the perinatal kidney to excrete an acid load (Fig. 24). All studies reveal a lower excretion of ammonium on acid loading in the immature than in the mature kidney. As mentioned previously, the ability of the tubular cells to secrete ammonia will depend on the ability of the kidney to synthesize ammonia and on the amount of free hydrogen ions present in the tubular lumen to trap the ammonia. One reason for the low ammonia secretion is the relatively high urinary pH of most acid-loaded perinatal animals. However, since ammonium excretion is also diminished in cases of good urinary acidification,[96] the low ammonium excretion must be related to decreased synthesis by renal tubular cells.

In favor of the hypothesis that the imparied response of the perinatal kidney to acid loading results from a limited ability to secrete hydrogen ions against a concentration gradient is the finding that, in most species, minimum urinary pH in perinatal animals is much higher than in the adult. This finding does not apply to all species under all conditions, however. The newborn dog, for example, is capable of lowering its urinary pH to 4.8,[96] a value approaching that of the adult. Moreover, when fetal lambs were infused with sodium sulfate, which resulted in increased delivery of sodium to distal hydrogen ion secreting nephron segments, and consequently in an enhancement of tubular sodium-hydrogen exchange, the urinary pH was lowered to a minimum of 4.7 and urinary titratable acidity and ammonium concentration were significantly enhanced.[105] These findings suggest that if the tubular cells of the perinatal kidney were presented with sufficient sodium ions for exchange with hydrogen, then they might be able to acidify the urine to the same or almost the same extent as the adult kidney. Further support for the hypothesis that poor response of the perinatal kidney to acid loading may be related to a limited tubular sodium-hydrogen exchange is the finding that in newborn infants, as the ability to excrete hydrogen ions increases with maturation, urinary sodium excretion decreases.[101]

Theoretically, deficient renal tubular carbonic anhydrase enzyme activity could impair the active secretion of hydrogen ions. Carbonic anhydrase activity is lower in the perinatal than in the adult kidney.[106] This lower enzyme activity may not contribute to the lower hydrogen ion secretion, however, since carbonic anhydrase activity may have to be decreased to levels much lower than those found in the perinatal animal before hydrogen ion secretion will be affected.[106] Moreover, inhibition of carbonic anhydrase results in significant urinary excretion of bicarbonate in fetal lambs[107] and neonatal dogs,[108] indicating that this enzyme is quite active in the kidney during the perinatal period.

Although hydrogen ion secretion appears to be limited in the perinatal kidney as the result of low reabsorption of exchangeable sodium ions, **there is no evidence that the bicarbonate reabsorptive capacity of the perinatal kidney is limited**. This may seem contradictory since renal tubular bicarbonate reabsorption is largely dependent upon active hydrogen ion secretion by renal tubular cells. However, hydrogen ion secretion must effect reabsorption of nearly all filtered bicarbonate before there can be any net acid secretion in the form of titratable acidity or ammonium and before urine pH is lowered. Thus, a modest limitation of hydrogen ion secretion may not affect bicarbonate reabsorption, but may have a pronounced effect on net acid excretion and the production of a maximally acid urine.

The plasma threshold for bicarbonate has been found to be lower in the newborn dog and human than in the adult of the species.[109,110] However, caution must be given to the utilization of plasma bicarbonate threshold as an index of bicarbonate reabsorptive capacity. Plasma threshold is a function not only of reabsorptive capacity, but also depends, as we have seen for glucose, on the degree of nephron heterogeneity. The large degree of nephron heterogeneity in the perinatal kidney would itself result in a low plasma threshold for bicarbonate.

Moreover, techniques used to measure threshold also influence the extracellular volume of the animal, which in turn influences bicarbonate reabsorption and consequently plasma threshold for bicarbonate. In newborn dogs, when extracellular volume expansion was kept at a minimum during threshold studies,[111] the plasma threshold for bicarbonate was 25 mmol/L compared with 18 mmol/L under standard experimental conditions where extracellular volume was increased.[109] Similarly, volume contraction raised the plasma threshold for bicarbonate excretion in fetal lambs.[112] Indeed, when extracellular volume was kept constant in neonatal dogs, as renal loads of bicarbonate were increased, renal tubular bicarbonate reabsorption increased to levels as high as 50 mmol/L GFR, a level more than double the baseline and equal to more than 98% of the renal tubular load of bicarbonate.[111] Thus, there is no evidence for any limitation in bicarbonate reabsorption capacity by the immature kidney.

In summary, **the kidney of the perinatal animal is well capable of handling the normal acid loads presented to the fetus and the newborn**. Hydrogen ion secretion is sufficiently effective to reabsorb all the bicarbonate filtered and to permit excretion of the normal metabolic acid production. Phosphate is filtered and ammonia is synthesized in amounts adequate to buffer hydrogen ion secretion, so that the acid may be excreted without taxing the secretory capacity of the tubular cells. **Under conditions of excessive acid load, however, the perinatal kidney cannot maintain acid-base homeostasis**. The tubules secrete enough hydrogen ions to reabsorb bicarbonate but they may not be able to secrete sufficient hydrogen ions as excretable acid because there is insufficient sodium available for exchange. In addition, there may not be sufficient phosphate filtered or ammonia synthesized to buffer the hydrogen ions that are secreted.

ACUTE PHASES OF RENAL ADAPTATION IN EXTRAUTERINE LIFE

In the majority of infants in the immediate postnatal period, acute changes in renal function are superimposed upon the more gradual maturational changes in renal function that have been the focus of most of this chapter. Although the primary physiologic mechanism(s) of these changes are unknown, they seem to be related to factors associated with the birth process itself rather than to maturation, since they occur after birth at a wide range of gestational ages. These changes are of particular importance for the clinician, since they have relevance to fluid and electrolyte management in infants in the first week of life (see Chapter 20).

Three phases of renal adaptation to extrauterine existence can be distinguished in the first week of life as summarized in Table 2.[113] Although these phases are based on observations in preterm infants, it is likely that they

TABLE 2.   Postnatal Phases of Water and Sodium Homeostasis

	PHASE I	PHASE II	PHASE III
Age	birth–36 hr	12–96 hr	after 2–4 days
Renal function	GFR is low	GFR increases abruptly	GFR decreases slightly, then continues to slowly increase with maturation
	FENa is low	FENa increases	FENa slowly decreases
Urinary output	Minimal regardless of intake—ability to excrete water and Na is most limited	Diuresis/natriuresis occurs independent of intake	Excretion of water and Na varies appropriately with intake
Balance	Water and Na balance remain unchanged on restricted intake	Water and Na balance become negative regardless of intake	Water and Na balance stabilize and then become positive with growth

*Time course is variable among infants and may be altered by disease. FENa = fractional excretion of sodium.

apply qualitatively to full term infants as well. During the first 12 to 36 hours of life, urine output is low (1–2 ml/kg/hr) and hypotonic to plasma. Glomerular filtration rate and fractional excretion of sodium are low. Urine flow rate during this phase is substantially lower than that reported in fetuses of corresponding gestational ages.[114,115] Studies in fetal and newborn lambs[116,117] suggest that a marked decrease in fractional sodium excretion may contribute significantly to this sharp fall in urine output. Whether or not the low GFR during this phase represents depression from prenatal values is not known. In any case, the combination of low fractional excretion of sodium and low GFR markedly limits the ability of the newborn to handle water and electrolyte loads during this phase.

Subsequently, a diuresis and natriuresis occurs spontaneously at 24 to 96 hours of age that is independent of fluid and electrolyte intake. This seems to be the result of an abrupt increase in glomerular filtration rate and modest increase in fractional sodium excretion, without a significant change in urine osmolality.[113] Management of fluid and electrolyte therapy during this time is hampered by a lack of understanding of the mechanism of this phenomenon. However, it is difficult,[118,119] and perhaps detrimental,[120,121] to prevent the net body water and sodium loss that is attendant to this diuresis/natriuresis.

Following the diuretic/natriuretic phase, GFR decreases slightly and fractional sodium excretion gradually falls after 2–4 days of age. Urinary water and sodium output begin to vary appropriately in response to intake to maintain

appropriate balance. Subsequently, the gradual maturational increase in GFR continues until the adult level is attained later in the first year of life.

SUMMARY AND CONCLUSIONS

The primary function of the kidney is to maintain water and electrolyte homeostasis within the body. The perinatal kidney has the ability to excrete loads of sodium, potassium, water and acid normally presented to it and can, thus, maintain water and electrolyte balance. When the perinatal kidney is taxed with excesses of water and electrolytes, it cannot compensate as well as can the adult kidney. Perinatal body water and electrolyte content are, therefore, thrown out of balance.

The relative inefficiency of the perinatal kidney to respond to water and electrolyte excesses should not necessarily be interpreted as a defect in its functional design. As we have discussed, an important factor in the inability of the perinatal kidney to respond to stresses is its low GFR. Yet, under most circumstances, the perinatal kidney requires a low rate of filtration to function properly. The tubules of the developing kidney have low active reabsorptive capacities due largely to their small size. Thus, **low GFR assures a reasonable degree of glomerular-tubular balance in the perinatal kidney,** a characteristic most important for proper functioning. If the immature tubular transport system were presented with excessive loads of water, glucose and electrolytes, as would occur if GFR were high, then excessive amounts of water, nutrient, and electrolyte would be lost in the urine. Under these conditions, the accretion of the substances necessary for growth could not occur.

Maintenance of glomerular-tubular balance, in turn, depends upon appropriate nephron-perfusion balance. Anatomically, the perinatal kidney exhibits glomerular preponderance. If hemodynamic factors were not such as to limit GFR, functional glomerular-tubular balance would not exist. Moreover, nephrons in the maturing kidney are at different stages of development. Juxtamedullary nephrons are more mature than those more peripheral. Selective distribution of blood flow to the juxtamedullary region maintains appropriate nephron-perfusion and glomerular-tubular balance. With maturation, relative blood flow to the cortex increases as nephrons in this region become functionally more capable.

Functional nephron-perfusion and glomerular-tubular balance then is a critical factor in the process of renal maturation. This balance is achieved partially by a fair degree of morphological correlation of glomerular and tubular size and largely hemodynamically by appropriate distribution of blood flow and limitation of glomerular filtration.

REFERENCES

1. Fetterman GH, Shuplock NA, Philipp FJ, Gregg HS. The growth and maturation of human glomeruli and proximal convolutions from term to adulthood. Pediatrics 1965; 35:601.
2. Fetterman GH, Shuplock NA, Philipp FJ, Gregg HS. The postnatal growth and maturation of the glomeruli and proximal convolutions in the human kidney with a note on cortical nephrons: studies by microdissection. In Excerpta Medica International Congr. Ser. No. 78, Proceedings of the Second International Congress of Nephrology (August 1963), p 32.
3. Aperia A, Herin P. Development of glomerular perfusion rate and nephron filtration rate in rats 17–60 days old. Am J Physiol (London) 1975; 228:1319.
4. Assali NS, Bekey GA, Morrison L. Fetal and neonatal circulation. In Assali NS (ed): Biology of Gestation, Vol. 2 New York, Academic Press, 1968; 51.
5. Behrman RE, Less MH. Organ blood flows of the fetal, newborn and adult rhesus monkey. Biol Neonate 1971;18:330.
6. Calcagno PL, Rubin, MI. Renal extraction of PAH in infants and children. J Clin Invest 1963; 43:1632.
7. Gruskin AB, Edelmann CM Jr, Yuan S. Maturational changes in renal blood flow in piglets. Pediatr Res 1970; 4:7.
8. Kleinman LI, Lubbe RJ. Factors affecting the maturation of glomerular filtration rate and renal plasma flow in the newborn dog. J Physiol (London) 1972; 223:395.
9. Weil WB Jr. Evaluation of renal function in infancy and childhood. Am J Med Sci 1955; 229:678.
10. Paton JB, Fisher DE, Delannoy CW, Behrman RE. Umbilical blood flow, cardiac output and organ blood flow in the immature baboon fetus. Am J Obstet Gynecol 1973; 117:560.
11. Rakusan K, Marciner H. Postnatal development of the cardiac output distribution in rat. Biol Neonate 1973; 22:58.
12. Robillard JE, Kulvinskas C, Sessions C, et al. Maturational changes in the fetal glomerular filtration rate. Am J Obstet Gynecol 1975; 122:601.
13. Kleinman LI, Reuter JH. Maturation of glomerular blood flow distribution in the newborn dog. J Physiol (London) 1973; 228:91.
14. Robillard JE, Weisman DN, Herin P. Ontogeny of single glomerular perfusion rate in fetal and newborn lambs. Pediatr Res 1981; 15:1248.
15. Granger P, Rojo-Ortega JM, Casado Perez S, et al. The renin-angiotensin system in newborn dogs. Can Physiol Pharmacol 1971; 49:134.
16. Kotchen TA, Strickland AL, Rice TW, Walters DR. A study of the renin-angiotensin system in newborn infants. J Pediatr 1972; 80:928.
17. Pipkin FB, Kirkpatrick SML, Lumbers ER, Mott JC. Renin and angiotensin-like levels in foetal newborn and adult sheep. J Physiol (London) 1974; 241:575.
18. Pipkin FB, Mott JC, Roberton, NRC. Angiotensin II-like activity in circulating arterial blood in immature and adult rabbits. J Physiol (London) 1971; 218:385.
19. Trimper LE, Lumbers ER. The renin-angiotensin system in foetal lambs. Pfluegers Arch 1972; 336:1.
20. Jose PA, Slotkoff LM, Lilienfield LS, et al. Sensitivity of neonatal renal vasculature to epinephrine. Am J Physiol 1974;226:796.
21. Spitzer A, Brandis M. Functional and morphological maturation of the superficial nephrons and relationship to total kidney function. J Clin Invest 1974; 53:279.
22. Kleinman LI. Developmental renal physiology. The Physiologist 1982; 25:104.
23. Rubin MF, Bruch E, Rapoport M. Maturation of renal function in childhood: clearance studies. J Clin Invest 1949; 28:1144.
24. Aperia A, Broberger O, Herin P. Maturational changes in glomerular perfusion rate and glomerular filtration rate in lambs. Pediatr Res 1974; 8:758.
25. Friis C. Postnatal development of renal function in piglets: glomerular filtration rate, clearance of PAH and PAH extraction. Biol Neonate 1979; 35:180.
26. Ichikawa I, Maddox DA, Brenner BM. Maturational development of glomerular ultrafiltration in the rat. Am J Physiol 1979; 236(Renal Fluid Electrolyte Physiol 5):F465.
27. Knutson DW, Chleu F, Bennett CM, Glassock RJ. Estimation of relative glomerular capillary surface area in normal and hypertrophic rat kidneys. Kidney Int 1978; 14:437.
28. Larsson L Maunsbach AB. The ulrastructural development of the glomerular filtration barrier in the rat kidney: a morphometric analysis. J Ultrastruct Res 1980; 72:392.
29. Tudvad F, Vesterdal J. The maximal tubular transfer of glucose and paraminohippurate in premature infants. Acta Paediatr Scand 1953; 42:337.
30. Hook JB, Williamson HE, Hirsch GH. Functional maturation of renal PAH transport in the dog. Can J Physiol Pharmacol 1970; 48:169.
31. Tudvad F. Sugar reabsorption in prematures and full-term babies. Scand J Clin Lab Invest 1949; 1:281.
32. Brodehl J, Franken A, Gellissen K. Maximal tubular reabsorption of glucose in infants and children. Acta Paediatr Scand 1972; 61:413.
33. Kurtzman NA, White MG, Rodgers PW, Flynn JJ III. Relationship of sodium reabsorption and glomerular filtration rate to renal glucose reabsorption. J Clin Invest 1972; 51:127.
34. Baker JT, Kleinman LI. Glucose reabsorption in the newborn dog kidney. Proc Soc Exp Biol Med 1973; 142:716.
35. Baker JT, Kleinman LI. Relationship between glucose and sodium excretion in the newborn dog. J Physiol (London) 1974; 243:45.
36. Kleinman LI. The kidney. In Stave U (ed): Perinatal Physiology, 2nd ed. New York, Plenum Medical Book Company, 1978.
37. Horster M, Valtin H. Postnatal development of renal function: micropuncture and clearance studies in the dog. J Clin Invest 1971; 50:779.
38. Solomon S. Absolute rates of sodium and potassium reabsorption by proximal tubule of immature rats. Biol Neonate 1974; 25:340.
39. Kleinman LI. Renal sodium reabsorption during saline loading and distal blockade in newborn dogs. Am J Physiol 1975; 228:1403.

40. Kleinman LI, Banks RO. Pressure natriuresis during saline expansion in newborn and adult dogs. Am J Physiol 1984; 246(Renal Fluid Electrolyte Physiol. 15):F828.

41. McCance RA, Widdowson EM. Hypertonic expansion of the extracellular fluids. Acta Paediatr Scand 1957; 46:337.

42. Aperia A, Broberger O, Thodenius K, Zetterstrom R. Development of renal control of salt and fluid homeostasis during the first year of life. Acta Paediatr Scand 1975; 64:393.

43. Aperia A, Broberger O, Thodenius K, Zetterstrom R. Development study of renal response to an oral salt load in preterm infants. Acta Paediatr Scand 1974; 63:517.

44. Kleinman LI, Reuter JH. Renal response of the newborn dog to a saline load: the role of intrarenal blood flow distribution. J Physiol (London) 1974; 239:225.

45. Haramati A, Kleinman LI. Chloride concentration gradient in newborn dogs in the presence of distal nephron blockade. Am J Physiol 1980; 239(Renal Fluid Electrolyte Physiol. 8):F328.

46. Kleinman LI, Banks RO. Segmental nephron sodium reabsorption in newborn and adult dogs during saline expansion. Proc Soc Exp Biol Med 1983; 173:231.

47. Larsson L. Ultrastructure and permeability of intercellular contacts of developing proximal tubules in the rat kidney. J Ultrastruct Res 1975; 52:100.

48. Horster M, Larsson L. Mechanisms of fluid absorption during proximal tubule development. Kidney Int 1976; 10:348.

49. Kleinman LI, Disney TA. Renal osmotic effect of mannitol in the neonatal and adult dog. Am J Physiol 1984; 247(Renal Fluid Electrolyte Physiol 16):F396.

50. Schmidt U, Horster M. Na-K-activated ATPase: activity maturation in rabbit nephron segments dissected in vitro. Am J Physiol 1977; 233(Renal Fluid Electrolyte Physiol 2):F55.

51. Rodriguez-Soriano J, Vallo A, Castillo G, Oliveros R. Renal handling of water and sodium in infancy and childhood: a study using clearance techniques during hypotonic saline diuresis. Kidney Int 1981; 20:700.

52. Malnic G, Klose RM, Giebisch G. Micropuncture study of renal potassium excretion in the rat. Am J Physiol 1964; 206:674.

53. Wright FS. Potassium transport by successive segments of the mammalian nephron. Fed Proc 1981; 40:2398.

54. Field MJ, Stanton BA, Giebisch GH. Differential acute effects of aldosterone dexamethasone, and hyperkalemia on distal tubular potassium secretion in the rat kidney. J Clin Invest 1984; 74:1792.

55. Stanton BA, Giebisch GH. Potassium transport by the renal distal tubule: effects of potassium loading. Am J Physiol 1982; 243(Renal Fluid Electrolyte Physiol 12):F487.

56. Malnic G, Mello-Aires M, Giebisch G. Potassium transport across renal distal tubules during acid-base disturbances. Am J Physiol 1978; 221:1192.

57. Mello-Aires M., Giebisch G., Malnic G. Kinetics of potassium transport across single distal tubules of rat kidney. J Physiol (London) 1973; 232:47.

58. Doucet A, Katz, A.I. Renal potassium adaptation: Na-K-ATPase activity along the nephron after chronic potassium loading. Am J Physiol 1980; 238 (Renal Fluid Electrolyte Physiol 7):F380.

59. Good DW, Wright FS. Luminal influences on potassium secretion: sodium concentration and fluid flow rate. Am J Physiol 1979; 236 (Renal Fluid Electrolyte Physiol 2):F192.

60. Stokes JB. Potassium secretion by cortical collecting tubule: relation to sodium absorption, luminal sodium concentration, and transepithelial voltage. Am J Physiol 1981; 241 (Renal Fluid Electrolyte Physiol 10):F395.

61. Sansom SC, O'Neil RG. Mineralocorticoid regulation of apical cell membrane Na^+ and K^+ transport of the cortical collecting duct. Am J Physiol 1985;248 (Renal Fluid and Electrolyte Physiol 17):F858.

62. Banks RO, Kleinman LI. Effect of amiloride on the renal response to saline expansion in newborn dogs. J Physiol (London) 1978; 275:521.

63. Lorenz JM, Kleinman LI, Disney TA. Renal response of newborn dog to potassium loading. Am J Physiol 1986; 251 (Renal Fluid Electrolyte Physiol 20):F513.

64. Tudvad F, McNamara H, Barnett HL. Renal response of premature infants to administration of bicarbonate and potassium. Pediatrics 1964; 13:4.

65. Ito Y, Goldsmith DI, Spitzer A. The role of aldosterone in renal electrolyte transport during development (abstract). Pediatr Res 1984; 18:370A.

66. Alexander DP, Nixon DA. The foetal kidney. Br Med Bull 1961; 17:112.

67. Ames RG. Urinary water excretion and neurohypophyseal function in full term and premature infants shortly after birth. Pediatrics 1953; 12:272.

68. McCance RA, Naylor NSB, Widdowson EM. The response of infants to a large dose of water. Arch Dis Child 1954; 29:104.

69. McCance RA, Widdowson EM. The response of puppies to a large dose of water. J Phyiol (London) 1955; 129:628.

70. Barnett HL, Vesterdal J, McNamara H, Lauson HD. Renal water excretion in premature infants. J Clin Invest 1952; 31:1069.

71. Dicker SE. Renal function in the newborn mammal. In Dicker SE(ed): Mechanism of Urine Concentration and Dilution in Mammals. Baltimore, Williams & Wilkins Co., 1970; 133.

72. Falk G. Maturation of renal function in adult rats. Am J Physiol 1955; 181:157.

73. McCance RA. Renal function in early life. Physiol Rev 1948; 28:331.

74. Valtin H. Renal Function: Mechanisms of Preserving Fluid and Solute Balance in Health, 2nd ed. Boston, Little, Brown and Co., 1983.

75. Sakai F, Endov H. Postnatal development of urea concentration in the newborn rabbit's kidney. Jpn J Pharmacol 1971; 21:677.

76. Stanier MW. Development of intrarenal solute gradients in foetal and post-natal life. Pfluegers Arch 1972; 336:263.

77. Trimble ME. Renal response to solute loading in infant rats: relation to anatomical development. Am J Physiol 1970; 219:1089.

78. Horster MF, Glig A, Lory P. Determinants of axial osmotic gradients in the differentiating countercurrent system. Am J Physiol 1984; 246(Renal Fluid Electrolyte Physiol. 15):F124.

79. Horster M. Principles of nephron differentiation. Am J Physiol 1978: 235 (Renal Fluid Electrolyte Physiol. 4):F387.

80. Boss JM, Dlouha H, Kraus M, Krecek J. The structure of the kidney in relation to age and diet in white rats during the weaning period. J Physiol 1963; 168:196.

81. Edelmann CM Jr, Barnett HL, Stark H. Effect of urea on concentration of urinary nonurea solute in premature infants. J Appl Physiol 1966; 21:1021.

82. Edelmann CM Jr, Barnett HL, Troupkov V. Renal concentrating mechanisms in newborn infants. Effect of dietary protein and water content, role of urea and responsiveness of antidiuretic hormone. J Clin Invest 1960; 39:1062.

83. Crawford JD, Doyle AP, Probst JH. Service of urea in renal water conservation. Am J Physiol 1959; 196:545.

84. Jose PA, Logan AG, Slotkoff LM, et al. Intrarenal blood flow distribution in canine puppies. Pediatr Res 1971; 5:335.

85. Kleinman, LI, Reuter JH. Maturation of glomerular blood flow distribution in the newborn dog. J Physiol (London) 1973; 228:91.

86. Obling H, Blauflox MD, Aschinberg LC, et al. Postnatal changes in renal glomerular blood flow distribution in puppies. J Clin Invest 1973; 52:2885.

87. Leake RD, Weitzman RE, Effros RM, et al. Maternal fetal osmolar homeostasis: Fetal posterior pituitary autonomy. Pediatr Res 1979; 13:841.

88. Leake RD, Weitzman RE, Weinberg JA, Fisher DA. Control of vasopressin secretion in the newborn lamb. Pediatr Res 1979; 13:257.

89. Pohjavouri M, Fyhrquist F. Hemodynamic significance of vasopressin in the newborn infant. J Pediatr 1980; 97:462.

90. Joppich R, Kiemann U, Mayer G, Haberle D. Effect of antidiuretic hormone upon urinary concentrating ability and medullary c-AMP formation in neonatal piglets. Pediatr Res 1979; 13:884.

91. McCance RA, Widdowson EM. The acid base relationships of the foetal fluids of the pig. J Physiol (London) 1960; 151:484.

92. McCance, RA, Widdowson EM. Renal aspects of acid base control in the newly born. I. Natural development. Acta Paediatr Scand 1960; 49:409.

93. Vaughn D, Kirschbaum TH, Bersentes R, et al. Fetal and neonatal response to acid loading in the sheep. J Appl Physiol 1968; 24:135.

94. Smith FG, Schwartz A. Response of the intact lamb fetus to acidosis. Am J Obstet Gynecol 1970; 106:52.

95. Daniel SS, Bowe ET, Lallemard R, et al. Renal response to acid loading in the developing lamb fetus, intact in utero. J Perinat Med 1975; 3:34.

96. Cort JH, McCance RA. The renal response of puppies to an acidosis. J Physiol (London) 1954; 124:358.

97. Goldstein L. Renal ammonia and acid excretion in infant rats. Am J Physiol 1970; 218:1394.

98. Hatemi N, McCance RA. Renal aspects of acid base control in the newly born. III. Response to acidifying drugs. Acta Paediatr Scand 1961; 50:603.

99. Kerpel-Fronius E, Heim T, Sulyok E. The development of the renal acidifying processes and their relation to acidosis in low-birth-weight infants. Biol Neonate 1970; 15:156.

100. McCance RA, Hatemi N. Control of acid base stability in the newly born. Lancet 1961; 1:283.

101. Sulyok E, Heim T, Soltesz G, Jaszai V. The influence of maturity on renal control of acidosis in newborn infants. Biol Neonate 1972; 21:418.

102. Svenningsen NW. Renal acid-base titration studies in infants with and without metabolic acidosis in the postnatal period. Pediatr Res 1974; 8:659.

103. Svenningsen NW, Lindquist B. Postnatal development of renal hydrogen ion excretion capacity in relation to age and protein intake. Acta Paediatr Scand 1974; 63:721.

104. Edelmann CM Jr, Soriano JR, Boichis H, et al. Renal bicarbonate reabsorption and hydrogen ion excretion in normal infants. J Clin Invest 1967; 46:1309.

105. Moore ES, DeLannoy LW, Patton JB, Ocampo M. Effect of Na_2SO_4 on urinary acidification in the fetal lamb. Am J Physiol 1972; 223:167.

106. Maren TH. Carbonic anhydrase: chemistry, physiology, and inhibition. Physiol Rev 1967; 47:595.

107. Robillard JE, Session C, Smith FG Jr. In vivo demonstration of renal carbonic anhydrase activity in the fetal lamb. Biol Neonate 1978; 34:253.

108. Kleinman LI, Disney TA. Effect of acetazolamide on renal tubular bicarbonate reabsorption in newborn dogs. Proc Soc Exp Biol Med 1979; 162:375.

109. Moore ES, Fine BP, Satrasook SS, et al. Renal absorption of bicarbonate in puppies: Effect of extracellular volume contraction on the renal threshold for bicarbonate. Pediatr Res 1972; 6:859.

110. Tudvad F, McNamara H, Barnett, HL. Renal response of premature infants to administration of bicarbonate and potassium. Pediatrics 1954; 13:4.

111. Kleinman LI. Renal bicarbonate reabsorption in the newborn dog. J Physiol (London) 1978; 281:487.

112. Robillard JE, Sessions C, Burmeister L, Smith FG Jr. Influence of fetal extracellular volume contraction on renal reabsorption of bicarbonate in fetal lambs. Pediatr Res 1977; 11:649.

113. Bidiwala KS, Lorenz JM, Kleinman LI. Renal function correlates of postnatal diuresis in preterm infants, in press.

114. Wladimiroff JW, Campbell S. Fetal urine production rates in normal and complicated pregnancy. Lancet 1974; 1:151.

115. Kurjak A, Kirkinen P, Latin V, Ivankovic D. Ultrasonic assessment of fetal kidney function in normal and complicated pregnancies. Am J Obstet Gynecol 1981; 141:266.

116. Iwamoto HS, Oh W, Rudolph AM. Renal metabolism in fetal and newborn sheep. Pediatr Res 1985; 19:641.

117. Robillard JE, Ramberg E, Sessions C, et al. Role of adosterone on renal sodium and potassium excretion during fetal life and newborn period. Dev Pharmacol Ther 1980; 1:201.

118. Lorenz JM, Kleinman LI, Kotagal UR, Reller MD. Water balance in very low-birth-weight infants: relationships to water and sodium balance and effect on outcome. J Pediatr 1982; 101:423.

119. Stonestreet BS, Bell EF, Warburton D, Oh W. Renal response in low-birth-weight infants. Am J Dis Child 1983; 137:215.

120. Bell, EF, Warburton D, Stonestreet BS, Oh W. Effect of fluid administration on the development of symptomatic patent ductus arteriosus and congestive heart failure in premature infants. N Engl J Med 1980; 302:598.

121. Stevenson, JG. Fluid administration in the association of patent ductus arteriosus complicating respiratory distress syndrome. J Pediatr 1977; 90:257.

5

Energy Requirements During Infancy

NANCY F. BUTTE, Ph.D.

"If the caloric intake is not sufficient to cover the energy output due to play and activity, the child will automatically restrict his activity so that the limited amount of food furnished will provide first for growth, primarily stature."

FRANCES G. BENEDICT

ABSTRACT

This chapter reviews the energy requirements of term and preterm infants during health and disease. In the first section the basic components of energy utilization are defined, namely, maintenance, the thermic effect of feeding, thermoregulation, and activity and growth. The second section deals with energy metabolism during the fetal and neonatal periods. In the third section energy balances of term and preterm infants are described. Special needs of total parenteral nutrition, infection, trauma, and other diseases are discussed. The last section reviews the consequences of energy deficiency and obesity.

INTRODUCTION

Although physically severed from their mothers at birth, infants are entirely dependent on nourishment provided by their mothers or surrogates. Adequate infant nutrition is required to promote optimal growth and development, to avoid illness, and to allow the infant to interact with and explore his environment. **Energy requirements are fundamental to all other nutrient needs.** Once energy requirements are fulfilled with a well-balanced diet, the intake of all other nutrients generally is ensured.

Energy is required for all vital functions of the body at the cellular and organ level. At the cellular level, heat production is associated with the continuous catabolism and anabolism cycles of body tissue turnover, with transport systems, and with the regulation of body temperature. At the systemic level, energy is required to meet circulatory, respiratory, neurological, and muscular demands.

ENERGY METABOLISM

COMPONENTS OF ENERGY UTILIZATION

Energy requirements during infancy may be partitioned into components of basal metabolism, thermic effect of feeding (TEF), thermoregulation at environmental temperatures above and below the zone of thermal neutrality, activity, and growth (Fig. 1).

Basal Metabolism

Basal metabolic rate (BMR) is defined as that energy expended to maintain cellular and tissue processes fundamental to the organism. Specifically, it is the energy needed to maintain body temperature, support the minimal work of the heart and respiratory muscles, and to supply the minimal energy requirements of tissues at rest. Some of the factors that affect basal metabolism are listed in Table 1. Conventionally, BMR is measured under standard conditions whereby the individual is at rest in a thermoneutral environment after a 12- to 18-hour fast. Heat production and heat loss are equal under thermoneutral conditions; body temperature is constant and maintained through control of skin circulation. The application of these criteria to infants would be impractical; thus investigators have adopted various approaches to measure "basal metabolism" in sleeping infants. Some investigators have used sedatives to induce sleep;[1] others have opted to feed the infant.[2] Sleep and some sedatives will lower BMR whereas feeding will augment it.

The basal metabolism of infants is accounted for primarily by the brain, liver, heart, and kidney. Holliday et al.[3] analyzed BMR in relation to body weight and organ weight, and noted that **oxygen consumption increased at**

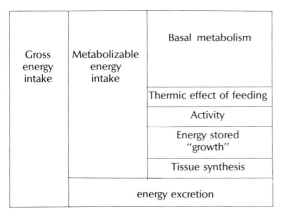

Gross energy intake	Metabolizable energy intake	Basal metabolism
		Thermic effect of feeding
		Activity
		Energy stored "growth"
		Tissue synthesis
	energy excretion	

FIGURE 1.   Partitioning of the energy requirements during infancy.

a rate greater than that of organ weight or body weight during the intrauterine and postnatal periods. The increased oxygen consumption was attributed to increased enzymatic activity during the transition to extrauterine life. Thereafter, the metabolic activity of these vital organs was proportional to increases in organ weight. The decline in BMR per kilogram of body weight observed during growth was due to the slower growth of these organs relative to body weight. The contribution of the brain to basal metabolism was exceptionally high in the newborn period (70%) and throughout the first years of life (60–65%).

Basal metabolism of term infants has been investigated extensively.[1,2] Reported BMR ranges from 43–60 kcal/kg/day. This wide range probably overestimates the true biological variability, due to differences in methodology and study conditions.

Basal metabolic rates of preterm infants are lower and increase at slower rates during the first month of extrauterine life than those of full-term infants. At thermoneutrality, metabolic rates did not exceed 40 kcal/kg/day in preterm infants weighing 1000–2000 gm and 2–31 days of age.[4] Due to their large brain size and higher growth rates, oxygen consumption is higher in small for gestational age (SGA) infants than in appropriate for gestational age (AGA) preterms.[5]

Thermic Effect of Feeding

The next component of energy production is the energy expended above basal metabolism in response to feeding and is referred to as

TABLE 1.   Factors That Affect Basal Metabolism

Age
Sex
Lean body mass
Temperature
Hormones, e.g., thyroxine
Drugs, e.g., anesthetics, epinephrine, caffeine
Nutritional status
Stress, e.g., thermal injury, infection

the thermic effect of feeding (TEF) or as diet-induced thermogenesis (DIT). The TEF amounts to approximately 10% of the daily energy expenditure.[6] The major part of the rise in energy expenditure after a meal is due to the metabolic costs of transporting and converting the absorbed nutrients into their respective storage forms; this component has been referred to as obligatory thermogenesis.

Since infants normally are fed frequently and not subjected to prolonged fasting, the residual effect of feeding will exert a continual, albeit variable, influence on energy expenditure.

Flatt[7] has calculated the metabolic cost of substrate storage from stoichiometric equations. Expressed as a percentage of the glucose calories ingested, the conversion of glucose to glycogen dissipates 7% of the energy, whereas conversion of glucose to fat expends 26%. The TEF associated with fat is approximately 2 to 4% depending on whether the absorbed fatty acids are oxidized or stored. With protein ingestion, approximately 25% of the energy is dissipated through peptide bond synthesis, gluconeogenesis, or ureagenesis.

The TEF in preterm infants[8] and in infants recovering from malnutrition[9] has been shown to be proportional to the rate of weight gain. These observations support the view that the increased energy expenditure is due to the metabolic costs of tissue synthesis.

The measured TEF is greater than that would be expected from theoretical calculations. The difference between what is observed empirically and what is calculated theoretically has been referred to as *facultative thermogenesis,* whereby heat is produced but no work is performed.[6] Possible calorigenic mechanisms include sympathetic nervous stimulation of brown adipose tissue, accelerated sodium pump, or activation of "futile cycles" of intermediate metabolism. **Faculta-**

tive thermogenesis presumably allows the individual to adapt to cold exposure and overfeeding. The role of facultative thermogenesis in energy regulation of infants is presently unknown.

Thermoregulation

Thermoregulation constitutes an additional energy cost when infants are exposed to temperatures below and above their zone of thermoneutrality. The environmental temperature at which oxygen consumption and metabolic rate are at their lowest is described as the critical temperature or *neutral thermal environment*.[10] In the first 24 hours after birth, this temperature is 34–36°C for the naked infant and falls to 30–32° by 7–10 days of age. The amount of energy required to maintain normal body temperatures is greater at lower than at higher temperatures. Basal oxygen consumption rates increase from 4.8 ml O_2/kg/min at 0–6 hours postpartum to 7.0 ml O_2/kg/min at 6–10 day of life and remain fairly constant thereafter throughout the first year of life.[11] At temperatures below the critical zone, energy expenditure increases proportionately to the drop in environmental temperature.

For preterm infants neutral thermal environmental temperatures vary according to gestational age, postnatal age, and body weight. Tables are available with which to adjust ambient temperatures accordingly.[12] Clothing and swaddling conserves body heat significantly. The energy expenditure of naked preterm infants maintained at 28–29°C exceeded that observed of swaddled infants maintained at 20–22°C (80 vs 58 kcal/kg/day.[4])

Activity

Activity represents an increasingly larger component of the total daily energy expenditure as the infant grows and develops. The energy costs of the activities of infants can only be estimated from a very limited set of data. Twenty-four hour measurements of energy expenditure were made on two term infants, 3 and 6 months of age.[13] Total daily energy expenditure was only 20–30% above basal. Maximum muscular activity corresponded to an increase of 70% above basal. Early observations by Murlin[14] demonstrated that crying increased metabolism by 49% in newborns. Talbot suggested adding 15%, 25%, and 40% to basal metabolic rates to cover the activity needs of very quiet, normally active, and extremely active infants, respectively.[13]

Based on calorimetric studies of 70 healthy, full-term infants, Benedict and Talbot[2] estimated that activity may represent as much as 40% of total daily energy expenditure. The peak of energy expenditure of activity occurred at 6 months; thereafter voluntary muscular control became more coordinated, and the energy expenditure more efficient.

From food intake and actometer records, Rose and Mayer[15] deducted that infants 4–6 months of age expended 27% of their energy intake on activity. Combining indirect calorimetry with heart rate monitoring, Spady[16] estimated that infants in the recovery stage of malnutrition expended 10 kcal/kg/day on activity; the average age of these children was 12.2 months.

Activity accounts for only a small proportion of the total heat production of low-birthweight infants. The contribution of activity to total energy expenditure in nongrowing preterm infants was 3 kcal/kg/day, which was consistent with their sedentary state.[17] Growth was accompanied by a three-fold increase in this compartment.

Growth

The energy cost of growth may be divided into two components: the energy content of the tissues and the energy needed for synthetic processes. The total cost of growth from nutrient balance and growth studies approximates 4–6 kcal/gm of tissue gained, of which 1.0 kcal/gm is oxidized for tissue synthesis.[16]

The amount of energy expended for growth decreases appreciably during the first year of life.[11] Between birth and 2 months the energetic equivalent of fat and protein laid down in the body is estimated at 33 kcal/kg/day. This value decreases to 7 kcal/kg/day at 4–6 months and to 3 kcal/kg/day at 10–12 months.

The energy requirement for maintenance takes precedence over protein synthesis. Protein synthesis is a high energy-requiring process, and the supply of energy influences the rate of whole body protein metabolism. Over the range of energy intake, 60–270 kcal/kg/day, energy intake and the rate of protein turnover are positively correlated.[18] When energy intake is below maintenance needs, growth will cease. **The more rapid the weight**

gain, the higher the protein:energy (P:E) ratio required. Growth rates of 10, 30, and 50 gm/day required P:E ratios of 5.6, 6.9, and 8.1% respectively, in infants recovering from malnutrition.[19] Standard infant formulas and human milk have P:E ratios of 12 and 8%, respectively.

FETAL AND NEONATAL ENERGY METABOLISM

Glucose is the major energy substrate of the fetus, although fatty acids are transported to a limited extent.[20] Even though most of the glucose is oxidized, the fetus has an enhanced ability to utilize glucose anaerobically and therefore is somewhat resistant to hypoxia. Lipogenesis is active in fetal tissues. In the last 2 months of gestation, body fat content increases from 3.5% to 16% of body weight.[20]

In the immediate postpartum period the infant mobilizes glucose from stored glycogen, until gluconeogenesis, fatty acid oxidation, and exogenous food intake are established. The hepatic glycogen stores of the term infant may be depleted rapidly within the first 24 hours.[20]

Hypoglycemia may develop in infants with low glycogen stores. Preterm infants are particularly vulnerable because of low reserves and limited gluconeogenesis. Infants of diabetic mothers have sufficient stores, but glycogenolysis is inhibited by elevated serum concentrations of insulin[20] and low serum concentrations of glucagon.

There are major shifts in the pattern of fuel utilization in the neonatal period. The proportions of carbohydrate, fat, and protein oxidized by the body under resting conditions are determined primarily by the amount and composition of the food consumed. Approximately 10, 40 and 50% of the energy in human milk or formula are derived from protein, carbohydrate and fat, respectively. Since 50% of the calories in milk are derived from fat, **fatty acid oxidation and ketone utilization emerge as major metabolic pathways in the neonatal period,** and carbohydrate oxidation continues to be substantial. Plasma concentrations of cholesterol, fatty acids, glycerol, and ketones rise after birth[21] and fall again at weaning when dietary carbohydrate levels increase.

Ketone body production and utilization are accelerated in the newborn even on a 4-hour feeding schedule.[22] Ketone bodies can yield approximately 10 kcal/kg/day during the first days of life, which may be utilized by skeletal and cardiac muscle, the renal cortex, as well as the brain.

ENERGY REQUIREMENTS OF TERM AND PRETERM INFANTS

ENERGY BALANCE

The energy balance of infants may be described simply as:

Gross energy intake = energy excreted + energy expended + energy stored.

Gross energy intake, measured by combustion in a bomb calorimeter, is greater than the energy available to the body when food is ingested, because **most foods are not completely absorbed and protein is oxidized incompletely.** Urea and other nitrogenous products are excreted in the urine. Fats in particular are not completely absorbed. The gross energy values (5.65 kcal/gm protein, 3.95 kcal/gm CHO, and 9.25 kcal/gm fat) may be used to estimate gross energy intake if a bomb calorimeter is not available.

Digestible energy refers to the energy absorbed by the individual, i.e., gross energy intake minus the heat of combustion of feces. Metabolizable energy is defined as digestible energy minus the heat of combustion of urine. **Atwater's fuel values of 4 kcal/gm protein or carbohydrate and 9 kcal/gm fat have been used incorrectly** to convert the macronutrient composition of infant formulas to metabolizable energy. These values derived from adult studies should not be applied to infants, because the infant excretory losses are higher than those of adults.

Energy expenditure and energy storage have been described in the previous section.

TERM INFANTS

Gross energy intakes of infants have been documented by many investigators.[23-30] A representative sample is presented in Table 2. The voluntary intakes of human milk-fed infants are notably less than those of formula-fed infants after the first month of life (Fig. 2). If the reported intakes are correct, energy utilization must differ between the two feeding groups. This is an area of current research and is discussed in Chapter 1.

The energy balance data in Table 3 demonstrate the fragmented and limited designs of the studies in term infants.[31-33]Metabolizable energy ranged betweeen 88 and 92% of in-

TABLE 2.   Gross Energy Intakes of Infants Fed Human Milk or Formula Supplemented with Solid Foods

METHODOLOGY	NO.	AGE (days)						REF.
		30	60	90	120	150	180	
Human milk (kcal/kg/day)								
Two 24-hr TW* (Assumed 70 kcal/dl)	363	101	103	94	87	—	72	23
Four 24-hr TW (Assumed 69 kcal/dl)								24
Males	27	—	104	97	91	89	87	
Females	20	—	101	94	93	90	88	
Two 24-hr TW	20	—	118	109	97	96	90	25
(Macronut. analysis Atwater conversion)		118	109	97	96	87	90	
One 24-hr TW (Bomb calorimetry)	40	110	83	74	71	—	—	26
Formula and Solid foods (kcal/kg/day)								
Interview (Dietary recall)	28	105	111	105	102	97	95	27
Weighed intake (67 kcal/dl)	154							28
Males	69	116	115	101	95	—	—	
Females	85	110	106	95	92	—	—	
Diet questionnaire	137							29
Males	66	—	139	—	—	118	—	
Females	61	—	130	—	—	126	—	
Dietary history	268							30
Males		109	120	120	101	108	103	
Females		111	116	100	114	101	96	

*Test weighing.
Energy intake/kg decreases with age.
Human milk energy intake is less than formula and solid food energy intake.

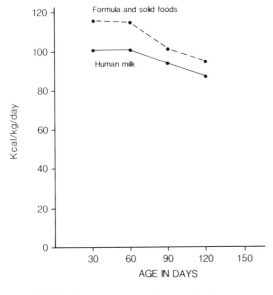

FIGURE 2.   Gross energy intakes of infants.

take. Energy storage was estimated at 26–27 kcal/kg/day in one study.[32]

Basal metabolism of term infants has been studied by numerous investigators[1,2] but 24-hour energy expenditure has been measured infrequently. In one study of two breastfed infants, 24-hour energy expenditure rates determined by indirect calorimetry were 74 and 70 kcal/kg/day.[13]

The recommended dietary allowances for infants are 115 kcal/kg/day for the first 6 months of life and 105 kcal/kg/day for the remainder of the first year.[34] These recommendations are based upon the median intakes of thriving, healthy infants. It is important to appreciate the normal range of intakes observed in these studies: 95–145 kcal/kg/day for 0–6 months, and 80–135 kcal/kg/day for 6 to 12 months. In determining an individual infant's energy requirement, appetite, activity and weight gain should be evaluated.

TABLE 3. Energy Balance Studies of Term Infants

	Southgate (1966)[31]*		Fomon (1969)[32]*		Meurling (1981)[33]*
			Formula		
	Human Milk	Formula	Male	Female	Human Milk + Formula
Gross energy intake (kcal/kg/day)	115	135			95.6
Absorption (%)	92	93			
Excretion (kcal/kg/day)	9.3	11.1			
Metabolizable energy[†] (percent)	91.8	91.9			88
(kcal/kg/day)	106	124	108	97	84
Energy expenditure (kcal/kg/day)			82	70	42 (RMR)[‡]
Energy storage (kcal/kg/day)			26	27	
(kcal/gm weight gained)					5.9
Age at study (days)	14		8–112		7
Numbers of subjects	10	10	37		5

*References in text.
†Metabolizable energy = gross energy intake minus fecal and urinary heat of combustion.
‡RMR = resting metabolic rate.

From limited balance studies on term infants it appears that metabolizable energy is 88–92% of gross energy intake.

PRETERM INFANTS

In recent years there has been a flurry of energy balance studies performed on preterm infants that has resulted in improved nutritional management of these infants (Fig. 3, Table 4A–B).

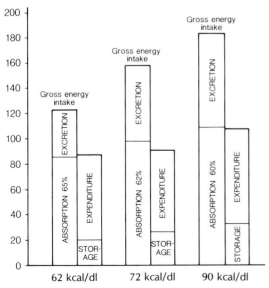

FIGURE 3. Energy balance in preterm infants (formula).

High Energy Formulas

In order to compensate for the preterm infant's intolerance of large intake volumes, the use of high-energy formulas (72–90 kcal/dl) was compared with that of a standard formula (62 kcal/dl) in one study (Table 4B).[35] Although the percentage of energy absorption declined, net retention increased. However, growth rate during periods of feeding high-density formula did not increase significantly. Apparently, greater amounts of adipose tissue were deposited. A further disadvantage of the high energy formulas was that fasting and postprandial metabolic rates increased 10.4 and 12.8% respectively, offsetting the higher retention of energy. It should be noted that the absorption rates reported in this study were low compared with those of other investigations. **The use of high-fat formulas cannot be recommended; metabolic rates were augmented at the expense of growth, offsetting the increase in digestible energy.**

Formulas Versus Human Milk

Combining nutritional balances with indirect calorimetry, Reichman[36] estimated the rates of protein and fat accretion (Table 4A). The very-

TABLE 4A.   Energy Balance Studies of Preterm Infants (Mean Values Given)

	Putet* (1984)[39]		Reichman* (1981)[36]	Reichman* (1983)[37]	Whyte* (1983)[38]	
	HM (pooled pasteurized)	F	SMA 20/24	HM (mother's own fresh)	HM (mother's own fresh)	F
Gross energy intake (kcal/kg/day)	103	126	149	111	117/136	123/129
Absorption (%)	84	94	88	90	84/86	87/87
Excretion (kcal/kg/day)	17	9	18	11	19/19	16/17
Energy expenditure (kcal/kg/day)	46	57	63	56	53	58
Energy storage (kcal/kg/day) (kcal/gm gained)	40 3.1	60 2.7	68 4.3	44 2.9	55 3.6	53 3.1
Weight gain (gm/kg/day)	14	23	16	15	15	17
Protein intake (gm/kg/day)	2.6	3.1	3.2	3.0	2.8/2.4	2.6/2.7
Birthweight (gm)	1318	1302	1155	1160	1320	1250
Gestational age (wk)	30	30	29	30	30	30
Postnatal age (d)	21/45	29/46	21	21	12	16

*References in text.
Abbreviations: HM = human milk; F = formula; SMA 20/24 = 20 kcal/oz or 24 kcal/oz.

TABLE 4B.   Energy Balance Studies of Preterm Infants (Mean Values Given)

	Brooke* (1980)[35]			Chessex* (1984)[40]		Sauer* (1984)[41]	Whyte* (1986)[42]		Freymond* (1986)[43]
	F (kcal/dl)			SMA 20/24			F		
	62	72	90	SGA	AGA	F	Hi Mct	Lo Mct	F
Gross energy intake (kcal/kg/day)	132	158	183	156	149	131	134	133	123
Absorption (%)	65	62	60	81	88	90	93	91	90
Excretion (kcal/kg/day)	46	60	74	30	18	13	9	12	12
Energy expenditure (kcal/kg/day)	67	71	75	67	63	67	63	63	68
Energy storage (kcal/kg/day) (kcal/gm gained)	20 —	26 —	33 —	58 3.0	68 4.3	50 2.7	59 2.8	57 2.6	41 2.5
Weight gain (gm/kg/day)	26	27	29	19	17	19	21	22	17
Protein intake (gm/kg/day)	3.8	3.7	3.5	3.3	3.2	3.1	3.0	3.0	3.0
Birthweight (gm)		1216		1120	1155	870–1850	1380		1740
Gestational age (wk)		31		33	29	29–34	31		33
Postnatal age (days)		18		26	21	1–58	15		21

*References in text.
Abbreviations: F = formula; SGA = small for gestational age; AGA = appropriate for gestational age; HiMct = high medium chain tryglycerides; lo Mct = low medium chain tryglycerides.

low-birthweight (VLBW) infant (less than 1500 gm at birth) retained protein at the intrauterine rate but accumulated fat at a rate three times that of the fetus. Undoubtedly, fat was accreted, as confirmed by skinfold thicknesses, but the exact amount is questionable. Frayn[44] has indicated that one cannot calculate the true rates of oxidation of either carbohydrate or fat from indirect calorimetry alone, when the rate of lipogenesis is high; glucose oxidation will be systematically overestimated and fat oxidation underestimated. Rates of fat deposition would be overestimated by this approach.

Reichman[37] examined energy partitioning in VLBW infants fed their own mothers' milk and compared these findings with those of his previous study on formula-fed infants (Table 4A).[36] Although metabolizable energy was lower in the human milk-fed group, growth rates were similar but the composition of the tissue gained was apparently different. The human milk-fed infants apparently accumulated less body fat.

In contrast, Whyte[38] found no significant differences in metabolizable energy intake or nitrogen retention between VLBW infants fed human milk or formula (Table 4A). Energy expenditure rates tended to be less in the human milk-fed infants, allowing more energy for storage. Energy stored per gram weight gain was significantly higher (p<0.02) among human milk-fed infants.

Pasteurized pooled human milk fed to preterm infants did not support adequate growth (Table 4A).[39] Energy absorption was relatively low. Poor fat absorption from pasteurized human milk may be caused by heat deactivation of bile-salt-stimulated lipase or heat removal of glycoproteins on the milk fat globule.

Small for Gestational Age Infants

Energy utilization of small for gestational age (SGA) and appropriate for gestational age (AGA) infants was compared using nutrient balance techniques and indirect calorimetry (Table 4B).[40] SGA infants had lower absorption rates of fat and slightly higher metabolic rates. **Somewhat surprisingly, the SGA infants tended to grow at rates higher than those of the AGA infants. However, the energy content of the newly formed tissues was less in the SGA infants (p<0.001), reflecting higher water and lower fat contents of the tissue gained.**

Fat and Protein Relationships

Energy balances of preterm infants fed formulas consisting of either a mixture of medium-chain triglycerides (MCT) and long-chain triglycerides (LCT) or predominantly LCT were compared, (Table 4B).[42] **The MCT afforded no advantage in terms of energy or nitrogen balance over the LCT.** Moreover, gastrointestinal problems, ketonemia, increased urinary excretion of dihydroxy and w-hydroxy fatty acids have been reported with MCT usage.[42]

The effect of varying protein and energy intakes on growth and metabolic parameters was examined in preterm infants.[45] A protein intake of 2.24 gm/kg/day was inadequate to support growth and normal plasma concentrations of albumin and prealbumin. Protein intakes of 3.5–3.6 gm/kg/day were well tolerated. Increasing energy from 115–150 kcal/kg/day did not improve protein utilization but promoted greater fat accretion. The lower energy intake 115 kcal/kg/day was sufficient for complete utilization of 3.5 gm/kg/day of protein.

In general when metabolizable energy exceeds 60 kcal/kg/day, energy storage will occur in preterm infants.[46] Further increases in metabolizable intake will result in increased excretion, expenditure, and storage. Increasing energy intake alone may result in higher rates of expenditure and storage without changes in weight gain, due to a disproportionate accretion of fat. Higher rates of weight gain can be obtained with energy supplementation if protein and possibly minerals are supplemented as well.

ALTERED ENERGY REQUIREMENTS AND ENERGY DEFICIENCY

TOTAL PARENTERAL NUTRITION

Total parenteral nutrition (TPN) is widely used to support the maintenance and growth needs of term and preterm infants who are unable to receive adequate nutrition enterally. The clinician must be knowledgeable of the choices of fuel sources and the appropriate caloric level to be administered.

Fuel Sources
Amino Acids. The amount of crystalline amino acids which may be administered is limited and the proportion oxidized will de-

pend on the rate of protein synthesis and the total amount of energy infused.

Glucose. Glucose may function as a fuel source for all cells in the body but it is essential for erythrocytes, the central nervous system, renal medulla, retina, and a few other tissues. If glucose is not available, glucose-dependent cells can adapt by using ketone bodies as an energy source. There are several disadvantages of using glucose as the sole nonprotein fuel source: essential fatty acid deficiency, increased basal metabolism, increased secretion of insulin, catecholamines, and cortisol, and lipid deposition in the liver.[47,48] Glucose administration exceeding the resting metabolic rate will result in lipogenesis with production of CO_2 exceeding that of consumed O_2. CO_2 retention will stimulate ventilation and potentiate respiratory distress in patients with respiratory difficulties.[47] Under these circumstances the respiratory quotient (CO_2 production/O_2 consumption) will rise.

Metabolic derangements of hyperglycemia and insulin resistance are observed in posttraumatic conditions depending on the clinical situation, and blood sugar concentrations may be normalized by decreasing the glucose concentrations in the TPN solution or by infusing insulin.

Fat. With use of fat emulsions it is possible to prevent essential fatty acid deficiencies and to provide adequate calories via the peripheral veins rather than the central route. Prior to the advent of fat emulsions it was not possible to deliver sufficient calories via peripheral veins. Alimentation solutions containing more than 12% glucose are associated with phlebitis and thrombosis.

Intralipid is most commonly used in the United States. It is an emulsion of soybean oil and egg yolk phospholipids, and consists of triglycerides of long-chain fatty acids.[47] Term infants tolerate and utilize intravenous fat (IVF) well, but preterm infants metabolize it slowly and are prone to hyperlipidemia.[49] **SGA infants utilize IVF slower than AGA infants.** Reduced oxidation rates have been observed in preterms with septicemia.[47] Relative fat intolerance may be related to decreased lipoprotein lipase activity and lower stores of adipose tissue. The serum lipid concentrations of infected or respiratory-distressed infants receiving fat emulsions should be monitored to avoid hyperlipidemia, which has been associated with dysfunction of the reticuloendothelial system and alveolar gas exchange.[50] Lipid administration should be limited to 2-3 gm/kg/

day. With caloric levels exceeding 80 kcal/kg/day, fat oxidation did not exceed 30% of total energy expenditure regardless of the fat level.[50]

Glucose Plus Fat. There is convincing evidence that the fuel source of choice is a combination of glucose and fat.[47] Most studies have demonstrated comparable nitrogen retention rates with glucose plus fat, or glucose alone.

Fat should provide 50% of the nonprotein calories when peripheral veins are used.[47] The ratio of glucose to fat may be increased if the central vein is utilized. In general, the amount of non-nitrogen energy should be derived from glucose and fat in equicaloric amounts.

Energy Requirements.. The term neonate consumes enterally approximately 105–115 kcal/kg/day[34] to support a weight gain of 20–30 gm/kg/day. The parenteral energy requirement should be approximately 95–105 kcal/kg/day.

The energy requirement of the VLBW infant is about 120 kcal/kg/day enterally and 110–120 kcal/kg/day parenterally.[51] Positive nitrogen balance was achieved with preterm infants infused with 60 kcal/kg/day but these infants were losing weight.[52] **Growth requires a minimum of 70 kcal/kg/day in the VLBW infant.** With a nonprotein energy intake of 80 kcal/kg/day and amino acid intakes of 2.7–3.5 gm/kg/day, nitrogen retention approaches the intrauterine rate.[53]

INFECTION AND TRAUMA

A characteristic response to infection and trauma is a rise in core body temperature and resting energy expenditure. Oxygen consumption was measured in adult patients with several febrile illnesses (i.e., tuberculosis, typhoid fever, malaria, bacterial pneumonia, and rheumatic fever).[54] These studies indicated that for each degree centigrade rise in body temperature the metabolic rate increased up to 13%.

During infection, fatty acids continue to be the major fuel source but utilization of ketone bodies is decreased.[54] Uptake and utilization of branched-chain amino acids are accelerated in skeletal muscles to fuel gluconeogenesis in the liver and kidney.

When the energy cost of measles was estimated in Kenyan children 28 months of age,[55] a 75% fall was seen in energy intake and a slight decrease in absorption during acute illness. BMR was similar during measles and after recovery. The energy density of the diet tolerated during illness declined from 0.9 kcal/gm to 0.6 kcal/gm. Inadequate intake, not elevated expenditure, resulted in an energy deficit with this infectious disease.

The degree of hypermetabolism with trauma varies with the extent of the injury, the most extensive being in burn patients.[56] A 50% total body surface burn may double the metabolic rate. If the burn patient's body temperature is regulated at a high set point, the patient must be kept warm and heat losses minimized during the febrile state. If heat production exceeds thermoregulatory needs, physical and pharmacological measures should be employed to lower body temperature. In either case energy requirements should be determined and met with vigorous nutritional support.

OTHER DISEASES

Bronchopulmonary dysplasia (BPD) typically is associated with slow growth. The impaired growth rate has been attributed to decreased intake during acute illness and increased work of respiration. Oxygen consumption was 25% higher in infants with BPD than that in controls.[57] The increased energy requirements should be supported with aggressive nutritional therapy.

The metabolic rates of infants with congenital heart failure (CHF) are elevated in proportion to their degree of growth retardation and heart failure. The oxygen consumption of infants with CHF was 9.4 ml O_2/kg/min compared with 6.5 ml O_2/kg/min in infants with cardiac heart disease (CHD) not in failure.[58] Infants with severe CHD who were markedly undergrown had abnormally high rates of oxygen consumption, whereas those with CHD whose growth was normal consumed oxygen at normal rates.[59]

NUTRITIONAL MARASMUS

Nutritional marasmus is due to extreme underfeeding. Classical clinical signs include growth retardation, severe wasting of muscle and subcutaneous fat, occasionally mild hair changes, and associated vitamin deficiencies.[60] Nonedematous protein energy malnutrition (PEM) or marasmus is primarily a deficiency of total calories. Unlike kwashiorkor (protein deficiency with variable reduction in energy), the marasmic child adapts to the insufficient intake. The edema, fatty liver, and abnormal serum concentrations of lipase, amylase, and cholesterol seen in kwashiorkor do not present in marasmus despite extreme emaciation.[61] Severe wasting does not preclude homeostasis; fat oxidation is intact despite depleted body fat. **The availability of fat is the major limiting factor in survival from infant malnutrition.**[62] Basal metabolic rates of marasmic infants were slightly elevated on admission (59.8 kcal/kg/day) and peaked during recovery (100.2 kcal/kg/day).[63]

The etiology of marasmus is multifactorial (Fig. 4): inadequate intake, increased energy requirements, reduced energy retention, and increased excretory losses.[64] Inadequate intake is associated with poverty, anorexia of ill-

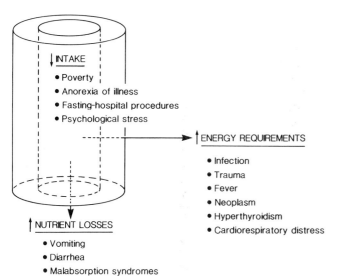

FIGURE 4.   Etiology of marasmus.

ness, fasting imposed by hospital procedures, and psychological stress. Energy requirements can be increased by infection, trauma, fever, neoplasm, hyperthyroidism, and cardiorespiratory distress. Vomiting, diarrhea, and malabsorption syndromes increase nutrient losses.

The prevalence of malnutrition among hospitalized pediatric patients has been reported to be 20 to 40%.[64] Risk factors for undernutrition include: weight less than 90% of standards, height less than 95% of standards, weight-for-height less than 90% of standards, rapid weight loss of 10% of usual weight, and no oral intake for greater than 3 days.

PEM predisposes the infant to increased morbidity and mortality. Surgical outcome and postoperative complications are related to nutritional status, although this relationship has not been studied specifically in infants.[64] The effect of malnutrition on the immune response significantly impairs the malnourished infant's ability to resist infection.

The energy requirements of the marasmic infant are elevated during the recovery period. Energy intake during catch-up growth (30 gm/kg/day) may need to be as high as 200 kcal/kg/day.[16]

OBESITY

Efforts to identify the infantile antecedents of nutritionally related diseases which persist later in life have focused much attention on infant obesity. Data conflict in regard to the persistence of infant obesity into childhood, but there is strong evidence to support the persistence of childhood obesity into adult years.

A prospective study in Switzerland showed no relationship between skinfold thicknesses at one year and at puberty.[65] Tracking of body fatness from 12 months to 5 years was demonstrated in one prospective study, but a history of excess weight accounted for only 30% of the variance in body fat.[66] In contrast, Huenenmann[67] found that none of the children with high weight-height ratios at age 3 years had been categorized as such at 6 months.

Rate of weight gain during infancy predicted subsequent obesity in some studies. Rapid weight gain during the first six months of life was related to excessive weight at school age.[66]

Suggested antecedents of infant obesity include genetic predisposition, excessive feeding, poor intake regulation, underactivity,

maternal attitudes toward infant feeding, and mother-child interactions.

Inappropriate infant feeding practices may result in infant obesity. The decline in breastfeeding, excessive consumption of formula, and early introduction of solid foods have been suggested as possible causal factors.

The ability to regulate food intake in the neonate may not be fully developed. Initially food consumption is controlled mainly by gastric filling and subsequently by additional regulatory mechanisms. Infants presented with two levels of formula density (67 or 133 kcal/dl) made some adjustment in total volume intakes, but only after 40 days of age were they able to make adjustments to control weight gain.[32]

In one of the few studies relating infant activity levels to obesity, Rose and Mayer[15] demonstrated **heavier infants to be less active than lighter ones.**

In order to identify antecedents of obesity in fants, Kramer[68,69] studied many clinical, sociodemographic and psychological factors (Table 5). The main determinants of weight at 12 months were birth weight, sex, duration of breastfeeding and age at introduction of solid foods. However, most of the variance in weight and adiposity remained unexplained. Maternal and paternal adiposity, beyond their effect on birth weight, were not predictive of infant size. At 24 months, the salient factors were birth weight, duration of breastfeeding, sex, and relative maternal weight. Breastfeeding and the later introduction of solid foods may offer a slight protective effect against obesity but seem to be overshadowed by factors yet to be identified.

Because of the deleterious effects of caloric restriction on growth, resistance to infection, and central nervous system development, specific caloric restriction is not recommended during infancy. Prophylactic measures for infant obesity can be implemented, however,

TABLE 5.   Determinants of Infant Adiposity

Maternal preconceptions of ideal body habitus
Maternal feeding attitudes
Socioeconomic status, e.g., mother's education, occupation of household head
Infant temperament questionnaire
Feeding history, e.g., breastfeeding, formula, introduction of solids
Anthropometry, e.g., weight, length, skinfold thicknesses
Paternal and maternal weights and heights

through parent education. Grossly inappropriate feeding practices should be corrected by pediatric health care providers.

SUMMARY OF REQUIREMENTS

The energy requirements of term and preterm infants have been discussed in regard to basal metabolism, thermic effect of feeding, thermoregulation, activity, and growth. Energy requirements decrease through the first year of life. It is estimated that the term infant requires 105–115 kcal/kg/day enterally and 95–105 kcal/kg/day parenterally. Energy allowances for preterm infants have been suggested at 120 kcal/kg/day enterally and 110-120 kcal/kg/day parenterally. Energy balances of term and preterm infants have been reviewed to evaluate energy utilization during infancy. Lastly, the effect of disease states on energy requirements has been addressed.

CASE REPORTS

Case A. A one-month-old male infant was admitted for failure to thrive. The infant was born prematurely at 34 weeks, birth weight 2.5 kg. The postnatal course was complicated by jaundice and treated with phototherapy. At one month the infant failed to demonstrate appropriate growth: weight 2.70 kg, height 47.5 cm, head circumference 33.2 cm. The diet consisted of Similac (Ross Laboratories), 3 oz every 4 hours. Despite failure-to-thrive, the infant had a voracious appetite. Physical examination revealed a wasted but otherwise normal infant. Laboratory data included: hemoglobin/hematocrit (Hgb/Hct) 8.6 gm/dl/25.0%, mean corpuscular hemoglobin/mean corpuscular volume (MCH/MCV) 33.5 pg/97.5 u³. White blood cell count 13200/mm³, urinalysis normal, SGOT/SGPT 113/46U/1, alkaline phosphatase 209 U/1, serum Ca/P 10.0/8.2 mg/dl, total protein/albumin (TP/AlB) 5.6/3.1 gm/dl, 72-hour stool fat 8.7 gm/day, stool weight 150 gm/day.

Diagnosis: cystic fibrosis with malabsorption and anemia.

Treatment: Portagen (formula consisting of maltodextrin, sodium caseinate, medium chain tryglycerides, corn oil, and lecithin) 3 oz every 4 hours; pancreatic enzyme supplement; multivitamin mineral supplement plus additional iron.

Q. What was the evidence for diagnosis of cystic fibrosis?
A. Despite an intake of 133 kcal/kg/day, this infant was only growing at a rate of 6.7 gm/day. The excessive amount of fat in the stool represented 44% of the fat intake or 22% of the total calories ingested. Poor growth associated with fat malabsorption suggested cystic fibrosis.

Q. What was the rationale for this diet prescription?
A. Medium-chain tryglycerides are readily absorbed by the portal circulation. Portagen together with the pancreatic enzyme supplement should increase fat absorption in the child. A caloric intake of 200 kcal/kg/day should support sufficient catch-up growth.

Case B. A three-week-old female was admitted for failure to thrive. Pregnancy was complicated by maternal drug abuse. The infant was born at term; birth weight 2.1 kg; length 45 cm. Postnatal course was uneventful. The diet consisted of Similac, 2 oz. every 4 hours. On admission the infant weighed 2.4 kg and measured 48 cm in length. Physical examination revealed no unusual findings. Laboratory data included Hgb/Hct 13/36, MCH/MCV 29/83, WBC 11400, urinalysis normal, serum Ca/P 10/5.5, TP/Alb 6.0/4.0.

Diagnosis: small for gestational age (SGA) infant with failure to thrive due to inadequate intake.

Treatment: Similac 3 oz every 3 hours.

Follow-up: weight at 2 months, 3.6 kg; length 52.5 cm.

Q. Describe the growth performance of this infant.
A. The child was below the 5th percentile in weight and height at birth and remained at this level after 3 weeks postpartum. The growth rate had been 14 gm/day during this interval. SGA infants usually have the potential for accelerated growth given a proper diet.

Q. What was the caloric intake of this infant at admission and what caloric intake was prescribed?
A. This child was receiving 100 kcal/kg/day on admission, which was probably inadequate for the relatively high energy requirement of SGA infants. The child was given the same formula at 200 kcal/kg/day after admission, and an appropriate growth rate of 34 gm/day was demonstrated on follow-up examination.

GLOSSARY

1. **Basal metabolic rate (BMR)** the energy expended to maintain cellular and tissue processes fundamental to the organism, measured in the fasted state (12–18hr postprandially) while at rest in a thermoneutral environment.
2. **Thermic effect of feeding (TEF)** the energy expended above basal metabolism in response to feeding primarily attributed to the transport and conversion of absorbed nutrients into their respective storage forms; also referred to as diet-induced thermogenesis (DIT) or specific dynamic action of foods (SDA).
3. **Energy balance** gross energy intake = energy excreted + energy expended + energy stored.
4. **Gross energy** heat of combustion of food determined by bomb calorimetry.
5. **Digestible energy intake** gross energy intake - heat of combustion of feces.
6. **Metabolizable intake** digestible energy intake - heat of combustion of urine.
7. **Calorie** the amount of heat necessary to raise the temperature of one gram of water from 14.5–15.5°C.
8. **Joule** the amount of energy expended when one kilogram weight is moved one meter's distance by one newton force. (1 cal = 4.184 joules).
9. **Indirect calorimetry** the measurement of oxygen consumption and CO_2 production to determine energy expenditure.

ACKNOWLEDGMENTS

I thank E. R. Klein for editorial advice and N. Hayley for secretarial assistance. This work is a publication of the USDA/ARS Children's Nutrition Research Center, Department of Pediatrics, Baylor College of Medicine, and Texas Children's Hospital. This project has been funded in part with federal funds from the U.S. Department of Agriculture, Agricultural Research Service under Cooperative Agreement #58-7MNI-6-100. The contents of this publication do not necessarily reflect the views or policies of the U.S. Department of Agriculture, nor does mention of trade names, commercial products, or organizations imply endorsement by the U.S. Government.

REFERENCES

1. Karlberg P. Determinations of standard energy metabolism (basal metabolism) in normal infants. Acta Paediatr Scand 1952;41:Suppl 89.
2. Benedict FG, Talbot FB. Metabolism of growth from birth to puberty. Carnegie Institution of Washington, Publication 302, Washington, DC, Carnegie Institute 1921;1-213.
3. Holliday M, Potter D, Jarrah A, Bearg S. Relation of metabolic rate to body weight and organ size. A review. Pediatr Res 1967;1:185-195.
4. Mestyan J, Jarai I, Fekete M. The total energy expenditure and its components in preterm infants maintained under different nursing and environmental conditions. Pediatr Res 1968;2:161-171.
5. Sinclair JC, Silverman WA. Relative hypermetabolism in undergrown neonates. Lancet 1964;2:49.
6. Danforth E. Diet and obesity. Am J Clin Nutr 1985;41:1132-1145.
7. Flatt JP. The biochemistry of energy expenditure. In Bray A (ed): Recent Advances in Obesity Research II, London, Newman Publishing Co., 1978;211-228.
8. Reichman BL, Chessex P, Putet G, et al. Partition of energy metabolism and energy cost of growth in the very low birth weight infant. Pediatrics 1982;69:446-451.
9. Ashworth A. Metabolic rates during recovery from protein-calorie malnutrition: the need for a new concept of specific dynamic action. Nature 1969;223:407-409.
10. Hill JR. The development of thermal stability in the newborn baby, In Jonxis JHP, Visses HKA, Troelstra JA (eds): The Adaptation of the Newborn to Extrauterine Life. Leiden, H.E. Stenfert Kroese N.V., 1964;223-228.
11. Widdowson EM. Nutrition. In Davis JA, Dobbing J (eds): Scientific Foundations of Pediatrics. Philadelphia, W.B. Saunders Co., 1974;44-55.
12. Scopes J, Ahmed I. Range of critical temperatures in sick and preterm newborn babies. Arch Dis Child 1966;41:417-419.
13. Talbot FB. Twenty-four-hour metabolism of two normal infants with special references to the total energy requirements of infants. Am J Dis Child 1917;14:25.
14. Murlin JR, Conklin MS, Marsh ME. Energy metabolism of normal new-born babies. With special reference to the influence of food and of crying. Am J Dis Child 1925;29:1-28.
15. Rose HE, Mayer J. Activity, calorie intake, fat storage and the energy balance of infants. Pediatrics 1968;41:18-29.
16. Spady DW, Payne PR, Picou D, Waterlow JC. Energy balance during recovery from malnutrition. Am J Clin Nutr 1976;29:1073-1078.
17. Rubecz I, Mestyan J. The partition of maintenance energy expenditure and the pattern of substrate utilization in intrauterine malnourished newborn infants before and during recovery. Acta Pediatr Acad Sci Hung 1975;16:335-350.
18. Golden M, Waterlow JC, Picou D. The relationship between dietary intake, weight change, nitrogen balance, and protein turnover in man. Am J Clin Nutr 1977;30:1345-1348.
19. Young VR. Protein-energy interrelationships in the newborn: a brief consideration of some basic aspects. In Lebenthal E (ed): Textbook of Gastroenterology and Nutrition in Infancy. New York, Raven Press, 1981;257-263.

20. Maniscalco WM, Warshaw JB. Cellular energy metabolism during fetal and perinatal development In Sinclair JC (ed): Temperature Regulation and Energy Metabolism in the Newborn. New York, Grune and Stratton, 1978;1-38.
21. Hahn P. Nutrition and metabolic development. Can J Physiol Pharmacol 1985;63:525-526.
22. Bougneres PF, Lemmel C, Ferre P, Bier DM. Ketone body transport in the human neonate and infant. J Clin Invest 1986;77:42-48.
23. Wallgren A. Breast milk consumption of healthy, full-term infants. Acta Paediatr Scand 1945;32:778-790.
24. Whitehead RG, Paul AA. Infant growth and human milk requirements. Lancet 1981;2:161-3.
25. Dewey KG, Lonnerdal B. Milk and nutrient intake of breastfed infants from 1 to 6 months: relation to growth and fatness. J Pediatr Gastroenterol Nutr 1983;2:497-506.
26. Butte NF, Garza C, Smith EO, Nichols BL. Human milk intake and growth performance of exclusively breast-fed infants. J Pediatr 1983;104:187-195.
27. Beal VA. Breast- and formula-feeding of infants. J Am Diet Assoc 1969;55:31-37.
28. Fomon SJ, Filer LJ, Thomas LN, et al. Relationship between formula concentration and rate of growth of normal infants. J Nutr 1969;98:241-254.
29. Maslansky E, Cowell L, Carol R, et al. Survey of infant feeding practices. Am J Pub Health 1974;64:780-785.
30. Ferris AG, Vilhjalmsdottir LB, Beal VA, Pellett PL. Diets in the first six months of infants in western Massachusetts. J Am Diet Assoc 1978;72:155-163.
31. Southgate DAT, Barrett IM. The intake and excretion of calorific constituents of milk by babies. Br J Nutr 1966;20:363-372.
32. Fomon SJ, Filer LJ, Thomas LN, et al. Relationship between formula concentration and rate of growth of normal infants. J Nutr 1969;98:241-254.
33. Meurling S, Arturson G, Zaar B, Eriksson G. Energy, fat, and nitrogen balance in healthy newborn infants during the first week after birth. Acta Chir Scand 1981;147:487-495.
34. Committee on Dietary Allowances. Food and Nutrition Board. Recommended Dietary Allowances. Washington DC, National Academy of Sciences, 1980.
35. Brooke OG. Energy balance and metabolic rate in preterm infants fed with standard and high energy formulas. Br J Nutr 1980;44:13-23.
36. Reichman B, Chessex P, Putet G, et al. Diet, fat accretion, and growth in preterm infants. N Engl J Med 1981;305:1495-1500.
37. Reichman B, Chessex P, Verellen G, et al. Dietary composition and macronutrient storage in preterm infants. Pediatrics 1983;72:322-328.
38. Whyte RK, Haslam R, Vlainic C, et al. Energy balance and nitrogen balance in growing low birth weight infants fed human milk or formula. Pediatr Res 1983;17:891-898.
39. Putet G, Senterre J, Rigo J, Salle B. Nutrient balance, energy utilization, and composition of weight gain in very-low-birth weight infants fed pooled human milk or a preterm formula. J Pediatr 1984;105:79-85.
40. Chessex P, Reichman B, Verellen G, et al. Metabolic consequences of intrauterine growth retardation in very low birthweight infants. Pediatr Res 1984;18:709-713.
41. Sauer PJJ, Dane HJ, Visser HKA. Longitudinal studies on metabolic rate, heat loss, and energy cost of growth in low birth weight infants. Pediatr Res 1984;18:254-259.
42. Whyte RK, Campbell D, Stanhope R, et al. Energy balance in low birth weight infants fed formula of high or low medium-chain triglyceride content. J Pediatr 1986;108:964-971.
43. Freymond D, Schutz Y, Decombaz J, et al. Energy balance, physical activity, and thermogenic effect of feeding in preterm infants. Pediatr Res 1986;20:638-645.
44. Frayn KN. Calculation of substrate oxidation rates in vivo from gaseous exchange. J Appl Physiol 1983;55:628-634.
45. Kashyap S, Forsyth M, Zucker C, et al. Effects of varying protein and energy intakes on growth and metabolic response in low birth weight infants. J Pediatr 1986;108:955-963.
46. Whyte RK, Bayley HS, Sinclair JC. Energy intake and the nature of growth in low birth weight infants. Can J Physiol Pharmacol 1985;63:565-570.
47. Ekman L, Wretlind A. Utilization of parenteral energy sources.

In Garrow JS, Halliday D (eds): Substrate and Energy Metabolism. London, John Libbey, 1985;222-231.

48. Shaw JCL. Parenteral nutrition in the management of sick low birthweight infants. Pediatr Clin North Am 1973;20:333-358.

49. Sunshine P, Kerner JA. The use of intravenous fat emulsions in preterm infants. In Kretchmer N, Minkowski A (eds): Nutritional Adaptation of the Gastrointestinal Tract of the Newborn. New York, Raven Press, 1983;163-175.

50. Committee on Nutrition, Academy of Pediatrics. Use of intravenous fat emulsions in pediatric patients. Pediatrics 1981;68:738-743.

51. Committee on Nutrition, Academy of Pediatrics. Nutritional needs of low-birth-weight infants. Pediatrics 1985;75:976-986.

52. Anderson TL, Muttart CR, Bieber MA, et al. A controlled trial of glucose versus glucose and amino acids in preterm infants. J Pediatr 1979;94:947-951.

53. Zlotkin SH, Bryan MH, Anderson GH. Intravenous nitrogen and energy intakes required to duplicate in utero nitrogen accretion in prematurely born human infants. J Pediatr 1981;99:115-120.

54. Beisel WR, Wannemacher RW, Neufeld HA. Relation of fever to energy expenditure. In Assessment of Energy Metabolism in Health and Disease. Columbus, Ohio, Ross Laboratories, 1980; 144-150.

55. Duggan MB, Milner, RDG. Energy cost of measles infection. Arch Dis Child 1986;61:436-439.

56. Aulick LH. Studies in heat transport and heat loss in thermally injured patients. In Assessment of Energy Metabolism in Health and Disease. Columbus, Ohio, Ross Laboratories, 1980; 141-144.

57. Weinstein MR, Oh W. Oxygen consumption in infants with bronchopulmonary dysplasia. J Pediatr 1981;99:958-61.

58. Krauss AN, Auld PAM. Metabolic rate of neonates with congenital heart disease. Arch Dis Child 1975;50:539-541.

59. Lees MH, Bristow JD, Griswold HE, Olmstod RW. Relative hypermetabolism in infants with congenital heart disease and undernutrition. Pediatrics 1965;36:183-191.

60. Jelliffe DB. The assessment of the nutritional status of the community. Geneva, WHO, 1966;187-189.

61. Hatch TF. Effects of protein-caloric malnutrition on the digestive and absorptive capacities of infants In Lebenthal E (ed): Textbook of Gastroenterology and Nutrition in Infancy. New York, Raven Press, 1981;767-776.

62. Kerr DS, Stevens CG, Robinson HM. Fasting metabolism in infants. I. Effect of severe undernutirtion on energy and protein utilization. Metabolism 1978;27:411-435.

63. Montgomery RD. Changes in the basal metabolic rate of the malnourished infant and their relationship to body composition. J Clin Invest 1962;41:1653-1663.

64. Baker SS. Protein-energy metabolism in the hospitalized pediatric patient. In Walker WA, Watkins JB (eds): Nutrition in Pediatrics: Basic Science and Clinical Application. Boston, Little, Brown and Co., 1985;171-181.

65. Hernesniemi I, Zachmann M, Prader A. Skinfold thickness in infancy and adolescence. A longitudinal correlation study in normal children. Helv Pediatr Acta 1974;29:523-530.

66. Mellies M, Glueck C. Infant nutrition and the development of obesity In Lebenthal E (ed): Textbook of Gastroenterology and Nutrition in Infancy. New York, Raven Press, 1981; 709-718.

67. Huenenmann RL. Environmental factors associated with preschool obesity. J Am diet Assoc 1974;64:480-491.

68. Kramer MS, Barr RG, Leduc DG, et al. Determinants of weight and adiposity in the first year of life. J Pediatr 1985;106:10-14.

69. Kramer MS, Barr RG, Leduc DG, et al. Infant determinants of childhood weight and adiposity. J Pediatr 1985;107:104-107.

6

Protein Needs for Term and Preterm Infants

KATHLEEN J. MOTIL, M.D., Ph.D.

ABSTRACT

Protein and amino acid requirements in the preterm and term infant remain controversial. Protein may be the most limiting nutrient in the rapidly growing animal and likewise in the human infant. The ability of the infant, particularly the prematurely born, to assimilate and utilize dietary protein is limited due to its functional immaturity. The dynamic assessment of the adequacy of the diet to meet the protein and amino acid needs of the infant is based on nitrogen balance, whole body protein turnover, growth rates in relation to dietary protein intakes, and the measurement of individual proteins or their metabolites in the body. The gold standard for the determination of protein and amino acid needs in preterm infants has been the accretion of nitrogen and amino acids in the body at rates comparable to intrauterine growth. Protein allowances for term and preterm infants are estimated to be 2.0–2.4 gm/kg/day and 3.5–4.0 gm/kg/day, respectively, when given as a casein- or whey-predominant protein source.

In the preterm infant, fortified human milk may be an appropriate source of protein; soy protein is not recommended for routine feeding in these infants. Protein allowances in parenterally-fed term and preterm infants are estimated to be 2–3 gm/kg/day and 2.7–3.5 gm/kg/day respectively, when administered as crystalline amino acids. Although specific amino acid needs for infants have been estimated in a similar manner, much less is known about individual requirements in the rapidly growing infant. Kwashiorkor is the clinical syndrome associated with dietary protein deficiency, while milk protein allergy and inborn errors of metabolism are diseases associated with dietary protein and amino acid "toxicities". A better understanding of developmental patterns and regulatory factors of body protein metabolism will permit more precise assessment of protein and amino acid needs of infants in health and disease.

INTRODUCTION

In 1784, in a book entitled, *A Treatise of the Diseases of Children*, Michael Underwood provided a comparative analysis of milk from women, cows, goats, asses, sheep, and mares. He concluded that "cow's milk, while adequate for healthy vigorous infants, is inferior to ass milk for the 'delicate' or 'sickly' infant." Although unknown to the physicians and midwives in the early 1900s, ass's milk is the only animal milk known to have a casein:whey content comparable to human milk.

In spite of the notable advances in infant feedings made during the past half century, many nutritional problems contributing to infant morbidity and mortality remain unsolved. Protein and amino acid requirements in the term and preterm infant remain controversial due to interindividual variability, nutrient interactions, and the technical difficulties associated with the precise determination of nutrient needs. The preterm infant presents with particular nutritional problems related to its physiologic and metabolic immaturity.

Protein is essential for the structural components of the cells during the process of maturation, remodeling, and growth, and for functional activity as synthetic and degradative enzymes and transport proteins for all body organs. The importance of protein in the diet is its source of nitrogen and amino acids. Nitrogen is not stored by the body and must be replenished to avoid irreversible consequences. The body has the ability to synthesize and interconvert some amino acids, but nine (histidine, isoleucine, leucine, lysine, methionine, phenylalanine, threonine, tryptophan, and valine) are considered to be essential. Objective criteria for the adequacy of dietary nutrients, particularly protein and amino acids, are lacking. **Some studies suggest that protein, rather than energy, is the most limiting nutrient in the young,** and that the quality of protein, i.e., the amino acid composition, is important in maintaining, regulating, and maturing developmental processes.[1]

This chapter focuses on the physiology of protein and amino acid utilization, the determination of protein and amino acid needs in the term and preterm infant, and deficiency and toxicity states associated with protein and amino acid metabolism. Ultimately, a better understanding of these aspects of protein and amino acid metabolism will permit a more optimal approach to the nutritional management of infants in health and disease.

PHYSIOLOGY

The infant is born with a body that is structurally immature and has organs that are functionally underdeveloped. This immaturity lends itself to special consequences in relation to protein and amino acid requirements during infancy. The organs most related to protein metabolism are the gut, liver, and kidneys.

John Clarke, in his writings of 1815, favored ass's milk if breastfeeding was impossible because cow's milk was "too rich, containing too much oil (fat) and cheesy (curd) matter." If ass's milk could not be found, skimmed cow's milk was mixed with barley, grits, rick, or arrow root in a ratio of two-thirds to one-third. If this mixture did not agree with the child, a weak broth of mutton, chicken, or beef was mixed with a "mucilaginous farinacous decoction" in a proportion of one to one.

GASTROINTESTINAL TRACT

Digestion and Absorption in the Adult

Protein digestion begins in the stomach where, in the adult, as much as 10–15% of the protein ingested is denatured by hydrochloric acid (HCl) or acted upon by gut enzymes such as pepsin.[2] At the same time, peptide hormones released by the gut trigger a series of reactions that facilitate the digestion of dietary proteins (Table 1, Fig. 1).

Thus, as the stomach contents enter the small intestine, gastrin, secretin, and cholecystokinin-pancreozymin stimulate the pancreas to release several precursor proteolytic en-

TABLE 1. Circulating Hormones of the Gastrointestinal Tract and Their Major Actions

Gastrin	Antrum	Acid secretion, mucosal growth, gastric motility
Secretin	Duodenum	Pancreatic bicarbonate secretion
Cholecystokinin	Jejunum	Gallbladder contraction, pancreatic enzyme secretion
Motilin	Jejunum	Upper gastrointestinal motor activity
Gastric inhibitory peptide	Jejunum	Insulin release
Neurotensin	Ileum	Inhibition of gastric motility and secretion
Enteroglucagon	Ileum	Mucosal growth, inhibition of transit
Pancreatic polypeptide	Pancreas	Inhibition of gallbladder and pancreatic enzyme secretions

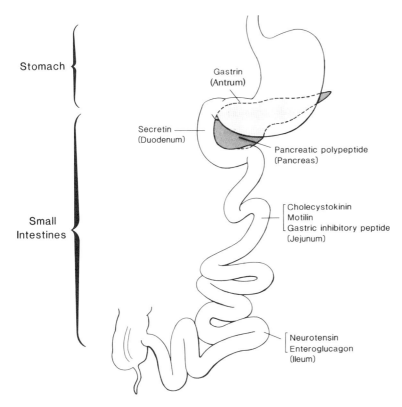

FIGURE 1. Sites of production of gastrointestinal hormones.

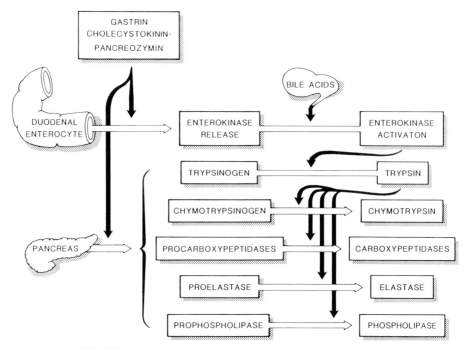

FIGURE 2.   Activation of the proteolytic enzymes of the pancreas.

zymes including trypsinogen, chymotrypsin-ogen, proelastase, and procarboxypeptidases (Fig. 2).

These precursors are activated directly by the intestinal enzyme enterokinase or indi-rectly through the action of trypsin. Each ac-tivated enzyme acts on specific peptide bonds of dietary and endogenous proteins in the small intestine (Table 2), resulting in the forma-tion of a mixture of approximately 30% neutral and basic amino acids and 70% small peptides.[3]

Protein also is secreted into the intestinal lumen during digestion; as much as 30% of postprandial protein products may be of en-dogenous origin. The majority of the peptides formed after hydrolysis by the pancreatic en-zymes may be hydrolyzed either at the surface of the cell by peptidases located within the brush border of the enterocytes with subse-quent transfer of amino acids and peptides across the mucosal cell membrane or they may be transported intact into the mucosal cell and hydrolyzed intracellularly in the soluble frac-tion of the cell (Fig. 3).[4] Amino acids and pep-tides are actively transported into the mucosal cells by carrier systems for dipeptides and for neutral, basic, and acidic amino acids. As the amino acids pass through the mucosal cells,

TABLE 2.   Actions of the Proteolytic Enzymes of the Pancreas

Enzyme	Site of Action
Trypsin	Hydrolyzes peptides at sites of basic (arginine, lysine) amino acids
Chymotrypsin	Hydrolyzes peptides at sites of aromatic (phenylalanine, tryptophan, tyrosine) amino acids; may act on leucine, methionine, and glutamine
Elastase	Hydrolyzes peptides at sites of aliphatic (alanine, leucine, serine, valine) amino acids
Carboxypeptidase a	Hydrolyzes aliphatic and aromatic amino acids from carboxyl site
Carboxypeptidase b	Hydrolyzes basic amino acids from carboxyl site

they are transported to the liver through the portal vein.

Neonatal Digestion and Absorption

The term infant is able to digest and absorb protein well, but the development of the vari-ous aspects of protein metabolism, particularly in the preterm infant, is not well-defined.[5,6]

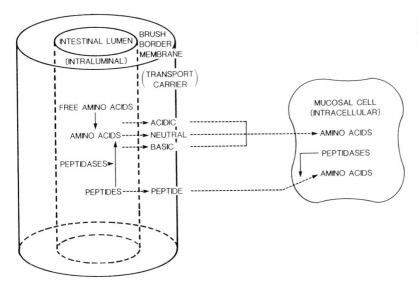

FIGURE 3. Peptide and amino acid absorption in the gut.

Detectable serum concentrations of gastrin, enteroglucagon, vasoactive inhibitory polypeptide (VIP), gastric inhibitory polypeptide (GIP), neurotensin, motilin, and pancreatic polypeptide (PP) are present and functionally active in term and preterm infants. [7,8]

After birth there are multiple gut hormone surges in both groups of infants. Basal plasma concentrations of all of these hormones rise significantly above adult values by 24 days of life. Plasma gastrin concentrations are elevated transiently above fasting adult values at birth and subsequently fall to adult values before the first feed at 2 to 6 hours postpartum.

With enteral feedings, the plasma concentrations of all of these hormones rise progressively in response to a meal. Moreover, the composition of the feed (e.g., glucose alone vs a mixed meal) also affects the endocrine response. Major differences in preprandial and postprandial hormone concentrations are found in breastfed and bottle-fed infants. Preprandial levels of enteroglucagon, PP, GIP, VIP, motilin, and neurotensin are much higher in bottle-fed infants. Although enteral feeding induces adaptive changes in the gastrointestinal tract of the newborn infant, the functional significance of these observations, particularly in relation to protein metabolism, is not well-defined.

The ability of the stomach to secrete HC1 in the neonate is established within 24 hours postpartum. Despite the relatively well-developed gastric parietal mass, the secretion of HC1 may be absent in the fasted state, may

TABLE 3.　Gastric Acid Secretion After Stimulation in Infancy*

Age (wk)	Volume (ml/hr)	Titratable Acid (mEq/hr)	Acid Output (mEq/kg/hr)
Birth	3	8	0.01
4	3	26	0.02
12	13	35	0.10
24	64	49	0.17
Adult	143	91	0.19

*Adapted from Grand RJ et al. Gastroenterology 1976; 70: 790–810.

decrease postprandially, and is lower in the infant compared with the pattern in the adult (Table 3, Fig. 4). [9] By six months of age, the term infant secretes as much HC1 as the adult. In the preterm infant, HC1 has been detected at 28 weeks' gestational age; however, the pH is less acidic than that in term infants. Secretion of gastric acid also may be lower in preterm than term infants after a meal or histamine stimulation.

Gastric pepsins are absent in preterm infants and present in decreased amounts in term infants. The pepsin concentrations do not attain adult levels until the infant is 2 years of age.

Pancreatic secretory cells have been noted in fetuses at 3 months' gestation and zymogen granules at 5 months' gestation. [10] Zymogen granules in the pancreas of the preterm infants are minimal in number but are present in adequate numbers in term infants. Enterokinase is detected at 26 weeks of gestation but

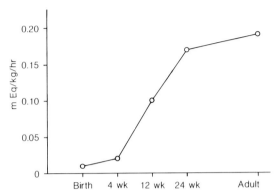

FIGURE 4. Stimulated gastric acid secretion. (Adapted from Grand RJ et al. Gastroenterology 1976;70:790–810.)

TABLE 4. Pancreatic Secretion After Stimulation in Infants and Children*

Parameter	Output†
Volume (ml)	3.9 ± 1.5
Bicarbonate (mEq)	0.19 ± 0.08
Trypsin (µg)	788 ± 549
Chymotrypsin (µg)	860 ± 456
Carboxypeptidase (IU × 10^3)	724 ± 540
Amylase (IU)	564 ± 434
Lipase (IU)	1424 ± 1100

*Adapted from Hadorn et al. J Pediatr 1968; 73; 39–50.
†Values expressed per kg per 50 min, mean ± SD, in children from 6 wk to 13 yr witwhout pancreatic disease; stimulation by secretin-pancreozymin.

at term is only one-fifth as active as that of older children.[11]

The activity of trypsin is detected at 16 weeks of intrauterine life, increases slowly to 28 weeks, then rises rapidly thereafter. The activity of trypsin and chymotrypsin in the basal and stimulated state is less in infants than that in older individuals, although when expressed per kilogram body weight, the rate of secretion of chymotrypsin is similar among all ages (Table 4).[12] The exocrine pancreatic function of the preterm infant is less well-developed than that in the term infant in the basal and stimulated state.[13]

Intestinal dipeptidase and tripeptidase activities have been detected in the brush border and cytoplasm of villous cells throughout the length of the small bowel between 8 and 11 weeks of gestation.[14] Specific dipeptidase activities mature to adult levels by four months gestation. **A carrier-mediated active transport system for amino acids and dipeptides and tripeptides is well-established in the fetal gut by 3 months' gestation.**[15,16]

Many mammalian species absorb intact proteins by pinocytosis. Macromolecular transport of intact protein by the human infant, however, has not been documented clearly.[17] Increased serum IgG concentrations have been found in infants fed colostrum, whereas lower levels were identified in those fed commercial formula.[18] Similarly, an immune response consisting of a rise in serum IgG and IgM has been noted in infants fed bovine albumin, whereas infants fed nonbovine albumin failed to show a response.[19]

Rotch was the authority on infant feeding from 1890 until 1915. His concept of percentage feeding was based on the premises that cow milk protein was difficult to digest, while cow milk fat was harmless. In modifying the infant's feeding, a certain percentage of each food element was to be administered, rather than giving a certain amount of food. Based on the available information on the composition of human milk, Rotch developed the following formula: ¼ part cream, ⅛ part milk, 1 part water, one measure (3⅜ drams) of lactose, and 1/16 part lime water for each 8 oz.

Rotch believed that the tolerance to cow milk varied enormously according to age, and as little as 0.1% variation in a single food element could make the difference of digestibility. As a result, milk was prescribed with the same accuracy and precision as dangerous drugs. Although Rotch's percentage method was adopted universally in America, interest waned quickly because of the mathematical gymnastics necessary to feed infants.

Functionally, the term neonate during the first month of life has an apparent ability to digest protein equal to at least 80% of its intake.[20-23] Casein and whey from human and cow milk is digested and absorbed readily by the newborn infant. The average coefficient of absorption is $83 \pm 5\%$ of intake for breastfed infants and $88 \pm 2\%$ for bottle-fed infants. Preterm infants have similar coefficients of absorption for dietary nitrogen.

Thus, the preterm infant has partially developed gastric, pancreatic, and intestinal function for the digestion and absorption of protein by 28 weeks' gestation. The induction of proteolytic enzyme activity long before substrates are fed to the human infant remains speculative, but may result from the swallowed amino acids in amniotic fluid and the proteins shed from the intestinal tract.[24] Further maturation occurs throughout the third trimester in utero and during the postnatal period in preterm and term infants. However, the complete patterns of development and the regulation of digestive and absorptive functions remain to be elucidated.

LIVER

The functionally important metabolic pathways of the liver that involve proteins and amino acids include the synthesis of nuclear and cytoplasmic structural components, the production of transport proteins, the metabolism of individual amino acids, gluconeogenesis, and urea formation. Much less is known about the developmental aspects of protein metabolism in the liver of the neonate compared with that in animals.[6] Rates of protein synthesis for structural components of the liver in the rat are high due to the rapid growth of the organ near term. Liver weight increases nearly seven-fold before birth and the rate of uptake of amino acids into peptides is more rapid than that in the adult.

With respect to transport proteins, albumin has been identified in the plasma of the human fetus by two months' gestational age. Plasma albumin concentrations increase from less than 2 gm/dl to near-adult levels at term. **By the eleventh week, human fetal plasma contains all major plasma proteins derived from liver after birth,** although several, such as ceruloplasmin, low density lipoproteins, and haptoglobin, are at concentrations below adult values.

Chronic stress to fetal sheep induced by ligation of the maternal side of the placental circulation results in increased plasma fibrinogen synthesis and reduced albumin synthesis, suggesting that the fetal liver is capable of synthesizing acute phase reactant proteins as does the mature liver.[25] During the first postnatal week, lipoproteins rise abruptly in response to the increase in serum lipids, while albumin and transferrin levels rise to adult concentrations after several months, and ceruloplasmin and complement factors rise to low normal adult levels by one year of age.

The metabolism of individual amino acids plays an important role in the developmental and regulatory aspects of body protein metabolism. **Cystathionase, the liver enzyme responsible for the conversion of methionine to cysteine, is absent in the preterm infant and barely measurable in the term infant.**[26] Thus, cysteine may be considered an "essential" amino acid for protein synthesis until maturation of the hepatic enzyme system has been achieved. Similarly, the metabolism of phenylalanine and tyrosine (Fig. 5) may be limited in the preterm infant, presumably due to the incomplete development of p-hydroxyphenylpyruvic acid oxidase.[27]

Removal of cystine or tyrosine from the diets of rats results in a decrease in growth rates and weight gain. No evidence of cystine deficiency has been identified in infants fed commercial formulas despite the presence of lower cystine concentrations in these preparations compared with those in human milk. In contrast, long-term follow-up of infants with transient tyrosinemia of prematurity demonstrated an inverse relationship between neonatal plasma tyrosine levels and scores on psychometric testing.[28]

The fetus depends on maternally-derived glucose and its own glycogen reserve for survival. **Gluconeogenesis becomes functionally important only after birth** (Fig. 6). In the adult, skeletal muscle provides the principal gluconeogenic precursor, alanine, which is transported to the liver and converted to pyruvate via the enzyme alanine transaminase. In an energy-requiring reaction, carbon dioxide is fixed to pyruvate by pyruvate carboxykinase to yield oxaloacetate. The rate-limiting enzyme in gluconeogenesis, phosphoenolpyruvate carboxykinase (PEPCK), converts oxaloacetate to phosphoenolpyruvate. Subsequent reverse conversions of the glycolytic pathway lead to the formation of glucose. Two additional enzymes, fructose-1,6-diphosphatase and glucose-6-phosphatase, facilitate the conversion of the substrates of the glycolytic pathway to glucose.

The major regulatory enzymes of gluconeogenesis, PEPCK and pyruvate carboxykinase, are virtually absent from the fetal rat liver and increase in activity only after birth when glucose is no longer available from the maternal circulation. In contrast, fructose-1,6-diphosphatase shows considerable activity in rat fetal liver and increases threefold by adulthood. During suckling, approximately 85% of the glucose metabolized by the rat is provided by gluconeogenesis.[29] In contrast to the adult rat, plasma alanine concentrations in the suckling rat remain unchanged in response to fasting and parallel the low activity of alanine amino transferase in the liver, suggesting that **lactate, an alternate energy source, is the major gluconeogenic substrate.**

Considerable glucose-6-phosphatase activity has been found in human fetal liver as early as 12 weeks' gestation. Pyruvate carboxylase activity also is measurable in early gestation at levels approximately two-thirds of adult values. Similarly fructose-1,6-diphosphatase activity is present in the early fetal stage, but at 20% of adult values, and increases gradually

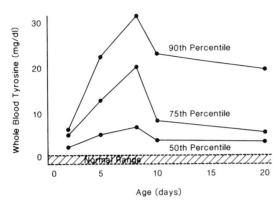

FIGURE 5. Plasma tyrosine concentrations in the premature infant. Immaturity of the liver leads to an imbalance of plasma amino acids in these infants.

during prenatal development. In contrast, the enzyme activity of PEPCK is only one-tenth that of adult activity, suggesting that the rate of gluconeogenesis is low before birth.[30]

The enzymes of the urea cycle are low in fetal rat liver, argininosuccinate synthetase being the lowest and therefore rate limiting (Fig. 7). Arginase is present in reduced amounts throughout fetal life whereas carbamyl phosphate synthetase appears later in fetal life. **The enzymes of the urea cycle increase in activity at birth in the rat to accommodate the induction of gluconeogenesis.**[31,32] Carbamyl phosphate synthetase activity rapidly reaches adult levels within three days of life. However, arginase, ornithine transcarbamylase, and particularly argininosuc-

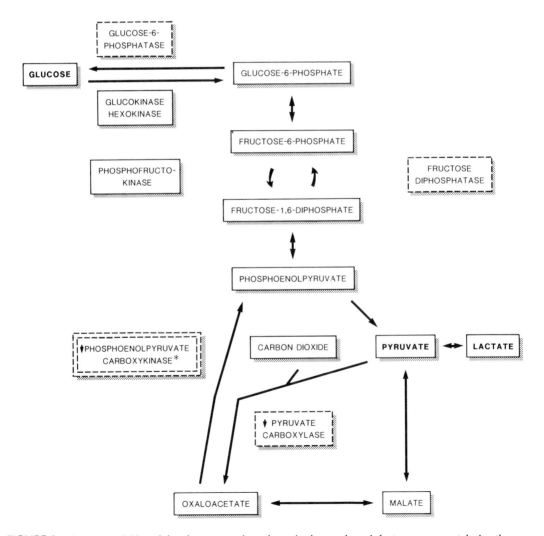

FIGURE 6. Enzyme activities of the gluconeogenic pathway in the newborn infant; enzymes catalyzing these reactions enclosed in dashed-line boxes; * = rate-limiting enzyme.

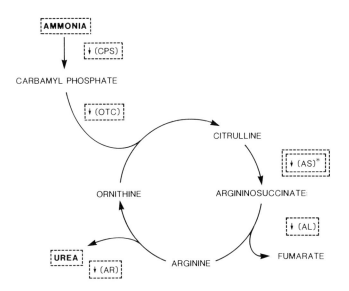

FIGURE 7.   Urea cycle enzyme activities in the newborn infant; CPS = carbamylphosphate synthetase, OTC = ornithine transcarbamylase, AS = argininosuccinate synthetase, AL = argininosuccinate lyase, AR = arginase.

cinate synthetase remain low for the first week of life, followed by an increase until adult levels are achieved at two weeks of age. Although adult enzyme activity patterns are present, urea synthesis slows down during suckling, presumably due to low rates of protein and amino acid degradation in the neonatal period.

In the human the activities of the urea cycle enzymes (Fig. 7), carbamyl phosphate synthetase, ornithine transcarbamylase, arginine synthetase, argininosuccinase, and arginase are present at 16 to 20 weeks of gestational age and incease one- to threefold at birth. Arginine synthetase has the lowest relative activity and is the rate-limiting enzyme of the urea cycle in the human infant. The activities of the urea cycle enzymes are lower in the infant at birth than those in the adult.[33]

After birth, blood urea nitrogen (BUN) and ammonia concentrations increase moderately in small for gestational age and preterm infants, presumably due to the consumption of dietary protein and metabolism of body protein for energy production, a reduction in free water for urine formation, and some reduction in urea clearance.[24] BUN concentrations subsequently fall after the first week of life, while plasma ammonia concentrations remain elevated for a longer period. The fall in BUN is associated in part with a reduction in the percent of body protein catabolized by the infant compared with that in the adult, averaging 4% in the former and 17% in the latter.

KIDNEYS

Approximately 90% of the protein nitrogen ingested by the human infant is incor-porated into newly synthesized body tissues and does not present itself for excretion as urea by the kidney. The functional capacity of the kidney to excrete urea nitrogen remains limited for the first two months of life as shown by the direct relationship between dietary protein intakes and BUN concentrations (Table 5, Fig. 8).[24] However, renal tubular maturation can be induced in conjunction with the provision of increased substrate loads such as dietary protein.[34]

Tubular reabsorption of amino acids has not been well-studied in the human neonate. However, short-term studies in infants less than four months of age have demonstrated increased rates of urinary excretion and lower net and percent tubular reabsorption of amino acids compared to those of older children.[35]

PROTEIN AND AMINO ACID NEEDS

The availability of protein, i.e., nitrogen, and amino acids is essential to the regulation of

TABLE 5.   Relationship Between Blood Urea Nitrogen and Protein Intakes in Premature Infants*†

	Birthweight (gm)		
	1000–1500		1500–2000
Dietary Protein (gm/kg/day)	Postnatal Age (Days)		
	1–3	7–12	7–12
2	7 ± 4	5 ± 3	4 ± 3
4	12 ± 5	13 ± 4	12 ± 5
6	26 ± 12	21 ± 9	23 ± 7

*Adapted from Smith CA. The Physiology of the Newborn Infant, 3rd ed. Springfield, IL, Charles C Thomas, 1976.
†Values expressed as mg/dl, mean ± SD.

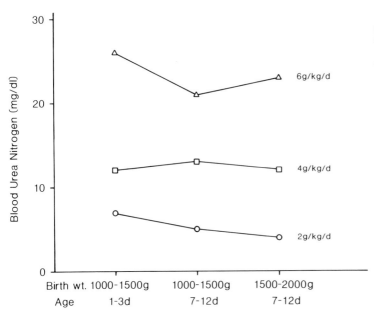

FIGURE 8. Blood urea nitrogen vs. protein intakes. (Adapted from Smith CA. The Physiology of the Newborn Infant, 3rd ed. Springfield, IL, Charles C Thomas, 1976.)

proper growth and development. Maximal rates of amino acid incorporation into newly synthesized proteins in the rat are observed only after suckling or weaning has become well-established. Furthermore, there is evidence to suggest that protein represents the most limiting nutrient for neonatal development.[1] **In the newborn rat, the rate of growth can be correlated with the concentration of protein in its mother's milk.** Moreover, protein requirements are highest during suckling and weaning, the periods when growth rates are highest. In contrast, weight gain is reduced proportionately with decreased dietary protein intake. The maintenance of the animal's growth potential and its regulation are protein dependent because the addition of dietary energy does not alter growth rates, while the addition of dietary protein restores normal weight gain.

Protein needs in the infant are determined primarily by the amount of dietary protein, i.e., nitrogen, and amino acids required to maintain body composition, promote growth, and support the functional aspects of body protein metabolism. Body protein accretion in the fetus increases from 1.7 gm/day (1.5 gm/kg) at 28 weeks' gestation to 2.0 gm/day (0.8 gm/kg) at 36 weeks' gestation (Fig. 9). From birth to four months of age, the average increase in body protein is 3.5 gm/day (1.0 gm/kg); thereafter, the infant accumulates approximately 3.1 gm of protein per day (0.6 gm/kg).[36] This amounts to increases in protein content from

9.0% at 28 weeks' gestational age to 11.4% at term, and to 17.5% at one year of age. Despite rapid accretion of body protein, plasma protein concentrations average 1 gm/dl lower in term neonates and 2 gm/dl lower in preterm infants than those in adults. In contrast, the accretion of individual amino acids in the body (Table 6) is relatively constant during fetal growth (Fig. 10).[37] Of the essential amino acids, methionine is present in the least quantity, while leucine and lysine contribute the greatest amount to body tissue proteins. Of the nonessential amino acids, glutamine and glycine are the most prevalent.

The studies that determined the changes in body composition form the basis for the estimates of protein and amino acid requirements. However, the body is not 100% efficient in the assimilation and utilization of

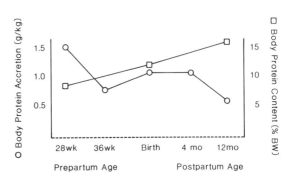

FIGURE 9. Body protein accretion in infancy.

TABLE 6.   Accretion of Essential Amino Acids and Nitrogen in the Fetus*

Amino Acid†	Average Fetal Weight (kg)			
	1.7	2.2	2.7	3.2
Histidine	1.0	1.1	1.0	1.1
Isoleucine	1.6	1.6	1.7	1.6
Leucine	3.5	3.5	3.5	3.5
Lysine	3.0	3.0	3.1	3.0
Methionine	0.7	0.7	0.7	0.7
Phenylalanine	1.5	1.5	1.5	1.6
Threonine	2.1	2.2	2.2	2.2
Valine	2.5	2.5	2.5	2.5
Nitrogen	400	475	550	650

*Adapted from Widdowson EM. In Assali NS (ed): Biology of Gestation, Vol. II. New York, Academic Press, 1968; 23.
†Values expressed as mmol amino acid per gm total nitrogen; excludes tryptophan.

dietary nutrients. Thus, protein and amino acid needs must be determined from the functional aspects of body protein and amino acid metabolism in the infant.

The most significant achievement in the field of infant nutrition came from Arthur V. Meigs. His contribution was the accurate analysis of human and cow milk. In 1882, Meigs read a paper before the Philadelphia Medical Society which stated that human milk contained 0.7% to 1.2% casein and 7% sugar. In a second paper, in 1893,

Meigs reiterated his findings and recommended a formula prepared as follows: 3 oz of top milk (7% fat), 3 oz of a 15% sugar solution, and 2 oz of lime water. This mixture provided a nutrient content of casein, 1.1%, fat, 4.7%, sugar 6.2%, and 21.7 kcal/oz. Meigs argued in favor of his formulation on the basis that this preparation was simple and that multiple formulations that inadvertently could lead to errors were unnecessary as the infant advanced in age. Although Meigs' formula closely resembled human milk, it was not widely popularized in part because sweetened condensed milk (Gail Borden, 1856) had become available.

Protein quality as well as quantity must be considered in the determination of protein and amino acid needs of infants. Protein quality refers to the relative nutritional adequacy of the protein source in the infant's diet. **The quality of a protein depends on its ability to supply essential amino acids in sufficient amounts to fulfill the requirements for the maintenance of body structure and function and for growth.** The evaluation of a protein source is based on the chemical analysis of its nitrogen and amino acid content and on biologic tests such as nitrogen balance, protein efficiency ratio which assesses weight gain in relation to protein consumption, biologic value, digestibility, and net protein utilization.[21]

The concept of the limiting amino acid is im-

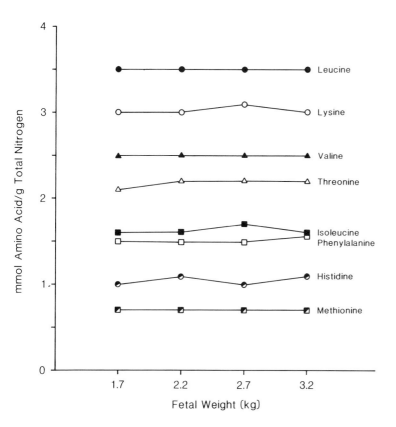

FIGURE 10. Fetal accretion—essential amino acids. (Adapted from Widdowson EM et al. In Assali NS (ed): Biology of Gestation, Vol. II. New York, Academic Press, 1968;23.)

portant for the determination of the nutritional quality of a protein on the basis of its constituent amino acids. In general, all amino acids must be provided simultaneously at the intracellular sites of protein synthesis. If deficits occur, rates of protein synthesis will be limited by the amino acid present in the least concentration relative to tissue needs.

The amino acid profile for the ideal protein has been established by the Food and Agriculture Organization/World Health Organization (FAO/WHO) based on the essential amino acid needs of the preschool child.[38] Thus, milk powder has a chemical score of 83 relative to the standard ideal protein and is considered to be a high quality protein source.

The variation of the amino acid composition in the protein of infant milk is of concern when feeding term, and particularly preterm, infants due to their biochemical immaturity. The limited ability of the immature infant to metabolize amino acids fully, e.g., phenylalanine and methionine, may lead to amino acid imbalances. Moreover, metabolic abnormalities such as elevated serum BUN concentrations may be seen in preterm infants who consume formulas of different protein and amino acid composition.[39,40] In the animal, amino acid imbalances lead to an arrest of normal growth rates.[41] The clinical implications of amino acid imbalances in human infants, however, remain to be elucidated.

METHODS TO DETERMINE NUTRIENT NEEDS

Nitrogen and amino acid needs in the infant are determined by research methods such as nitrogen balance and whole body protein turnover, or by clinical methods such as the correlation of rates of growth with actual nutrient intakes and the measurement of individual proteins or their metabolites in the body.

Research Methods and Concepts

Nitrogen balance determines the quantity of dietary nitrogen retained by the infant after obligatory urinary, fecal, and other miscellaneous losses have been measured. The protein content of food is estimated by chemical analysis for nitrogen content and by assuming that nitrogen accounts for 16% of protein by weight. The nitrogen balance technique has its limitations.[42] The variability of nitrogen balance among individuals averages 15%, and may lead to wide ranges in "requirement"

TABLE 7.   Factors that Affect Nitrogen Balance

Diet
    Protein quantity
    Protein quality
    Energy intake
    Energy source
Nutritional status
    Malnutrition
Growth
    Infant/adolescent "spurts"
    Catch-up growth
Stress
    Physiologic status
    Psychologic abnormality
    Pathologic diseases

values. Factors that contribute to the variability of nitrogen balance among individuals are listed in Table 7.

Increasing the amount of high quality protein in the diet leads to a nonlinear response in nitrogen balance. At lower intakes, the improvement in nitrogen balance is proportional to the amount of protein in the diet, but as intake increases further, the efficiency of utilization decreases by 30%; thus, a greater amount of dietary protein is needed to achieve nitrogen balance. If the dietary protein is of poor biologic quality, i.e., an amino acid imbalance, the amount of dietary protein needed to replace body protein will be increased proportionately.[43]

Nitrogen balance also is influenced by dietary energy intake, i.e., **the level of dietary protein needed to maintain nitrogen balance is lower with excessive dietary energy intakes due to the metabolic efficiency of utilization.** The nutritional status of the individual influences nitrogen balance, i.e., the more malnourished the infant, the greater the level of nitrogen retained.[44] Infants have an additional nitrogen need for growth that is reflected in a persistently positive nitrogen balance. Finally, the efficiency of utilization of dietary protein is affected by conditions such as psychologic stress and the presence of disease. All of these factors must be considered when estimating nitrogen needs for the term and preterm infant.

More recently, protein needs in the neonate have been estimated from whole body protein turnover studies using stable isotope techniques.[45,46] In these studies the ^{15}N enrichment of urinary urea or ammonia is measured during the oral administration of [^{15}N] glycine. Net protein retention is calculated from the differences between the rates of body protein synthesis and breakdown estimated during the administration of the isotopically labeled amino acid.

The kinetic isotope technique has limitations similar to those identified for nitrogen balance, as well as additional assumptions and errors inherent in the methods, such as the heterogeneity of the metabolic pools of the body for protein synthesis, the instantaneous distribution of substrate to the metabolic sites of protein synthesis, the establishment of steady-state conditions for the determination of the synthetic rates of body protein metabolism, and the functional similarity of the isotopically labeled and unlabeled amino acid substrates. Despite these problems, the kinetic isotope technique serves as an additional method to corroborate the findings of the nitrogen balance studies.

Clinical Measurements of Protein Adequacy

Growth rates in conjunction with measured amounts of formula consumption have been monitored in preterm and term infants to assess the adequacy of dietary protein intakes and to estimate dietary protein requirements.[22,39,47-49] Although this technique permits a general assessment of dietary protein adequacy, the approach has several limitations.

Growth studies require a large number of individuals who can be followed for extended periods. Such studies assume that growth occurs at a constant rate, although variations in length and weight velocities are known to occur. Bias may be introduced because the participants generally are a healthy group of infants rather than those who are failing to thrive. Despite participant self-selection, correlations between linear growth rates or weight gains and dietary intakes may be difficult to ascertain due to the heterogeneity of the population studied.

The measurement of formula consumption, and hence dietary nutrient intakes, provides an overestimate of "requirements" because the nutrients being consumed are not present in limiting amounts. Moreover, if failure to thrive becomes apparent, the identification of the limiting nutrient may be difficult due to the number of nutrients being monitored. Finally, the relationship between weight gain

and the composition of the tissue deposited is unknown in dietary intake studies.

In the clinical setting, selected laboratory tests may be useful to determine dietary protein adequacy. The quantity of dietary nitrogen ingested may be reflected by the BUN concentration and by the rate of urine total nitrogen and urea excretion.[50] Urine total nitrogen excretion correlates well with dietary nitrogen intake; however, the methods required to obtain this information in the neonate are impractical. Urinary urea accounts for 80% of the total urinary nitrogen excreted in the well-fed individual. In individuals receiving low intakes of dietary protein, the proportion of urea nitrogen relative to total urinary nitrogen may fall to 50%. Therefore, as a measure of recent dietary nitrogen intake, urinary urea may be a useful clinical indicator of protein needs when monitored sequentially.

BUN concentrations serve as a useful predictor of recent dietary protein intake by the infant. Concentrations less than 3.5 mg/dl reflect a low intake of dietary nitrogen. Conversely, high BUN values may be found in preterm infants who receive feedings in which 20% or more of their energy content is derived from protein, or may reflect dehydration despite low dietary protein intakes.

Serum concentrations of amino acids or ratios among selected amino acids may be utilized to assess the quality of the dietary protein source. **Plasma amino acid patterns respond promptly to alterations in dietary protein intake.** Low protein intakes are associated with an increased ratio of nonessential to essential amino acids due to a fall in plasma lysine and branched-chain amino acids and a concomitant rise in glycine and serine levels.[51,52]

More recently, the rapid turnover transport proteins, prealbumin and retinol-binding protein, have been utilized for the assessment of visceral protein status and the response to nutritional intervention in infants.[53-56] In contrast to serum albumin and transferrin, prealbumin and retinol-binding protein may reflect more accurately the response of visceral protein metabolism to nutrient intake because of their short half-lives (2 days and 10 hours, respectively). However, several factors including gestational age (Table 8) and dietary intake (Table 9) influence the serum concentrations of prealbumin and retinol-binding protein in infants (Fig. 11).[54]

TABLE 8.   Serum Prealbumin and Retinol Binding Protein Concentrations in Preterm and Term Infants*†

Number of Infants	Gestational Age (wk)	Postpartum Age (wk)	Weight (kg)	Prealbumin (mg/dl)	Retinol Binding Protein (mg/dl)
50	Term	Birth	NA	12.8 ± 4.2	2.1 ± 0.6
31	37–40	Birth	NA	12.0 ± 3.9	2.3 ± 0.8
37	34–37	Birth	NA	8.8 ± 2.3	1.8 ± 0.5
12	27	Birth	<1.0	7.7 ± 0.7	2.2 ± 0.2
14	30	Birth	1.0–1.5	8.5 ± 0.7	1.9 ± 0.2
17	33	Birth	>1.5	9.2 ± 0.7	2.1 ± 0.1
10	AGA, 38 ± 4	4 ± 5	3.0 ± 0.8	9.1 ± 3.7	1.6 ± 0.5
15	SGA, 35 ± 4	5 ± 6	2.2 ± 0.5	8.3 ± 2.9	1.8 ± 0.6

*Values expressed as mean ± SD; NA = information not available.
†Adapted from references 53–56.

TABLE 9.   Influence of Dietary Protein and Energy Intakes on Prealbumin and Retinol Binding Protein in Infants*

Daily Dietary Intake	Visceral Proteins† Prealbumin Nutritional Therapy		Visceral Proteins† Retinol Binding Protein Nutritional Therapy	
	Before	After	Before	After
Protein				
≤2 gm/kg	7.4 ± 3.9	6.9 ± 2.7	1.7 ± 0.3	1.5 ± 1.0
>2 gm/kg	8.7 ± 3.5	12.8 ± 4.3‡	1.7 ± 0.7	2.7 ± 1.1‡
Energy				
≤100 kcal/kg	7.7 ± 3.6	10.9 ± 4.7‡	1.5 ± 0.4	2.2 ± 1.0
>100 kcal/kg	9.5 ± 3.4	12.5 ± 4.8‡	1.0 ± 0.7	2.8 ± 1.2‡

*Adapted from Helms RA et al. J Pediatr Gastroenterol Nutr 1986;5:586–592.
†Values expressed as mg/dl, mean ± SD.
‡$p < 0.05$ from baseline.

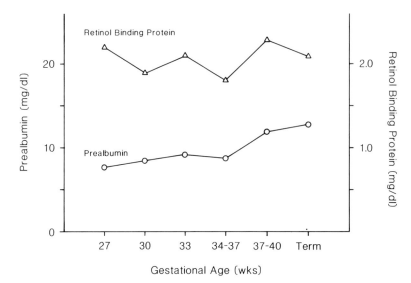

FIGURE 11.   Serum protein concentrations at birth. (Adapted from references 53–56.)

The role of protein in infant feeding was not an issue except for the presence of curd. Thomas Rotch pointed out that curds were difficult for the infant to digest, and Abraham Jacobi advocated the addition of cereals to milk to prevent the formation of large casein curds. Thomas S. Southworth and Oscar M. Schloss demonstrated that there were two types of curd: **soft** curds derived from fat and **large hard** curds derived from casein. Joseph G. Brennemann contended that the physical state of the casein curd was the important factor related to protein digestibility. This observation ultimately led to the process of homogenation.

TABLE 10. Estimates of Amino Acid Requirements in Infancy*

Amino Acid	Estimate of Requirement		
	mg/kg/day	mg/gm protein	mg/100 kcal
Histidine	25	14	26
Isoleucine	111	35	66
Leucine	153	80	132
Lysine	96	52	101
Methionine + cysteine	50	29	47
Phenylalanine + tyrosine	90	63	57
Threonine	66	44	59
Tryptophan	19	8	16
Valine	95	47	83

*Adapted from references 21, 38, 58.

ESTIMATES OF PROTEIN AND AMINO ACID NEEDS IN INFANTS

The initial estimates of dietary protein requirements in healthy term infants were made by Fomon and coworkers.[21] In their studies, protein requirements were determined primarily from the volume of milk consumed and the composition of the milk source, during which time they monitored the rate of growth of the infants and the levels of nitrogen retained.[20,22,23,47,48,57] From birth to six months of age, healthy infants received nitrogen intakes of 390 to 230 mg/kg/day as human or cow milk, respectively. At these levels, 50% to 25%, respectively, of the dietary nitrogen intake was retained by the infant. In addition, all infants grew normally.

In similar studies, a soy-protein formula supplemented with methionine promoted growth and comparable nitrogen retention without metabolic complications to nearly the same extent as did the cow-milk-based formula.[20,48,57] Based on these observations, recommended daily protein allowances are estimated to be 2.0–2.5 gm/kg/day for the first month of life and to fall gradually to 1.5 gm/kg/day by six months of age for healthy term infants.[38,58]

Estimates of amino acid requirements in infants were determined by Holt and Snyderman[38,58] and Fomon and coworkers.[21] In the former studies variable levels of individual amino acids were administered to infants while nitrogen balance and growth rates were monitored. In the latter studies, the amount of individual amino acids consumed by normally growing infants fed a variety of formulas was determined. When expressed per kilogram of body weight, the need for each essential amino acid declined progressively with increasing age. However, the requirements for essential amino acids decreased much more extensively than did those for total protein. Consequently, **the proportion of total protein needs represented by essential amino acids fell from 43% in infants to 36% in older children, and to 19% in adults.**

The nonessential nitrogen component of protein is equally important. Supplementation of protein-deficient diets with nonessential nitrogen restores positive nitrogen balance and promotes growth in malnourished infants.[59] Glycine, another source of nonessential nitrogen, may become "essential" to meet the needs of growth in preterm infants.[45] The estimates for amino acid requirements in infancy were reviewed by an Ad Hoc expert committee of the FAO/WHO (Table 10). The derived pattern of requirements for infants, expressed as mg of amino acid per gm of protein, resembles the composition of human milk and is thought to reflect an appropriate amount of amino acids to meet the needs of growing infants.

The protein and amino acid requirements of the preterm infant are subject to debate due to the functional immaturity of the preterm infant and interindividual variability.[60] The optimal level of protein intake was studied in preterm infants fed human or cow-milk formula; protein intakes ranged from 2–9 gm/kg/day and energy intakes averaged 120 kcal/kg/day.[61-67] In general, linear growth and weight gain were greater and approximated intrauterine growth rates in those infants who received the higher protein intakes. Furthermore, nitrogen retention was greater (218 vs 520 mg/kg/day) with increased dietary protein intakes (2 vs 9 g/kg/day, respectively). Protein intakes of 2 gm/kg/day or less were inadequate for growth. Moreover, edema, hypoproteinemia, and depressed BUN concentrations were seen more frequently in infants on the low protein intakes.

Infants who received protein intakes greater than 6 gm/kg/day also gained poorly and manifested symptoms of "protein intoxication," i.e., increased frequency of fever, lethargy, poor nipple feeding, higher plasma protein and BUN concentrations, and less edema.[68] Long-term follow-up demonstrated an increased prevalence of strabismus and lower IQ scores in infants given the higher dietary protein intakes.[69]

More recently, protein needs in preterm infants have been estimated to be 3.5–4 gm/kg/day, based on the accretion rates of the reference fetus.[70] In support of the theoretical estimates, Foman et al. studied the preterm infant fed human milk.[71] These studies estimated protein requirements in the very low birth-weight infant to be 3 gm/kg/day.

In a series of studies by Räihä, Gaull, and coworkers,[39,40,72,73] preterm infants received protein intakes of 2.2 or 4.5 gm/kg/day from casein- or whey-predominant formulas. Growth in weight and length and metabolic responses were compared with similar measurements in preterm infants fed pooled human milk. These studies demonstrated that all infants grew equally well regardless of the dietary protein quantity or quality.

However, in these studies, BUN, blood ammonia, and serum albumin concentrations were higher in those infants fed the high-protein formula. Similarly, plasma methionine and cystine concentrations were higher in the groups fed the high-protein formula regardless of the type of protein. Plasma taurine concentrations decreased steadily in infants who received a casein-predominant formula but not in those who received a whey-predominant formula devoid of this amino acid. Elevated plasma phenylalanine and tyrosine concentrations were observed, particularly with the high-protein, casein-predominant formula, but not in the other groups. Amid much controversy,[74] the authors concluded that there was no apparent growth advantage, but rather a metabolic "price," when preterm infants were fed high-protein formulas compared with those fed pooled human milk.

In subsequent studies, preterm infants were fed a casein-predominant formula at protein intakes of 1.5–4.4 gm/kg/day and energy intakes of 60–175 kcal/kg/day.[46] From regression analysis of the growth and nitrogen balance data (Fig. 12), the authors suggested that protein requirements for maintenance and growth were 1.1 and 2.7 gm/kg/day, respec-

tively. These estimates were supported by comparable values for rates of net protein retention based on [15N] glycine turnover studies. Remarkably similar values were obtained by other investigators using nitrogen balance, [15N] glycine, and L-[1-13C] leucine turnover techniques.[75,76]

Additional studies were performed in preterm infants using a soy protein formula supplemented with methionine.[77] Protein and energy intakes averaged 3.6 gm/kg/day and 120 kcal/kg/day, respectively. Although the growth rates of these infants were comparable with those of infants fed a casein-based formula, nitrogen retention was less than that in the casein-fed group. Moreover, phosphorus absorption was diminished in the soy-fed group and resulted in a relative hypophosphatemia. Accordingly, **the use of soy-protein formulas for the routine feeding of preterm infants is not recommended currently.**[78]

Recent interest has focused on the use of human milk as the nutrient source for preterm infant feedings. Human milk confers many advantages on the infant, including low renal solute load, easily digestible fat, desirable pro-

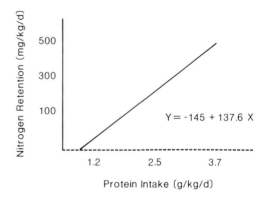

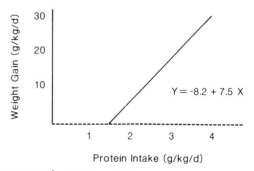

FIGURE 12.   Relationship between nitrogen retention or weight gain and protein intake in premature infants.

tein composition with respect to amino acid content, immunologic properties, and the psychologic effects of maternal-infant bonding.[79] However, the adequacy of term and preterm human milk has been questioned in relation to estimated nutritional requirements for the preterm infant.

Current studies have shown that preterm infants fed their own mothers' milk have a more rapid rate of growth than those fed pooled term human milk.[80-83] Moreover, the composition of weight gain in preterm infants fed their own mothers' milk is similar to that of fetuses of similar postconceptional age.[84] Metabolic complications, such as hypoproteinemia, associated with the use of pooled human milk feedings did not develop in these infants.[85] Milk from mothers of preterm infants has higher concentrations of protein than that in pooled term milk. Thus, the higher protein concentration of preterm milk may account for better growth rates.

Human milk contains taurine, an amino acid thought to be important for the rapidly growing preterm infant. Although taurine may be necessary for the functional aspects of the brain, retina, heart, and liver, its role in human preterm infant nutrition is not clear. Recent studies of preterm infants receiving taurine-supplemented, whey-predominant commercial formulas have not demonstrated enhanced growth, fat absorption, or production of taurine-conjugated bile acids.[83,86-88] A taurine deficiency has not been identified and its essentiality has not been established. Further studies are necessary to determine if the preterm infant has a dietary requirement for taurine.

The use of protein fortifiers for infant feedings may be an alternative method to establish optimal growth in the preterm infant. Recent studies have assessed growth and nutrient balances in preterm infants fed their mothers' milk fortified with skim and cream components derived either from mature human milk or commercial formulas of similar composition.[89] With dietary protein intakes of 2.9 gm/kg/day, apparent nitrogen retention was similar between both groups and equivalent to estimates of intrauterine nitrogen accretion (325 mg/kg/day). Moreover, all infants maintained adequate growth when fed their mothers' fortified milk. Studies are currently in progress that compare growth and nutrient balances in infants fed their mothers' milk fortified with commercially prepared products derived from cow-milk-based formula.

Parenteral nutrition is frequently an essential part of the total care of older infants with intractable diarrhea, short bowel syndrome, or severe malnutrition. Similarly, the high incidence of respiratory problems, limited gastric capacity, and intestinal hypomotility often precludes the use of the gut for enteral feedings in the preterm infant. Although none of the parenteral nutrition solutions available in the United States has a composition that is qualitatively similar to human milk, nutritional requirements can be met for prolonged periods by the intravenous route alone.

The nitrogen source in parenteral solutions currently is derived from crystalline amino acids. The nitrogen in these solutions is better utilized than that in protein hydrolysates and is associated with a low incidence of hyperammonemia, unless parenteral amino acids are given at a rate exceeding 3.5-4 gm/kg/day. Metabolic complications related to amino acids in solutions, including azotemia and acidosis, occur with intravenous intakes of more than 4 gm/kg/day of protein equivalents. The commercial solutions do not contain cysteine, although separate additive preparations are available. Taurine and carnitine, both thought to be essential nutrients for the preterm infant, are absent from commercial nutritional preparations.

The recommended intake of protein equivalents for term infants is 2-3 gm/kg/day.[90,91] In the preterm infant parenteral amino acid intakes of 2.5-3 gm/kg/day and nonprotein energy intakes of 60 kcal/kg/day have been associated with positive nitrogen balance.[92,93] However, with increased amino acid and nonprotein energy intakes (2.7-3.5 gm/kg/day and 80-85 kcal/kg/day, respectively), nitrogen retention rates approximate fetal accretion rates.[94,95] The ideal amino acid composition of these solutions for the preterm infant is unknown. Whether enteral amino acid requirements extend to parenteral amino acid needs is unclear. For example, although cysteine is thought to be an essential amino acid in infants, cysteine supplementation of cysteine-free parenteral amino acid solutions did not improve nitrogen balance or growth in preterm and term infants.[96]

In summary, nitrogen and amino acid "requirements" in term and preterm infants remain controversial at best. Protein "allowances" have been estimated for term and preterm infants fed enterally or parenterally and are summarized in Table 11. Amino acid

TABLE 11.   Protein "Allowances" in Infants*

Group of Infants	Type of Protein	Recommended Protein Intake (gm/kg/day)
Enteral		
Term	Casein/soy	2.0–2.4
Preterm	Casein	3.5–4.0
Preterm	Fortified, human	2.9
Parenteral		
Term	Parenteral amino acids	2.0–3.0
Preterm	Parenteral amino acids	2.7–3.5

*Adapted from references 20, 38, 46, 58, 75, 90, 91, 93.

"allowances" also have been derived from limited information and are summarized in Table 10. Further studies are necessary to elucidate more precisely the parenteral nitrogen and amino acid needs of infants in health and disease.

DEFICIENCY

Kwashiorkor is the clinical syndrome that results from dietary protein deficiency.[97] Kwashiorkor develops in settings where infants are fed a low-protein, high-carbohydrate diet for prolonged periods or may be precipitated by acute episodes of infections during periods of chronic protein-energy malnutrition (marasmus) and stress.

Neonates and infants less than one year of age are at risk for the development of malnutrition secondary to protein deficiency. The prevalence of protein-energy malnutrition in hospitalized preterm and term infants less than three months of age is 63%.[98] Among infants who require acute intensive care, most preterm infants and nearly two-thirds of term infants may demonstrate clinical or biochemical features of malnutrition. **Among infants requiring chronic intensive care, 90% of all preterm infants, and at least one-third of term infants may be malnourished.** In preterm infants whose birth weight was less than 1200 gm, serum albumin concentrations of 2 gm/dl or less were observed in 85% of the group studied. None of these very-low birthweight infants achieved intrauterine growth rates and steady weight gain did not occur until acceptable dietary intakes were achieved.[99]

The classic features of kwashiorkor include the findings of irritability, edema, hypoproteinemia, hypoalbuminemia, and skin abnormal-

ities such as hyperpigmentation, hyperkeratosis, desquamation, and ulcerated lesions. The hair becomes sparse, depigmented, and is plucked easily from the scalp. The cheeks become prominent, leading to a "moon-face" appearance. Hepatomegaly due to fatty infiltrates of the liver also is present. Anthropometric measurements such as weight may not reflect nutritional deficits due to the preserved subcutaneous fat stores and peripheral edema. In the neonate, the classic features of kwashiorkor may not be apparent due to the presence of generalized protein-energy malnutrition and specific organ disease.

Serum albumin concentrations are the most frequently monitored laboratory values to make the diagnosis of kwashiorkor. Depressed serum albumin concentrations are a sensitive indicator of visceral protein status and are associated with an increased risk of infection, prolonged hospital stay, increased morbidity (particularly after surgery), and increased mortality.[100] However, the use of the serum albumin concentration as a diagnostic index for kwashiorkor has its limitations because "normal" values in preterm infants remain undefined. Despite these uncertainties, serum albumin concentrations less than 3.0 and 2.5 mg/dl in term and preterm infants, respectively, suggest the presence of kwashiorkor.[101] From more recent studies, it has been suggested that serum transferrin, prealbumin, and retinol binding protein measurements may be more sensitive indicators of body protein status due to their shorter half-lives and may hold promise as a more accurate guide for the assessment of the nutritional status of the infant (Table 9).[102]

The goals of nutritional therapy in kwashiorkor include the attainment of maximal rates of weight gain within the shortest period in a safe manner. Maximal rates of weight gain have been seen in infants receiving protein and energy intakes of 4–5 gm/kg/day and 200 kcal/kg/day, respectively, once the acute problems of protein-energy malnutrition have resolved.[97]

TOXICITY

Milk-Protein Allergy

Allergy to cow milk is the most common "toxic" response to dietary protein, but occurs in only 2% of infants.[103] **Approximately 25% of those infants with cow milk protein al-**

lergy also have an intolerance to soy proteins. The pathogenesis of this syndrome has not been elucidated, although an immunologic mechanism is suspected.

Cow-milk-protein allergy usually presents before six months of age. The clinical features include vomiting, diarrhea, failure to thrive, atopic dermatitis, and bronchial wheezing. A more subtle manifestation of milk-protein allergy is the presence of occult intestinal bleeding with or without diarrhea, iron deficiency anemia, hypoproteinemia, and hypoalbuminemia.[104] Intestinal bleeding is seen most frequently after severe bouts of acute infectious gastroenteritis or in infants with a family history of atopy.

Although there are no laboratory tests that make the diagnosis of cow-milk or soy-protein allergy, a complete blood count with differential white cell counts, serum total protein, albumin, and IgE concentrations, and stool guaiac measurements should be obtained. Small bowel biopsies may show an intestinal lesion with shortening of villous height, lengthening of the crypts, and increased intraepithelial lymphocytes. Colonic biopsies may demonstrate inflammation with eosinophilic infiltrates of the mucosa.[105]

The diagnosis is made by the disappearance of symptoms when milk products are withdrawn from the diet and by the recurrence of symptoms when the milk product is reintroduced.[106] Human milk serves as a preventive measure, although potential allergens may be transferred through maternal milk, thereby sensitizing the infant.[107] Soy-protein formulas may or may not be an allergen-free milk substitute, and in severely sensitized infants, protein hydrolysate formulas or amino acid preparations may be necessary. **Tolerance to cow milk usually develops around 2 years of age.**

Toxicity to individual amino acids is manifested as inborn errors of metabolism. The most common inborn errors include phenylketonuria and the hyperphenylalaninemias, histidinemia, disorders of branched-chain amino acids, and disorders of urea cycle enzymes (Table 12). Most inborn errors of metabolism are associated with severe clinical manifestations. Mental retardation, seizures, and other neurologic and behavioral manifestations such as irritability, hyperkinesis, hypertonicity, tremors, and microcephaly are seen in the untreated patient. Many of the inborn errors of metabolism are fatal when metabolic complications such as hypoglycemia and hyperammonemia develop. Nutritional therapy provides the mainstay for the treatment of children with inborn errors of metabolism.[108] Protein and amino acid requirements have been estimated for selected inborn errors of metabolism (Table 13).

TABLE 12.   Common Inborn Errors of Amino Acid and Protein Metabolism

Type	Defect	Dietary Treatment
Hyperphenylalaninemias		
Phenylketonuria	Phenylalanine hydroxylase	↓ Phenylalanine
Hyperphenylalaninemias	Phenylalanine hydroxylase, tyrosine enzymes	↓ Phenylalanine
Dihydropteridine	Cofactor	↓ Phenylalanine; 5-OH-tryptophan supplement
Hereditary tyrosinemia	Several enzymes of tyrosine metabolism	↓ Tyrosine
Transient neonatal tyrosinemia	p-OH-phenylpyruvate oxidase	↓ Phenylalanine, tyrosine; vitamin C supplement
Histidinemia	?	? Histidine
Maple syrup urine disease	Branched-chain ketoacid dehydrogenase complex	↓ Leucine, isoleucine, valine
Urea cycle defects		
Hereditary urea cycle defects	Ornithine transcarbamylase, argininosuccinate synthetase, argininosuccinate lyase, arginase	↓ Protein; ketoanalogues of essential amino acids, arginine supplements
Transient hyperammoniemia of infancy	Several urea cycle enzymes	↓ Protein; ketoanalogues of essential amino acids, arginine supplements

TABLE 13.   Recommended Amino Acid and Protein Intakes in Some Inborn Errors of Metabolism of Infancy*

| Age (mo) | Phenyl-ketonuria | Tyrosinemia | | Maple syrup urine disease | | | Urea cycle defects | | |
| | | | | Amino Acid/Protein Allowance† | | | | | |
	PHE	TYR	MET	LEU	ISO	VAL	PRO	CIT	ARG
0–2	65	70	40	75	80	85	1050	180	550
2–6	50	70	40	75	80	85	—	—	—
6–12	40	40	20	—	—	—	—	—	—

*Adapted from Caballero B. Clin Nutr 1985;4:85–95.
†Values expressed as mg/kg/day; PHE = phenylalanine, TYR = tyrosine, MET = methionine, LEU = leucine, ISO = isoleucine, VAL = valine, PRO = protein, CIT = citrulline, ARG = arginine.

CASE REPORTS

Case 1. The patient is a 4-week-old preterm infant born at 28 weeks' gestational age. His hospital course was complicated by hyaline membrane disease requiring prolonged ventilatory support and high concentrations of oxygen. When ventilatory support was no longer necessary, fluid intakes were limited to 90 ml/kg/day. The infant also had sepsis but was on day 6 of appropriate antibiotic therapy. In order to maintain his nutritional status, the infant was given total parenteral nutrition by a "central" venous line. Protein intake by this route was estimated to be 2.5 gm/kg/day. Energy intake (20% dextrose and 10% Intralipid) averaged 75 kcal/kg/day. Routine laboratory monitoring of this patient revealed a blood urea nitrogen (BUN) of 52 mg/dl (normal ≤ 20) and a triglyceride level of 310 mg/dl (normal ≤ 150). You have been consulted to explain these abnormalities and to recommend an appropriate treatment regimen.

Questions and Answers

Q.   What are protein and energy "requirements" versus "allowances" in the newborn infant and in children in general?
A.   **"Requirements"** represent absolute values of nutrients that meet the metabolic need of the individuals. **"Allowances"** are estimates of nutrient needs of the body based on obligatory losses and the amount of the nutrient required to keep the individual in metabolic equilibrium. Absolute nutrient requirements are difficult to ascertain. Recommended daily allowances for protein and energy in bottle-fed infants less than 1 year of age are 2.0–2.2 gm/kg/day and 100–120 kcal/kg/day.

Q.   Why are the BUN and triglyceride concentrations elevated? What metabolic pathways may be involved?
A.   BUN and triglycerides are elevated because of an inadequate supply of nonprotein energy source. Excess protein is catabolized via gluconeogenesis and utilized for glucose formation. Nitrogen from endogenous protein breakdown is converted to urea because nitrogen is toxic; however, urea cannot be excreted quickly by the infant's immature kidney. Serum triglycerides are not metabolized in the face of inadequate dietary protein and energy in-

takes due to inadequate synthesis of the enzyme lipoprotein lipase.

Q.   What role does the theory of the limiting nutrient have in this case?
A.   Energy is a limiting nutrient for protein metabolism.

Q.   What treatment program would you institute?
A.   Liberalize intravenous fluids and supply additional nonprotein energy as carbohydrate and lipid. These changes result in resolution of the metabolic disturbances.

Case 2. A 3-month-old infant was admitted for evaluation of failure to thrive. On admission the infant's weight was 4.08 kg. Poor weight gain was noted since one month of age. The infant was breastfed for the first two months of life, then supplemented with a soy protein formula. On physical examination the infant appeared proportionate in size, but somewhat floppy in its activity. Laboratory screening revealed a blood hemoglobin of 8.0 gm/dl (normal ≥ 11.0) and serum albumin of 3.0 gm/dl (normal ≥ 3.5). A sweat test was consistent with the diagnosis of cystic fibrosis. You have been consulted to explain the apparent discrepancy between the clinical appearance of this child and the laboratory findings and to provide recommendations for therapeutic management.

Questions and Answers

Q.   What is the nutritional diagnosis in this infant? What other physical findings help to make this diagnosis?
A.   The nutritional diagnosis is kwashiorkor. The etiology is due to a protein deficiency rather than energy. Clinical findings include edema, hypoproteinemia, hypoalbuminemia, and skin rashes in contrast to general wasting seen in marasmus.

Q.   Why do you think this child failed to gain weight while receiving human milk and a soy formula? What is the relationship between these milk sources and protein quantity and quality?

A.   Human milk contains 0.9 mg/dl protein nitrogen and may have been limited in quantity rather than overall quality. The quality of a protein is assessed by its amino acid composition. **Soy formulas have trypsin inhibitors.** In an infant who has limited trypsin due to pancreatic insufficiency, these formulas often do not support growth in infants with cystic fibrosis.

Q.   What would happen if you treated this child's anemia with oral iron therapy?
A.   **Anemia would not resolve with iron therapy alone in a protein-deficient patient** because hemoglobin must be synthesized from proteins to carry iron.

Q.   What therapeutic approach would you take in this child and what laboratory measurements would you obtain to monitor the infant's progress?
A.   Change the infant's formula to a casein- or whey-based preparation and provide pancreatic enzyme replacement. Albumin can be measured to monitor the infant's progress, but the turnover time is 10 days. More rapidly turning-over proteins such as prealbumin, retinol-binding protein, or transferrin may reflect recovery earlier.

Case 3. A 9-month-old infant was admitted because of recurrent vomiting, diarrhea, pallor, and weight loss. The infant was breastfed for the first six months of life, then weaned to whole cow milk. On physical examination the infant was irritable and pale; minimal weight loss was apparent. Laboratory examination revealed a blood hemoglobin of 10.0 gm/dl (normal ⩾ 11.0), a serum albumin of 3.0 gm/dl (normal ⩾ 3.5), and guaiac-positive stools. An upper gastrointestinal x-ray evaluation was negative for gastroesophageal reflux and outlet obstruction. Serum electrolytes failed to demonstrate a metabolic disorder. While in the hospital, the infant was noted to have projectile vomiting and worsening diarrhea. As an afterthought, the infant's mother commented that she was fed goat milk as an infant.

Questions and Answers

Q.   What is the nutritional diagnosis in this child? What etiologic factor is thought to cause this problem?
A.   The diagnosis is milk-protein allergy. The etiologic factor is thought to be due to the presence of beta-lactoglobulin, a protein present in cow milk but not in human milk.

Q.   How does this clinical problem relate to lactose intolerance? In what other situations might you see this problem and lactose intolerance combined?
A.   Milk-protein allergy is a clinical syndrome thought to be IgE mediated. Carbohydrate intolerance is a clinical syndrome related to altered intestinal absorptive capacity or the genetic background of the individual. The latter is not IgE mediated and is not an "allergy." Both of these entities may be seen in severe diarrheal disease due to a rotavirus infection.

Q.   What is the relationship between cow milk, soy formula, and goat milk in this clinical entity?
A.   There may be cross reactivity among cow milk and goat milk proteins; 30% of children with cow milk sensitivity will be "allergic" to soy protein.

Q.   How would you treat this infant?
A.   Change the infant's formula to a protein hydrolysate-based preparation or provide human milk. In severely sensitized infants an amino acid/dipeptide preparation may be necessary.

REFERENCES

1. Miller SA. Nutrition in the neonatal development of protein metabolism. Fed Proc 1970;29:1497-1502.
2. Sunshine P. Digestion and absorption of proteins. In Bloom RS, Sinclair JC, Warshaw JB (eds): Selected Aspects of Perinatal Gastroenterology. Evansville, Mead Johnson, 1977;17-21.
3. Gray GM, Cooper HL. Protein digestion and absorption. Gastroenterology 1971;61:535-544.
4. Matthews DM, Adibi SA. Peptide absorption. Gastroenterology 1976;71:151-161.
5. Grand RJ, Watkins JB, Torti FM. Development of the human gastrointestinal tract. A review. Gastroenterology 1976; 70:790-810.
6. Lebenthal E. Textbook of Gastroenterology and Nutrition in Infancy, Vol I. New York, Raven Press, 1981;109-184.
7. Aynsley-Green A. Hormones and postnatal adaptation to enteral nutrition. J Pediatr Gastroenterol Nutr 1983;2: 418-427.
8. Lucas A, Aynsley-Green A, Bloom SR. Gut hormones and the first meals. Clin Sci 1981;60:349-353.
9. Euler AR, Byrne WJ, Cousins LM, et al. Increased serum gastrin concentrations and gastric acid hyposecretion in the immediate newborn period Gastroenterology 1977;72: 1271-1273.
10. Cozzi F, Wilkinson AW. Intrauterine growth rate in relation to anorectal and oesophageal anomalies. Arch Dis Child 1969;44:59-62.
11. Antonowicz I, Lebenthal E. Developmental patterns of small intestine enterokinase and disaccharidase activities in the human fetus. Gastroenterology 1977;72:1299-1303.
12. Hadorn B, Zoppi G, Shmerling DH, et al. Quantitative assessment of exocrine pancreatic function in infants and children. J Pediatr 1968;73:39-50.
13. Lebenthal E, Lee PC. Development of functional responses in preterm exocrine pancreas. Pediatrics 1980;66: 556-560.
14. Heringova A, Koldovský O, Jirsova V, et al. Proteolytic and peptidase activities of the small intestine of human fetuses. Gastroenterology 1966;51:1023-1027.
15. Levin RJ, Koldovský O, Hošková J, et al. Electrical activity across human foetal small intestine associated with absorption processes. Gut 1968;9:206-213.
16. Matthews DM. Intestinal absorption of peptides. Physiol Rev 1975;55:537-608.
17. Walker WA, Isselbacher KJ. Uptake and transport of macromolecules by the intestine. Possible role in clinical disorders. Gastroenterology 1974;67:531-550.
18. Iyengar L, Selvaraj RJ. Intestinal absorption of immunoglobulins by newborn infants. Arch Dis Child 1972;47: 411-414.
19. Rothberg RM. Immunoglobulin and specific antibody synthe-

sis during the first weeks of life of premature infants. J Pediatr 1969;75:391-399.

20. Fomon SJ. Comparative study of human milk and a soya bean formula in promoting growth and nitrogen retention by infants. Pediatrics 1959;24:577-584.

21. Fomon SJ. Infant Nutrition. Philadelphia: W.B. Saunders Co., 1974;118-151, 542-548.

22. Fomon SJ, Filer LJ Jr, Thomas LN, et al. Relationship between formula concentration and rate of growth of normal infants. J Nutr 1969;98:241-254.

23. Fomon SJ, Owen GM. Retention of nitrogen by normal fullterm infants receiving an autoclaved formula. Pediatrics 1962;29:1005-1011.

24. Smith CA. The Physiology of the Newborn Infant, 3rd ed. Springfield, Charles C. Thomas, 1976;416-553.

25. Pickart LR, Creasy RK, Thaler MM. Hyperfibrinogenemia and polycythemia with intrauterine growth retardation in fetal lambs. Am J Obstet Gynecol 1976;124:268-271.

26. Sturman JA, Gaull G, Raiha NCR. Absence of cystathionase in human fetal liver: is cystine essential? Science 1970; 169:74-76.

27. Avery ME, Clow CL, Menkes JH, et al. Wasserman BP. Transient tyrosinemia of the newborn: dietary and clinical aspects. Pediatrics 1967;39:378-384.

28. Menkes JH, Welcher DW, Levi HS, et al. Relationship of elevated blood tyrosine to the ultimate intellectual performance of premature infants. Pediatrics 1972;49:218-244.

29. Snell K. Regulation of protein metabolism during postnatal development. Biochem Soc Trans 1981;9:367-368.

30. Räihä NCR, Lindros KO. Development of some enzymes involved in gluconeogenesis in human liver. Ann Med Exp Biol Fenn 1969;47:146-150.

31. Jones ME, Anderson AD, Anderson C, Hodes S. Citrulline synthesis in rat tissue. Arch Biochem Biophys 1961;95:499-507.

32. Räihä NCR, Kekomäki MP. Studies on the development of ornithine-keto acid amino transferase activity in the liver. Biochem J 1968;108:521-525.

33. Räihä NCR, Suihkonen J. Development of urea-synthesizing enzymes in human liver. Acta Pediatr Scand 1968;57:121-124.

34. Edelmann CM Jr, Wolfish NM. Dietary influence on renal maturation in premature infants. Pediatr Res 2:421-422, 1968.

35. Brodehl J, Gellissen K. Endogenous renal transport of free amino acids in infancy and childhood. Pediatrics 1968;42:395-404.

36. Widdowson EM. Growth and composition of the fetus and newborn. In Assali NS (ed): Biology of Gestation, Vol II. New York, Academic Press, 1968;23.

37. Widdowson EM, Southgate DAT, Hey EN. Body composition of the fetus and infant. In Visser HKA (ed): Nutrition and Metabolism of the Fetus and Infant. The Hague, Martinus Nijhoff Publishers, 1979:169-174.

38. Food and Agriculture Organization/World Health Organization. Energy and Protein Requirements. WHO Tech. Rpt. No. 522. Geneva, World Health Organization, 1973; 40-73.

39. Räihä NCR, Heinonen K, Rassin DK, Gaull GE. Milk protein quality and quantity in low-birthweight infants. I. Metabolic responses and effects on growth. Pediatrics 1976;57:659-674.

40. Rassin DK, Gaull GE, Heinonen K, Räihä NCR. Milk protein quantity and quality in low-birth-weight infants. II. Effects on selected aliphatic amino acids in plasma and urine. Pediatrics 1977;59:407-422.

41. Harper AE, Benevenga NJ, Wohlheuter RM. Effects of ingestion of disproportionate amounts of amino acids. Physiol Rev 1970;50:428-557.

42. Munro HN, Crim MC. The proteins and amino acids. In Goodhart RS, Shils ME (eds): Modern Nutrition in Health and Disease. Philadelphia, Lea and Febiger, 1980;51-98.

43. Arroyave G. Amino acid requirements and age. In Olson RE (ed): Protein-Calorie Malnutrition. New York, Academic Press, 1975;1-22.

44. Hanson JDL, Schendel HE, Wilkins JA, Brock JF. Nitrogen

45. Jackson AA, Shaw JCL, Barber A, Golden MHN. Nitrogen metabolism in preterm infants fed human donor breast milk: the possible essentiality of glycine. Pediatr Res 1981;15:1454-1461.

46. Pencharz PB, Steffee WP, Cochran W, et al. Protein metabolism in human neonates: nitrogen-balance studies, estimated obligatory loss of nitrogen and whole-body turnover nitrogen. Clin Sci Mol Med 1977;52:485-498.

47. Filer LJ Jr, Fomon SJ, Thomas LN, Rogers RR. Growth and serum chemical values of normal breastfed infants. Acta Paediatr Scand 1970; 202(Suppl):1-20.

48. Fomon SJ, Thomas LN, Filer LJ Jr, et al. Food consumption and growth of normal infants fed milk-based formulas. Acta Paediatr Scand 1971; 223(Suppl):1-36.

49. Järvenpää A-L, Räihä NCR, Rassin DK, Gaull GE. Milk protein quantity and quality in the term infant. I. Metabolic responses and effects on growth. Pediatrics 1982;70:214-220.

50. Waterlow JC. The assessment of protein nutrition and metabolism in the whole animal with special reference to man. In Munro HN (ed): Mammalian Protein Metabolism, Vol III. Academic Press, New York, 1969;325-390.

51. Alleyne GAO, Hey RW, Picou DI, et al. Protein-energy malnutrition. London, Edward Arnold Ltd., 1977;154.

52. Snyderman SE, Holt LE Jr, Norton PM, et al. The plasma aminogram. I. Influence of the level of protein intake and a comparison of whole protein and amino acid diets. Pediatr Res 1968;2:131-144.

53. Giacoia GP, Watson S, West K. Rapid turnover transport proteins, plasma albumin, and growth in low birth weight infants. J Parent Ent Nutr 1984;8:367-370.

54. Helms RA, Dickerson RN, Ebbert ML, et al. Retinol-binding protein and prealbumin: Useful measures of protein repletion in critically ill, malnourished infants. J Pediatr Gastroenterol Nutr 1986;5:586-592.

55. Sasanow SR, Spitzer AR, Pereira GR, Heaf L, Watkins JB. Effect of gestational age upon prealbumin and retinol binding protein in preterm and term infants. J Pediatr Gastroenterol Nutr 1986;5:111-115.

56. Vahlquist A, Rask L, Peterson A, Berg T. The concentration of retinol binding protein, prealbumin, and transferrin in the sera of newly delivered mothers and children of various ages. Scand J Clin Lab Invest 1975;35:569-575.

57. Fomon SJ, Thomas LN, Filer LJ Jr, et al. Requirements for protein and essential amino acids in early infancy. Studies with a soy isolate formula. Acta Paediatr Scand 1973;62:33-45.

58. Food and Nutrition Board/National Research Council. Recommended Daily Allowances, 8th ed. Washington DC, National Academy of Sciences, 1974;37-48.

59. Snyderman SE, Holt LE Jr, Dancis J, Roitman E, Boyer A, Balis ME. "Unessential" nitrogen: a limiting factor for human growth. J Nutr 1962;78:57-72.

60. Snyderman SE. The protein and amino acid requirements of the premature infant. In Jonxis JHP, Vesser HRA, Troelstra JA (eds): Metabolic Processes in the Foetus and Newborn Infant. Lieden, Stenfert Kroese, 1971.

61. Babson SG, Bramhall JL. Diet and growth in the premature infant. J Pediatr 1969;74:890-900.

62. Davidson M, Levine SZ, Bauer CH, Dann M. Feeding studies in low-birth-weight infants. I. Relationships of dietary protein, fats, and electrolyte to rates of weight gain, clinical courses, and serum chemical concentrations. J Pediatr 1967;70:695-713.

63. Gordon HH, Levine SZ, McNamara H. Feeding of premature infants. Arch Dis Child 1947;73:422-452.

64. Kagan BM, Hess JH, Lundeen E, et al. Feeding premature infants—a comparison of various milks. Pediatrics 1955; 15:373-382.

65. Omans WB, Barness LA, Rose CS, Gyorgy P. Prolonged feeding studies in premature infants. J Pediatr 1961;59:951-957.

66. Pincus JB, Gittleman IF, Schmerzler E, Brunetti N. Protein levels in serum of premature infant fed diets varying in protein concentrations. Pediatrics 1962;30:622-628.

67. Snyderman SE, Boyer A, Kogut MD, Holt LE Jr. The protein requirement of the premature infant. I. The effect of protein intake on the retention of nitrogen. J Pediatr 1969;74:872-880.

68. Goldman HI, Freudenthal R, Holland B, Karelitz S. Clinical effect of two different levels of protein intake on low birth weight infants. J Pediatr 1969;74:881-889.

69. Goldman HI, Liebman OB, Freudenthal R, Reuben R. Effect of early dietary protein intake on low-birth-weight infants: evaluation at 3 years of age. J Pediatr 1971;78:126-129.

70. Ziegler EE, O'Donnell AM, Fomon SJ. Body composition of the reference fetus. Growth 1976;40:329-341.

71. Fomon SJ, Ziegler EE, Vazques HD. Human milk and the small premature infant. Am J Dis Child 1977;131: 463-467.

72. Gaull GE, Rassin DK, Räihä NCR, Heinonen K. Milk protein quantity and quality in low-birth-weight infants. III. Effects on sulfur amino acids in plasma and urine. J Pediatr 1977;90:348-355.

73. Rassin DK, Gaull GE, Räihä NCR, Heinonen K. Milk protein quantity and quality in low-birth-infants. IV. Effects on tyrosine and phenylalanine in plasma and urine. J Pediatr 1977;90:356-360.

74. Fomon SJ, Ziegler EE. Protein intake of premature infants: interpretation of data. J Pediatr 1977;90:504-506.

75. De Benoist B, Abdulrazzak Y, Brooke OG, et al. The measurement of whole body protein turnover in the preterm infant with intragastric infusion of L-[1-13C] leucine and sampling of the urinary leucine pool. Clin Sci 1984;66:155-164.

76. Schutz Y, Catzeflis C, Gudinchet F, et al. Energy expenditure and whole body protein synthesis in very low birth weight infants. Experientia [Suppl] 1983;44:45-56.

77. Shenai JP, Jhaveri BM, Reynolds JW, et al. Nutritional balance studies in very low-birth-weight infants: role of soy formula. Pediatrics 1981;67:631-637.

78. Mauer AM, Dweck HS, Holmes F, et al. Soy protein formulas: recommendations for use in infant feedings. Pediatrics 1973;72:359-363.

79. Newton N, Newton M. Psychologic aspects of lactation. N Engl J Med 1967;277:1179-1188.

80. Atkinson SA, Bryan MH, Anderson GH. Human milk feeding in premature infants: protein, fat, and carbohydrate balances in the first two weeks of life. J Pediatr 1981;99: 617-624.

81. Davies DP. Adequacy of expressed breast milk for early growth of preterm infants. Arch Dis Child 1977;52: 296-301.

82. Gross SJ. Growth and biochemical responses of preterm infants fed human milk or modified infant formula. N Engl J Med 1983;308:237-241.

83. Järvenpää A-L, Räihä NCR, Rassin DK, Gaull GE. Preterm infants fed human milk attain intrauterine weight gain. Acta Paediatr Scand 1983;72:239-243.

84. Chessex P, Reichman B, Verellen G, et al. Quality of growth in premature infants fed their own mothers' milk. J Pediatr 1983;102:107-112.

85. Rönnholm KAR, Sipilä I, Siimes MA. Human milk protein supplementation for the prevention of hypoproteinemia without metabolic imbalance in breast-milk fed, very low-birth weight infants. J Pediatr 1982;101:243-247.

86. Järvenpää A-L. Feeding the low-birth-weight infant. IV. Fat absorption as a function of diet and duodenal bile acids. Pediatrics 1983;72:684-689.

87. Järvenpää A-L, Räihä NCR, Rassin DK, Gaull GE. Feeding the low-birth-weight infant. I. Taurine and cholesterol supplementation of formula does not affect growth metabolism. Pediatrics 1983;71:171-178.

88. Järvenpää A-L, Rassin DK, Kuitunen P, et al. Feeding the low-birth-weight-infant: III. Diet influences bile acid metabolism. Pediatrics 1983;72;677-683.

89. Schanler RJ, Garza C, Nichols BL. Fortified mothers' milk for very low birth weight infants: results of growth and nutrient balance studies. J Pediatr 1985;107:437-445.

90. American Academy of Nutrition Committee on Nutrition. Commentary on Parenteral Nutrition. Pediatrics 1983;71: 547-552.

91. Kanarek KS, Williams PR, Curran JS. Total parenteral nutrition in infants and children. Adv Pediatr 1982;29: 151-181.

92. Anderson TL, Muttart CR, Bierber MA, et al. A controlled trial of glucose versus glucose and amino acids in premature infants. J Pediatr 1979;947-951.

93. Rubecz I, Mestyán J, Varga P, Klujber L. Energy metabolism, substrate utilization, and nitrogen balance in parenterally fed postoperative neonates and infants. J Pediatr 1981; 98:42-46.

94. Duffy B, Gunn T, Collinge J, Pencharz P. The effect of varying protein quality and energy intake on the nitrogen metabolism of parenterally fed very low-birth-weight (<1600 g) infants. Pediatr Res 1981;15:1040-1044.

95. Zlotkin SH, Bryan MH, Anderson GH. Intravenous nitrogen and energy intakes required to duplicate in utero nitrogen accretion in prematurely born human infants. J Pediatr 1981;99:115-120.

96. Zlotkin SH, Bryan MH, Anderson GH. Cysteine supplementation to cysteine-free intravenous feeding regimens in newborn infants. Am J Clin Nutr 1981;34:914-923.

97. Suskind RM. Textbook of Pediatric Nutrition. New York, Raven Press, 1981;189-228.

98. Cooper A, Jakobowski D, Spiker J, et al. Nutritional assessment: an integral part of the preoperative pediatric surgical evaluation. J Pediatr Surg 1981; 16(Suppl 1):554-561.

99. Baker S. Protein-energy malnutrition in the hospitalized pediatric patient. In Walker WA, Watkins JB, (eds): Nutrition in Pediatrics: Basic Science and Clinical Application. Boston, Little, Brown and Co., 1985;171-181.

100. Blackburn GL, Bistrian BR, Harvey K: Indices of protein-calorie malnutrition as predictors of survival. In Levenson SM, McBean LD, Redfern DE (eds). Nutritional Assessment: Present Status, Future Directions and Prospects. Columbus, Ohio, Ross Laboratories, 1981;131-137.

101. Hey RW, Whitehead RG, Spicer CC. Serum albumin as a prognostic indicator in oedematous malnutrition. Lancet 1975;2:427-429.

102. Georgieff MK, Sasanow SR. Nutritional assessment of the neonate. Clin Perinatol 1986;13:73-89.

103. Halpern SR, Sellars WA, Johnson RB, et al. Development of childhood allergy in infants fed breast, soy, or cow milk. J Allergy Clin Immunol 1973;51:139-151.

104. Wilson JF, Lahey ME, Heiner DC. Studies on iron metabolism. V. Further observations on cow's milk-induced gastrointestinal bleeding in infants with iron deficiency anemia. J Pediatr 1974;84:335-344.

105. Powell GK. Milk- and soy-induced enterocolitis of infancy. J Pediatr 1978;93:553-560.

106. Goldman AS, Anerson DW Jr, Sellers WA, Saperstein S, Kniker WT, Halpern SR. Milk allergy. I. Oral challenge with milk and isolated milk proteins in allergic children. Pediatrics 1963;32:425-443.

107. Lake AM, Whittington PF, Hamilton SR. Dietary protein-induced colitis in breast-fed infants. J Pediatr 1982;101: 906-910.

108. Caballero B. Dietary management of inborn errors of amino acid metabolism. Clin Nutr 1985;4:85-94.

7

Carbohydrate Needs in Preterm and Term Newborn Infants

CARLOS H. LIFSCHITZ, MD

ABSTRACT

Carbohydrates are the most abundant and least expensive of the three major nutrients. Birth drastically changes the nutriture of the infant from an exclusive intravenous infusion of glucose to a process that requires sucking, swallowing, digestion, and absorption of carbohydrates, protein, and fat. The newborn infant, particularly the preterm infant, depends on carbohydrates for caloric and metabolic needs. Hypoglycemia and hyperglycemia can occur with the administration of minimal or excessive amounts of carbohydrate, respectively; however, neither specific deficiencies nor toxicities have been described in *normal* subjects. Fewer problems are encountered with the enteral and parenteral administration of carbohydrates in the term, well-nourished infant than in the preterm and/or malnourished child. In this chapter, we will review aspects related to enteral and parenteral administration of sugars and the development of carbohydrate digestion and utilization.

INTRODUCTION

Dr. John Rodman of Paisley, Scotland reported a case of an infant born on 19 April 1815 with a gestation of less than 19 weeks (?) "The nourishing heat with the mother in bed was relied on . . . the child was kept regularly and comfortably warm by the mother and two females alternately lying in bed with him for more than two months. . . . " At three weeks of age, the infant's length was 13 inches and his weight, clothes and all, was 2 pounds and one half; the weight of the clothes was 11 ounces. But "it was extremely difficult to get the child to swallow nourishment the first week and that which was principally used was toasted loaf bread boiled in water, with the addition of a little sugar and strained or passed through a fine linen. He was frequently applied to the breast in order to encourage the formation of milk and also to give him a chance of some falling into his mouth."[1]

Dietary carbohydrates provide 24 to 50% of the infant's energy needs and, in addition, constitute a form of energy storage (see chapter 5). The percentage of energy provided by carbohydrates, however, can be as high as 100% in the intravenously-fed infant. Although glucose is the major source of energy at the cellular level, carbohydrate is rarely ingested as such. The infant who is fed milk exclusively receives mainly disaccharides and, in certain cases, nonbranch glucose polymers. Disaccharides are hydrolyzed by intestinal brush border enzymes and the constituent carbohydrates are then absorbed and metabolized. More complex carbohydrates (starches) are introduced to the infant's diet with the addition of cereal. The newborn infant is not prepared developmentally to swallow semisolids or to digest starch.

In addition to the caloric contribution, carbohydrates are needed for the synthesis of nucleic acids. **Moreover, glucose is the principal nutrient that the brain of the neonate utilizes.** There is evidence that ketone bodies also can be utilized as a source of energy by the brain of newborns.[2]

The minimal amount of carbohydrates needed is determined by the metabolic requirements; theoretically, calories required for maintenance or growth could be provided by other nutrients. In general, carbohydrates are inexpensive and abundant sources of energy. Although energy requirements would be extremely difficult to meet during severe carbohydrate restriction, the intake of subminimal amounts of carbohydrates ordinarily would not lead to specific deficiencies as would occur with that of other nutrients. Hypoglycemia does occur, however, when the amount of carbohydrate is inadequate. Although toxicity from excessive carbohydrate intakes is unknown in *normal* individuals, diarrhea or hyperglycemia may result when the amount of carbohydrates delivered is too large to be absorbed or metabolized. The excessive intake of carbohydrates will lead to obesity but generally will not result in overt toxicity.

The nutrition of the fetus is similar to that of a patient who receives a constant intravenous infusion of glucose. At birth, the infant passes abruptly to periodic oral feedings. From a nutritional point of view, cutting the umbilical cord is equivalent to writing the order "DC IV" (discontinue intravenous). Based on studies of rats during early gestation and of fetal animals, birds, reptiles, and invertebrates at maturity, carbohydrate is the primary fetal nutrient.[3] With nutrients no longer delivered passively, the newborn undergoes a profound nutritional adaptation. In extrauterine life, protein and fat are introduced into the diet, although carbohydrates continue to provide the major source of calories, approximately 25 to 50% of the energy. The carbohydrate concentration of feedings in the neonatal period is constant; human milk and most infant formulas contain 7% lactose, and cow milk contains 5% lactose.

Dietary carbohydrate was considered an innocuous compound until the early part of this century when the German pediatrician Finkelstein captured the attention of other physicians by suggesting that carbohydrates caused gastrointestinal disturbances. He attributed the acute form of infantile disease characterized by stupor, melituria, and fever as the result of dietary sugar. In agreement with other physicians of the time, Finkelstein considered lactose "extremely pyrogenic." These authors also blamed the mineral salts in cow milk for causing fever in both ill and healthy infants. Emphasis was later placed on the damage caused by bacterial fermentation of lactose in the intestine rather than on direct toxicity. The Finkelstein school of thought in 1910 suggested that fermenting lactose injured the permeability of the intestinal wall permitting the absorption of an abnormal quantity and quality of salts which alone or in combination with sugar produced poisoning.

PHYSIOLOGY

Glucose, Fructose and Galactose. The products that result from the digestion of dietary carbohydrates, i.e., glucose, fructose, and galactose, are absorbed through the intestinal mucosa into the portal venous system.

Absorption occurs by three mechanisms: active transport, simple diffusion, and facilitated diffusion. Both glucose and galactose are absorbed from the lumen of the intestine by active transport. Glucose and sodium bind to separate sites of a mobile carrier[4] which transports them into the cytoplasm of the intestinal cell and returns for another "load." Sodium is transported down its concentration gradient, simultaneously causing the carrier to transport glucose against its concentration gradient. The free energy required to activate the carrier is obtained from the hydrolysis of ATP, which is linked to a sodium pump that expels sodium from the cell.

Glucose. Active transport of glucose occurs in the jejunum of 10-week-old human fetuses and increases with the length of gestation (Fig. 1).[5] Glucose absorption, however, is incompletely developed in the term infant, and the 12-month-old infant has a limited capacity to absorb glucose, compared with children older than 2 years of age (Fig. 2).[6]

Fructose. Fructose, like glucose, is a hexose. It is found in some fruit juices and in honey, and can result from the hydrolysis of sucrose, a reaction that also produces glucose. The metabolism of fructose leads to the formation of glycogen and pyruvate.[4] The absorption of fructose through the intestinal mucosa is an energy-independent mechanism, proceeds slower than that of glucose and galactose, and occurs by facilitated diffusion along a concentration gradient.[7]

Galactose. Galactose, which is not found in the diet, is produced by the intestinal hydrolysis of lactose. The mechanism for intestinal absorption of galactose is the same as that for glucose.[4]

Sucrose. Sucrose is formed by one molecule each of glucose and fructose. The disaccharidase, sucrase, hydrolyzes both sucrose and maltose (Table 1). Sucrase activity occurs in the fetal intestine at levels comparable with those found in the mature intestine (Fig. 2). Maximal specific activity, however, is found in

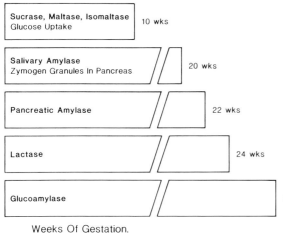

Sucrase, Maltase, Isomaltase Glucose Uptake	10 wks
Salivary Amylase Zymogen Granules In Pancreas	20 wks
Pancreatic Amylase	22 wks
Lactase	24 wks
Glucoamylase	24-28 wks

Weeks Of Gestation.

FIGURE 1. Appearance during gestation of different carbohydrate digestive and absorptive processes. (Adapted from published data.[5-7])

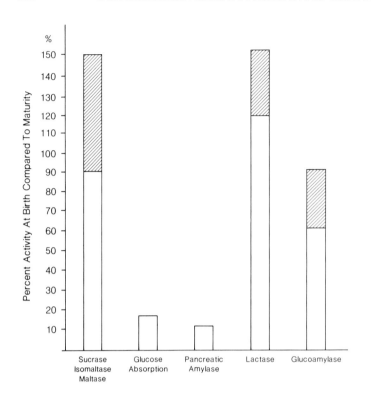

FIGURE 2. A comparison of the activity levels of several carbohydrate digestive and absorptive processes at birth and during mature function. Each bar represents the percentage or range at birth compared to that when the mature function is achieved. Shaded area represents range. (Adapted from the published data.[5-7])

the proximal jejunum of 17- to 24-week-old fetuses (see Figs. 1-4).[8] The sucrase-isomaltase enzyme complex is produced as a single high-molecular weight protein and becomes a dimer at the microvillous membrane. The dimer consists of two subunits that can be separated readily from each other and act independently upon a different substrate.[9]

Lactose. Lactose, a disaccharide formed by glucose and galactose, is the only dietary galactoside that man can digest (Table 1). Lactose is hydrolyzed selectively by a brush border enzyme called lactase, which is located predominantly in the tip of the intestinal villi (Fig. 3). Digestion of lactose is the rate-limiting step in its absorption.

Low activity levels of lactase are present in

the small bowel of fetuses younger than 24 weeks of gestation (Fig. 1).[10] **Lactase activity develops later in fetal life than that of other disaccharidases,** is greatest in the proximal jejunum, and decreases distally (Figs. 1 and 4). Lactase levels increase progressively as gestation proceeds, reaching concentrations at term 2 to 4 times those found in infants 2 to 11 months of age (Fig. 2). However, preterm infants who survive more than 24 hours have higher intestinal lactase levels independent of milk intake than those who die on the first day.[10] Cicco et al. have shown that 2- to 3-week-old preterm infants achieve plasma-reducing substance levels similar to those of term infants after the feeding of glucose polymers or lactose.[11]

TABLE 1.   Dietary Carbohydrate Digestion

Carbohydrate	Enzyme	Appearance in Fetal Life (wk)	Products of Digestion
Lactose	Lactase	>24	Glucose and galactose
Glucose polymers	Amylase		
	Human milk	—	Shorter glucose polymers
	Salivary	>20	Shorter glucose polymers
	Pancreatic	>22	Shorter glucose polymers
	Glucoamylase	>24	Glucose monomers
	Maltase	>14	Glucose monomers
Sucrose	Sucrase-Isomaltase	>10	Glucose and fructose

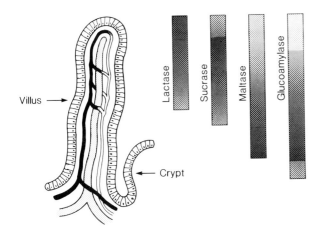

FIGURE 3. Distribution of disaccharidases along the intestinal villus. The darker markings indicate greater concentrations. This graph is an approximation and does not correspond to actual enzyme concentrations.

Glucose Polymers. Glucose polymers are composed of 5 to 10 glucose units joined linearly (with few lateral chains) by 1-4 alpha linkages. For glucose polymers to be absorbed, they first must be hydrolyzed to their glucose components by amylase, maltase, or glucoamylase (Table 1 and Fig. 5).

Amylase is present in human milk, saliva, and the pancreas. The content of amylase in human milk is 10 to 50 times higher than that in adult serum.[12] Salivary and pancreatic amylases can be detected in the fetus at 20 and 22 weeks of gestation, respectively (Fig. 1). Amylase activity in pancreatic homogenates from term neonates is approximately 10% of that in adults. Mature levels of pancreatic amylase often are not achieved until after birth (Fig. 2).[10] Amylase is not contained in the duodenal fluid of preterm and term infants; its production cannot be stimulated by administering pancreozymin and secretin.[13] At one month of age, the response to hormonal stimulation is minimal; maximal response is not achieved until two years of age.

Maltase hydrolyzes oligomers which contain two glucose units (maltose) and three glucose units (maltriose). Maltase is present in the fetus at the tenth week of gestation and reaches adult levels by 6 to 8 months (Fig. 1).[10] The development of maltase activity does not appear dependent on the time of birth or feeding time.

Glucoamylase is a brush border enzyme which acts predominantly upon glucose oligomers containing 4 to 9 glucose units. Located predominantly at the base of the villi (Fig. 3), glucoamylase appears to survive partial intestinal villous atrophy which may result from enteritis. Glucoamylase activity in neonates and infants ranges from 50 to 100% that

of adults (Fig. 2)[14] and is present in the intestine of fetuses of 28 weeks' gestation.

Glucose polymers are utilized as sources of carbohydrates for caloric supplementation and as substitutes for lactose in special formulas. Because of their structure, **glucose polymers produce a lower osmolar load than an equimolar amount of glucose.** Several studies have demonstrated an inverse relationship between polymer chain length and digestibility.[15]

Starch. Infants consume starch usually in the form of cereal, although small amounts can be found in certain special infant formulas (see chapter 24). The two major forms of starch are amylose (molecular weight of 100,000 or greater), which is composed of a linear chain of glucose units joined by alpha 1-4 linkages, and amylopectin (molecular weight of 1,000,000), which is composed of linear 1-4 linked chains and lateral chains joined by alpha 1-6 linkages.[7]

Starch hydrolysis begins in the duodenum with the action of pancreatic amylase. Breakdown of the interior bonds of amylose results in two oligosaccharides, maltose and maltotriose (Fig. 5). The alpha 1-6 linkages, and the 1-4 bonds which are close to the 1-6 links or terminal on carbohydrate chains, are resistant to cleavage by alpha amylase.[16] The products of starch hydrolysis, therefore, are glucose units joined in a linear manner and in a branched manner (alpha-limit dextrins). The alpha 1-6 linkages are digested by a-dextrinase (isomaltase) and converted into glucose units joined linearly (alpha 1-4). Only small amounts of free glucose are released by the action of salivary and pancreatic amylases.[16] Finally, the products of starch digestion are hydrolyzed by intestinal enzymes located

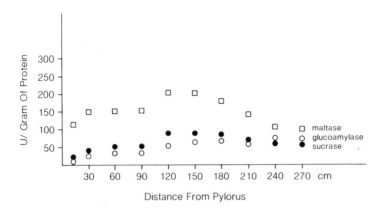

FIGURE 4. Disaccharidase distribution along the small bowel of a full-term newborn infant. Note that sucrase and lactase activities are higher in the jejunum while glucoamylase activity increases distally and is highest near the ileocecal valve. Maltase activity is intermediate between sucrase and glucoamylase. (Adapted from the data of Auricchio et al.[7])

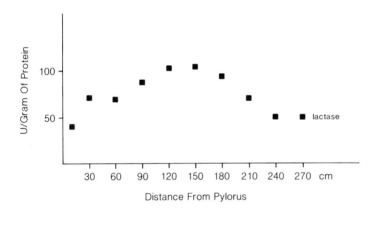

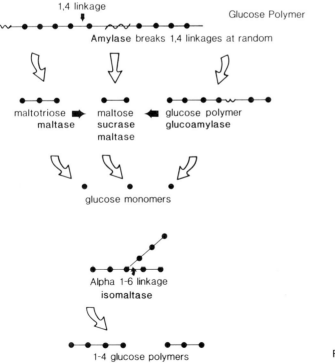

FIGURE 5.   Digestion of glucose polymers.

in the brush border, i.e., maltase, sucrase, isomaltase, and glucoamylase.

Fiber. Dietary fiber comprises carbohydrate compounds resistant to enzyme degradation in the gastrointestinal tract. The suggestion that dietary fiber may help to prevent certain diseases in the older adult population has stimulated a great deal of interest and research. The utilization of fiber may diminish the risk for diverticulosis, obesity, atherosclerosis, coronary heart disease, and cancer of the colon.[17] The addition of fiber to the diet results in softer and more frequent stools, which are direct advantages to the pediatric population. In the United States, 75% of children have been estimated to eat less than the recommended amount of fiber, contained mainly in fruits, vegetables, legumes, and whole grain cereals and breads.

However, use of fiber in the diet of infants and young children has attracted criticism. Objections include early satiety produced by the ingestion of fiber, which is low in calories, and interference with the absorption of certain minerals that are essential to the diet, i.e., calcium, copper, iron, magnesium, phosphorus, and zinc.[17] The mechanism by which fiber diminishes mineral bioavailability is the formation of insoluble compounds with phytate. The possibility exists that infants under one year of age do not require fiber in the diet.[17]

Effect of Carbohydrate on Osmolality. Glucose used as a source of dietary carbohydrate in infant formulas increases osmolality. Human milk and lactose-containing formulas have an osmolality of 290 mOsm/kg. An isocaloric amount of glucose substituted for lactose in a formula increases the osmolality by 200 mOsm/kg. If glucose were used as a caloric supplement, every gram of glucose added to 100 ml of formula in excess of 7 gm/100 ml would increase the osmolality 58 mOsm/kg. Even though the addition of glucose increases the osmolality of a formula, glucose may be the ideal carbohydrate for infants with severe sugar intolerance. Glucose is recommended particularly if the formula is delivered as a constant gastric drip, in which case a higher osmolality may be tolerated more easily.

Effects of Carbohydrates in the Regulation of Gastric Emptying. Although the number of studies on gastric emptying in newborn infants is limited,[18] extensive work has been performed in adults. Results indicate that the carbohydrate concentration and osmolality influence the rate of gastric emptying, which is approximately 2 kcal/min in healthy adults.[19] Gastric emptying is delayed by hyperosmolar and hypercaloric solutions.

Siegel et al. studied gastric emptying in ten premature infants who were fed formula at varying caloric concentrations.[18] **A significant inhibition of gastric emptying was related to increasing caloric density,** despite the fact that feedings of greater caloric density were associated with the emptying of more calories over comparable periods.

CARBOHYDRATE NEEDS

In 1848, an infant born after 26 weeks of gestation who weighed 680 grams at 7 days survived. The infant was wrapped in folds of cotton wool and covered with flannel. An earthenware bottle, filled with warm water, was placed behind the cushion. Dr. Anan reports: "As the infant showed more signs of vitality, the lips and mouth were gently moistened with a mixture of one part of cream, three parts of warm water, and sweetened with sugar. At first it was observed to swallow, but in the evening when I returned, there could be little doubt that this had been the case from the minute quantities of mixture, given from time to time, not having been rejected. On the following day, to this mixture from 3 to 4 drops of sherry wine were added and continued to be used as yesterday. On the third day the deglutition was very perceptible . . . on the seventh day, the child was weighed and found, including a small flannel roller, to be 24 ounces. The roller was under one ounce in weight. . . . Occasionally a small portion of magnesia usta or castor oil was given, so as to ensure regularity in the bowels. About the end of the third week very fine oatmeal gruel, sweetened with sugar, was alternated with the cream and water, the quantity of wine being gradually increased."[1]

In contrast to protein and other nutrients, i.e., vitamins and minerals, no recommended daily allowance has been established for carbohydrates in normal individuals. A relatively low amount of carbohydrate is needed for metabolic requirements; otherwise, energy could be supplied by protein and fat. In the unstressed subject, extremely low or high intakes of carbohydrates may result in "malnutrition" (undernutrition or obesity, respectively) but generally not in specific deficiencies or toxicity. However, the stressed patient, e.g., the preterm infant, the asphyxiated newborn, or the septic, burned, or postoperative patient, requires well-defined amounts of carbohydrates in order to meet his nutritional needs. Specifically, hypoglycemia can result from an inadequate glucose supply and hyperglycemia can occur with an excessive glucose supply.

Enteral Needs

Term Infants. For the majority of healthy neonates, lactose is the only source of carbohydrates; both human milk and special infant formulas have a concentration of 7.1 gm/dl. Therefore, a breastfed infant who ingests 150 ml of milk/kg/day receives 10 gm of lactose/kg/day, while a bottle-fed infant who ingests 200 ml of formula/kg/day receives about 14 gm of lactose/kg/day. If lactose digestion and absorption are complete, this intake assures the normal, unstressed infant at least 4 mg/kg/min of glucose, which is the rate of glucose utilization in such infants as measured by non-radioactive isotopes.[20]

The normal term infant regulates glucose homeostasis without much difficulty and, therefore, is able to feed every three to four hours after birth. The term newborn infant has a storage of 34 gm of glycogen, of which 6 gm is in the liver. In the postprandial period, the glucose that has not been utilized (oxidized) immediately is stored as glycogen in the liver. By a reverse mechanism and under appropriate hormonal stimuli, the infant can transform glycogen into glucose (glycogenolysis) and therefore maintain adequate serum glucose concentrations. A carbohydrate intake less than 4 mg/kg/min will lead to gluconeogenesis (the process by which glucose is generated from noncarbohydrate sources).[20] During the first 48 hours of life, however, the infant's capacity for gluconeogenesis is limited.

Diets that provide less than 10% of the calories as carbohydrates will produce ketosis, a condition more likely to occur in children than in adults.[20] Ketone bodies, however, constitute an alternate source of energy. Although the brain of the newborn infant can utilize ketone bodies,[2] preterm infants in particular may be unable to produce sufficient ketone bodies to support all of their energy needs.[21] In the presence of hypoglycemia, they would be left without metabolizable energy. Mainly for this reason, **newborns should receive 40 to 45% of the calories as carbohydrates.**

Based on the amount of lactase present in the intestine, the estimated amount of lactose that term newborn infants can digest is 8 gm/kg/day. The quantity is contained in approximately 114 ml of human milk or formula per kg weight. Soon after birth, however, formula-fed infants ingest a quantity of lactose greater than 8 gm/kg/day. Auricchio et al. speculated that the larger lactose load in the diet of the healthy term infant exceeded the capacity of the small intestine to hydrolyze the sugar.[10] MacLean and coworkers, however, studied term infants and concluded that they absorb lactose in the small bowel almost completely.[22] **The small amounts of carbohydrate "malabsorbed" in the small bowel reach the colon where they are digested** by intestinal bacteria and produce gases (e.g., carbon dioxide and hydrogen) and short-chain ("volatile") fatty acids (e.g., acetate, butyrate, and propionate).[23] Lifschitz et al. studied a group of exclusively breastfed infants and determined that incomplete small bowel absorption of carbohydrate could persist for several months, although weight gain remained normal and the infants were asymptomatic and healthy.[24]

Preterm Infants. The preterm infant has a very high brain-to-body weight ratio, and estimates have indicated high brain glucose requirements. Therefore, the major site of glucose consumption by the preterm infant is most likely the brain.[25] Hypoglycemia in the newborn and particularly the preterm or malnourished infant can have catastrophic effects.

More than thirty years ago sugar absorption in premature infants was demonstrated to be virtually complete.

MacLean et al. studied lactose assimilation in preterm infants and concluded that they normally malabsorb substantial amounts of lactose.[26] Metabolic acidosis, observed in growing preterm infants and in malnourished infants recovering from diarrhea, has been attributed to colonic absorption of volatile fatty acids (see above).[27] The acidosis usually can be corrected by diminishing the oral carbohydrate intake, using simpler carbohydrates, using a combination of carbohydrates, e.g., glucose and glucose polymers, or administering the formula by constant intragastric drip through a tube. An intragastric drip may facilitate the small bowel digestion and absorption of formula when small amounts of formula are delivered constantly rather than in a bolus (see chapter 19).

Parenteral Needs

Term Infants. Glucose is presently the only carbohydrate available for intravenous use and constitutes the major source of calories for patients fed parenterally. The general concepts mentioned above for enteral carbohydrate administration also are valid for parenteral carbohydrates. The newborn infant may not tolerate intravenously infused glucose as well as the older infant or adult. Although a certain degree of glucose intolerance can be found even in older children under stress conditions,[28] fairly high concentrations (20%) of intravenously infused glucose generally are well tolerated due to an appropriate insulin response.[29] The amount of carbohydrates administered to the stressed infant, however, must be calculated carefully. The intravenous administration of glucose to term newborns can begin at a rate of 8 mg/kg/min and probably increased without problems to 12 to 14 mg/kg/min.[30]

During the first three days of life, the disappearance rate of glucose from the circulation is about 1% per minute, after which it increases steadily.[31]

Because glycogen stores are limited in newborn infants, sudden discontinuation of intravenously administered glucose may result in sudden hypoglycemia, especially if concentrations are high and stimulation of insulin release is maximal.

Preterm Infants. The use of intravenous infusions of 10% glucose in low birthweight preterm infants was reported more than 20 years ago to decrease mortality. It also was shown that the same intervention resulted in decreased catabolism. These reports initiated serious attempts at successful intravenous alimentation of the preterm infant.

The intolerance to intravenous carbohydrates is even greater in preterm infants. Hyperglycemia is frequent and may lead to osmotic diuresis and dehydration.[32] Several reasons may account for this problem, among which insulin resistance, decreased insulin production, and abnormal insulin receptors probably are the most important.[33] Simultaneous administration of insulin may be used to overcome some of the problems related to hyperglycemia. **However, the preterm infant's response to insulin can be unpredictable.**[33,34]

The disappearance rate of glucose from the circulatory system in slightly preterm infants under one day of age is similar to that of term infants.[31,35] Following the initial day of life, the progressive increase in glucose tolerance correlates with postnatal age.[31,35] The capacity to clear glucose in the very low birthweight infant, however, is not as efficient. In contrast to the pattern of increasing glucose tolerance demonstrated by 1-day-old term and preterm infants with birth weights over 1000 gm, the very low birthweight infant of the same age will clear the second of two successive intravenous

loads of glucose slower than the first.[36]

Glucose infusions begun at 6 mg/kg/min are recommended for infants weighing less than 1000 gm, and infusions not exceeding 8 mg/kg/min are recommended for infants weighing between 1000 and 1500 gm. Increments of the infusion should be made with caution and the infant should be monitored closely for the presence of glycosuria,[30] which may lead also to sodium and calcium losses.

Infusions high in carbohydrates will increase CO_2 production, which may result in CO_2 retention and respiratory acidosis in children with pulmonary problems. This problem can be resolved by administering the same amount of calories from a combination of carbohydrates and lipids (see chapter 7). Considerable amounts of carbohydrates infused over a long period will lead to fatty infiltration of the liver.[37]

CARBOHYDRATE DEFICIENCIES

At the beginning of this century, early feeding of premature infants within the first 12 hours of birth was encouraged because it was generally held that small infants could not tolerate starvation. However, delaying the first feeding until the second or third day or even longer in sick or very small infants became the custom in the 1940s. In 1954 E. Cross wrote, "In recent years, the survival rate has been improved by giving *nothing* by mouth for several days." In her nursery, the smallest infants were submitted to the longest periods of starvation, for example, four to five days for infants weighing 2 pounds and less. In 1955, Gleiss reported a lower mortality (28%) in premature infants who were given their first feeding between 12 and 24 hours compared with that of infants who were fed initially at 36 hours (41%).[1]

Pathologic Carbohydrate Malabsorption

We have mentioned above that some dietary carbohydrate remains unabsorbed by the small bowel and reaches the colon. In certain abnormal cases (Table 2), however, the amount of carbohydrate malabsorbed is much larger. The intestinal capacity to absorb glucose is limited by the total absorptive surface area and is dependent on intestinal transit time.[38] **The capacity to absorb lactose is limited by the rate of hydrolysis of the sugar.** Greater amounts of carbohydrates will reach the colon consequent to excessive intake, incomplete digestion, or incomplete absorption. Excessive intakes of carbohydrates, rare in breastfed infants, can occur in bottle-fed infants and cause sugar malabsorption that results in diarrhea. Incomplete digestion and

TABLE 2.   Pathologic Carbohydrate
Malabsorption

Excessive intake
Incomplete absorption:
  Rapid transit time
  Impaired digestion:
    Disaccharide deficiency (congenital or acquired)
    Pancreatic insufficiency
  Reduced absorptive surface area:
    Mucosal atrophy (acute or chronic diarrhea)
    Short bowel (congenital or acquired)

absorption are caused by a congenital or acquired deficiency of disaccharidases, or by very rapid intestinal transit time which decreases the exposure of the carbohydrates to digestive enzymes. Absorption also may be impaired if the intestinal surface is decreased, as in small bowel villous atrophy following gastroenteritis or in congenital or acquired short bowel, e.g., following resection for necrotizing enterocolitis (Table 2).[38] An equilibrium normally exists between the small bowel "malabsorption" of dietary carbohydrates and the colonic bacterial fermentation of unabsorbed dietary carbohydrates. The disruption of equilibrium may result in diarrhea, acid stools, and/or the presence of undigested sugars in feces. Bacterial fermentation of malabsorbed carbohydrates from the small bowel is absent or incomplete in newborn infants with an incompletely developed colonic flora, those treated with antibiotics, and those with ileostomies. In such circumstances, carbohydrate that arrives in the colon will not be metabolized and diarrhea is likely to occur.[39]

CARBOHYDRATE EXCESS

Excessive intakes of carbohydrates do not occur in the exclusively breastfed infant and cannot occur as an isolated problem in the exclusively bottle-fed infant in whom an excessive carbohydrate intake is accompanied by excessive fat ingestion, ultimately leading to obesity. Diarrhea can result from an excessive milk intake (more than 190 to 230 ml of formula or cow milk/kg/day), particularly if additional carbohydrates are administered in the form of sucrose or starch (cereal).

Carbohydrate Toxicity

Carbohydrates ingested in nutritionally appropriate quantities do not lead to toxicity in normal subjects. Excessive enteral intakes of carbohydrate can result in diarrhea and meteorism. Excessive amounts of intravenously administered carbohydrates can lead to hyperglycemia and hypertriglyceridemia.

In subjects with congenital intolerance to galactose (see chapter 21) or fructose,[40] intake of these carbohydrates can result in toxic effects.

Congenital fructose intolerance is due to a deficiency in the enzyme fructose-1, 6-diphosphatase. Although these patients develop fasting hypoglycemia, hepatomegaly, and lactic acidosis following the ingestion of fructose, they can lead normal lives if they refrain from ingesting that sugar.

PRACTICAL CONSIDERATIONS FOR TERM AND PRETERM INFANTS

Carbohydrates are a major source of calories in infant nutrition (Table 3). In healthy preterm and term infants, lactose is well tolerated at 7% concentration in milks and provides approximately 40 to 50% of the calories. If an increase in caloric density is necessary, addition

TABLE 3.   Comparison of Carbohydrate Content of Infant Formulas

Trade name	Carbohydrate (g/L)	Lactose (%)	Glucose Polymers (%)	Energy (cal/oz)	Protein whey/casein
Similac 20* (Ross)	72	100	—	20	18:82
Enfamil 20†					
(Mead-Johnson)	72	100	—	20	60:40
SMA (Wyeth)	72	100	—	20	60:40
Similac 24 LBW (Ross)	85	50	50	24	18:82
Similac Special Care 20‡					
(Ross)	72	50	50	20	60:40
Enfamil Premature Formula§					
(Mead-Johnson)	89	40	60	24	60:40
Preemie SMA (Wyeth)	86	50	50	24	60:40

*13, 24, and 27 cal/oz also available.
†13, 24, and 40 cal/oz also available.
‡24 cal/oz also available.
§20 cal/oz also available.

of glucose polymers rather than glucose is preferable, since carbohydrates and particularly monomers such as glucose contribute substantially to the osmolality of formula. Hyperosmolar feedings may not be well tolerated.[41] Therefore, the amount and concentration of carbohydrates present in the formula must be calculated with attention, particularly in high-risk newborns, as **carbohydrate concentrations above 9% can lead to intolerance.**

Another factor to consider when calculating the carbohydrate intake of small infants is their *glycogen stores*. Liver storage of glycogen in small malnourished and stressed infants is limited; therefore, maintenance of normal glycemia is difficult. Infants to whom carbohydrate cannot be provided enterally, such as in cases of ileus, severe vomiting, or diarrhea, should receive intravenous supplementation.

Because sucrose is generally the sweetest carbohydrate, infants who have been fed a sucrose-containing formula (such as Isomil) may refuse one containing a less sweet carbohydrate, such as lactose or glucose polymers. The temporary addition of a noncaloric edulcorant may solve the problem of formula rejection.

tion of the infusate was decreased but glycosuria persisted. Later, nasal flaring, tachypnea, and poor peripheral perfusion were noted. A chest radiograph and several complete blood counts were normal. A gram-negative organism was grown from a urine culture. One day after antibiotic treatment was started, the infusate glucose concentration was increased to previous levels and was well tolerated.

Comment. The sudden intolerance to previously well-tolerated intravenous glucose infusion is an alarm for sepsis. In such cases, a sepsis "workup" is indicated initially rather than the addition of insulin to the infusate.

Questions and Answers

Q.   Under what circumstance would insulin infusion be used to control hyperglycemia?
A.   If sepsis can be ruled out or is being treated, the addition of insulin is pertinent when an increase in the amount of glucose administered results in glycosuria.

Q.   Couldn't one just lower the glucose concentration of the infusate?
A.   The glucose concentration could be lowered; however, care should be exercised when concentrations of glucose are less than 5%, because *hypoosmolar* infusions can easily lead to severe hemolysis in infants. If glucose concentrations are less than 5%, iso-osmolar concentrations should be maintained by addition of electrolytes. In addition, it would be difficult to provide adequate calories with low glucose concentrations.

CASE REPORTS

Case 1. A 25-day-old, bottle-fed infant developed gastroenteritis and was fed a diluted lactose formula for two days. On the third day, when full-strength formula was administered, the child developed watery stools and dehydration. Following rehydration, he was given lactose-free formula containing glucose polymers as the source of carbohydrate. The infant tolerated the formula and regained his pre-illness weight in a few days. A week later the lactose-containing formula was reintroduced progressively without any problems.

Comment. Many infants develop *lactose malabsorption* following an episode of acute gastroenteritis. Substitution of lactose with other carbohydrates may solve this temporary problem and, therefore, may prevent malnutrition.

Question and Answer

Q.   How long should such infants be on a lactose-free formula?
A.   The length of time depends on many factors such as severity of diarrhea, etiology, and nutritional status of the child. In moderate cases, bottle-fed infants usually can resume lactose-containing formulas three to seven days after the initiation of the diarrheal episode.

Case 2. An 1100-gram preterm infant was placed on total parenteral nutrition because he had developed necrotizing enterocolitis. The infant had tolerated the infusion well for five days when suddenly glycosuria was noted. The serum sugar was 198 mg/dl. The glucose concentra-

ACKNOWLEDGMENT
This work is a publication of the USDA/ARS Children's Nutrition Research Center, Department of Pediatrics, Baylor College of Medicine and Texas Children's Hospital, Houston, TX. This project has been funded in part with federal funds from the U.S. Department of Agriculture, Agricultural Research Service under Cooperative Agreement number 58-7MNI-6-100. The contents of this publication do not necessarily reflect the views or policies of the U.S. Department of Agriculture, nor does mention of trade names, commercial products, or organizations imply endorsement by the U.S. Government.

REFERENCES

1. Cone TE Jr. History of the Care and Feeding of the Premature Infant. Boston, Little, Brown and Co., 1985;18,20,73.
2. Denne SC, Kalhan SC. Glucose carbon recycling and oxidation in human newborns. Am J Physiol 1986;251:E71-E77.
3. Hay WW Jr, Sparks JW, Quissell BJ, et al. Simultaneous measurements of umbilical uptake, fetal utilization rate, and fetal turnover rate of glucose. Am J Physiol 1981;240:E662-E668.
4. Harper HA, Rodwell VW, Mayes PA. Digestion and absorption from the gastrointestinal tract. In Harper HA, Rodwell VW (eds): Physiological Chemistry, 16th ed. Los Altos, CA, Lange Medical Publications, 1977;202-217.
5. Koldovsky, O. Development of the functions of the small intestine in mammals and man. Basel, Switzerland, S Basel and AG Karger, Publishers, 1969;168.
6. Younoszai MK. Jejunal absorption of hexose in infants and children. J Pediatr 1974;85:446-448.

7. Gray GM. Carbohydrate absorption and malabsorption. In Johnson LR (ed): Physiology of the Gastrointestinal Tracts. New York, Raven Press, 1981;1063-1072.

8. Grand R, Watkins J, Torti F. Development of the human gastrointestinal tract. Gastroenterology 1976;70:790-810.

9. Hauri H, Quaroni A, Isselbacher K. Monoclonal antibodies to sucrase/isomaltase: probes for the study of postnatal development and biogenesis of the intestinal microvillus membrane. Proc nat Acad Sci 1980;77:6629-6633.

10. Auricchio S, Rubino A, Murset G. Intestinal glycosidase activities in the human embryo, fetus, and newborn. Pediatrics 1965;35:944-954.

11. Cicco R, Holzman IR, Brown DR, Becker DJ. Glucose polymer tolerance in premature infants. Pediatrics 1981;67:498-501.

12. Jones JB, Mehta NR, Hamosh M. Alpha amylase in preterm human milk. J Pediatr Gastroenterol Nutr 1982;1:43-48.

13. Hadorn B, Zoppi G, Shmerling DH, et al. Quantitative assessment of exocrine pancreatic function in infants and children. J Pediatr 1968;73:39-50.

14. Lebenthal E, Lee PC. Glycoamylase and disaccharidase activities in normal subjects and in patients with mucosal injury of the small intestine. J Pediatr 1980;97:389-393.

15. Kerzner B, Sloan HR, Haase G, et al. The jejunal absorption of glucose oligomers in the absence of pancreatic enzymes. Pediatr Res 1981;15:250-253.

16. Fogel MR, Gray GM. Starch hydrolysis in man: an intraluminal process not requiring membrane digestion. J Appl Physiol 1973;35:263-267.

17. Carbohydrate and Dietary Fiber, Pediatric Nutrition Handbook, Committee on Nutrition, American Academy of Pediatrics, G.B. Forbes (ed), Elk Grove Village, IL, 1985;97-104.

18. Siegel M, Lebenthal E, Krantz B. Effect of caloric density on gastric emptying in premature infants. J Pediatr 1984;104:118-122.

19. Brener W, Hendrix T, McHugh P. Regulation of the gastric emptying of glucose. Gastroenterology 1983;85:76-82.

20. Kalhan SC, Savin SM, Adam PAJ. Measurement of glucose turnover in the human newborn with glucose-1-13C. J Endocrinol Metab 1976;43:704-707.

21. Heird WC, Anderson TL. Nutritional requirements and methods of feeding low birth weight infants. Curr Probl Pediatr 1977;7(8):13.

22. MacLean Jr WC, Fink BB, Schoeller DA, et al. Lactose assimilation by full-term infants: relation of (^{13}C) and H$_2$ breath tests with fecal (^{13}C) excretion. Pediatr Res 1983;17:629-633.

23. McNeil NI, Cummings JH, James WPT. Short chain fatty acid absorption by the human large intestine. Gut 1978;19:819-822.

24. Lifschitz CH, Smith EO, Garza C. Delayed complete functional lactase sufficiency in breast-fed infants. J Pediatr Gastroenterol Nutr 1983;2:478-482.

25. Hay WW Jr. Fetal neonatal glucose homeostasis and their relation to small for gestational age infant. Semin Perinatol 1984;8:101-116.

26. MacLean Jr WC, Fink BB. Lactose malabsorption by premature infants: magnitude and clinical significance. J Pediatr 1980;97:383-388.

27. Lifshitz F, Diaz-Bensussen S, Martinez-Garza V, et al. Influence of disaccharides on the development of systemic acidosis in the premature infant. Pediatr Res 1971;5:213-225.

28. Seashore JH. Metabolic complications of parenteral nutrition in infants and children. Surg Clin North Am 1980;60:1239-1312.

29. Das JB, Filler RM, Rubin VG, Eraklis AJ. Intravenous dextrose amino acids feeding: the metabolic response in the surgical patients. J Pediatr Surg 1970;5:127-135.

30. Kerner JA, Jr. Carbohydrate requirements. In Kerner, JA, Jr (ed): Manual of Pediatric Parenteral Nutrition. New York, John Wiley and Sons, 1983;79-88.

31. Falorni A, Fracassini F, Massi-Benedetti F, Maffei S. Glucose metabolism and insulin secretion in the newborn infant: comparisons between the responses observed the first and seventh day of life to intravenous and oral glucose tolerance tests. Diabetes 1974;23:172-181.

32. Cowett RM, Oh W, Pollack A, et al. Glucose disposal of low weight infants. Steady state hyperglycemia produced by constant intravenous glucose infusion. Pediatrics 1979;63:389-396.

33. Goldman SL, Hirata T. Attenuated response to insulin in very low birth weight infants. Pediatr Res 1980;14:50-53.

34. Brans YW. Parenteral nutrition of the very low birth weight neonate: a critical review. Clin Perinatol 1977;4:367-373.

35. Cornblath M, Wybregt SH, Baens GS. Studies of carbohydrate tolerance in premature infants. Pediatrics 1963;32:1007-1024.

36. Dweck HS, Brans YW, Summers JE, Cassady G. Glucose intolerance in infants of very low birth weight. II. Intravenous glucose tolerance tests in infants of birth weights 500-1380 g. Biol Neonate 1976;30:261-267.

37. McDonald ATJ, Phillips MJ, Jeejeebhoy KN. Reversal of fatty liver by Intralipid in patients on total parenteral alimentation. Gastroenterology 1973;64:885-890.

38. Klish WJ, Udall JN, Rodriguez JT, et al. Intestinal surface area in infants with acquired monosaccharide intolerance. J Pediatr 1978;92:566-571.

39. Bond JH, Curtier BE, Buchwalk H, Levitt HD. Colonic conservation of malabsorbed carbohydrate. Gastroenterology 1980;78:444-447.

40. Cornblath M, Rosenthal IM, Reisner SH, et al. Hereditary fructose intolerance. N Engl J Med 1963;269:1271-1278.

41. Graham GG, Klein GL, Cordano A. Nutritive value of elemental formula with reduced osmolality. Am J Dis Child 1979;133:795-797.

8

Fat Needs for Term and Preterm Infants

MARGIT HAMOSH, Ph.D.

ABSTRACT

Fats supply more than 40% of the total calories in Western industrial societies. Fat digestion and absorption is very efficient (greater than 95%) and there is no feedback regulation to reduce its deposition. Adult American intake of fat averages approximately 150 gm/day and this high intake level correlates with high incidences of atherosclerosis and cancer. Absorption of fat permits the efficient assimilation of a great number of hydrophobic (fat-soluble) chemicals, some beneficial (such as the fat-soluble vitamins) and some detrimental (such as hydrophobic xenobiotics, drugs, food additives, carcinogens and chemicals produced during cooking). Fats are vital for normal growth and development. They provide 40-50% of total calories in human milk or infant formulas, and in addition to being the main energy source, are essential for brain development and for cellular structure and function.

INTRODUCTION

The aim of this chapter is to provide a concise overview of fat composition, digestion and metabolism, especially as related to the newborn infant. The main topics discussed are (1) fat structure, (2) fat composition of human milk, (3) fat digestion and absorption, (4) transport of lipid in the circulation, (5) lipoproteins, (6) uptake of lipoprotein-fatty acids by tissues, (7) role of carnitine in fatty acid catabolism, (8) importance of ketone bodies in infancy, and (9) recommendations for infant feeding.

Fats supply more than 40% of the total calories in Western industrial societies. Fat digestion and absorption are very efficient (greater than 95%) and there is no feedback regulation to reduce its deposition. Adult American intake of fat averages approximately 150 gm/day,[1] and this high intake level correlates with high incidences of atherosclerosis[2] and cancer.[3] Absorption of fat permits the efficient assimilation of a great number of hydrophobic (fat-soluble) chemicals, some beneficial (such as the fat-soluble vitamins) and some detrimental (such as hydrophobic xenobiotics, drugs, food additives, carcinogens and chemicals produced during cooking).

Fats are vital for normal growth and development. Fat is the main energy source of the newborn infant. In addition to providing 40-50% of the total calories in human milk or formula, fats are essential to normal development because they provide fatty acids necessary for brain development, are an integral part of all cell membranes and are the sole vehicle for fat-soluble vitamins and hormones in milk. Furthermore, **these energy-rich lipids can be stored in the body in nearly unlimited amounts in contrast to the limited storage capacity for carbohydrates and proteins.** Before birth, glucose is the major energy source whereas the fetal requirement for fatty acids is supplied mainly as free acids from the maternal circulation. After birth, fat is supplied chiefly in the form of milk or formula triglycerides.

Lipids are nonpolar or amphipathic substances that are insoluble in aqueous media (Fig. 1). The major lipid classes comprise fatty acids, glycerides, phospholipids, and sterols.

Fats and oils have always played an important part in human history, not only because of their role in nutrition (which was perhaps the last to be recognized), but because they were the chief lighting materials and because soap was important in hygiene.[4] The manufacture of soap by boiling fat with various forms of alkali was practiced by the early Germans as reported by Pliny (23-79 AD).[4]

The chemical nature of fats, as esters of glycerol, was recognized by Chevreul in the first part of the 19th century.[4] Chevreul conducted extensive studies on the chemistry of fats during his long life (1786-1889). Among his many important observations are that (1) the character of a fat depends upon the properties of the fatty acids in the glycerides; (2) butyric acid loses its pungency when esterified; and (3) the difference in the odor of butter prepared from the milk of different species is due to differences in short-chain fatty acid composition. Most important was the fact that he recognized that the fats found in the bodies of different species were all composed of fatty acids and that the difference between the properties of human fat and mutton tallow was the result of mixtures of fatty acids of different melting points.[4]

The early studies were mainly qualitative. Quantitation of the component fatty acids of glycerides started with the work of Hilditch and associates.[4] These studies really "took off" with the introduction of new techniques such as gas chromatography (1952).[5] We are indeed reminded of Claude Bernard's remark, **"Every**

133

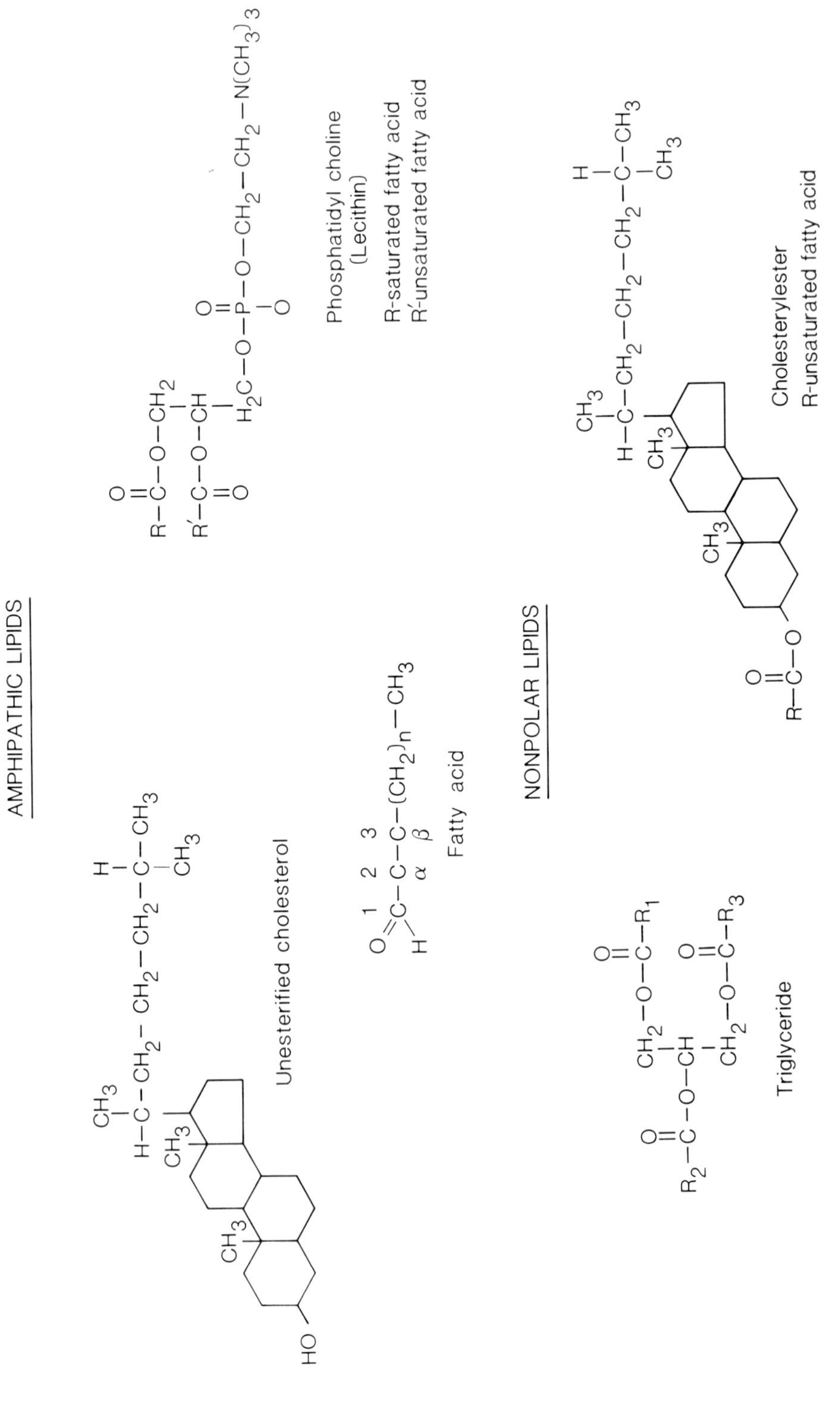

FIGURE 1. Principal dietary lipid components. (From Hamosh M, Hamosh P: Lipoprotein lipase: its physiological and clinical significance. Molec Aspects Med 1983; 6:199, with permission.)

advance in science is first preceded by an advance in technique.[6]

DEFINITIONS

Glycerides

Glycerides are non-phosphorus-containing lipids that result from the esterfication of glycerol and fatty acids (Fig. 1). Three forms occur in nature. Triglycerides (neutral fat) are the most abundant lipids in animal tissue and serve as an important energy source. In triglycerides all three of the carbon molecules of glycerol are esterified with fatty acids. Monoglycerides and diglycerides are compounds resulting from ester links between glycerol and one or two fatty acids, respectively.

Phospholipids

Phospholipids, phosphorus-containing lipid compounds, may be subdivided into three classes: derivatives of glycerol-3-phosphate (phosphatidyl choline, phosphatidyl ethanolamine, phosphatidyl serine and phosphatidyl inositol), sphingosine, and the glycolipids.

Phospholipids are found as structural components of all biologic membranes. They are important in oxidative phosphorylation, in transport across cell membranes, and in electron transport reactions.

Sterols

Sterols are alcohols with the cyclopentanoperhydrophenanthrene skeletal structure. The principal sterol is cholesterol, the parent compound of the steroids, including the adrenocortical, ovarian, and testicular hormones. The bile acids, degradative products of cholesterol, are important in gastrointestinal absorptive processes.

Fatty Acids

Fatty acids of animal origin are usually unbranched, monocarboxylic acids containing an even number of carbon atoms, varying from 2 to 24 in chain length. The fatty acid chains may be either saturated or unsaturated (Table 1). Most biologically important fatty acids are esterified with glycerol, while a small portion are linked with other compounds or are free. The

TABLE 1.   Structure of Fatty Acids

Descriptive Name	Systematic Name	Carbon Atoms	Double bonds	Position of double bonds*	Unsaturated fatty acid class†
Acetic		2	0		
Butyric		4	0		
Caproic	Hexanoic	6	0		
Caprylic	Octanoic	8	0		
Capric	Decanoic	10	0		
Lauric	Dodecanoic	12	0		
Myristic	Tetradecanoic	14	0		
Palmitic	Hexadecanoic	16	0		
Palmitoleic	Hexadecanoic	16	1	9	n-7
Stearic	Octadecanoic	18	0		
Oleic	Octadecanoic	18	1	9	n-9
Linoleic	Octadecadienoic	18	2	9,12	n-6
Linolenic	Octadecatrienoic	18	3	9,12,15	n-3
Linolenic	Octadecatrienoic	18	3	6,9,12	n-6
Homolinolenic	Eicosatrienoic	20	3	8,11,14	n-6
Arachidonic	Eicosatrienoic	20	4	5,8,11,14	n-6
‡	Eicosatrienoic	20	5	5,8,11,14,17	n-3
‡	Docosahexaenoic	22	6	4,7,10,12,19,19	n-3

Adapted from Montgomery R, Dryer RL, Conway TW, Spector AA. Biochemistry: A Case-oriented Approach, 4th ed. St. Louis, C.V. Mosby Co., 1983.
*Position of the one or more double bonds listed according to the Δ numbering system. In this numbering system, only the first carbon of the pair is listed: that is, 9 means position 9, 10, starting from the *carboxyl end*.
†In the n numbering system, only the first double bond from the *methyl end* is listed and, as above, only the first carbon of the pair is written.
‡No commonly used descriptive name.

Fatty acids are classified according to structure as follows: *medium-chain fatty acids*—chain length < C12 carbon atoms; *long-chain fatty acids* > C12 are divided into saturated (no double bonds) and unsaturated ($\leqslant$6 double bonds). Saturated fats are considered atherogenic, whereas unsaturated fats have the opposite effect.

TABLE 2. Fatty Acid Composition (%) of Various Cooking Oils and Fats

Fatty Acid	Sesame Oil*	Corn Oil*	Coconut Oil*	Cottonseed Oil*	Olive Oil*	Peanut Oil*	Safflower Oil*	Soybean Oil*	Cocoa Butter	Butter*	Cow Milk†
4:0											3.6
6:0			0.8							2.0	0.9
8:0			5.4							0.5	0.8
10:0			8.4							2.3	2.5
12:0 Lauric			45.4					0.2		2.5	3.3
14:0		1.4	18.0	1.4	Trace			0.1		11.1	10.4
16:0 Palmitic	9.1	10.2	10.5	23.4	6.9	8.3	6.8	9.8	24.4	29.0	32.0
18:0	4.3	3.0	2.3	1.1	2.3	3.1		2.4	33.4	9.2	14.5
20:0	0.8		0.4	1.3	0.1	2.4		0.9		2.4	
16:1		1.5		2.0				0.4	38.1	4.6	2.7
18:1 Oleic	45.4	49.6	7.5	22.9	84.4	56.0	18.6	28.9	2.1	26.7	23.4
18:2 Linoleic	40.4	34.3	Trace	47.8	4.6	26.0	70.1	30.7		3.6	3.5
18:3 Linolenic							3.4	6.5			0.8
Other			1.3	0.1	1.7	4.2	1.1	0.1		2.5	5.2

Adapted from Drash AL. Lipids in Nutrition. In Kelly VD (ed): Practice of Pediatrics, Vol. 6. Baltimore, Harper and Row, 1983; 56, ch. 9.

*Data from Altman PL, Dittmer DS (eds) Biology Book, Washington, D.C., Federation of American Societies for Experimental Biology, 1964; 380.

†Averages of milk fatty acid composition of Guernsey, Holstein, and Jersey Cows. Data from Stull JW, Brown WA. Fatty acid composition of milk. II. Some differences in common dairy breeds. J Dairy Sci 1964; 47:142. From Scheir R. In Bondy PK, Rosenberg LE (eds): Duncan's Diseases of Metabolism, 7th ed. Philadelphia, W.B. Saunders Co.,1974: 350.

Among the various cooking oils the coconut oil and cocoa butter are highly saturated, olive oil contains mainly monounsaturated fatty acids, whereas the other oils contain both mono- and polyunsaturated fatty acids.

fatty acid composition of the most commonly used fats is listed in Table 2 (see also Fig. 2). The fat composition of commercially available infant formulas is listed in Table 3 and shown in Figure 3. The composition of lipids in human milk will be discussed in detail in this chapter. The functions of the above listed lipid classes are listed in Table 4. **Storage lipid contains higher amounts of saturated fatty acids than do structural lipids** (Fig. 4).

Essential Fatty Acids

According to Duell, linolenic acid was first isolated from hempseed oil in 1887.[7]

In higher plants, animals, protozoa, and fungi, saturated fatty acids are acted upon by disaturases to introduce double bonds, usually of the cis configuration. The introduction of the first double bond, a process occurring in both plants and animals, takes place in the cytosol. The resulting oleyl-CoA can be converted to CoA derivatives of linoleic, linolenic and other polyenoic acids by desaturation reactions that take place in the endoplasmic reticulum of plant cells and require NADPH and light-generated ferredoxin as well as O_2.[7] Because the conversion of oleyl-CoA to linoleyl-CoA does *not* occur in animals, polyenoic

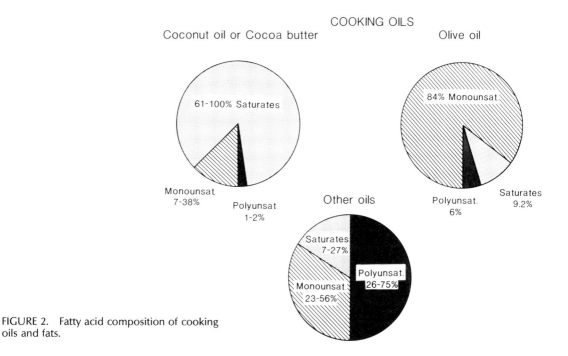

FIGURE 2. Fatty acid composition of cooking oils and fats.

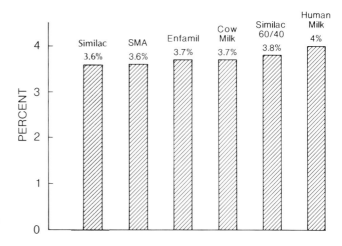

FIGURE 3. Percentage of fat in standard U.S. formulas versus milks.

TABLE 3. Principal Fat Sources for
Milk and Infant Formulas

Milks and Formulas	Fat (%)	Source
Milks		
Human*	4.0*	
Cow	3.7	Butterfat
Formulas		
Enfamil 20	3.8	Coconut and soy oils
Similac 20	3.6	Coconut and soy oils
Similac PM 60/40	3.8	Coconut and corn oils
SMA	3.6	Oleo, coconut, safflower and soy oils
Lonalac	3.5	Coconut oil
ProSobee	3.6	Coconut and soy oils
Soyalac	4.0	Soybean oil
Isomil	3.6	Coconut and soy oils
Nutramigen	2.6	Corn oil
Portagen	3.2	88% MCT oil, 12% corn oil
Pregestimil	2.7	60% corn oil, 40% MCT oil

*The composition of human milk fat is given in Tables 5 and 6.
MCT = medium-chain triglyceride.

TABLE 4. Function of Lipids in Mammals

Lipid Class	Function
Glycerides	Fatty acid storage, metabolic intermediates
Phospholipids	Membrane structure, lung surfactant
Sterols:	
Cholesterol	Membrane and lipoprotein structure; precursor of steroid hormones; degradation products are bile salts important in fat digestion and absorption
Cholesteryl ester	Storage and transport
Fatty acids	Major energy source, components of most lipids precursors of prostaglandins

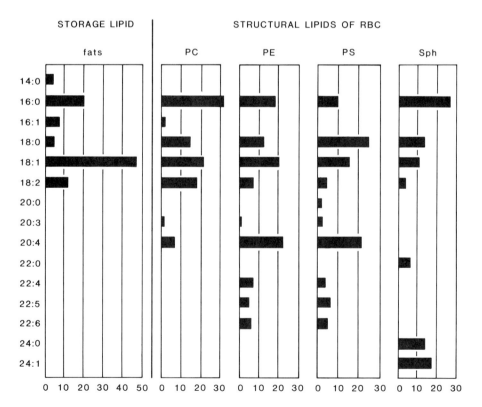

FIGURE 4.   Fatty acid composition of storage and of structural lipids. Storage lipid is triglyceride, whereas structural red blood cell (RBC) lipids are phospholipids and sphingomyelin: PC, PE, PS are phosphatidylcholine, phosphatidylethanolamine, and phosphatidylserine, respectively, Sph is sphingomyelin. (From McGilvery RW, Goldstein GW. Biochemistry: A Functional Approach. Philadelphia, W.B. Saunders 1983, with permission.)

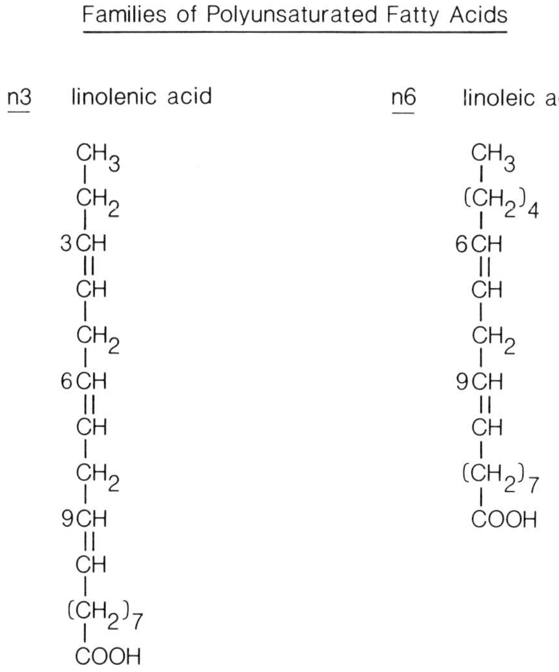

Families of Polyunsaturated Fatty Acids

n3   linolenic acid   n6   linoleic acid

CH_3 | CH_2 | 3 CH ‖ CH | CH_2 | 6 CH ‖ CH | CH_2 | 9 CH ‖ CH | $(CH_2)_7$ | $COOH$

CH_3 | $(CH_2)_4$ | 6 CH ‖ CH | CH_2 | 9 CH ‖ CH | $(CH_2)_7$ | $COOH$

Source :   vegetable oils, leaves   vegetable oils

Derivatives : $C_{20:5\ n3}$ marine oils $C_{20:4\ n6}$ animal fats

                $C_{22:6\ n3}$ marine oils

FIGURE 5.   Families of fatty acids derived from the essential fatty acids.

fatty acids such as linoleic and linolenic acid have to be provided in the diet.

Essential fatty acids include two families distinguished by the position of the double bond closest to the methyl terminal group of the fatty acid chain: n-6 fatty acids, including linoleic acid (18:2 n6) and its longer-chain derivatives, and n-3 fatty acids, comprising α-**linolenic acid** (18:3 n3) and its derivatives (Fig. 5). These fatty acids are important to brain development, cell proliferation, myelination,[8] and retinal function.[9]

It was thought until recently that the structural lipids (which contain most of the essential fatty acids) are much more resistant to change (in fatty acid composition) than the storage fats (which are mainly adipose tissue triglycerides). Recent studies in primates maintained on diets deficient in n-3 essential fatty acids show that brain with an abnormal fatty acid composition ($C_{22:5}$, n-3, no descriptive name available) has a remarkable capacity to change its fatty acid

content and composition ($C_{22:6}$, n-3 docosahexaenoic) after ingestion of fish oil, implying a greater lability of the fatty acids of brain phospholipids than previously assumed.[10]

Phosphoglycerides of brain contain high levels of docosahexaenoic acid (22:6, n-3). Recent studies show that human brain lipids change during development, from very little 22:6 n-3 (docosahexaenoic) at 6-12 weeks post conception to 4% and 18% of total fatty acids in phosphatidylethanolamine at 17-18 weeks and later during the second trimester, respectively. Similar increases were observed in the other brain phospholipid classes.[11] These long-chain polyenoic fatty acids accumulate rapidly in the fetal brain during the last trimester of pregnancy, 43 mg n-6 and 22 mg n-3 polyenoic fatty acids per week.[11]

We and others have shown that polyenoic fatty acids are present in the milk of women who deliver prematurely or at term (Table 5; Fig. 6). Thus, human milk is able to meet the

TABLE 5. Fatty Acid Composition (%) of Human Milk
Comparison of milk* from mothers who delivered at 26 to 30 weeks (VPT), 31 to 36 weeks (PT), and 37 to 40 weeks (T) of pregnancy.

	Fatty acid	VPT† 26-30 WK	PT 31-36 WK	T 37-40 WK
	10:0	1.37±0.17	1.27±0.18	0.97±0.28
Lauric	12:0	7.47±0.72	6.55±0.77	4.46±1.17
Myristic	14:0	8.41±0.83	7.55±0.89	5.68±1.36
	15:0	0.23±0.04	0.27±0.05	0.31±0.07
Palmitic	16:0	20.13±1.40	23.16±1.49	22.20±2.28
	16:1	2.56±0.24	2.92±0.26	3.83±0.39
	17:0	0.34±0.22	0.60±0.24	0.49±0.36
	18:0	7.24±1.13	7.25±1.21	7.68±1.85
Oleic	18:1	33.41±1.67	33.74±1.79	35.51±2.73
Linoleic	18:2	15.75±1.22	13.83±1.30	15.58±1.99
	18:3	0.76±0.13	0.76±0.14	1.03±0.21
	20:0	0.17±0.07	0.09±0.08	0.32±0.11
	20:2	0.35±0.13	0.33±0.13	0.18±0.20
	20:3	0.51±0.09	0.43±0.10	0.53±0.15
	20:4	0.55±0.18	0.58±0.19	0.60±0.29
	20:5	0.04±0.05	00	00
	21:0	0.05±0.07	0.07±0.08	0.17±0.12
	22:4	0.13±0.10	0.24±0.11	0.07±0.16
	22:5w6	0.11±0.05	0.04±0.05	0.03±0.08
	22:5w3	0.42±0.09	0.12±0.10	0.11±0.15
	22:6	0.24±0.09	0.21±0.09	0.23±0.14

†Means ± SE.
*Milk was collected at 6 weeks of lactation. Data from Bitman J, Wood DL, Hamosh M, et al. Comparison of the lipid composition of breast milk from mothers of term and preterm infants. Am J Clin Nutr 1983; 38:300.

Fatty acids account for more than 80% of milk fat. The long-chain fatty acids (C_{20}-C_{22}) are essential to brain development; these fatty acids are not provided in formula fat.

MAJOR FATTY ACIDS IN HUMAN MILK

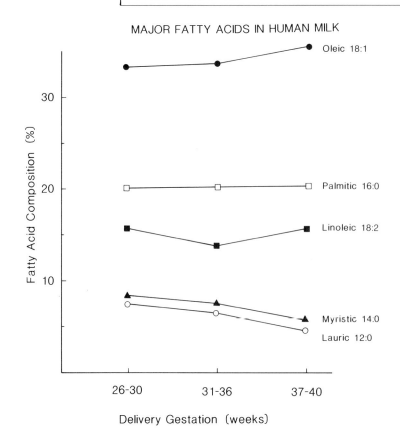

FIGURE 6. Fatty acid composition of human milk in mothers of term and preterm infants.

needs for these fatty acids in preterm infants and to efficiently substitute for the placental supply of these fatty acids to the fetus.

The American Academy of Pediatrics has recommended that infant formulas should contain a minimum of 3.3 gm/100 cal of fat (30% of calories) and 300 mg/100 cal of 18:2 (about 1.7% of total calories).[12] The Academy was concerned that excess 18:2 would produce peroxidation (because of the presence of double bonds which are easily oxidized) and increase the vitamin E requirements (to act as antioxidant) but did not set an upper limit on the 18:2 content of the diet. In human milk, linoleic acid amounts to 12-15% of total fatty acids.[13] Preterm infants who received fat-free parenteral nutrition showed rapid onset of essential fatty acid deficiency. Recent observations suggest that linolenic acid should amount to about 0.50% of calories.[14]

Fish Oils

Most common animal and vegetable fats are devoid of n-3 fatty acids, especially of the 20 and 22 carbon series. High concentrations of these fatty acids are present in fish oils. Fish oil consumption has been linked to reduced rates of atherosclerosis in Eskimos. Indeed, a diet high in n-3 fatty acids significantly reduced plasma cholesterol and triglyceride levels, improved fat tolerance and reduced platelet counts and adherence. Thus, n-3 fatty acids appear to have two antiatherogenic effects: a hypolipidemic action and an antithrombotic action upon platelets, and can be helpful in the prevention and treatment of atherosclerosis.[15,16]

Prostaglandins

Prostaglandins (PG) are derivatives of arachidonic acid (20:4) present in membrane phospholipids. Arachidonic acid is present in phosphatidylcholine and phosphatidylinositol and is released from the former through the action of phospholipase A_2, and from the latter by phospholipase C.

Oxygenation of arachidonic acid through the lipoxygenase pathway gives rise to leukotrienes and SRS-a (slow reacting substance of anaphylaxis), whereas oxygenation by the cylooxygenase pathway gives rise in different cells to different prostaglandins (PGs) and thromboxane end products.[17] The leukotrienes are powerful mediators of inflammatory and delayed hypersensitivity responses.[18] Among the many functions of prostaglandins, the production of thromboxane A_2 in platelets and PGI_2 in the endothelial cell is particularly important for the regulation of hemostasis.

PGE_2 and $PGF_{2\alpha}$ are present in human milk in concentrations 100-fold higher than in adult plasma.[19] As does the lipid content of milk, PG levels increase during each feed from low levels in fore milk to highest concentration in hind milk.[19] Recent studies show that PGE_2 and PGF_2 are absorbed after oral administration and they appear in intact form in the liver and other organs of suckling rats. Although the amount of intact PGs detected in various organs is small, the fact that a certain amount is absorbed unchanged probably is important for the suckling mammal. There seem to be changes in the metabolism of prostaglandins during early development, because the metabolites of prostaglandins in the liver are different in suckling and weanling animals.[20]

Milk PGs might exert a cytoprotective effect in the gastrointestinal tract of the newborn. Recent studies show that gastrointestinal ulceration does not occur in suckling rats following indomethacin administration, while similar inhibition of prostaglandin synthesis leads to jejunoileal ulceration in weaned and adult rats.[21] PGs in milk promote healing of peptic ulcers and protect the gastroduodenal mucosa from experimentally induced ulcers.[22] Oral admininstration of PGE_2 protects the gastrointestinal mucosa from indomethacin-induced blood loss in the human,[23] inhibits gastric secretion in man,[24] and has a trophic effect on rat intestinal mucosa.[25] The PG-induced cytoprotection might be mediated by localized increases in phospholipid concentration.[26,27]

PHYSIOLOGY

FAT COMPOSITION OF HUMAN MILK

Mature human milk has a fat content of 3.5-4.5%. The fat in milk is contained within membrane-enclosed milk fat globules. The core of the globules consists of triglycerides (98-99% of total milk fat), whereas the globule membrane is composed mainly of phospholipids, cholesterol and proteins (Table 6). The packaging of triglyceride within the core of the globules permits the dispersion of these nonpolar lipids in the aqueous environment of

TABLE 6. Composition of Human Milk Fat*

Glycerides		3.0–4.5 gm/dl	
Triglycerides	98.70%†		Major component
Diglycerides	0.01%		of the core of milk fat
Monoglycerides	0		globules
Free Fatty Acids	0.08%		
Cholesterol		10–15 mg/dl	
			Major component of milk fat globule
Phospholipids		15–20 mg/dl	membrane
Sphingomyelin	37%†		
Phosphatidylcholine	28%		
Phosphatidylserine	9%		
Phosphatidylinositol	6%		
Phosphatidylethanolamine	19%		

Data from Hamosh M, Bitman J, Wood DL, et al. Lipids in milk and the first steps in their digestion. Pediatrics 1985; 75(Suppl):146.
*Mature milk from mothers of term infants.
†Percent in lipid class (glycerides and phospholipids, respectively).

milk and also protects them from hydrolysis by milk lipases.[28]

Milk fat content and composition change during lactation. These changes are most pronounced during early lactation (colostrum, secreted 1-3 days postpartum), during the transition to mature milk (within the following 2-3 days), and again during weaning. Mature milk, however, maintains a constant fat composition.

Lipid Classes

Total fat content increases gradually from colostrum (2.0%) through transitional (2.5-3.0%) to mature milk (3.5-4.5%).[13] Cholesterol content is highest in colostrum and decreases to lower levels in transitional and mature milks; it is distributed as 87% free cholesterol and 13% cholesteryl esters (see Table 6). Phospholipids show a similar decrease from high levels in colostrum to lower levels in mature milk (Table 7). **The decline in phospholipid and cholesterol levels agrees well with an increase in the fat globule size**[29] and thus a decrease in the amount of membrane lipids (containing about 60% of milk phospholipid and 85% of milk cholesterol).

Fatty Acid Composition

Over 98% of the fat in human milk is present in 11 major fatty acids from $C_{10:0}$ to $C_{20:4}$ (Table 5). Medium-chain fatty acids (MCFA) amount to 10% of total fatty acids in mature milk of mothers of term infants but contribute 17% of total fatty acids in milk produced by mothers of preterm infants.[13]

Saturated fatty acids constitute 42% and unsaturated fatty acids account for 57% of total lipid in human milk. Linoleic acid concentrations are higher in recent studies[13] than in earlier reports[30] and reflect the higher intake of polyunsaturated fats by the American population. Essential fatty acid contents are higher in colostrum and transitional milk than in mature milk.[13] Long-chain polyunsaturated fatty acids derived from linoleic acid (20:2 n6, 20:3, 20:4, 22:5 n6) and from linolenic acid (20:5, 22:5 n3, 22:6) show a similar decrease throughout lactation. The level of these fatty acids is significantly higher in colostrum and milk of mothers of preterm infants than mothers of full-term infants.[13]

The increasing survival of very low birth-weight infants recently has led to the study of the developmental accretion of essential fatty acids during the last trimester of fetal development through the early weeks of life. These studies have shown that, during the last trimester, brain levels of linoleic acid were low, whereas substantial accretion of long-chain polyunsaturated essential fatty acids (22:4n6, 22:5n3 and 22:6n3) occurred.[31]

Postnatal brain development is characterized by an increase in brain linoleic acid content. Increase in chain elongation-desaturation products did not occur for several weeks postnatally.[31] These results suggest that placental transfer of these fatty acids is of primary importance in accretion of these fatty acids in the fetus. Based on quantitation of these fatty acids in human milk, these studies show that

TABLE 7.   Changes in Human Milk
Composition During Lactation

Lipid Class	Lactation Day				
	3	7	21	42	84
Total Fat (g/dl)	2.04	2.89	3.45	3.19	4.87
Triglyceride (%)*	97.60	98.50	98.70	98.90	99.00
Cholesterol (%)	1.30	0.70	0.50	0.50	0.40
Phospholipid (%)	1.10	0.80	0.80	0.60	0.60

Data from Hamosh M, Bitman J, Wood DL, et al. Lipids in milk and the first step
in their digestion. Pediatrics 1985; 75(Suppl):146.
*Lipid class % of total lipid. Data are means of 8-41 term milk specimens at dif-
ferent lactation times.

**preterm infants fed their own mother's milk
receive adequate amounts of long-chain
polyunsaturated fatty acids** that are sufficient
to meet the estimated requirements for neural
tissue synthesis.[31] Among all the lipid classes
(neutral lipid, phospholipid and cholesteryl
ester), cholesteryl ester has the highest content
of unsaturated fatty acids (70% of which is
linoleic acid).[32]

Factors That Affect the Amount and Composition of Milk Fat

**Fat is the most variable component of
milk.** In addition to the changes in the concentration and composition of milk fat that are
associated with the stage of lactation and the
length of pregnancy, there are diurnal and in-
feed variations of fat concentration. The rise in
fat content during the feed led to the suggestion that this change might regulate food
intake in breastfed infants, resulting in a lower
incidence of obesity than in formula-fed infants. This interesting hypothesis was, however, not supported by cross-feeding studies in
newborn infants, who consumed equal
amounts of high-fat or low-fat-containing
human milk (for recent review of these studies
see reference 33). Fat content rises during the
day, early morning milk having the lowest fat
content. Minerals, trace elements, and enzymes associated with the cream fraction of
milk have similar diurnal variations. Nutrient
content might also vary in the milk secreted
from the right or left breast at the same
feeding.

In contrast to the changes in fat concentration, the fat composition of mature human
milk is remarkably constant. Only drastic
changes in the diet, such as consumption of excessively large amounts of polyunsaturated
fats, carbohydrates, or severe limitation of total
food intake, result in the increase of linoleic

acid, palmitic acid and medium-chain fatty
acid levels, respectively.[33] Recent studies show
that the amount of eicosapentaenoic acid or of
trans fatty acids (geometric isomers of cis fatty
acids, formed during partial hydrogenation of
fat) rises markedly in milk of women who consume large amounts of fish oil[34] or hydrogenated fats,[35,36] respectively. The greatest
increase in milk trans fatty acids occurred in
women who were losing weight and consuming hydrogenated fat.[36] From these data it appears that trans fatty acids from the diet and
from the mother's fat depots contribute to
milk trans fatty acids.

FAT DIGESTION, ABSORPTION AND TRANSPORT

The mechanism of fat absorption has been a
controversial subject in the physiological and
biochemical literature for nearly 200 years.[37]
In 1856 Claude Bernard observed that the
lymphatics just distal to the pancreatic duct of
the rabbit became cloudy after a fat meal.[38] He
suggested that fat was absorbed via the lymphatic system and proposed the involvement
of the pancreatic juice in this process. Furthermore, earlier Bernard noted that "when mixed
with pancreatic juice at 20-40°C, olive oil, butter or fat was found to be immediately emulsified and chemically modified...We examined the products and we could easily
recognize that the fat had been split into fatty
acids and glycerol."[39]

Toward the end of the last century, Munk
and Pfluger each proposed different theories
for the absorption of dietary fat. According to
Munk the major part of ingested fat is finely
dispersed and transported across the intestinal
epithelium into the lymph without need for
prior hydrolysis of the triglyceride,[40,41] whereas
according to Pfluger, ingested fats must be
completely hydrolyzed to free fatty acids before absorption.[42] The controversy between

these two champions of the "particulate theory" and the "lipolytic theory" and their respective followers became very acrimonious and degenerated at times into personal attacks.[43] An example of the "dialogue" between these highly respected investigators follows:

E. Pfluger: "I agree with I. Munk that these facts are of importance for my interpretation. But by no means can I admit that I. Munk is the discoverer of these facts. In the entire field of fat physiology no new idea or any new important fact can be attributed to him, although invariably he presents his research as if a new star had risen while it is actually only a matter of repeating the investigations of his predecessors. These repetitious experiments are usually imperfect, and sometimes only slightly modified."

I. Munk: "... the memorable E. du Bois Reymond lamented in his academical speech of 1882: 'Have not the last two years become witnesses of a movement whose disgrace we thought as impossible in our time as torture, witch trials and slave trade?' But up to a few weeks ago, this practice was confined to the streets and to the beer halls and the doors of science resisted its admission with dignity. It is Pfluger's sorry achievement to have transplanted the jargon of the street into science. With it he has irreparably lowered the ethical level of his Archive. Such poisoned arrows fly back at the marksman."

Progress was made in the late 1920s when Verzar and associates pointed to the importance of bile salts in the solubilization and absorption of fatty acids,[44] and suggested that glycerophosphate is important in the resynthesis of triglycerides.[45] In 1938 Frazer reopened the question of particulate fat absorption.[46] Basically, Frazer suggested that some of the fat is hydrolyzed to partial glycerides and free fatty acids, whereas the remainder was emulsified and absorbed without prior hydrolysis. This theory known as the "partition theory" suggested that the glycerides passed into the lymphatic circulation, whereas the free fatty acids were absorbed via the portal circulation. It was only in the early 1950s that Chaikoff and associates showed that long-chain fatty acids are absorbed through the lymphatics whereas medium- and short-chain fatty acids pass directly into the portal circulation.[47] The mechanism of fat digestion and absorption was elucidated in large measure by the elegant studies of Borgstrom and associates.[48]

In addition to the above listed controversies on the mechanism of fat absorption, it is interesting that several of the steps of fat digestion described at the turn of the century were afterwards completely forgotten and had to be "rediscovered" again recently! The role of the stomach in fat digestion, the function of colipase and the activity of human milk lipase in neonatal fat digestion are examples of early observations that fell into oblivion.

Although many current textbooks of physiology discuss the role of gastric lipolysis with comments such as: "dietary triglycerides are not appreciably affected by any of the enzymatic processes involved in the gastrointestinal tract until the fat reaches the duodenum,"[49] the first report on gastric lipolysis appeared in 1885,[50] and in 1901 Volhard suggested that the stomach is an important site of fat digestion.[51] Intragastric lipolysis was recently shown to be an important compensatory mechanism in physiologic and pathologic pancreatic insufficiency,[52] and nonpancreatic lipases to be of major importance in this process in the human.[53]

In 1971, two laboratories reported that pancreatic lipase is inactive in the intestinal milieu in the absence of a polypeptide cofactor named "colipase."[54,55] An examination of the older literature[56] reveals, however, that in 1910 Rosenheim published a paper entitled "On pancreatic lipase III, the separation of lipase from its coenzyme."[57] This study showed that when a glycerol extract of porcine pancreas is diluted with water, one obtains a precipitate and a clear filtrate. Each fraction is lipolytically inactive, but after mixing, the full activity of the glycerol extract is restored. Rosenheim noted that the factor in the clear filtrate was thermostable and concluded that "pancreatic lipase is a complex enzyme which can be separated into two inactive fractions, a fact which has so far not been observed with any other enzyme."

Milk bile salt stimulated lipase, an enzyme present in human milk, was studied extensively between 1927 and 1953 by Freudenberg, who published his findings in a superb monograph "Die Frauenmilch Lipase" (Human Milk Lipase) in 1953.[58] Freudenberg attributed to this enzyme an important function in the digestion of milk fat. As with the other early observations, however, this lipase had to be rediscovered in 1974.[59]

Fat Digestion, Absorption, and Transport

More than 95% of dietary fat (including that in human milk and infant formula) is triglyceride (see Fig. 1; Table 6). Digestion and absorption of dietary fat involve essentially the transport of water-insoluble molecules from one water phase, the lumen of the gastrointestinal tract, to another water phase, the lymph and plasma.[60] This process can be divided into three steps: The luminal phase involves the solubilization and hydrolysis of triglycerides to

FIGURE 7.   Changes in the composition of human milk during lactation. (Data from Hamosh M et al. Lipids in milk and the first step in their digestion. Pediatrics 1985; 75(Suppl): 146.)

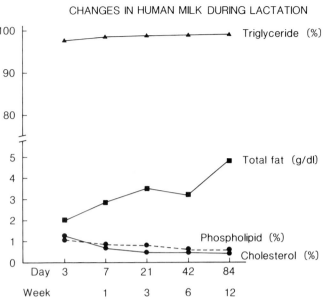

CHANGES IN HUMAN MILK DURING LACTATION

free fatty acids, monoglycerides, and glycerol, prior to their uptake by the intestinal mucosa. The mucosal phase involves the reesterification of free fatty acids to form triglycerides, which are assimilated into chylomicrons and very low density lipoproteins (VLDL) prior to their release from the mucosal cell into the blood via the lymphatics. In the transport and delivery phase, the fatty acids within chylomicrons and VLDL are taken up by the individual tissues for their metabolic needs.

1. Luminal Phase.   Fat digestion requires adequate lipase activity and bile salt concentrations, the former for the breakdown of triglycerides and the latter for emulsification of fat prior to and during lipolysis.[60] The lipases,

TABLE 8.   Lipase Available for Nutrient Lipid Digestion

Source	Enzyme	Substrate	Site of Luminal Action*
Food			
Milk (primates, carnivores)	Milk lipase (BSSL)	TG, lipovitamins	Small intestine
Oral			
Glands (von Ebner)	Lingual lipase	TG exclusively	Stomach (intestine)
Gastric mucosa	Gastric lipase	TG	Stomach (intestine)
Pancreas	Pancreatolipase -Colipase	TG	Small intestine
	Phospholipase A₂	Phospholipid Biliary and dietary	Small intestine
	Cholesteryl esterase Nonspecific lipase	CE, MG, TG Lipovitamins	Small intestine
Intestinal mucosa	Intestinal lipase	? TG†	Small intestine
Microbes	Alkaline lipases and phospholipases	TG + ? other	Colon, feces

Adapted from Patton JS. Gastrointestinal lipid digestion. In Johnson LR (ed): Physiology of the Gastrointestinal Tract. New York, Raven Press, 1981; 1123 and Watkins JB. Lipid digestion and absorption. Pediatrics 1985; 75(Suppl):151.
*Enzymes known to act in the small intestine probably also function in the large intestine to some degree.
†No data
BSSL = bile salt stimulated lipase; TG = triglycerides; CE = cholesterol ester; MG = monoglycerides.

Recent studies show that the milk lipase and the pancreatic cholesteryl esterase are identical enzymes produced in the lactating mammary gland and in the pancreas. Because the oral (lingual) lipase and the gastric lipase act in the same milieu (the stomach) they have identical characteristics. Partial fat hydrolysis in the stomach is essential to normal intestinal fat digestion.

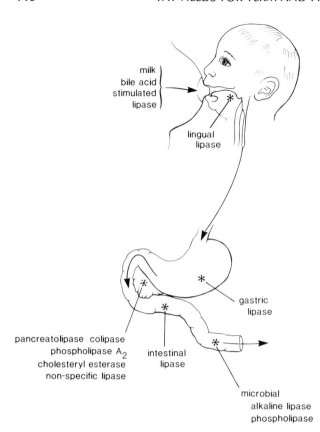

FIGURE 8.   Lipase activity in nutrient lipid digestion. See text for details.

significant for fat digestion, are listed in Table 8. Fat digestion begins in the stomach with the action of lingual lipase, an enzyme secreted from lingual serous glands,[61,62] and of gastric lipase secreted from glands within the gastric mucosa.[63] Further digestion takes place in the small intestine through the action of pancreatic lipase (Fig. 8).

The Stomach.   Initial hydrolysis of fat in the stomach leads to the formation of partial glycerides and free fatty acids.[52,53] This critical step is necessary for efficient fat absorption in the adult with adequate pancreatic function.[63,64] In the newborn and especially the preterm infant, pancreatic lipase and intraduodenal bile acid concentrations (the major components of intestinal fat digestion) are low.[65] Therefore, efficient fat absorption in the newborn depends on alternate mechanisms for the digestion of dietary fat.

Of special importance is intragastric lipolysis in which lingual and gastric lipases compensate for low pancreatic lipase (Table 8).[53,66] In addition, the products of intragastric lipolysis (fatty acids and monoglycerides) compensate for low bile salt concentrations by emulsifying the lipid mixture.[61] As much as 10-30% of dietary fat is hydrolyzed in the stomach

of the newborn.[66] Indeed, lingual and gastric lipases appear before 26 weeks' gestation and have high activity levels at birth.[66] Furthermore, in pancreatic insufficiency the lower pH in the duodenum enables these lipases (which have a pH optimum under 6.5) to continue the hydrolysis of fat in the upper small intestine.[67,68]

Lingual lipase has a special function in the hydrolysis of milk fat. **Milk fat globules are resistant to the action of pancreatic lipase but are readily hydrolyzed by lingual lipase, which penetrates into the core of the fat particles** and hydrolyzes the triglyceride without disrupting the globule membrane.[69] Indeed, as much as 15% of core triglyceride is hydrolyzed without producing any change in the microscopic appearance of milk fat globules (Fig. 9).[69] Lingual and gastric lipases hydrolyze medium- and short-chain triglycerides at higher rates than long-chain triglycerides. Short- and medium-chain fatty acids are absorbed directly through the gastric mucosa and these products of intragastric lipolysis appear rapidly in the circulation.

Intragastric hydrolysis of milk fat produces relatively large amounts of monolauryl glyceride,[70] a substance with antibacterial, an-

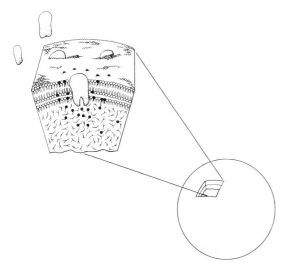

FIGURE 9. Hydrolysis of milk fat globule triglyceride by lingual lipase. Schematic drawing based on data that show that although as much as 15% of triglyceride is hydrolyzed to FFA and partial glycerides, there is no change in the appearance of the milk fat globules. (Patton JS, et al. Biochim Biophys Acta 1982; 712:400-407.) Enzyme molecules penetrate the trilayer member of the globule and hydrolyze the triglycerides in the core oil (shown as forked sticks) to fatty acids (black tipped sticks) and diglycerides (darkened sticks) which remain associated with the droplet. (From Hamosh M. Lingual Lipase. In Borgstrom B, Brockman HL (eds): Lipases. Amsterdam, Elsevier, 1984; p. 49, with permission.)

tiviral and antifungal activity, indicating that anti-infective agents are formed in the infant's stomach during fat hydrolysis. Fat digestion in the stomach is probably quantitatively much more important for the newborn than for the healthy adult: the stomach is a large receptacle where food is well mixed with enzyme through churning and squirting movements. Gastric pH is higher than in adults and stomach emptying is slower in the newborn, allowing for longer periods of food digestion than in adults. High fat concentration in gastric contents further delays gastric emptying.

The Duodenum. The hydrolysis of fat in the intestine is catalyzed primarily by pancreatic lipase in a complex interaction between the lipase, colipase, bile salts, and the triglyceride substrate (Fig. 10).[71,72] The colipase is necessary to provide higher affinity for lipase attachment at the surface of a bile-salt covered, triglyceride-water interface. Bile salts enhance the hydrolysis by promoting the formation of a colipase-lipase complex, which then adheres to the triglyceride molecules at the region of the ester bonds.

Pancreatic phospholipase A_2 hydrolyzes phospholipids, including those in the surface layer of milk fat globules or formula fat emulsions.[71] The enzyme has an absolute requirement for calcium and bile salts for the hydrolysis of long-chain phospholipids. Pan-

TABLE 9. Compensatory Digestive Lipases in the Newborn

	Lipase in Gastric Aspirates	Milk Bile Salt Stimulated Lipase
Origin	Lingual serous glands; gastric mucosa	Mammary gland (human, gorilla and carnivores)
Ontogeny	Present from 24 weeks' gestation	Present after term and preterm (26-36 weeks) delivery and in prepartum mammary secretions
Site of action characteristics	Stomach (duodenum)	Intestine
pH Optimum	3.0–6.5	7.0–9.0
pH Stability	>2.2	>3.5
Rate	MCT > LCT FA unsaturated > saturated	MCT = LCT Water-soluble esters
Reaction products	FFA, DG, MG	FFA, glycerol
Bile salts	20-40% stimulation	Obligatory
Molecular weight	46,000–48,000	90,000–125,000
Function	Hydrolysis of 50–70% of ingested fat	Hydrolysis of 30–40% of milk fat

Data from Hamosh M, Bitman J, Wood DL, et al.: Lipids in milk and the first steps in their digestion. Pediatrics 1985; 75(Suppl):146.
MCT = medium-chain triglyceride; LCT = long-chain triglyceride; FA = fatty acids, FFA = free fatty acids; DG = diglycerides; MG = monoglycerides.

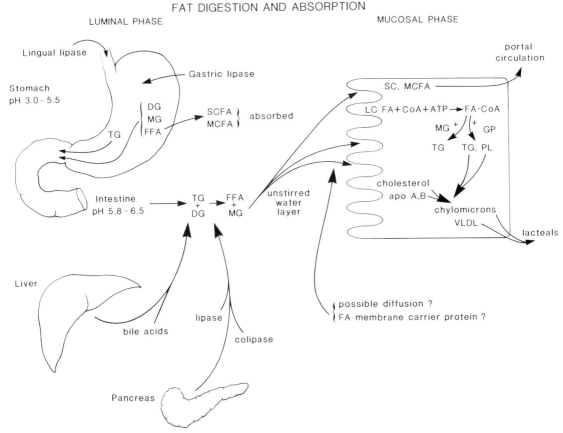

FIGURE 10.   Fat digestion and absorption. Abbreviated scheme of major steps in fat hydrolysis in the lumen of stomach and intestine and reesterification in the intestinal mucoas. TG - triglyceride, DG - diglyceride, MG - monoglyceride, FFA - free fatty acids, GP- αglycerophosphate; apo A, apoB - apoproteins A and B, PL - phosholipid.

creatic cholesterol ester hydrolase hydrolyzes cholesteryl esters, monoglycerides, and fat-soluble vitamins (see Table 8).[71]

Little is known about these processes in the newborn except that, as mentioned, pancreatic lipase and bile salt levels are low (<CMC) and that the secretory response to exogenous and endogeous stimuli is diminished.[65] The newborn benefits, however, from the extensive intragastric lipolysis. The products of this process (protonated fatty acids and diglycerides) facilitate the action of pancreatic lipase; and fatty acids increase lipase-colipase binding and the binding of colipase to bile salts.

The breastfed infant depends on an additional digestive enyzme, the bile salt stimulated lipase of human milk.[58] The characteristics of this lipase are decribed in Table 9. Because of low substrate specificity, the en-zyme hydrolyzes a large variety of triglycerides completely to free fatty acids and glycerol, thus continuing, in the intestine, the lipolytic process started in the stomach (Fig. 10).

Thus, even with very low pancreatic lipase the newborn is able to absorb 90-95% of dietary fat through the combined action of gastric lipolysis and intestinal lipolysis by human milk lipase. Recent studies show that bile salt stimulated lipase activity levels are similar in preterm and term milk and that the enzyme is stable at low temperatures, indicating that preterm infants fed their own mothers' milk receive adequate digestive lipase even when fed previously stored milk.[73,74]

2. Mucosal Phase. The products of luminal lipolysis pass into the enterocyte by passive diffusion.[75] Recent studies suggest, however, that fatty acid transport across the enterocyte could be facilitated by a specific membrane fatty acid binding protein.[76] Once inside the enterocyte the fatty acids are transported to the reesterification site (the endoplasmic reticulum) by means of a soluble intracellular fatty acid binding protein.[77]

After the fatty acids are activated to acyl-CoA (a step that is catalyzed by acyl-CoA ligase and occurs in the mitochondria), the reesterification to triglyceride occurs by two mechanisms, the monoglyceride and the phosphatidic acid pathways. In the first mechanism the acceptor of fatty acids is monoglyceride, whereas in the second pathway the acceptor is α-glycerophosphate produced from glucose metabolism. The monoglyceride pathway accounts for the reesterification of about 70% of absorbed fatty acids, whereas the phosphatidic acid pathway is the only mechanism for phospholipid synthesis in the intestinal mucosa (see Fig. 10).[78]

Studies in developing animals show that the mucosal phase of fat absorption is well developed and keeps pace with the higher fat intake of the neonatal period.[79]

3. Transport and Delivery Phase. The newly synthesized triglyceride, together with phospholipid, cholesterol and protein, are assembled into lipoproteins, namely chylomicrons and very low density lipoproteins. The large particles are released into the intercellular space by reverse pinocytosis and move across the basement membrane into the lymphatics.[80] Chylomicrons are released into the lacteals on the first day after birth, suggesting that this phase of fat assimilation is well developed in the newborn.

TRANSPORT OF LIPID IN THE CIRCULATION

Lipids are nonpolar or polar amphipathic substances (see Fig. 1) that are insoluble in aqueous media and can be transported in the circulation only in association with specific proteins. Polar lipids, such as free fatty acids and lysolecithin, bind to plasma albumin, whereas nonpolar lipids are transported within much larger particles—the lipoproteins. The nonpolar lipids (triglycerides and cholesteryl ester) form the hydrophobic core of the lipoproteins, while amphipathic lipids (phospholipids, cholesterol, small amounts of free fatty acids and partial glycerides) combine with apoproteins to form the surface film (Fig. 11).

The lipoproteins are generally divided into four categories: chylomicrons, very low density lipoproteins (VLDL), low density lipoproteins (LDL) and high density lipoproteins (HDL). The primary function of the lipoproteins is the transport of lipids, chiefly triglyceride (chylomicrons and VLDL) and cholesterol (LDL and HDL). In addition to their transport function—the solubilization of hydrophobic lipid in the aqueous environment of blood—the protein component of lipoproteins, the apolipoproteins, have important metabolic functions.

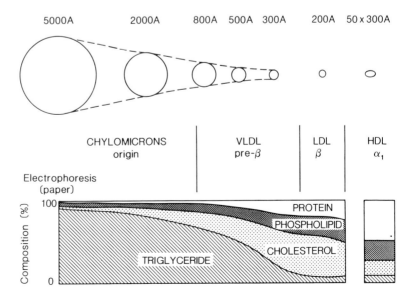

FIGURE 11. Classification of plasma lipoprotein by physical and chemical characteristics. (From Bierman EL. Hyperlipoproteinemia. Scope Monograph, Kalamazoo, MI, Upjohn Co., 1973, with permission.)

TABLE 10.   Composition of Intravenous Fat Emulsions

	Soybean Oil		Safflow Oil
	Intralipid*	Travamulsion †	Liposyn ‡
Fatty acid content (%)			
Palmitic acid C16:0	9	11	7
Stearic acid C18:0	3	3	2.5
Oleic acid C18:1w9	26	23	13
Linoleic acid C18:2w6	54	56	77
Linolenic acid C18:3w3	8	6	0.5
Egg yolk phospholipids (%) (Lecithin)	1.2	1.2	1.2
Glycerol (%)	2.25	2.25	2.5
Kcal/ml	1.1	1.1	1.1
Osmolarity (mOsm/L)	280	280	300
Fat particle size (microns)	0.5	0.4	0.4

*Cutter Laboratories
†Baxter-Travenol Laboratories
‡Abbott Laboratories

Some apoproteins (apo B and apo AII) have a primary role in lipid transport, whereas others (apo CII and AI) are specific activators of enzymes involved in lipolysis (lipoprotein lipase) and interconversion of lipoproteins (lecithin cholesterol acyl transferase, LCAT).

Improvement in the clinical nutritional management of very-low birthweight infants has been largely dependent on methods of nutrient delivery. The addition of lipids to total parenteral nutrition has markedly advanced the growth of very tiny babies.

In a review on the development of fat emulsions[81] Wretlind credits Courten with the first attempt to administer fat parenterally.[82] This first attempt in 1678 resulted in the death of the experimental animal, and later studies, giving the lipid by subcutaneous infusion, showed that administration by that route caused severe pain.[83]

Studies to produce a stable fat emulsion that resembles natural chyle were started in the 1920s and continued for several decades.[81,83] The result of these studies was the production of stable emulsions containing long-chain triglycerides and egg yolk lecithin.

TABLE 11.   Plasma Lipoproteins: Composition and Function

Lipoprotein	Protein*	Lipid †				Origin	Half-life	Function
		TG	CE	C	PL			
Chylomicrons	2.0	85	5.0	2.0	8.0	Intestine	5 min	TG transport
VLDL**	8-10	56	13.0	8.0	20.0	Intestine[a+b] Liver[b]	hours	TG transport
LDL***	25	10	50.0	10.0	30.0	Circulation from VLDL	hours	Cholesterol transport to tissue (anabolic)
HDL++	41-55	1-8	28.0	6.5-9.0	50.0	Intestine Liver Circulation[c]	Days	Cholesterol transport to liver (catabolic)

Adapted from Hamosh M, Hamosh P. Lipoprotein lipase: its physiological and clinical significance. Molec Aspects Med 1983; 6:199.
*Weight percent per particle.
†Weight percent of total lipid.
TG = triglyceride; CE = cholesteryl ester; C = cholesterol; PL = phospholipid; **VLDL = very low density lipoprotein; LDL = low density lipoprotein; HDL = high density lipoprotein; a = dietary fat; b = endogenous fat; c = surface coat of chylomicrons and VLDL during lipolysis.

The lipoprotein profiles differ markedly between cord blood and postnatal blood specimens. Very little is known about the factors that modulate these rapid postnatal changes.

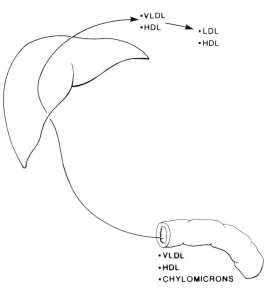

FIGURE 12. The function of the major lipoprotein classes—VLDL, LDL, HDL, and chylomicrons—is graphically depicted.

Intralipid (Cutter Laboratories), a 10% soybean oil emulsion that provides 1.1 calories/ml, was the first and remains the most widely used preparation for total parenteral nutrition (TPN) of the newborn. The composition of fat emulsions for intravenous use is given in Table 10. The fat particles of the Intralipid emulsion are similar in size to chylomicrons and, like the latter, are cleared from the circulation by similar mechanisms.[84]

The composition and function of the major lipoprotein classes are summarized in Table 11 and depicted in Figure 12. The properties of the apoproteins of the major lipoproteins are listed in Table 12.

The catabolism of chylomicrons, VLDL or Intralipid, occurs by a stepwise reduction of the triglyceride core through the action of lipoprotein lipase, an enzyme that hydrolyzes lipoprotein-triglyceride at the luminal surface of the capillary endothelium (Fig. 13).[85] Concomitantly with triglyceride hydrolysis, surplus surface constituents (apoproteins and polar lipids, 60% of free cholesterol, 90% of phosphatidylcholine and 100% of sphingomyelin) are removed from VLDL.[86] These surface constituents are released in particulate form that associate into disk-shaped structures similar to HDL precursors ("nascent" HDL) isolated from intestinal lymph or from rat liver perfusate.[86]

The hydrolysis of chylomicrons and VLDL by lipoprotein lipase reduces the core of the lipoprotein particles producing chylomicron remnants and LDL from chylomicrons and VLDL, respectively. The surplus surface constituents are the precursors of HDL (nascent HDL) (Figs. 13 and 14).

A second lipase that hydrolyzes lipoprotein-triglyceride is hepatic lipase, located in the endothelium of liver capillaries. The enzyme acts on VLDL triglyceride as well as on HDL phospholipids. Another enzyme with a key role in lipoprotein metabolism is lecithin-cholesterol

TABLE 12.   Properties and Functions of Apoproteins of Plasma Lipoproteins

Apoprotein	Structure*	Molecular Weight	Function‡	Site of Synthesis
Apo AI	Single chain, 245AA	28,000	Activates LCAT	Intestine, liver
Apo AII	Two identical chains 77AA each	17,000	?	
Apo AIV	?	46,000		Intestine, liver
Apo B†	?	264,000	TG transport	Intestine
		549,000	TG transport	Liver
Apo CI	Single chain, 57AA	6,331	Activates LCAT	Liver
Apo CII	Single chain, 78AA	8,837	Activates LPL	Liver
Apo CIII	Single chain, 79AA	8,764	Inhibits LPL	Liver
Apo D	?	22,000	Transfer protein	?
Apo E	?	33,000	Binds to specific liver and endothelial receptors	Liver, intestine?

Adapted from Hamosh M, Hamosh P. Lipoprotein lipase: its physiological and clinical significance. Molec Aspects Med 1983; 6:199.

*Peptide chain and number of amino acids (AA).

†Very hydrophobic protein, marked heterogeneity according to organ or species. The molecular weight listed is for human Apo B. Rat Apo B has a molecular weight of 240,000 (intestine) and 353,000 (liver).

‡LCAT = lecithin:cholesterol acyl transferase; LPL = lipoprotein lipase.

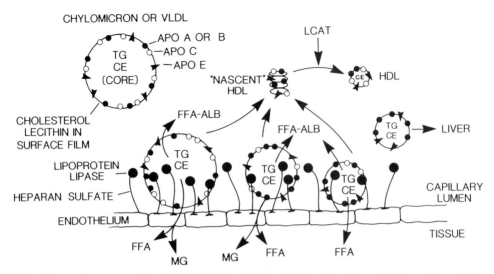

FIGURE 13.   Schematic representation of the hydrolysis of triglyceride in chylomicrons, VLDL, and Intralipid emulsion by endothelial lipoprotein lipase. Triglyceride-rich lipoproteins are represented schematically as large particles containing a neutral lipid core of triglyceride (TG), and cholesteryl ester (CE), and a surface film composed of lecithin, cholesterol, and apoproteins. VLDL are smaller than chylomicrons and contain different amounts of apoproteins. Lipoprotein lipase, bound to the endothelial surface through heparan sulfate, hydrolyzes lipoprotein triglyceride (TG) to monoglyceride (MG) and free fatty acids (FFA); the latter are taken up by the tissues or are released into the circulation where they bind to albumin (ALB). Shrinking of the particle core by lipolysis leaves an excess of surface components (broken line), which break off as disks similar to "nascent" high density lipoprotein (HDL). These newly formed particles acquire cholesteryl ester via the LCAT (lecithin-cholesterol acyl transferase) reaction, becoming spherical HDL particles. (From Hamosh M, Hamosh P: Lipoprotein lipase: its physiological and clinical significance. Molec Aspects Med 1983; 6:199-289.

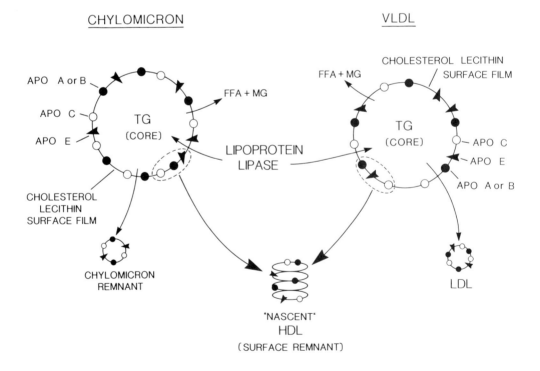

FIGURE 14.   Central role of lipoprotein lipase in the formation of low density and high density lipoproteins.

acyl transferase (LCAT). LCAT is released from the liver into the circulation, where it acts specifically on plasma HDL by converting the lecithin and unesterfied cholesterol of HDL to lysolecithin and cholesteryl ester.[87] Once esterified, the cholesteryl ester leaves the surface coat and moves into the non-polar lipid core in the center of the particle, leading to the transformation of disk-shaped "nascent" HDL into spherical "mature" HDL.

Lipoprotein lipase, the key enzyme in removal of lipoprotein triglyceride, is thus important in the formation of both LDL and HDL lipoprotein. Lecithin-cholesterol acyl transferase (LCAT) catalyzes the synthesis of almost the entire cholesterol ester of circulating lipoproteins. These two key enzymes differ in one important respect: **lipoprotein lipase is active at the capillary wall and under normal conditions is completely absent from the circulation.** This specific location probably facilitates the uptake of lipolytic products (FFA and monoglycerides) into tissue. **LCAT, on the other hand, acts exclusively in plasma,** where it accomplishes its function of continuous modulation of the cholesteryl ester content of circulating lipoproteins.

Lipid is administered to infants on an empirical basis; it is generally advised that it be given in amounts that do not cause lipemia (plasma triglycerides in excess of 100-150 mg/dl).[88,89] The widespread use of lipid in parenteral nutrition is in marked contrast to the limited knowledge of the enzymes and cofactors active in the lipid clearing process in low birthweight infants.[90,91]

Recent studies indicate that infusion period and infusion rate affect the clearing of lipid in low birthweight infants maintained on total parenteral nutrition.[92,93] Furthermore, the presence of heparin in solutions prepared for intravenous (IV) use (even the low concentration of 1 U/ml IV fluid, added to prevent clotting of catheters) might affect the lipid clearing process.[94,95] We have recently reviewed the enzymes and cofactors active in the mechanism of lipid clearing[85] with special emphasis on the developmental period.[90,91]

Low birthweight (LBW) infants have lower levels of lipolytic enzymes (lipoprotein lipase[94]) and LCAT[96] than full term infants. This is probably the reason for the hyperlipemia that develops in very-low birthweight (VLBW) infants maintained on total parenteral nutrition with lipids in excess of 2 gm/kg/day.[97] **The ability to synthesize lipoprotein lipase in response to the administration of heparin seems to be well developed even in preterm infants.**[91,98] The presence of high levels of free fatty acids and triglycerides in preterm infants who clear the infused Intralipid well[91,93,95] suggests that free fatty acids are produced in excess of the infant's ability for their catabolism.

Uptake by Tissues

Normally, the infused lipid would be rapidly removed from the circulation by uptake into adipose tissue or by oxidation in muscle. Lack of a critical mass of adipose tissue in LBW infants, as well as the low tissue level of carnitine (required for the oxidation of FFA in muscle or liver),[99,100] prevents the efficient uptake of fatty acids. A major part of the circulating FFAs are therefore probably reincorporated into triglycerides in the liver and will return to the circulation in the form of VLDL.

The final step in the catabolism of long-chain fatty acids, oxidation to H_2O and CO_2 occurs in mitochondria and depends upon the presence of carnitine. Long-chain fatty acids can cross mitochondrial membranes only in the form of acyl-carnitine. Carnitine is thus an essential cofactor for fatty acid oxidation, and acyl-CoA carnitine transferases are the key enzymes in fatty acid oxidation. The characteristics of the enzymes participating in lipid clearing and fatty acid oxidation are listed in Table 13.

Carnitine (γ-trimethylamino-β-hydroxybutyrate) is essential for the catabolism of long-chain fatty acids. All the enzymes for β-oxidation of fatty acids are localized in the matrix of the mitochondria; the inner mitochondrial membrane is, however, impermeable to fatty acids. Long-chain fatty acids are transported into the mitochondrial matrix by a system involving carnitine and several specific enzymes (carnitine palmitoyl transferase I, carnitine transferase and carnitine palmitoyl transferase II). Carnitine is synthesized in human liver and kidney from the essential amino acids lysine and methionine; cardiac and skeletal muscle cannot synthesize carnitine and receive it from the blood. The metabolism and function of carnitine[101] as well as its special role in the newborn[102] have been reviewed recently.

There are two acyl transferases: one for acetyl and short-chain fatty acids and one palmitoyl transferase. An additional octanoyl transferase has been isolated from liver perox-

TABLE 13.   Enzymes, Cofactors, and Sites of Lipid Clearing and Catabolism

Enzyme	Cofactor	Substrate	Site of Activity	Function
Lipoprotein lipase (LPL)	Apoprotein C-II	Chylomicrons, VLDL, Intralipid	Endothelium of extra-hepatic tissues	Hydrolysis* to TG to FFA and MG
Hepatic lipase (HL)		VLDL, HDL	Endothelium of liver	Hydrolysis of triglycerides and phospholipids
Lecithin: cholesterol Acyl transferase (LCAT)	Apoprotein AI	Lecithin, cholesterol	Plasma	FA transfer; synthesis of cholesteryl ester
Acyl carnitine transferase (ACT)	Carnitine	Long-chain fatty acid	Mitochondria	Transfer of FA across mitochondrial membrane for oxidation

Data from Hamosh M, Dhanireddy R, Zaidan H, Hamosh P. Total parenteral nutrition with lipid in the newborn: the enzymes and cofactors active in the clearing of circulating lipoprotein triglyceride. In Stern L, Xanthou M, Friis-Hansen B (eds): Physiologic Foundations of Perinatal Care. New York, Praeger, 1985; 178.

isomes. The carnitine dependent transport of acyl-CoA across the mitochondrial membrane is a regulated process. Malonyl CoA inhibits this process in all tissues.

In liver, the activity of palmitoyl transferase in the outer mitochondrial membrane appears to be regulated by the nutritional state of the animal and by hormones (3, 5, 3-triiodothyronine). The sensitivity of the transferase to malonyl CoA also seems to vary with nutritional state.

Inborn errors of carnitine metabolism and function are known. In some patients the activity of carnitine palmitoyl transferase is decreased and they suffer fatigue and myoglobulinuria. In severe cases the liver has a reduced capacity to oxidize FA to ketone bodies. Carnitine deficiency in tissues is also a recognized disorder. In some cases the condition is limited to skeletal muscle. Patients having this deficiency suffer from muscle fatigue and muscle lipidosis. In the systemic deficiency all tissues seem to lack carnitine, and fatal cases have been reported. The cause may be an inability of the tissues to concentrate and retain carnitine. Conditions are also recognized in which the loss of carnitine from tissues (or lack of carnitine in the diet) is part of the pathogenic mechanism.

Because fatty acid oxidation and ketogenesis are critical to the survival of newborn infants, an adequate supply of carnitine is of major importance for the newborn. Recent studies[102] show that (1) the newborn has a critical need for carnitine; (2) plasma and tissue concentrations of carnitine are low in the newborn; (3) the biosynthesis of carnitine is not fully developed in the newborn; and (4) the

lack of dietary carnitine results in significantly lower plasma carnitine concentrations.

Newborn infants receive adequate amounts of carnitine from their mother's milk or current U.S. cow-milk-based formulas. Carnitine concentrations are similar in colostrum and in mature milk (approximately 60 nmol/ml), but are slightly higher during the first two weeks postpartum (80-100 nmol/ml). Mothers of full term and preterm infants secrete milk with similar carnitine concentrations.[102] Until recently soy-based formulas did not contain carnitine.

Total parenteral nutrition (TPN) is usually given without carnitine supplements, leading in some cases to carnitine deficiency. Conflicting data on the plasma concentrations of carnitine during total parenteral nutrition[91] suggest that additional studies are needed to clearly define whether L-carnitine should be administered to infants who receive total parenteral nutrition with lipid.

Ketone bodies give rise to acetoacetate. Acetoacetate is reduced by a specific innermembrane mitochondrial β-hydroxybutyric acid dehydrogenase to yield β-hydroxybutyrate. The release of acetoacetate and hydroxybutyrate from the liver into the blood and their uptake by peripheral tissues are a constant, normal process.

Recent studies suggest that the capacity for ketone synthesis by the liver is low in the immediate neonatal period in the human[103] and the guinea pig.[104] Developmental changes in ketogenesis in the perinatal period have been reported also in other species.[105,106]

The activity of the enzymes of ketone body utilization (such as 3-oxoacid-CoA transferase) in adult rat tissue is highest in kidney, heart, brown adipose tissue and adrenal gland; followed by submaxillary gland, lactating mammary gland and brain. The liver has low activity of 3-oxoacid-CoA transferase and this means that ketone bodies synthesized by the liver are not utilized by the liver but directed to peripheral tissues. The enzymes of ketone body utilization show marked changes in activity during development of the rat and the pattern varies in different tissues. In the suckling rat, activity is very high in brain and low in heart and kidney, resulting in channeling of ketone bodies to the developing brain in the suckling rat.

Although fatty acid oxidation does not occur in adult brain, it is present in fetal and neonatal brain,[107] contributing as much as 25% of the metabolites entering the Krebs (TCA) cycle.[108] Ketone bodies are a major source of energy for the developing brain in many species, including humans, in whom ketone bodies can be metabolized as early as 12-21 weeks' gestation. Such activity remains high during the remainder of gestation as well as postnatally.[109]

In rat brain, permeability for 3-hydroxybutyrate is sevenfold higher during suckling than either at birth or in the adult.[110] Milk fatty acids are the source of ketone bodies during this period. The brain is the major ketone-body-using tissue in suckling mammals;[111] activity of the enzymes that convert ketone bodies to acetyl-CoA increases rapidly after birth, reaches peak activity before weaning, and decreases thereafter.[112] There is a direct relationship between neurological immaturity at birth and the extent of ketone-body utilization.[113]

Because medium-chain fatty acids can enter mitochrondria without the need for carnitine-mediated transfer, they are a good source of ketone bodies. Indeed, the milk produced by mothers of preterm infants contains an almost twofold higher level of medium-chain fatty acids than the milk of women who deliver at term.

REQUIREMENTS FOR TERM AND PRETERM INFANTS

Long-term follow-up studies would be the only way to assess the effects of early nutrition on child development and health in adult life. Such studies are difficult to carry out and indeed follow-up of the effects of early fat nutrition is available only up to the end of the first decade of life.[33]

Several important questions have to be answered such as: Is obesity associated with bottle feeding, i.e., formula, rather than breast-feeding? Does early nutrition with cholesterol, present in human milk but only in trace amounts in formulas, affect cholesterol synthesis and catabolism in adult life? Should long-chain polyunsaturated fatty acids (C_{20}-C_{22}) be added to infant formula? Fat needs in preterm infants are complicated by the special nature of the questions. Survival of very preterm newborns is limited to the human; indeed premature delivery rarely occurs in other species. Milk of different species varies greatly in amount and composition of fat. Size and composition of fat depots as well as fetal and postnatal growth rates vary greatly among species. Thus, animal studies often cannot be used specifically to extrapolate to humans.[33]

The composition of milk possibly is the result of an "evolutionary adaptation" that aims to keep the diad of mother and infant in reasonably good health, i.e., nutrients might be in somewhat lower concentration than needed to achieve maximal potenial growth in order to avoid depriving the mother of her nutritional requirements.[116] Recognizing, however, that the human race has survived by rearing its young (like all other species) on mother's milk, one must recommend that during the early postnatal period infants be fed their own mother's milk or formula closely resembling human milk.

Preterm infants should be fed either their own mother's milk (which contains higher concentrations of protein, medium-chain fatty acids, and long-chain polyunsaturated fatty acids) or specially prepared formulas. Banked term human milk is inadequate for optimal growth of the preterm infant.[114] Although medium-chain triglycerides are more readily absorbed and metabolized than long-chain triglycerides, it might not be advisable to feed large amounts to infants because of an increased frequency of intestinal disturbances (such as loose stools).[89,115] Recommendations for lipid nutrition of the newborn are provided in Table 14.

DEFICIENCY

It is important to monitor the amount and type of dietary lipid as well as the extent of fat absorption in the infant in order to prevent deficiencies. Special attention should be given to provide sufficient essential fatty acids

TABLE 14.   Requirements for Newborn Infants

Fat Content	3.3-6.0 gm/100 Kcal (30-54% of calories)

Fat Composition
   Essential fatty acids $C_{18:2}$ 0.3 gm/100 kcal
   Polyunsaturated fatty acids C_{20}, C_{22} should be added
      in amounts present in human milk.
   Saturated fatty acids C_{12}, C_{14} should be kept at levels
      present in human milk.
   **Fat absorption should be at least 85% in full-term
   infants at 1 month of age.**
   Cholesterol
   Phospholipids $\searrow$ should be present in amounts
                    similar to that in human milk, i.e.,
                    10-20 mg/dl

(linoleic acid, 0.3 gm/100 cal). In light of the special role of n-3 fatty acids in neonatal brain development, and in normal nerve function at all ages, linolenic (C18:3, n-3) acid should be provided as well as the long-chain fatty acids eicosapentaenoic and docosahexaenoic. The latter should be provided because of clinical evidence of the inability of the newborn (especially the premature) infant to chain elongate and desaturate the parent compounds of this fatty acid family—linolenic acid.

EXCESS

Excess consumption of fat will lead to obesity. However, because diets high in carbohydrates will also result in excessive fat deposition, the intake of both fats and carbohydrates should not be excessive. Overfeeding, even to limited excess, will lead to an increase in the size and number of adipocytes, resulting in excessive weight. The critical period of increase in the cellularity of adipose tissue is the period between birth and two years of age. It is therefore important not to overfeed infants or toddlers.

SUMMARY AND NEEDS

As with many other nutrients, the needs and requirements for specific fats change as our understanding of their exact role improves. Another aspect that is important is the increased survival of infants of very low birth weight. Their specific nutritional needs are different from those of full term infants. A good knowledge of the metabolic differences as a function of gestational and postnatal age is essential in providing the proper nutrition for the newborn infant.

CASE REPORT

A six-year-old girl, previously in good health, who lost 300 cm of intestine following a gunshot wound, was maintained on TPN with a preparation rich in linoleic but low in linolenic acid. After 5 months on this nutritional regimen, she experienced episodes of distal numbness and paresthesias, and infrequent episodes of weakness that left her unable to ambulate for 10-15 minutes. The numbness began distally on the bottom of the feet, involved the dorsum of the feet, spreading centrally to the midlateral thigh areas. A vague pain accompanying these episodes was described in the lower extremities. Symptoms were worse at night and were associated with a pale appearance and a mottled discoloration of the distal lower extremities. Episodes of visual blurring increased from weekly to almost daily occurrence. Two months after the onset of symptoms she was admitted for evaluation. Neurological examination at that time was normal except for decreased peripheral vibratory sensation and a mild tremor of the left upper extremity. Findings, in addition, included a normal complete blood count, sedimentation rate, 20 channel chemistry analysis, T_4, folate, zinc, vitamin B_{12}, electroencephalogram, electromyogram. Nerve conduction velocities measured in the left peroneal and the left posterior tibial nerves were 48.9 and 47.3 m/s, respectively. These latter values were considered within normal limits. The ophthalmological examination was normal. The serum selenium level was less than 10 pg/ml (normal greater than 12 pg/ml). Height and weight were normal for age. FA patterns of serum lipids were measured in an effort to diagnose the cause of these abnormalities. The analysis, indeed, showed a deficiency of n-3 fatty acids. One month later the lipid source for the TPN was changed to a preparation containing higher levels of linolenic acid. Over the next 12 weeks, she experienced gradual and complete resolution of the paresthesias and episodes of weakness.

Careful analysis of the fatty acid composition of serum lipids revealed marginal linolate deficiencies and significant deficiency of linolenate. The metabolites derived from linolenic acid were significantly decreased. The nutritional change from TPN containing 0.66% linolenic acid (provided during the first 5 months of treatment) to a different lipid preparation containing 6.9% linolenic acid led, after several weeks, to normal serum fatty acid profile and disappearance of all symptoms.

The onset of neurological symptoms associated with n-3 fatty acid deficiency and their resolution upon provision of linolenic acid ($C_{18:3}$ n-3) suggest that the latter is a required dietary nutrient in humans and that n-3 long-chain polyunsaturated fatty acids are required for normal nerve function.

This classical report (Holman et al, Am J Clin Nutr 35:617-623, 1982) led to changes in the composition of lipid preparations for TPN use. Furthermore, it stressed the need for careful nutritional evaluation of patients maintained on TPN for long periods of time.

Acknowledgments

The skillful secretarial assistance of Mrs. Barbara Runner-Avery is greatfully acknowledged.
This work was supported by NIH Grants HD-10823, HD-15631, and NIH Contract HD-2-2816.

REFERENCES

1. Klis JB (ed). Scientific status summary of the Institute of Food Technologists. Fats in the diets. Why and where? Food Tech Dec 1981; 33-38.
2. Stamler J. Population studies. In Levy RI, Rifkind BM, Bennis N (eds): Nutrition, Lipids, and Coronary Heart Disease: A Global View. New York, Raven Press, 1979; 25-88.
3. Kritshevsky D (ed). Workshop of fat and cancer. Cancer Res 1981; 41:3677-3826.
4. McCay CS. Notes On The History of Human Nutrition. Bern, Switzerland, Hans Huber, 1973; 34-56.
5. James AT, Martin ATP. Gas-liquid partition chromatography: The separation and microestimation of volatile fatty acids from formic acid to dodecanoic acid. Biochem J 1952; 50:679-690.
6. Lindgren FT. The plasma lipoproteins: historical developments and nomenclature. Ann NY Acad Sci 1980; 348:1-15.
7. Tinoco J. Dietary requirements and functions of α-linoleic acid in animals. Progr Lipid Res 1982; 21:1-45.
8. Crawford MA, Hassam AG, Rivers JPW. Essential fatty acid requirements in infancy. Am J Clin Nutr 1978; 31:2181.
9. Neuringer M, Connor WE, Van Petten C, Barstad L. Dietary omega-3 fatty acid deficiency and visual loss in infant rhesus monkeys. J Clin Invest 1984; 73:272-276.
10. Connor WE, Neuringer M, Lin D, Neuwelt E. The incorporation of docosahexoenoic acid into the brain of monkeys deficient in W-3 fatty acids. XIII Internatl. Congr. Nutr. Abstracts 1985; 104.
11. Clandinin MT, Chappell JE, Heim T, et al. Fatty acid utilization in perinatal de novo synthesis of tissues. Early Human Dev 1981; 5:355-366.
12. American Academy of Pediatrics Committee on Nutrition. Commentary on breast feeding and infant formulas including proposed standards for formulas. Pediatrics 1976; 57:278.
13. Bitman J, Wood DL, Hamosh M, et al. Comparison of the lipid composition of breast milk from mothers of term and preterm infants. Am J Clin Nutr 1983; 38:300-313.
14. Holman RT, Johnson SB, Hatch TF. A case of human linolenic acid deficiency involving neurological abnormalities. Am J Clin Nutr 1982; 35:617-623.
15. Harris WS, Connor WE, Goodnight SH Jr.. Dietary fish oils, plasma lipids and platelets in man. Progr Lipid Res 1981; 20:75.
16. Phillipson BE, Rothrock DW, Connor WE, et al. Reduction of plasma lipids, lipoprotein and apoproteins by dietary fish oils in patients with hypertriglyceridemia. N Engl J Med 1985; 312:1210-1216.
17. Moncada S, Vane JR. Arachidonic acid metabolism and the interactions between platelets and blood vessels. N Engl J Med 1979; 300:1142-1147.
18. Samuelsson B. Leukotrienes: mediators of allergic reactions and inflammation. Int Arch Allergy Appl Immun 1981; 66(Suppl I): 98.
19. Lucas A, Mitchell MD. Prostaglandins in human milk. Arch Dis Child 1980; 55:950.
20. Koldovsky O, Bedrick A, Thornberg W. Hormones in milk: effect on the developing gastrointestinal tract in weanling and suckling rats. J Pediatr Gastroenterol Nutr 1986; 6:172-196.
21. Bedrick AD, Holtzapple PG. Indomethacin fails to induce ulceration in the gastrointestinal tract of newborn and suckling rats. Pediatr Res 1986; 20:598-601.
22. Materia A., Jaffe BM, Money SR, et al. Prostaglandins in commercial milk preparations. Their effect in the prevention of stress-induced gastric ulcer. Arch Surg 1984; 119:290-292.
23. Johansson C, Kollberg B, Nordemar R, et al. Protective effect of prostaglandin E₂ in the gastrointestinal tract during indomethacin treatment of rheumatic diseases. Gastroenterology 1980; 78:479-483.
24. Befrits R, Johansson C. Oral PGE₂ inhibits gastric acid secretion in man. Prostaglandins. 1980; 29:143-152.
25. Johansson C, Aly A, Kollberg B, et al. Trophic action of oral E₂ prostaglandins on the rat gastrointestinal mucosa.
Adv Prostagland Thrombox Leukotrien Res 1983; 12:403-407.
26. Lichtenberger LM, Graziani LA, Dial EJ, et al. Role of surface-active phospholipids in gastric cytoprotection. Science 1983; 219:1327-1329.
27. Dial EJ, Lichtenberger LM. A role of milk phospholipids in protection against acid. Studies in adult and suckling rats. Gastroenterology 1984; 87:379-385.
28. Hamosh M. Physiological role of human milk lipases. In Lebenthal E (ed): Gastrointestinal Development and Infant Nutrition. New York, Raven Press 1981; 473-482.
29. Ruegg M, Blanc B. The fat globule size distribution in human milk. Biochem Biophys Acta 1981; 666:7-13.
30. Jensen RG, Clark RM, Ferris AM. Composition of the lipids in human milk: A review. Lipids 1980; 15:345.
31. Clandinin MT, Chappell JE, Heim T. Do low birth weight infants require nutrition with chain elongation—desaturation products of essential fatty acids? Progr Lipid Res 1982; 20:901.
32. Bitman J, Wood DL, Mehta NR, et al. Comparison of the cholesteryl ester composition of breast milk from preterm and term mothers. J Pediatr Gastroenterol Nutr 1986; 6:780-786.
33. Hamosh M, Hamosh P. Does nutrition in early life have long term metabolic effects? Can animal models be used to predict these effects in the human? In Goldman AS, Atkinson AS, Hanson LA (eds): Human Lactation, Vol 3: The Effect of Human Milk Upon the Recipient Infant. New York, Plenum Press, 1987; 37-55.
34. Harris WD, Conner WE, Lindsey S. Will dietary W-3 fatty acids change the composition of human milk? Am J Clin Nutr 1984; 40:780-785.
35. Craig-Schmidt MC, Weete JD, Faircloth SA, et al. The effect of hydrogenated fat in the diet of nursing mothers on lipid composition and prostaglandin content of human milk. Am J Clin Nutr 1984; 39:778-786.
36. Chappell JE, Clandinin MT, Kearney-Volpe C. Trace fatty acids in human milk lipids: influence of maternal diet and weight loss. Am J Clin Nutr 1985; 42:49-56.
37. Johnston JM. Mechanism of fat absorption. In Code CF, Heidel W (eds): Handbook of Physiology, Section 6: Alimentary Canal, Vol III; Intestinal Absorption. Washington DC, American Physiological Society, 1968; 1353-1375.
38. Bernard C. Memoire sur le pancreas et sur le role du suc pancreatique dans les phenomenes digestifs, particulierement dans la digestion des matieres grasses neutres. Compt Rend Suppl 1856; 43:379-563.
39. Bernard C. Recherches sur les usages du suc pancreatique dans la digestion. CR Acad Sci 1849; 28:249-253.
40. Munk I. Zur Kenntniss der Bedeutung des Fettes und seiner Componenten fur den Stoffwechsel. Arch Pathol Anat Physiol 1980; 80:10-47.
41. Munk I. Zur Frage der Fettresorption. Z. Physiol 14:155-156, 1900.
42. Pfluger E. Uber die Resorption kunstlich gefarbter Fette. Arch Ges Physiol 1900; 81:375-400.
43. Munk I. Die Frage der Fettresorption und Herr E. Pfluger. Z Physiol 1900; 14:409-412.
44. Verzar F, McDougal EJ. Absorption from the Intestine. London; Longmans, 1936; 150-211.
45. Verzar F, Laszt L. Untersuchungen uber die Resorption von Fettsauren. Biochem Z 1934; 270:24-34.
46. Frazer AC. Fat absorption and metabolism. Analyst 1938; 63:308-314.
47. Bloom B, Chaikoff IL, Reinhard WO. Intestinal lymph as pathway for transport of absorbed fatty acids of different chain lengths. Am J Physiol 1951; 166:451-455.
48. Borgstrom B, Dahlquist A, Lundh G, Sjovall J. Studies on intestinal digestion and absorption in the human. J Clin Invest 1957; 36:1521-1536.
49. Johnston JM, Intestinal absorption of dietary fat. Compr Biochem 1970; 18:1-18.
50. Willis ED. Lipases. Adv Lipid Res 1965; 3:197-240.
51. Volhard. Uber das fettspaltende Ferment des Magens. Z Clin Med 1901; 42:414-429.
52. Hamosh M. Fat digestion in the newborn: role of lingual lipase and preduodenal digestion. Pediatr Res 1979; 13:615-622.

53. DeNigris SJ, Hamosh M, Kasbekar DK, et al. Human gastric lipase: Secretion from dispersed gastric glands. Biochim Biophys Acta 1985; 836:67-72.

54. Borgstrom B, Erlanson C. Pancreatic juice colipase: physiological importance. Biochim Biophys Acta 1971; 242:509-513.

55. Maylie MF, Charles M, Gache C, Desnuelles P: Isolation and partial identification of a pancreatic colipase. Biochim Biophys Acta 1971; 229:286-289.

56. Borgstrom B, Erlanson-Albertsson C. Pancreatic colipase. In Borgstrom B, Brockman HL (eds): Lipases. Amsterdam, Elsevier, 1984; 151-183.

57. Rosenheim O. On pancreatic lipase III. The separation of lipase from its co-enzyme. J Physiol 1910; 15:XIV-XVI.

58. Freudenberg E. Die frauenmilch Lipase. Basel, Karger, 1953.

59. Hernell O, Olivecrona T. Human milk lipases. II. Bile salt stimulated lipase. Biochim Biophys Acta 1974; 369:234-244.

60. Patton JS. Gastrointestinal lipid digestion. In Johnson LR (ed): Physiology of the gastrointestinal tract. New York; Raven Press, 1981; 1123-1146.

61. Hamosh M, Klaeveman HL. Wolf RO, Scow RO. Pharyngeal lipase and digestion of dietary triglycerides in man. J Clin Invest 1975; 55:908-913.

62. Hamosh M, Burns WA: Lipolytic activity of human lingual glands (Ebner). Lab Invest 1977; 37:603-608.

63. Roy CC, Roulet M, Lefebre D, et al. The role of gastric lipolysis in fat absorption and bile acid metabolism in the rat Lipids 1979; 14:811-814.

64. Plucinski TM, Hamosh M, Hamosh P. Fat digestion in the rat: role of lingual lipase. Am J Physiol 1979; 237:E541-E547.

65. Watkins JB. Mechanism of fat absorption and the development of gastrointestinal function. Pediatr Clin North Am 1975; 22:721-730.

66. Hamosh M. Lingual and breast milk lipases. Adv Pediatr 1982; 29:33-67.

67. Abrams CK, Hamosh M, Hubbard VS, et al. Lingual lipase in cystic fibrosis. Quantitation of enzyme activity in the upper small intestine of patients with exocrine pancreatic insufficiency. J Clin Invest 1984; 73:374-382.

68. Abrams CK, Hamosh M, Dutta SK, et al. Role of nonpancreatic lipolytic activity in exocrine pancreatic insufficiency. Gastroenterology 1987; 92:125-129.

69. Patton JS, Rigler MW, Liao TH, et al. Hydrolysis of triacylglycerol emulsions by lingual lipase—a microscopic study. Biochim Biophys Acta 1982; 712:400-407.

70. Jensen RG, Clark RM, de Jong FA, et al. The lipolytic triad: human lingual, breast milk and pancreatic lipases: physiological implications of their characteristics in digestion of dietary fat. J Pediatr Gastroenterol Nutr 1982; 1:243-255.

71. Carey MC, Small DM, Bliss CM: Lipid digestion and absorption. Ann Rev Physiol 1983; 45:651-677.

72. Watkins JB. Lipid digestion and absorption. Pediatrics 1985; 75(Suppl):151-155.

73. Mehta NR, Jones JB, Hamosh M. Lipases in human milk: ontogeny and physiologic significance. J Pediatr Gastroenterol Nutr 1982; 1:317-326.

74. Hamosh M, Bitman J, Fink CS, et al. Lipid composition of preterm human milk and its digestion by the infant. In Schaub J (ed): Composition and Physiological Properties of Human Milk. Amsterdam, Elsevier, 1985; 153-164.

75. Johnston JM, Borgstrom B. The intestinal absorption and metabolism of micellar solution of lipids. Biochim Biophys Acta 1964; 84:412-423.

76. Stremmel W, Lotz G, Strohmeyer G, Berk PD. Identification, isolation and partial characterization of a fatty acid binding protein from rat jejunal microvillus membranes. J. Clin Invest 1985; 75:1068-1076.

77. Ockner RK, Manning JM. Fatty acid binding protein in small intestine: identification, isolation and evidence for its role in cellular fatty acid transport. J Clin Invest 1974; 54:326-338.

78. Johnston JM. Triglyceride biosynthesis in the intestinal mucosa. In Rommel K, H. Goebell H, Bohmer R (eds): Lipid Absorption: Biochemical and Clinical Aspects. Lancaster, UK, MTP, 1976; 85-94.

79. Holzapple PG, Smith G, Koldowsky O. Uptake, activation,

and esterification of fatty acids in the small intestine of the suckling rat. Pediatr Res 1975; 9:786-791.

80. Tso P, Balint JA. Formation and transport of chylomicrons by enterocytes to the lymphatics. Am J Physiol 1986; 250:G715-G726.

81. Wretlind A. Development of fat emulsions. J Parent Ent Nutr 1981; 5:230-235.

82. Courten W. Experiments and observations of the effect of several sorts of poisons upon animals. Ecc. made at Montpellier in the years 1678-1679. Phil Trans Roy Soc (Lond) 1710; 27:485-499.

83. Geyer R. Parenteral nutrition. Physiol Rev 1960; 40:150-186.

84. Olegard R, Gustafson A, Kjellmer I, Victorin L. Nutrition in low birth weight infants. III. Lipolysis and free fatty acid elimination after intravenous administration of fat emulsion. Acta Pediatr Scand 1975; 64:745-751.

85. Hamosh M, Hamosh P. Lipoprotein lipase: Its physiological and clinical significance. Molec Aspects Med 1983; 6:199-289.

86. Eisenberg S. Very low density lipoprotein metabolism. Progr. Biochem Pharmacol 1979; 15:139-165.

87. Glomset JA. Lecithin: cholesterol acyltransferase. An exercise in comparative biology. Progr Biochem Pharmacol 1976; 15:41-46.

88. American Academy of Pediatrics, Committee on Nutrition. Use of intravenous fat emulsions in pediatric patients. Pediatrics 1981; 68:739-743.

89. American Academy of Pediatrics, Committee on Nutrition. Nutritional needs of low-birth-weight infants. Pediatrics 1985; 76:976-986.

90. Hamosh M, Dhanireddy R, Zaidan H, Hamosh P. Total parenteral nutrition with Intralipid in the newborn: the enzymes and cofactors active in the clearing of circulating lipoprotein-triglyceride. In Stern L, Xanthou M, Friis-Hansen B (eds): Physiologic Foundations of Perinatal Care. New York, Praeger, 1985; 176-195.

91. Stahl GE, Spear ML, Hamosh M. Intravenous administration of lipid emulsion to premature infants. Clin Perinatol 1986; 13:133-162.

92. Kao LC, Cheng MH, Warburton D. Triglycerides, free fatty acids, free fatty acid/albumin molar ratio, and cholesterol levels in serum of neonates receiving long-term lipid infusions: controlled trial of continuous and intermittent regimens. J Pediatr 1984; 104:429-435.

93. Berkow S, Spear ML, Gutman A, et al. Lipid clearing in premature infants. Response to increasing doses of Intralipid (IL): I-Circulating lipoprotein lipase (LPL) and hepatic lipase (HL). Pediatr Res 1984; 18:136A.

94. Dhanireddy R, Hamosh M, Sivasubramanian KN, et al. Postheparin lipolytic activity and Intralipid clearance in very low birth weight infants. J Pediatr 1981; 98:617-622.

95. Zaidan H, Dhanireddy R, Hamosh M, et al. Effect of continous heparin administration on Intralipid clearing in very low birth weight infants. J Pediatr 1982; 101:599-602.

96. Papadopolous A, Hamosh M, Scanlon JW, et al. Lipid clearing in premature infants: lecithin-cholesterol acyl transferase activity. Pediatr Res 1985; 19:256A.

97. Griffin E, Breckenridge WC, Kuksis A, et al. Appearance and characterization of lipoprotein-X during continuous Intralipid infusion in the neonate. J Clin Invest 1979; 64: 1703-1712.

98. Rovamo L, Nikkila EA, Taskinen MR, Raivio KO. Postheparin plasma lipoprotein and hepatic lipases in preterm neonates. Pediatr Res 1984; 18:1104-1107.

99. Schmidt-Sommerfeld E, Penn D, Wolf H. Carnitine deficiency in premature infants receiving total parenteral nutrition: effect of L-carnitine supplementation. J Pediatr 1983; 102:931-935.

100. Shenai JP, Borum PR, Mohan P, et al. Carnitine status at birth of newborn infants of varying gestation. Pediatr Res 1983; 17:579-582.

101. Brennen J. Carnitine metabolism and function. Physiol Rev 1983; 63:1420.

102. Borum PR. Carnitine. Ann Rev Nutr 1983; 3:233-259.

103. Stanley CA, Anday E, Baker L, Delivoria-Papadopoulos M. Metabolic fuel and hormone responses to fasting in newborn infants. Pediatrics 1979; 64:613-619.

104. Stanley CA, Gonzales E, Baker L. Development of hepatic fatty acid oxidation and ketogenesis in the newborn guinea pig. Pediatr Res 1983; 17:224-229.
105. Warshaw JB. Cellular energy metabolism during fetal development. IV. Fatty acid activation, acyl transfer and fatty acid oxidation during development of the chick and rat. Develop Biol 1972; 28:537.
106. Yeh YY, Zee P. Fatty acid oxidation in isolated rat liver mitochrondria. Developmental changes and their relation to hepatic levels of carnitine and glycogen and to carnitine acyltransferase activity. Arch Biochem Biophys 1979; 197:560.
107. Yoshida T, Roux JR. In vitro metabolism of palmitic acid in human fetal tissue. Pediatr Res 1972; 6:675.
108. Spitzer JJ. Application of tracers in studying free fatty acid metabolism of various organs in vitro. Fed Proc 1975; 34:2242.
109. Gonzales LW, Geel SE. Enhanced cerebral protein synthesis in developing hypothyroid rats: Evidence of delayed maturation. J Neurochem 1978; 31:1239.
110. Moore TJ, Lione AP, Sugden MC, Regen DM. Hydroxy-

butyrate transport in rat brain: Developmental and dietary modulations. Am J Physiol 1976; 230:619.
111. Meisami E, Timiras PS. Normal and abnormal biochemical development of the brain after birth. In Jones CT (ed): Biochemical Development of the Fetus and Neonate. New York, Elsevier 1982; 759.
112. Page MA, Williamson DH. Enzymes of ketone-body utilization in human brain. Lancet 1971; 2:66.
113. Booth RFG, Patel TB, Clark JB. The development of enzymes of energy metabolism in the brain of precocial (guinea pig) and nonprecocial (rat) species. J Neurochem 1980; 34:17.
114. Gross SJ. Growth and biochemical response of preterm infants fed human milk or modified infant formula. N Engl J Med 1983; 308:237-241.
115. Okamoto E, Muttart CR, Zucker CL, et al Use of medium chain triglycerides in feeding the low birth weight infant. Am J Dis Child 1982; 136:418-431.
116. Dugdale AE. Evolution and breast feeding. Lancet 1986; 1:670-673.

9

Requirements for Sodium Chloride and Potassium and Their Interrelation with Water Requirement

MALCOLM A. HOLLIDAY, M.D.

ABSTRACT

The basis for determining sodium chloride (NaCl) and water requirements for very-low birth weight (VLBW) infants is uncertain because physiological and pathological variables alter requirements and tolerances so that there is no safe general range. Requirements are based on the amount of NaCl and water needed to sustain an effective circulating volume; intolerances are based on amounts that cause signs of circulatory overload. A review of the signals of circulatory deficiency and overload are the best specific guides for determining a safe intake in individual cases. In VLBW infants without major complicating factors, the NaCl provided by conventional milks, 1-1.5 mM/kg/day, commonly appears to be insufficient. Supplements to increase intake to 3-5 mM/kg/day for the first 2-3 weeks of life appear to meet the requirements for NaCl without clinical signs of overload. Intakes of NaCl provided by conventional milks may limit nitrogen retention and growth, whereas slightly more—2-3 mM/kg/day—appears to suffice. VLBW infants who have major complications require individual assessment. The intake of water usually is determined by calorie requirement because water is the vehicle for all nutrients; its intake ranges between 100-200 ml/kg/day. To sustain water balance on this intake, 50-150 ml will be excreted as urine. The renal capacity to excrete free water (C_{H_2O}/100 ml GFR) usually will be sufficient; if antidiuretic hormone (ADH) release is effected by stress, including the stress of inadequate circulation, free water excretion is impaired. When this occurs, free-water excretion may not balance free-water intake without hyponatremia developing. The incidence of hyponatremia is less in salt-supplemented infants.

The need for potassium (K) is equal to the K retained for growth and the obligate renal and extrarenal losses. All milks used provide enough K for the growth and usual maintenance requirements based on the K:N ratios in these milks. Unusual renal losses of K from drugs, alkali therapy, steroid administration or secondary hyperaldosteronism may increase the requirement for K and may necessitate supplementation.

INTRODUCTION

Sodium (Na), chloride (Cl) and potassium (K) are the principal electrolytes of body fluids: Na and Cl for extracellular fluid (ECF), and K for intracellular fluid (ICF).

For adults in normal health, the requirement of each is very low and the range of intake tolerated is great because a complex set of feedback controls regulates the balance of each. **The requirement for NaCl is related to the maintenance of an effective circulating volume and an interstitial fluid (ISF) volume,** which interact with these feedback controls to effect NaCl balance. Water balance is regulated by feedback controls that usually are sensitive to changes in osmolarity; under most conditions water balance is regulated by ADH and the same controls that govern NaCl balance. Hence the requirement for water is considered in relation to the requirement for NaCl. Illness or stress that is associated with large extrarenal loss or sequestration of ECF creates an acute need for NaCl and water to restore the effective circulating volume; the capacity to excrete water alone is impaired when circulating volume is reduced. Renal disease that limits excretion or conditions associated with hypervolemic edema create a need for restricting NaCl and water intake or promoting their removal.

Determining appropriate intakes of NaCl and water for low birthweight (LBW) and very-low birthweight (VLBW) infants is based on these same principles. However, defining and monitoring effective circulating and ISF volumes are difficult and hence there is uncertainty about how much NaCl and water to give. This chapter approaches the definition of NaCl and water requirement and tolerance from the perspective of describing signs of deficiency and excess of circulating and ISF volume.

Determining the appropriate intake of K is

based on anticipated losses—renal and non-renal—which in LBW and VLBW infants are related to a variety of physiological abnormalities or treatment plans more than they are to conventional nutritional requirements. The requirement for K and the factors affecting requirement are discussed in a subsequent section. Deficiency of either NaCl or K will limit growth.

For the purposes of this chapter, term infants are defined as infants who are generally appropriate for gestational age (AGA) and weigh more than 2500 gm; low birthweight (LBW) infants weigh between 1500 and 2500 gm and are AGA; very-low-birthweight (VLBW) infants are AGA infants who weigh between 800 and 1500 gm and are less than 32 weeks' gestation. Small for gestational age (SGA) infants generally are more mature than LBW or VLBW infants of the same weight. They appear to function closer to their gestational age than to their weight when compared with AGA infants. This chapter focuses on VLBW and term infants in relation to normal adults. In general LBW infants behave more like term infants but are more likely than term infants to experience vicissitudes common to the VLBW infants.

SODIUM CHLORIDE AND WATER

PHYSIOLOGY

The physiology of NaCl and water is related to control of distribution of ECF and excretion of NaCl and water. The common experience is that intake exceeds minimal losses, i.e., that intake is in excess of need and excess is excreted in urine. It is appropriate to consider physiology in terms of intake, body composition and excretion of excess. Deficiency invokes redistribution of the circulation, and renal-conserving mechanism.

Intake

The intake of NaCl by adults among different cultures varies from 10–1000 mM/day. The intake of infants varies from 10 to 100 mM/day.[5] In neither case does difference in intake cause a signifiant difference in Na or Cl concentration in plasma or ECF; ECF volume is only slightly affected; excess intake is generally excreted by the kidney. Individuals on high intakes show fluctuations in ECF volume that do not occur in those on low intakes. The former show a circadian change in ECF volume with a frequency of 4-8 days.[19] The latter have higher plasma renin and aldosterone concentrations that reflect the slight contraction of ECF volume.[30]

The intake of NaCl by infants fed human milk is low compared with intakes of infants fed cow milk formulas. However gain in weight is the same or only slightly greater in the infants fed more NaCl.[25] LBW infants also appear to do well over a comparable range of intakes (Table 1). For both term and LBW infants, 1 mM/kg/day suffices as long as extrarenal losses are normal.

The range tolerated by VLWB infants is in dispute. Conventional intakes, 1-1.5 mM/kg/day, suitable for term and LBW infants have consequences in VLBW infants that have led some to recommend intakes of 3-5 mM/kg/day.[1] Others feel that these higher intakes are harmful because they are associated with an increased prevalence of patent ductus arteriosus and respiratory distress.[9,44]

The intake of water by adults varies from 1-4 L/day in response to changes in solute intake, extrarenal fluid losses or, more commonly today, because of personal preferences. The extreme range of tolerance is 0.5-20 L/day. The range of intake by infants is less—100-200 ml/kg/day—because infant formulas have similar calorie densities; differences in milk composition result in two-to-threefold differences in renal solute load. Urine volume in

TABLE 1. Sodium and Water Exchange of Infants Fed Different Milks

	Na*		Water		
	Intake	Renal excretion	Intake	Excretion	Urine Osmolality
	(mEq/kg/day)		(ml/kg/day)		(mOsm/L)
Human milk	1.0	0.5	160	110	70
Most formulas	1.5	1.0	160	110	120
Cow milk	3.5	3.0	160	110	250

*Values for Cl run higher by 30-50%.

BLOOD CAPILLARY

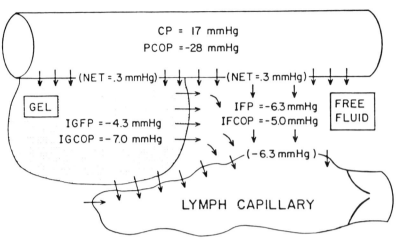

FIGURE 1. The microcirculation. Pressures that regulate the exchange of fluid between capillaries, interstitial fluid and lymph are shown. The forces moving fluid out in mm Hg are capillary pressure (CP = 17) plus negative interstitial fluid pressure (IFP = −6.3) plus interstitial fluid colloid oncotic pressure (IFCOP = −5) totaling 28.3. The force moving fluid into capillaries is the plasma colloid oncotic pressure (PCOP = −28). The net difference = .3; there results a net gain of fluid by the interstitial space and this is moved back to the circulation via lymphatics. (From Guyton AC. Capillary dynamics and exchange of fluid between the blood and interstitial fluid, In Guyton AC: Textbook of Medical Physiology, 6th ed. Philadelphia, W.B. Saunders Co., 1981, with permission.)

these infants also tends to be the same unless there is a change in effective circulating volume that causes water retention. Urine osmolarity varies directly in relation to solute load (see Table 1). Water intake relative to body water is higher in infants than it is in adults. An intake of 100-200 ml/kg/day exceeds the minimum intake by two-to-fourfold and, in the absence of stress that causes release of antidiuretic hormone or vasopressin, is well below the limits of tolerance.[24]

The water intake of VLBW infants also tends to vary between 100–200 ml/kg/day and is largely determined by the perceived need for nutrients such as human milk or infant formula. Both extrarenal and renal excretion of water in VLBW infants is subject to wide changes that are independent of intake, and these changes may lead to water retention (hyponatremia) or deficit (hypernatremia), which is common in VLBW infants.[28]

Body Composition

More than 90% of NaCl is distributed in the extracellular phase of the body. A small percent of exchangeable Na and a smaller percent of Cl is intracellular. The extracellular phase includes bone, connective tissue, interstitial space and plasma. There are also the transcellular fluids—gastrointestinal and cerebrospinal—and other secreted fluids including sweat, which contain Na and Cl. The ECF in adults is 20% of body weight;[23] in infants it is 40% of body weight (see below).

Plasma and ISF volume are the two physiologically critical variables of the extracellular phase. The exchange of fluid between plasma and ISF is controlled by the Starling forces, which regulate the flux of fluid between capillaries and the interstitium, and by lymph flow. The efflux of fluid from capillaries is mediated by capillary hydraulic pressure (which, in adults, is approximately 28 mm Hg at the arterial end of the capillary, around 20 at the venous end), and the negative interstitial free-fluid pressure, which is -6 mm Hg. The influx is mediated by the oncotic pressure of plasma proteins which, in adults, is 28 mm Hg minus the oncotic pressure of ISF (5 mm). The efflux in adults at rest averages 16 and the influx 14-15 ml/min. The difference is the net transfer of fluid from plasma to the interstitium. This is returned to plasma as lymph by the lymphatics (Fig. 1).[21] When this exchange is not balanced, either circulating or ISF volumes or both may be compromised. This is much more likely to happen in VLBW infants.

Body water in adults is 50-60% of body weight; it is freely permeable across cells and therefore is distributed between ECF and ICF according to the solute content of each. The commonest factors causing a change in osmolarity are extrarenal or renal water loss, water intake that is not excreted, or a change in body NaCl that affects the osmolar content of ECF.[22] These also are much more likely to occur in VLBW infants.

The ECF phase of term infants at birth when expressed as percent of body weight is high—approximately 40%. There is a normal decrease in ECF in the first few days of life that accounts for most of the postnatal weight loss of 5-8% of body weight. Thereafter, ECF volume as a percent of body weight decreases slightly until 1-2 years of age when it reaches a stable percent of body weight.[49]

The ECF of VLBW infants as a percent of body weight is even larger than that of term infants. ECF is 70% of body weight in a 23-week fetus and it declines so that it is 50% in the 28–32-week fetus. The higher ECF phase of VLBW infants, given the same intake as term infants, decreases following birth by an amount that equals 12-15% body weight. Whereas the loss in the term infant has no measurable adverse effects, this may not be the case for VLBW infants. In fact, the evidence cited below indicates that these losses compromise circulating volume in the VLBW infant.

Circulating volume is compromised in adults when there is a deficiency of NaCl due either to losses (renal or extrarenal) exceeding intake, e.g., dehydration secondary to gastroenteritis, or its sequestration as edema following tissue injury. Reduced lymph return or lymphatic obstruction leads to an accumulation of fluid in the interstitium and contraction of plasma volume. A reduction in plasma protein as occurs with "capillary leak" decreases plasma oncotic pressure; influx of fluid into the circulation is reduced so that there is a net shift of fluid from plasma to the interstitium. Capillary pressure drops as a result of the loss of fluid from plasma.[21] In these three examples, the decrease in circulating volume initiates vasoconstrictor, antinatriuretic and antidiuretic responses. These are the signs of NaCl and water deficiency for which NaCl and water intake should be increased, or factors causing shifts of fluid from plasma should be corrected, so that circulating volume is sustained.

Sodium chloride and water overload (isotonic expansion) as occurs with saline infusion is distributed proportionally between plasma and the interstitium. This initiates vasodilatory responses, suppression of vasconstrictive hormones such as renin and angiotensin, a release of atrial natriuretic peptide (ANP) and a saline diuresis.[40] Retention of NaCl in renal failure is similarly distributed but it is less readily excreted.[11] The concentration of Na in ECF remains normal in both instances either because the fluid is administered and

excreted at that concentration or because water is ingested in response to thirst so that Na and Cl concentration and effective osmolarity remain normal. Lymph flow adjusts so that distribution between plasma and ISF is balanced. In these instances vasodilator and natriuretic factors are released, and vasoconstrictor and antidiuretic factors are suppressed.[27] There is a sustained release of these factors in renal failure when intake exceeds excretory capacity, leading to a chronically expanded ECF volume.

ECF volume contraction and overload occur with few clinical signs in LBW and VLBW infants. As a consequence, it is difficult to gauge effective circulating volume from clinical signs. Therefore it is necessary to find indicators for circulating volume status that can be used to indicate NaCl deficiency or excess (Fig. 2).

Controls Affecting Distribution of Blood Flow and Renal Excretion

Both distribution of blood flow and the renal excretion of NaCl and water are regulated by a series of integrated feedback loops (see Fig. 2).[8] These systems have been the subject of intense study in adults in the last decade, and their responses to volume contraction and expansion can be described in some detail. Some work has been carried out in term and even in VLBW infants. Knowledge of how the systems operate in adults is a valuable prerequisite for interpreting the data obtained from VLBW infants in response to different levels of NaCl and water intake.

The Afferent Limbs. There are two kinds of afferent limbs of these loops:

1. The osmoreceptors. The osmoreceptors located in the hypothalamus respond to change in the osmotic gradient between ECF and ICF. A rise in extracellular osmolarity activates the powerful drive for water intake and the efferent limbs of the feedback loop that concentrate urine and reduce urinary water loss; a drop in extracellular osmolarity does the reverse. As a result **the osmolarity of body water is kept relatively constant**—around 290 mOsm/L—unless stimuli from baroreceptors override this loop.[36]

2. The baroreceptors. The baroreceptors located throughout the vascular system respond to change in pressure. A decrease in pressure activates the efferent limbs of the loop that initiate vasoconstrictor responses in a progressive sequence to maintain peripheral resistance and cardiac output, which sustain

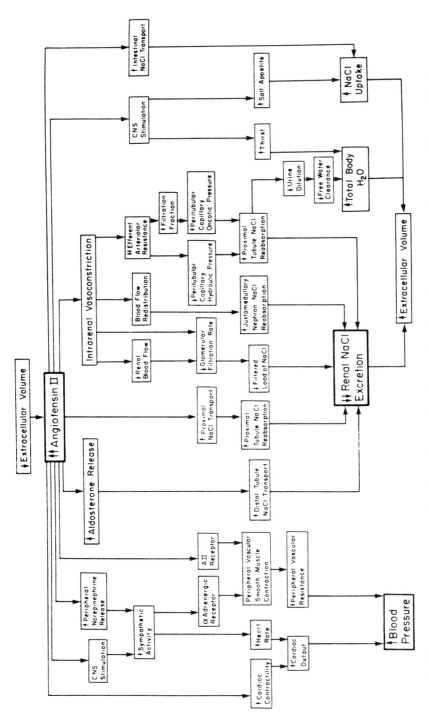

FIGURE 2.   A schematic depiction of the forces that regulate Na excretion with particular emphasis on how these integrate with changes in effective circulating volume. Critical areas are shaded. (From Ballarmann BJ, Levenson DJ, Brenner BM. Renin-angiotensin, kinins, prostaglandins and leukotrienes. In Brenner BM, Rector FC (eds): The Kidney, 3rd ed. Philadelphia, W.B. Saunders Co., 1986, p. 294, with permission.)

blood pressure. Blood flow is redistributed. These same responses change renal hemodynamics and renal tubular function to conserve NaCl and water. An increase in pressure has the opposite effects.[22]

The Efferent Limbs. The following systems are included in the efferent limbs of the loop:[22]

1. Sympathetic nervous system—norepinephrine, and dopamine. The sympathetic nervous system, through direct action and release of norepinephrine and epinephrine, causes an increase in cardiac output and a vasoconstrictor response that increases vascular resistance, particularly in the skin and splanchnic area. Blood pressure rises; blood flow is shunted from the periphery and splanchnic area, including the kidneys, to the heart, brain and muscle. Stimulation of beta-adrenergic receptors causes renin release and decreased NaCl excretion.[32] Urinary excretion of catecholamines increases. Dopaminergic stimuli released from alpha-adrenergic stimulation decrease renal resistance and increase renal blood flow and NaCl excretion.[12]

2. The renin-angiotensin aldosterone system (RAAS). The renin-angiotensin system produces the potent vasoconstricter angiotensin II. Release of renin in response to stimuli from the juxtaglomerular (JG) apparatus, which is located at the neck of the glomerulus, initiates the sequence. The juxtaglomerular apparatus is sensitive to change in afferent and efferent glomerular arteriolar tone and to tubular fluid flow through the distal convolution where it passes adjacent to the JG apparatus (Fig. 3).[33] Renin initiates release of angiotension I from renin substrate in plasma, and this in turn is transformed into angiotension II—the active vasoconstrictor. Its action upon arterioles raises peripheral resistance and sustains blood pressure in response to blood volume contraction. This action increases afferent and efferent glomerular arteriolar resistance and maintains glomerular capillary blood flow; reduced NaCl excretion results but there is little or no reduction in glomerular filtration rate (GFR). Angiotensin II also stimulates release of aldosterone.[8,33]

3. Arginine vasopressin (AVP) or antidiuretic hormone (ADH). AVP (or ADH) acts to regulate free water clearance (C_{H_2O}) or its reabsorption. Hyperosmolality (295-300 mOsm/L) stimulates AVP release, which stimulates thirst and reabsorption of free water; hypoosmolality (288-295 mOsm/L)

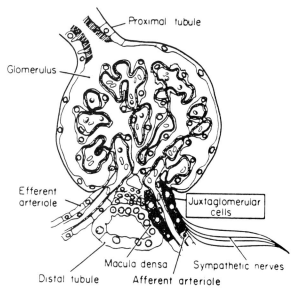

FIGURE 3. The relation of the juxtaglomerular cells to the afferent and efferent arterioles of the glomerulus and the distal tubule in the mammalian kidney. Change in resistance of afferent and efferent arteriole alters glomerular capillary flow and pressure. (From Rauh W. Renin angiotensin system. In Holliday MA, Barratt TM, Vernier R (eds): Pediatric Nephrology, 2nd ed. Baltimore, Williams and Wilkins, 1987, p. 228, with permission.)

suppresses AVP release. When AVP is totally suppressed, C_{H_2O}* may attain values of 10-15 ml per 100 ml of GFR even in LBW infants.[37] With maximum antidiuretic activity (plasma AVP concentrations greater than 5 pg/ml), urine is concentrated to where urine osmolality is approximately 1200 mOsm/L in older infants, children and adults,[36] but only approximately 400 mOsm/L in LBW and VLBW infants.[37]

The pressor or vasoconstrictor effect of AVP occurs at higher plasma concentrations (greater than 30 pg/ml), which are attained in adults when blood pressure or volume is reduced by 10-15%.[36] Smaller changes in blood pressure and blood volume affect the magnitude of response of AVP release to osmotic stimuli (Fig. 4). Stress reactions of a more specific type and a number of drugs also cause release of AVP independent of osmotic

---

*Free water clearance is defined conventionally by the equation $C_{H_2O} = V \cdot C_{osm}$ where V equals urine volume (ml/min), C_{osm} is the volume of urine needed to excrete solute as isotonic urine (300 mOsm/L), and C_{H_2O} is "free water." C_{H_2O} is also used to define the degree of Na reabsorption in the distal convolution.[37]

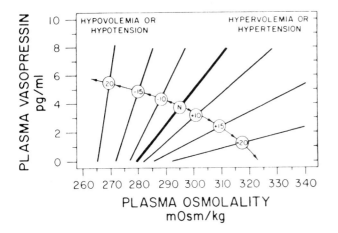

FIGURE 4. The interdependent relation of osmolarity with pressure-volume changes in regulating plasma AVP concentrations. Note that changes in volume modulate but do not obviate the effect of osmolarity upon AVP release. Circled numbers indicate percent change in plasma volume from normal. (From Robertson GL, Berl T. Water metabolism. In Brenner BM, Rector FC (eds): The Kidney, 3rd ed. Philadelphia, W.B. Saunders, 1986, p. 390, with permission.)

or pressure stimuli and may limit the rate of free water excretion (C_{H_2O}).[36] AVP is filtered and a large fraction is catabolized in the kidney; a smaller fraction appears in urine and its rate of excretion is a semiquantitative indication of its plasma concentration.[35]

4. *Prostanoids.* This class of compounds regulates renal hemodynamics and affects tubular reabsorption of NaCl in a number of ways. The prostaglandins act with renin as part of a **negative** feedback loop. **Prostaglandins are released by angiotensin and in general act as vasodilators, countering the vasoconstrictor effects of A II, particularly by decreasing afferent arteriolar resistance.**[8] At the same time prostaglandin release stimulates release of renin. Because of the action of the prostaglandins, the vasoconstrictor role of A II usually does not result in decreased GFR.[43] However suppression of prostaglandin synthetase coincident with renin stimulation does lead to a decrease in renal blood flow and GFR. While the acute effects of prostaglandin synthetase inhibition on patients with cirrhosis are profound, the effect of chronic therapy in patients with renal disease is marginal.[15] Thromboxane, a prostanoid of the cyclo-oxygenase pathway of the arachidonate cascade, acts principally to cause arteriolar constriction, particularly of the efferent glomerular arterioles. It also increases platelet aggregation.[43]

5. *Atrial Natriuretic Peptide (ANP).* A class of peptides released from the atria in response to volume expansion has the property of stimulating vasodilation and increasing GFR. This leads to a *"hyperfiltration" natriuresis that is associated with inhibition of renin release*, with resultant reduced effects of angiotensin and vasopressin on renal hemody-

namics.[27] With NaCl loading or volume expansion, ANP is released and a brisk natriuresis follows.[40] Such an expansion comes with retention of infused saline or with the retention of water sufficient to cause hyponatremia in response to stress-induced AVP (ADH) release. **The natriuresis seen with water retention, as is characteristic of the syndrome of inappropriate secretion of ADH, may be mediated by ANP.**[29]

Interaction of Controls. This system of feedback loops in adults, children and even term infants is highly integrated and effective.[22] Much of its effect on vascular resistance and renal hemodynamics depends on relative changes in resistance of afferent and efferent glomerular capillaries (see Fig. 3). Increasing afferent resistance raises total peripheral resistance, lowers renal blood flow (RBF) and GFR, and decreases NaCl excretion. Increasing efferent resistance, relative to afferent, raises glomerular pressure, GFR and renal tubular fluid flow. Relaxing the afferent resistance also increases glomerular capillary pressure and GFR, whereas relaxing efferent resistance increases peritubular blood flow and usually initiates a saline diuresis.[10]

The different feedback loops have both positive or reinforcing limbs and negative or modulating limbs. The reinforcing limbs, exemplified by sympathetic nerve stimulation, renin, and aldosterone, may seem redundant, but together they provide a several-layered backup system that can tolerate failure of one limb and still regulate vasomotor tone and NaCl excretion in response to volume change. **Renin and PGE_2 act together as vasoconstrictor-vasodilator effectors, respectively.** As a result the renin effect, which is to increase renovascular resistance and raise blood pressure by its vasoconstriction effect on the efferent glomerular arteriole, is counterbalanced by a PGE_2 vasodilatory effect on the afferent arteriole; GFR remains unaffected. However, when the same stimulus is applied to individuals receiving indomethacin, which inhibits PGE_2 synthesis, afferent vasoconstriction is predominant and renal blood flow and GFR decrease.[15]

Adaptations in the Neonatal Period

Glomerular Filtration Rate and Tubular Function. GFR in term infants (surface area = 0.23 m²) measured in the first days of life is 4-7 ml.min (1-2 ml/kg/min); the average during the first month is 5-9 ml/min.[20] After delivery in the term infant there is an abrupt increase in GFR (Fig. 5).[6,20] GFR in LBW and VLBW infants is lower. **In (AGA) LBW infants, postconception age has an overriding influence upon GFR.** GFR in the first week of life in infants of 28-33 weeks' gestation weighing 1500 gm and having a SA of approximately 0.13 m² is approximately 1 ml/min (0.7 ml/kg/min).[17] Between 34 and 40 weeks of conceptual age, irrespective of postnatal age, GFR increases from 2 to 4-7 ml/min. When infants studied in the first week of life are compared with those studied after the first week, there is an increase of 20-30% as the infant adapts to extrauterine life. This increase is greater in infants with a conceptual age that is greater than 34 weeks (see Fig. 5).[20]

The factors that increase GFR during development are increases in glomerular capillary pressure and increases in glomerular plasma flow.[50] In experimental animals and, by inference, in humans, **the increase in GFR early in life is due to a rise in blood pressure and glomerular capillary pressure.** The increases that come later are principally a result of an increase in renal plasma flow that is secondary to changes in afferent and efferent arteriolar resistance.[50]

The loss of ECF by VLBW infants in the early days post-delivery is associated with a high fractional excretion of Na (Fe Na—3%). The loss of NaCl is 3 mM/kg/day for infants of 27-29 weeks' gestational age. **Within 10 to 15 days following birth, Fe Na decreases to less than 1% and urinary loss of NaCl is approximately 1 mM/kg/day.** LBW infants greater than 33 weeks' gestational age have a low Fe Na (less than 1%) and excrete less than 1 mM/kg/day.[1] Coincident with the fall in Fe Na with advancing postconceptional age, GFR is increasing fivefold (Fig. 6).

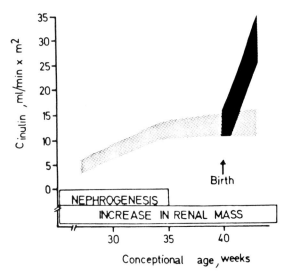

FIGURE 5. The differing effects of gestational age and postnatal age upon glomerular filtration rate (GFR). Hazed area indicates GFR in the first week at various conceptual ages. Blackened area indicates GFR of term infants followed periodically. (From Guignard JP. Adaptation of the kidney to extrauterine life. In Strauss J (ed): Neonatal Kidney and Fluid-Electrolytes. Boston, Martinus Nijhoff, 1983, p. 102, with permission.)

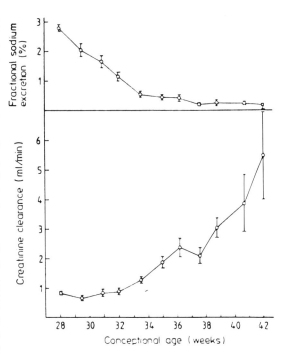

FIGURE 6. Change in fractional excretion of Na and in creatinine clearance in VLBW infants as a function of postconceptional age. (From Al Dahhan J, Haycock GB, Chantler C, Stimmler L. Sodium homeostasis in term and preterm neonates. I Renal aspects. Arch Dis Child 1983; 58:338, with permission.)

TABLE 2.   Changes in Weight, Surface Area (SA), Glomerular Filtration Rate (GFR), and Tubular Function with Maturation*

	Less Than 35 wks	More Than 35 wks
Weight (kg)	1.40	2.30
SA m^2	0.13	0.18
GFR† ml/min	2.00	4.80
$C_{H_2O} + C_{Na} + K$‡ (ml/100 ml GFR)	17.10	12.20
C_{H_2O}** (ml/100 ml/GFR)	13.90	10.90
$C_{H_2O} + C_{Na} + K$ (ml/min)	0.34	0.59
C_{H_2O} (ml/min)	0.28	0.52

Adapted from reference 37.

*Note that $C_{H_2O} + C_{Na}$ and C_{H_2O} both decrease as a fraction of GFR but increase in absolute amounts.

†GFR estimated from creatinine clearance (Cr) measured on days 6-7 and adjusted to the average surface area of the infants studied using average for body weight and normal length for weight. (Adapted from reference 37.)

‡$C_{H_2O} + C_{Na} + K$ is used to define the volume of fluid delivered from the proximal tubule, i.e., distal delivery. C_{H_2O} is used to define free water clearance and NaCl reabsorption, which take place in the distal nephron.

The high Fe Na seen in VLBW infants appears to be a result of decreased proximal and distal tubular Na reabsorption. The changes in tubular handling of Na that occur with maturation have been studied by clearance techniques in infants at 6-7 days of age.[37] Those less than 35 weeks' gestational age were compared with those greater than 35 weeks. Delivery of fluid to the distal nephron and reabsorption of NaCl from this segment were greater relative to GFR in the less mature infants. However, because GFR in infants more than 35 weeks was more than twice that of the smaller infants, the absolute rate of fluid delivery to, and NaCl reabsorption from, the distal nephron increased (Table 2).

Vasomotor Tone and Excretion of NaCl and Water

Control of vasomotor tone and excretion of NaCl and water in infants is mediated by the same factors that operate in adults; the interaction of the regulatory feedback loops is less well-studied. Term infants have high plasma renin and aldosterone concentrations at birth, which appear to be a result of birth. Within a few days concentrations decrease to approach those seen in older infants and adults[14] despite a 5-8% loss of body weight owing to a contraction of the ECF space. Quickly the infant, fed human milk, adapts to a low NaCl and high water intake (see Table 1), and growth proceeds. The loss of ECF is not accompanied by signs of contraction of circulating volume.

The VLBW infant on the standard NaCl intake, 1 to 1.5 mM/kg/day, has a similar but exaggerated course. The saline diuresis is much larger in proportion to body size so that weight loss is 13-15% of body weight and ECF loss is greater than that of LBW infants.[28] These losses in VLBW infants are associated with hormonal responses characteristic of circulating and ISF volume depletion,[16,45-47] which are not seen in comparable infants given 3-5 mM/kg/day of NaCl. The latter have an increase in ANP when compared with the former (Table 3).[48] However clinical signs, readily observed with ECF volume contraction in older infants and adult, are less evident than in later life.

Although the feedback loops described for adults and older infants in general operate in a similar manner in VLBW infants, the greater susceptibility of the VLBW infant to shifts of fluid between circulating and ISF volume, and the lower renal functional capacity limit tolerances to variations in intake.

When term infants are challenged during a water diuresis with an oral NaCl load, the fraction of the load that is excreted is less than that seen when more mature infants are challenged.[7] This finding, if projected over days and applied to VLBW infants, would lead to cumulative retention of NaCl and water. Clinical reports of an association of higher NaCl intakes with patent ductus arteriosus and respiratory distress in VLBW infants have raised questions about the safety of giving extra NaCl to these infants.[9,45] Controlled trials have not found this association (see below).

TABLE 3.   Hormonal Differences Between NaCl-Supplemented (S) and Nonsupplemented (NS) Infants Studied Between 1-5 Weeks of Age Relative to Concentrations Seen During the First Week*

	S	NS
Plasma renin	↓	↑
Urinary aldosterone	↓	↑
Urinary noradrenalin	↓	↑
Urinary dopamine	↓	↑
Urinary serotonin	no difference	no change
Urinary PGE_2	↓	no change
Urinary PGF_2	↓	no change
Urinary AVP	low	+/- elevated
Plasma ANP	↑	↓

*Adapted from references 16, 45, 46, 47 and 48.

Hyponatremia in VLBW Infants

Hyponatremia is due to retention of water relative to solute and usually occurs when there is a strong stimulus to AVP release from contraction of circulating volume or from some stress, e.g., a painful procedure or use of certain drugs. NaCl deficiency is a cause of the former; intubation or morphine is a cause of the latter. AVP secretion and physiologic responses to it develop during fetal life.[18] The renal capacity for free water clearance in VLBW infants is sufficient to excrete more than 150 ml/kg/day. Since this capacity exceeds the urine volume of most infants receiving water intake of 100-200 ml/kg/day, the occurrence of hyponatremia usually is not due to limited renal capacity. Rather, hyponatremia often appears to be due to stress, e.g., respiratory distress and manipulation of respirators, causing AVP release sufficient to prevent appropriate water excretion. Salt supplementation lowers the incidence of hyponatremia, indicating that AVP release often is due to volume contraction; however, it does not abolish it, indicating that non-volume-dependent AVP release does contribute to the incidence of hyponatremia.[38]

Hyponatremia occurs in VLBW infants in the first week of life from one set of circumstances and in the second to fifth weeks from another. In the first week of life it appears to be due to the stress of adaptation[34] and is not demonstrably influenced by giving more NaCl and water parenterally.[28] Hyponatremia in the first week of life has been related to a diminished ability to excrete free water secondary to release of AVP as a consequence of stress.[34]

A high incidence of hyponatremia between the second and fifth weeks of life in infants fed 1-1.5 mM/kg/day of NaCl is often called late hyponatremia.[38,46] A slower rate of growth has been associated with hyponatremia.[13] High urinary AVP excretion, which reflects high plasma AVP[35] that is associated with increased urinary aldosterone, provides additional evidence that NaCl deficiency contributes to the hyponatremia.[46] As noted, the potential for C_{H_2O} of these infants (Table 2)[37] makes it reasonable to assume that the inability to excrete free water intake is not from renal incapacity. Because Na balance in this period is positive, the role of Na deficiency in AVP secretion is less readily separated from the role of stress, e.g., hypoxia, intracranial hemorrhage, pneumothorax and intubation itself. While the incidence of late hyponatremia is lower when NaCl supplements are given,[38,46] the fact that hyponatremia does occur with NaCl supplementation is evidence that other stresses stimulate AVP secretion and contribute to late hyponatremia.

NaCl Supplementation: Results of Controlled Trials

Several controlled clinical trials have evaluated the effects of NaCl supplementation in VLBW infants. In an early study,[13] NaCl supplementation (3 mM/kg/day) of VLBW infants from 14 days of age until they reached a weight of 1.8 kg was associated with a reduced rate of hyponatremia and hyperkalemia. Sulyok,[45] reporting the effects of NaCl supplementation in VLBW infants on urinary catecholamine excretion, noted that NaCl-supplemented infants cumulatively gained 68 gm by

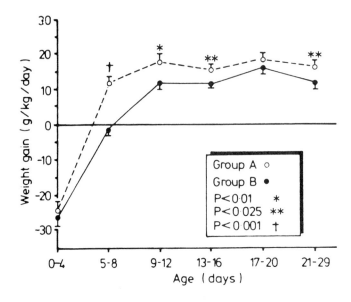

FIGURE 7. The difference in cumulative weight gains in salt-supplemented infants (from days 4 to 14, Group A) and unsupplemented infants (Group B). Note that the difference in weight gain was sustained after the supplement was discontinued. (From Al Dahhan J, Haycock GB, Nichol B, et al. Sodium homeostasis in term and preterm infants. Arch Dis Child 1984; 59:948, with permission.)

6 weeks of age, whereas non-supplemented infants gained 54 gm by that age.

Al-Dahhan and colleagues[2] compared results of VLBW infants given 1-1.5 mM/kg/day through the first 25 days of life with those of infants given a NaCl supplement of 4-5 mM/kg/day from days 4-14; from days 15-25 these latter infants received 1-1.5 mM/kg/day. The infants supplemented from days 4-14 gained more weight over the full 25-day period (Fig. 7), had higher C_{Cr} values in the post-supplemented period (15-25 days), and had greater retention of K, which was interpreted as evidence of greater growth. The supplemented infants experienced no greater frequency of patent ductus arteriosus, necrotizing enterocolitis or intracranial hemorrhage.

A recent report[26] compares the failure of infants in an earlier study[31] to improve nitrogen retention when protein intake was increased and Na intake was limited to 1.2 mM/kg/day with results in which a similar increase of protein intake associated with an increase in Na intake to 2.2 mM/kg/day was associated with greater nitrogen retention. Gain in weight, length and head circumference also was greater when protein and NaCl intakes were greater. The inference drawn from these observations is that a NaCl intake of 1.2 mM/kg/day limited nitrogen retention and growth when protein intake was 3.6 gm/kg/day, whereas twice that NaCl intake did not.

NEEDS

For term infants on oral intake the requirement for NaCl is met in most instances when human milk or formulas containing 7-10 mM/l of NaCl are given ad libitum. This provides an average of 1-1.5 mM/kg/day. The formulas meet the minimum recommendation of the Committee on Nutrition of the American Academy of Pediatrics.[3] The quantity provided by these formulas is sufficient throughout the first 6-12 months of life. Infant foods now sold without added salt have little impact on NaCl intake. It is relevant to note that formulas containing inadequate chloride (less than 3 mEq/L or less than 0.5 mM/kg/day) stop growth and cause contraction alkalosis.[39]

For most LBW infants weighing between 1500-2000 gm the same recommendations usually apply. In either group signs of circulating volume overload (hypertension, edema) associated with high NaCl and water intakes by intravenous or oral route should lead to a decrease in NaCl intake and may justify diuretic therapy to induce negative NaCl balance. Conversely, signs of circulating and/or ISF volume contraction (see below) should lead to increases in NaCl intake (3-5 mM/kg/day) and may require acute volume expansion with intravenous saline.

For most VLBW infants (those weighing less than 1500 gm or having a postconceptional age less than 35 weeks) who are on oral feedings, an intake of NaCl of 1.5 mM/kg/day from 4-14 days of life appears to be inadequate as judged from clinical results,[2] from the response of the vasoactive hormones,[16,44,47,48] the tendency to hyponatremia and hyperkalemia[28] and poor growth.[26,38] Infants supported by continuous parenteral nutrition probably have the same needs, but circumstances that lead to the use of parenteral nutrition often are associated with changes in circulating volume, either toward excess or deficiency.

DEFICIENCY OF NaCl

NaCl deficiency may be inferred from the presence of hyperkalemia, hyponatremia, or failure to gain weight satisfactorily when intake is less than 3 mM/kg/day. The diagnosis is not readily established. It may be made from noting their response to a supplement of NaCl 1-2 mM/kg/day. In the future, the use of renin, aldosterone, and PGE_2 concentrations in plasma or blood may provide a more accurate assessment of need.

Sodium and chloride are considered together in this discussion because Na as $NaHCO_3$, or sodium salt of any anion other than Cl, is poorly reabsorbed by the renal tubule and therefore is excreted. When sodium is given with any anion other than chloride to a person who is volume contracted, there is a stimulus for Na reabsorption with bicarbonate so that metabolic alkalosis develops: there is a deficiency of chloride often termed contraction alkalosis.[39] Aldosterone secretion increases in response to the ECF volume contraction and mediates the effect. Consequently metabolic alkalosis not related to a hyperadrenocortical state, such as Cushing's syndrome or glucocorticoid therapy, is likely a result of Cl deficiency or ECF volume contraction. Under these conditions, giving NaCl leads to excretion of an alkaline urine and retention of chloride until ECF volume is normal.

Water intake of 150 ml/kg/day usually is well tolerated. One study noted no increase in hyponatremia when 200 ml/kg/day was given.[28] The risk for hyponatremia or water excess appears to be related more to the coexistence of NaCl deficiency and stress, either of which stimulates release of AVP independent of hypoosmolarity.

The question of what constitutes a safe average level of intake is unresolved. As mentioned, intakes of NaCl 2.2 mM/kg/day were associated with improved weight gain and growth in length and head circumference of VLBW infants when milk protein was increased to improve nitrogen retention.[26] Intakes of NaCl 4-5 mM/kg/day are associated with an increase in ANP,[48] which may be a signal for excess retention. From current information, the range of uncertainty regarding NaCl requirements and tolerance has narrowed. Hormonal signals may provide the clinician with a more accurate assessment of NaCl status than any of the currently used indices. Appropriate studies are needed to test this hypothesis. **The author recommends an intake of 2-4 mM/kg/day of NaCl for the period of 4-15 days after birth unless clinical signs mandate an increase or decrease from this level. After 15 days 1-1.5 mM/kg/day appears to suffice but more—up to 2-3 mM/kg/day—may be needed to support optimal growth.[2]**

DEFICIENCY OF WATER

Deficiency of water is defined by an increase in sodium concentration in ECF (S_{Na}). Hyperosmolarity due to hyperglycemia that is more than transient also defines water deficiency; that due to uremia is not. The deficiency occurs either because there is a failure in the thirst mechanism or, as may be the case in VLBW infants, insufficient free water is given. Water deficiency is more prone to occur when either renal or extrarenal losses of water are increased. Increased renal losses occur with renal disease associated with obligatory hyposthenuria, an increase in solute excretion as occurs with glycosuria or the receiving of x-ray contrast medium. Increased skin losses are common with radiant heat therapy. AVP is elevated. The treatment of water deficiency is to correct the reason for excess loss, if practical, and to give more free water. Approximately 70 ml of water *retained* per kg will lower S_{Na} by approximately 10 mM/L.

EXCESS NaCl

The signs of excess NaCl are those of overexpansion of the cirulating volume. These develop when intake of NaCl and water exceeds the upper limits of tolerance. An increase in pulmonary vascular markings and peripheral edema are early signs. Pulmonary edema, heart failure and, in VLBW infants, the development of respiratory distress, patent ductus arteriosus and necrotizing enterocolitis are suggestive. Peripheral edema per se may be due to a deficiency in circulating volume as occurs with hypoalbuminemia or alteration in the Starling forces, which regulate the distribution of ECF.

The treatment of excess NaCl is the restriction of NaCl intake and diuretic therapy. The restriction of water intake will depend on whether there exists, at the same time, hypo-natremia or other factors that might inhibit free water excretion once NaCl intake is restricted.

EXCESS WATER

The presence of excess water relative to solute is defined by the finding of hypos-molarity or hyponatremia. It may arise because there is a deficiency of extracellular solute—NaCl—or because the capacity for free water clearance is less than the intake of free water required to assure water balance. This may be due either to renal disease or to AVP release.

The treatment of hyponatremia consists of giving NaCl sufficient to correct the NaCl deficit, reducing the stimulus to AVP release, where that is possible, or restricting water intake. Discontinuing the use of diuretic therapy often is necessary.

SUMMARY

The requirement of NaCl for VLBW infants is that amount needed to sustain an effective circulating volume; this appears to be between 2-3 mM/kg/day during the first 2 weeks of life for those VLBW infants who do not have major complicating illnesses. Water requirement is that amount needed to maintain Na within a normal range. Intake, usually determined by the need for other nutrients, is between 150-200 ml/kg/day. Hypernatremia is an indication for increasing free water intake; hyponatremia is a cause for reducing free water intake or correcting the factors that limit free water excretion.

POTASSIUM

PHYSIOLOGY

Body Composition

Potassium is the principal cation in intracellular fluid (ICF); its concentration in cell fluid is 160 mM/L. The ICF is 35-40% of total body weight in adults and this is approximately the case for children and for infants after 1 year of age. During early development concentration of K in ICF is slightly lower. Concentration of K in ECF is between 3.5-5 mM/L. The ratio of ICF:ECF potassium is maintained by the permeability characteristics of cell membranes and a Na-K exchange pump that ex-

trudes Na in exchange for K. This pump—Na, K-ATP'ase—requires energy and maintains an electrochemical gradient between ECF and ICF.[42]

Intake

The intake of K in adults varies between 40-200 mM/day. The lower intakes represent those receiving low K diets that meet the general requirements of normal subjects;[5] the high intakes are by vegetarians who subsist on low Na, high K foods.[30] Within this intake range, total body K and serum K values remain normal.

Definition of Deficiency and Excess

K deficiency is defined as a lowering of total body K associated with a reduction in intracellular K concentrations. It arises when dietary K is insufficient, which for normal adult individuals occurs only under experimental conditions in which K intake is less than 20 mM/day.[42]

Deficiency usually results from endocrine or metabolic abnormalities, such as Cushing's syndrome, aldosteronism or Bartter's syndrome, or from therapy that causes renal K "wasting," such as diuretic therapy, steroid toxicity, or chloride deficiency states in which alkali is given. In these instances there is usually a state of metabolic alkalosis and either primary or secondary hyperaldosteronism. Gastroenteritis with large stool losses, diabetic ketoacidosis, and distal renal tubular acidosis also cause K deficiency that can be profound. In these conditions there is also a state of ECF volume contraction and metabolic acidosis.

Hypokalemia (serum K less than 3.5 mM/L) usually is associated with K deficiency but may occur independently when there is a stimulus to shift K from ECF to ICF. The latter usually occurs with a sudden change in acid-base status in which serum pH increases, or with the action of insulin and glucose increasing glycogen storage as occurs with the treatment of diabetic ketoacidosis.

Potassium excess is manifested by hyperkalemia. There is no demonstrable rise in intracellular K above normal, although hyperkalemia may arise from aggressive K therapy in which intracellular K is increasing from deficiency levels toward normal. **By far the most common cause of hyperkalemia is the**

breakdown of glycogen and protein, leading to a release of K into ECF. Any catabolic state can cause acute hyperkalemia. Other causes are aldosterone deficiency or target organ (kidney) unresponsiveness to aldosterone.

Excretion

The excretion of K is regulated by the kidney, usually in response to intake. K appears in urine predominantly as a result of tubular secretion in exchange for Na in the distal nephron, which is regulated in part by aldosterone. **Aldosterone is sensitive to K intake through effects of hyperkalemia or K uptake by adrenal cells.** This fairly simple feedback loop provides for the considerable range in tolerance to K intake. Stimulation of aldosterone secretion independently, as occurs with hyperreninemia from any cause, can lead to exaggerated aldosterone action and K deficiency. Diuretic therapy using "loop" diuretics is a good example.

K excretion is also increased when there is a large anion load other than chloride that is excreted. $NaHCO_3$, sodium penicillin and sodium given with other poorly reabsorbed anions are capable of causing K deficiency and hypokalemia by increasing K excretion.

DEFICIENCY

Hypokalemia and K Deficiency. Hypokalemia develops when intake fails to meet requirement, e.g., when total intake is predominantly glucose, or glucose and amino acids, given with no maintenance K.

Other factors that may cause hypokalemia and K deficiency are those that stimulate aldosterone secretion, or those that entail a high rate of Na excretion due to the administration of furosemide or sodium salts of anions other than Cl, e.g., $NaHCO_3$ or Na penicillin. Contraction alkalosis or chloride deficiency often is associated with hypokalemia and K deficiency. While it is appropiate to give KCl under these conditions, it is also imperative to review therapy in an effort to amend the physiological factors causing hypokalemia.[41]

EXCESS

Hyperkalemia. Hyperkalemia is a sign of a shift of K from cells to ECF, as occurs with metabolic acidosis, a state of hypoaldosteronism, or a catabolic state. Occasionally it occurs in association with giving too much K. Remedy for the hyperkalemia is discontinuing K intake and reversing the process that is causing it. Diagnosis of deficiency of aldosterone or target organ insensitivity to aldosterone is difficult to establish in a timely manner. Giving supplemental NaCl and $NaHCO_3$ may be beneficial as long as renal function and urine volume are satisfactory.[41]

Hyperkalemia associated with renal failure is managed as a part of the treatment of renal failure, which is beyond the scope of this chapter.

NEEDS

For adults the requirement for K is that amount lost in urine, stool and skin secretions, and detritus—about 20 mM/day or 0.3 mM/kg/day. These may be exaggerated by high Na intakes, particularly when Na is given with an anion other than chloride, or by hyperadrenocortical states.

For children over 1 year of age there are no studies that evaluate a minimum requirement. Extrapolating from adults using metabolic rate, renal function or surface area as a reference, 1 mM/100 kcal/day or 20 mM/1.73 m^2/day would almost certainly suffice to meet maintenance losses. Translated to body weight, 1 mM/kg/day would be generous for maintenance of K status. Because growth rate is slow at this age, less than 1 gm/kg/day, the requirement for growth would be less than 0.1 mM/kg/day. For infants under 1 year of age who grow at a maximum rate (7 gm/kg/day), 0.5 mM/kg/day is required for growth. By convention, 2.0 mM/kg/day is recommended.

For VLBW infants who may gain 15 gm/kg/day, the requirement for growth is 1.0 mM/kg/day, and a safe allowance is 2.5 mM/kg/day.

The ratio of K to energy in human milk is 1.5 mM/100 kcal and the K:N ratio is 5. The ratio of K energy in special formulas is higher—2.5 mM/100 kcal—but the K retention is associated with greater weight gains and obligate K losses.

REFERENCES

1. Al Dahhan J, Haycock GB, Chantler C, Stimmler L. Sodium homeostasis in term and preterm neonates. I. Renal aspects. Arch Dis Child 1983;58:335-342.
2. Al Duhhan J, Haycock GB, Nichol B, et al. Sodium homeostasis in term and preterm infants. Arch Dis Child 1984; 59:945-950.
3. American Academy of Pediatrics Committee on Nutrition. Commentary on breast feeding and infant formulas, including proposed standards for formulas. Pediatrics 1976;57:278.
4. American Academy of Pediatrics Committee on Nutrition.

Nutritional needs for low-birth-weight infants. Pediatrics 1985;75:976-986.

5. American Academy of Pediatrics Committee on Nutrition. Salt intake and eating patterns of infants and children in relation to blood pressure. Pediatrics 1974;53:115-121.

6. Aperia A, Broberger O, Elinder G, et al. Postnatal changes in glomerular filtration rate in preterm and full-term infants. In Spitzer A (ed): The Kidney During Development. New York, Masson, 1980;133-137.

7. Aperia A, Broberger O, Thodenius K, Zetterstrom R. Developmental study of the renal response to an oral salt load in preterm infants. Acta Paediatr 1974;63:517.

8. Ballarmann BJ, Levenson DJ, Brenner BM. Renin-angiotension kinins, prostaglandins, and leukotrienes. In Brenner BM, Rector FC (eds): The Kidney, 3rd ed. Philadelphia, W.B. Saunders Co., 1986.

9. Bell EF, Warkerton D, Stonestreet BS, Oh W. Effects of fluid administration on the development of symptomatic patent ductus arteriosus and congestive heart failure in premature infants. N Engl J Med, 1980;302:598-604.

10. Brenner BM, Dworkin LD, Ichikawa I. Glomerular ultrafiltration. In Brenner BM, Rector FC (eds): The Kidney, 3rd ed. Philadelphia, W.B. Saunders Co., 1986.

11. Cole BR, Kuhnline MA, Needleman P. Atriopeptin III. A potent natriuretic, diuretic, and hypotensive agent in rats with chronic renal failure. J Clin Invest 1985;76:2413-2415.

12. Davis BB, Walter MJ, Murdaugh HV. The mechanisms of the increase in sodium excretion following dopamine infusion. Proc Soc Exp Biol 1968;129:211-213.

13. Day GM, Radde SC, Balfe JW, Chance GW. Electrolyte abnormalities in very low birth weight infants. Pediatr Res 1976; 10:522-526.

14. Dillon MJ, Gillen ME, Ryness JM, de Sweet M. Plasma renin activity and aldosterone concentration in the human newborn. Arch Dis Child 1976;51:537-540.

15. Donker AJM, Arisz L, Brentgens JRH, et al. The effect of indomethacin on kidney function and plasma renin activity in man. Nephron 1976;17:288-296.

16. Ertle T, Sulyok E, Neweth M, et al. The effect of sodium chloride supplementation on the postnatal development of plasma prostaglandin E and F_2 values in premature infants. J Pediatr 1982;101:761-763.

17. Fawer CL, Torrado A, Guignard JP. Maturation of renal function in full term and premature neonates. Helv Paediatr Acta 1979;34:11.

18. Fisher DA, Robillard JE, Leake RD, et al. Maturation of the vasopressin secretion control mechanism in the fetus and newborn. In Spitzer A (ed): The Kidney During Development. New York, Masson, 1980;215-221.

19. Gamble JL. Chemical anatomy physiology and pathology of extracellular fluid. Cambridge, MA, Harvard University Press, 1947;33.

20. Guignard JP. Adaptation of the kidney to extrauterine life. In Strauss J (ed): Neonatal Kidney and Fluid–Electrolytes. Boston, MA, Martinus Nijhoff, 1983;101-111.

21. Guyton AC. Capillary dynamics and exchange of fluid between the blood and interstitial fluid. In Guyton AC (ed): Textbook of Medical Physiology, 6th ed. Philadelphia, W.B. Saunders Co., 1981.

22. Haycock GB. Sodium and water. In Holliday MA, Barratt TM, Vernier R (eds): Pediatric Nephrology, 2nd ed. Baltimore, Williams and Wilkins, 1987;84-89.

23. Holliday MA. Body composition, metabolism and growth. In Holliday MA, Barratt TM, Vernier R (eds): Pediatric Nephrology, 2nd ed. Baltimore, Williams and Wilkins, 1987;1-11.

24. Holliday MA. Maintenance and deficit therapy: a perspective. In Holliday MA, Barratt TM, Vernier R (eds): Pediatric Nephrology, 2nd ed. Baltimore, Williams and Wilkins, 1987; 173-180.

25. Kagan BM, Hess JH, Lundeen E, et al. Feeding premature infants—comparison of various milks. Pediatrics 1955; 15:373.

26. Kashyap S, Forsyth M, Zucker C, et al. Effects of varying protein and energy intakes on growth and metabolic response in low birth weight infants. J Pediatr 1986;108:955-963.

27. Laragh JH. The endocrine control of blood volume, blood pressure and sodium balance: atrial hormone and renin system interactions. J Hypertension 1986;4 (Suppl 2):S-143-S156.

28. Lorenz JM, Kleinman LI, Kotagal UR, Reller MD. Water balance in very low birth weight infants: relationship to water and sodium intake and effect on outcome. J Pediart 1982; 101:423-432.

29. Manning P, Schwartz D, Katsube NC, et al. Vasopressin-stimulated release of atriopeptin: endocrine antagonists in fluid homeostasis. Science 1985; 229:395-397.

30. Oliver WJ, Cohen EL, Neel JV. Blood pressure, sodium intake and sodium related hormones in the Yanamamo Indians, a "no-salt" culture. Circulation 1975;52:146-151.

31. Raiha NCR, Heinonen K, Rassin DK, Gaull GE. Milk protein quantity and quality in low birth weight infants. I. Metabolic responses and effect on growth. Pediatrics 1976;57:659-674.

32. Rascher W. Catecholamines. In Holliday MA, Barratt TM, Vernier R (eds): Pediatric Nephrology, 2nd ed. Baltimore, Williams and Wilkins, 1987;242-247.

33. Rauh W. Renin angiotensin system. In Holliday MA, Barratt TM, Vernier R (eds): Pediatric Nephrology, 2nd ed. Williams and Wilkins, Baltimore, 1987;227-231.

34. Rees L, Brook GGD, Shaw JCL, Forsleng ML. Hyponatremia in the first week of life in preterm infants. I. Arginine vasopressin secretion. Arch Dis Child 1984;59:414-422.

35. Rees L, Forsling ML, Brook CGD. Continuous urine collection in the study of vasopressin in the newborn. Hormone Res 1983;17: 134-140.

36. Robertson GL, Berl T. Water metabolism. In Brenner BM, Rector FC (eds): The Kidney, 3rd ed. Philadelphia, W.B. Saunders Co., 1986;385-342.

37. Rodriguez-Soriano J, Vallo A, Oliveros R, Castillo G. Renal handling of sodium in premature and full-term neonates: a study using clearance methods during water diuresis. Pediatr Res 1983;17:1013-1016.

38. Roy RN, Chance GW, Radde IC, et al. Late hyponatremia in very low birth weight infants (less than 1.3 kg). Pediatr Res 1976;10:526-531.

39. Roy S, Stapleton FB, Arant BS. Hypochloremic metabolic alkalosis in infants fed a chloride deficient formula. Pediatr Res 1980;14:509.

40. Sagnella GA, Markandu ND, Shore AC, MacGregor GA. Changes in plasma immunoreactive atrial natriuretic peptide in response to saline infusion or to alterations in dietary sodium in normal subjects. J Hypertension 1986;4 (Suppl 2):S115-S118.

41. Schwartz GJ, Feld LG. Potassium. In Holliday MA, Barratt TM, Vernier R (eds): Pediatric Nephrology, 2nd ed. Baltimore, Williams and Wilkins, 1987;114-127.

42. Schwartz WB. Potassium and the kidney. N Engl Med 1955; 253: 601.

43. Seyberth H. Prostaglandins. In Holliday MA, Barratt TM, Vernier R (eds): Pediatric Nephrology, 2nd ed. Baltimore, Williams and Wilkins, 1987;232-241.

44. Stevenson JG. Fluid administration in the association of patent ductus arteriosus complicating respiratory distress syndrome. J Pediatr 1977;90:257-261.

45. Sulyok E, Gyodi G, Ertl T, et al. The influence of NaCl supplementation on the postnatal development of urinary excretion of noradrenalin, dopamine and serotonin in premature infants. Pediatr Res 1985;19:5-8.

46. Sulyok E, Kovacs L, Lichardus B, et al. Late hyponatremia in premature infants: role of aldosterone and arginine vasopressin. J Pediatr 1985;106: 990-994.

47. Sulyok E, Nemeth M, Tenyi I, et al. Relationship between the postnatal development of the renin angiotension-aldosterone system and electrolyte and acid-base status of the NaCl supplemented premature infants. In Spitzer A (ed): The Kidney During Development. New York, Masson, 1980.

48. Tulassay T, Rascher W, Seyberth HW, et al. Role of atrial natriuretic peptide in sodium homeostasis in premature infants. J Pediatr 1986;109:1023-1027.

49. Widdowson EM, Dickerson JWT, McCance RA. Chemical composition of the body. In Comar CL, Bronner F (eds): Mineral Metabolism, Vol II, Part A. New York, Academic Press, 1962;1-247.

50. Yared A, Ichikawa I. Renal blood flow and glomerular filtration rate. In Holliday MA, Barratt TM, Vernier R (eds): Pediatric Nephrology, 2nd ed. Baltimore, Williams and Wilkins, 1987; 45-58.

10

Calcium, Magnesium and Phosphorus

WINSTON W.K. KOO, M.B.B.S., F.R.A.C.P.
REGINALD C. TSANG, M.D.

ABSTRACT

Calcium (Ca), magnesium (Mg) and phosphorus (P) are three minerals essential for tissue structure and function. This chapter deals specifically with physiologic and practical aspects of the nutritional needs of Ca, Mg and P in infancy. For healthy infants born at term, the Ca, Mg and P content of human milk is the reference for determination of requirements for these minerals. For cow milk formula fed infants, Ca intake should be higher because of differences in intestinal Ca absorption. In infants of very-low birthweight (< 1500 gm) receiving conventional vitamin D supplementation (400 IU/day), chronic deficiency of Ca and P appears to be a major problem with resultant bone demineralization and/or rickets. For infants who are unable to tolerate intestinal feeding, early commencement of parenteral nutrition with meticulous attention to details of fluid, electrolyte, glucose and amino acid infusion, and subsequent introduction of intestinal feeding at the earliest opportunity, should minimize disturbances of Ca, Mg and P metabolism.

INTRODUCTION

The word calcium (Ca) is derived from the Latin *calx*, limestone, from Greek, *khalix*, pebble. Magnesium (Mg) is derived from Latin *magnesia*, from Greek *magnesia*, name of various minerals, from *Magnesia*, a metalliferous region of Thessaly. Phosphorus (P) is derived from Latin and Greek, *phosphoros*, "light bearing" (so named because white phosphorus is phosphorescent in air); *phos* indicates the presence of light; *phoros* indicates pherein, to bear. (The American Heritage Dictionary of the English Language, 1975.)

Calcium, magnesium and phosphorus are three minerals essential for tissue structure and function. Descriptions of clinical symptoms and signs of calcium-related disorders and research on this subject around the turn of this century indicated a keen appreciation of the importance of these minerals in tissue function and structure. Even in 1879, Routh described:

Phosphate of lime in breast milk: *deformity of every kind in the skeleton may depend on an insufficient quantity of*

this salt in the blood for it should be remarked first that not only is it useful because it is itself appropriated into the system, but secondly, phosphate of lime, when present in a fluid which in the present case is milk and by subsequent assimilation becomes blood, has the property of enabling that fluid to take up more carbonic acid. Now, when carbonic acid in its turn is in excess, it dissolves carbonate of lime, hence the quantity of carbonate of lime held in solution in the blood is thereby made greater and is in this way from time to time more easily and largely *deposited in bone. Infant Feeding and Its Influence on Life, 3rd ed.*

CHF Routh

Howland and Marriott's paper "The Calcium Content of the Blood in Rachitis and Tetany" showed that in the former disease there was no more than a "very slight" reduction in calcium, but that in tetany (seven cases) the reduction was marked during the active stage, returning to normal with recovery. They had devised a method applicable to 1 to 2 cc of serum, a significant step in the direction of microchemistry. (Proceedings 31st Meeting of the American Pediatric Society, Atlantic City, NJ, June 1919.)

The physiology and metabolism of the minerals Ca, Mg and P are frequently inter-related; they are in turn modulated by other nutrients and hormones. Several comprenesive reviews on the function, regulation and physiologic requirements of these minerals are available.[1-4]

PHYSIOLOGY

Body Content

In the fetus, Ca, Mg and P accretion increase exponentially from 24 weeks to term gestation. This accretion reaches a peak of approximately 117 mg Ca, 2.7 mg Mg and 7.4 mg P/ kg/day at 34 to 36 weeks' gestation.[5-7] After birth, infancy is the period of most rapid mineral accretion. Bone mineral accretion continues until the third decade.[8]

Calcium is the most abundant mineral in the body. At all ages, 98% of the total body Ca is in bone. In adults, the total body Ca is approximately 1.3 kg. In newborn infants the total body Ca content is approximately 28 gm. The bone of the infant is less densely mineralized than that of adults, there being approximately 4 and 19 gm of Ca per kg of body weight in the infant and adult, respectively.

Magnesium is the fourth most abundant metal in the body. In contrast to the low concentrations of intracellular Ca, **Mg is the second most common intracellular electrolyte in the body.** In adults, the total body Mg is reported to be between 21 and 28 gm. In newborn infants the total body Mg is approximately 0.8 gm. The body Mg content increases between infancy and adulthood, there being approximately 0.22 and 0.39 gm of Mg per kg of body weight, respectively. About 60% of the body's magnesium is in bone, 20% in muscle and most of the remainder is found in intracellular space of other tissues.

Phosphorus and Ca are the major minerals contributing to the supportive structures of the body. In adults, the total body P is approximately 700 gm. In the newborn infant, total body P is approximately 16 gm. The body P content increases between infancy and adulthood, there being approximately 2.4 and 10.6 gm of P per kg of body weight, respectively. About 80% of total body P is in bone, 9% in skeletal muscle, and the remainder in viscera and extracellular fluid.

In 1771 Scheele and also Gahn discovered that the earthy matter of bone consisted of calcium phosphate. When Thomas Thompson's *Chemistry* appeared in 1817, the chief constituents of bone were analyzed as fat, earthy salts, gelatin and cartilage. The inorganic part of bones was known to be largely calcium phosphate with a small amount of carbonate and some magnesium. Some sulfate was also found if bone ash was dissolved in acid and treated with barium nitrate. This probably came from ashing the protein of bone. Since calcined bones gave off some carbon dioxide when dissolved in acid, it was assumed that some calcium carbonate was present. (Verzar F (ed). Clive M. McCay: Notes on the History of Nutrition Research, Berne, Hans Huber Publishers, 1973; 172.)

Although the principal part of the Ca, Mg and P in the body is found in the skeleton, all three elements are essential to the function of soft tissues.

Serum Concentration

Circulating fractions of Ca, Mg and P are < 1% of their total body content and serum concentrations of these elements may not reflect tissue content. However, serum concen-

trations beyond the normal ranges for each of these elements may be associated with disturbances in physiologic function. The differences between plasma and serum values of these minerals are minimal and of no practical significance.

Total serum Ca concentration is maintained within narrow limits between 8 and 11 mg/dl;[9,10] the diurnal range of serum Ca in an individual is $< \pm 0.3$ mg/dl.[11] Forty to 45% of total serum Ca is bound to protein. Fifty-five to 60% of total serum Ca is ultrafilterable; 85 to 90% of this fraction exists in an ionized form, and 10 to 15% exists as complexes of Ca to anions such as phosphate, lactate and citrate. Serum ionized Ca concentration is the best indicator of physiologic calcium activity.

In a population survey,[12] serum total Mg apparently is higher in infants and early childhood than in adults, being 2.2 ± 0.3 mg/dl (M $\pm$ 2SD), and 2.1 ± 0.3 mg/dl (M $\pm$ 2SD), respectively. The ultrafilterable portion of serum Mg is greater than that for serum Ca, being approximately 70 to 80%. Of the ultrafilterable Mg, only 70 to 80% is believed to be in the ionic form, the remainder being largely complexed to anions, particularly phosphate, citrate and oxalate.[13,14] There is as yet no specific ion electrode for successful measurement of Mg ion.

The total phosphorus in plasma can be divided into an acid-insoluble fraction comprising mainly phospholipids, and an acid-soluble fraction comprising a small amount of organic ester phosphate and all of the inorganic phosphate.[15] Inorganic phosphate consists predominantly of orthophosphate, and > 90% of the inorganic phosphate is diffusible.[13,16,17] About 75% of orthophosphate ions in plasma exist as HPO_4^{2-} and $H_2PO_4^{-}$. The ratio of the 2 moieties is governed by blood pH. Using a pK of 6.8, the ratio of HPO_4^{2-} and $H_2PO_4^{-}$ at a plasma pH of 7.4 is 4:1. However, no direct measurements of free phosphate ion concentrations in biologic fluids are available. **There is a rough correlation between the rate of skeletal growth and serum P concentrations during development.** Thus in human beings, the serum P concentration is high during infancy (4 to 7.1 mg/dl, compared with values in adults of 2.7 to 4.5 mg/dl) and during pubertal growth spurts.[18,19]

Acute and transient fluctuation of serum concentrations of Ca, Mg and P may occur in response to compartmental shifts of these elements but may not reflect tissue changes. Chronic and severely lowered serum concentrations of these minerals may reflect the presence of a deficiency state.[1,4,20]

Serum Ca concentrations are high in infants at birth but fall to a nadir between 24 to 48 hours of age.[21] The fall in serum Ca concentrations is accentuated in preterm infants, infants of insulin-dependent diabetic mothers and infants with birth asphyxia.[22] Thereafter, serum Ca concentrations increase and stabilize generally above 8.5 mg/dl. In infants exclusively fed human milk, a recent study demonstrated that, over a 6-month period, "physiologic hypercalcemia" and "physiologic hypermagnesemia" appear to develop, in concert with a gradual fall in serum P concentration.[23] By 6 months of age, serum Ca concentrations have increased from 9.2 to 10.5 mg/dl and serum Mg from 1.9-2.5 mg.dl, whereas serum P concentrations have decreased from 7.9-5.7 mg/dl (Fig. 1). Presumably, the physiologic hypercalcemia and hypermagnesemia, associated with the fall in serum P concentration, are important in mineral metabolism of infancy but the exact significance is currently unclear.

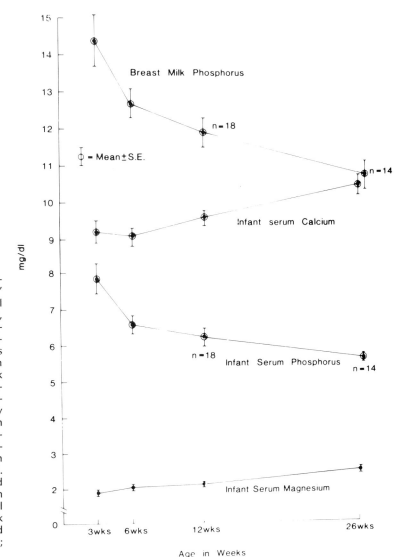

FIGURE 1. "Physiologic hypercalcemia and hypermagnesemia" of infancy, seen by longitudinal measurements of serum calcium, phosphorus and magnesium concentrations in exclusively breast-fed infants. Serum phosphorus concentrations fall significantly in parallel with falling breast milk phosphorus content. Infant serum calcium and magnesium concentrations increase significantly over the 6-month period to reach "hypercalcemia" and "hypermagnesemia" ranges. Values depicted are M± SEM (From Greer FR, Tsang RC, Levin RS, et al. Increasing serum calcium and magnesium concentrations in breast-fed infants: longitudinal studies of minerals in human milk and in sera of nursing mothers and their infants. J Pediatr 1982; 100:59-64, with permission.)

In a recent study of 198 infants less than 18 months of age, no sex differences were observed in serum Ca, Mg, P, parathyroid hormone or calcitonin concentrations. However, the mean serum P concentration was slightly but significantly lower in black infants (by approximately 0.3 mg/dl) compared with white infants. During winter, serum P, parathyroid hormone and calcitonin concentrations were lower (by approximately 0.4 mg/dl, 0.2 ng/ml and 29 pg/ml, respectively) and serum Ca and Mg concentrations were higher (by approximately 0.5 mg/dl and 0.1 mg/dl, respectively) compared to summer. Infants fed cow-milk formula had increased serum P (by 0.5 mg/dl) and decreased ionized Ca and parathyroid hormone concentrations (by 0.1 mg/dl and 0.3 ng/ml respectively), compared with infants fed human milk. Thus, age, race, season and diet appear to exert significant effects on serum minerals and calcium-regulating hormones in infancy (Table 1).[24]

Hess, in his classic work "Rickets Including Osteomalacia and Tetany," states, "the old conception was shown to be erroneous which held that deficiency of calcium is the essential disturbance in rickets, and it was shown that a disturbance of *phosphorus* must also be included in the metabolic picture.... Indeed, it was shown later that there is what may be termed a 'phosphate tide' in the blood of infants, an ebb during the winter months followed by a flood in the spring with advent of sunshine." (Hess AF. Rickets Including Osteomalacia and Tetany. Philadelphia, Lea & Febiger, 1929; 20.)

Intestinal Absorption (Table 2)

The regulation of body Ca content is primarily by way of the gastrointestinal tract. Ca absorption occurs by *active* transport primarily in the duodenum; there is also absorption by *passive* diffusion. Normally, the colon plays no

TABLE 1.   Summary of Factors Related to Serum Minerals and Calcium-Regulating Hormones in Infants Less Than 18 Months of Age*

	Race	Age	Season	Diet
Ionized calcium	No	Yes (decreases with age)	No	Yes (lower in formula-fed)
Total calcium	No	No	Yes (lower in summer)	No
Phosphorus	Yes (lower in blacks)	Yes (decreases with age)	Yes (lower in winter)	Yes (lower in human milk-fed)
Magnesium	No	No	Yes (lower in summer)	No
Parathyroid hormone	No	No	Yes (lower in winter)	Yes (lower in formula-fed)
Calcitonin	No	No	Yes (lower in winter)	No

*Adapted from Specker et al. Pediatrics 1986; 77:891-896.

TABLE 2.   Sites of Intestinal Absorption and Effects of Some Nutrients on the Absorption of Ca, Mg, and P in Infancy

	Ca	Mg	P
Major site of absorption	Duodenum	Jejunum, ileum	Jejunum
Active	++	+	+
Passive	++	+	+
Endogenous intestinal secretion	++	+	?

Effect on mineral absorption from various nutrients in amounts greater than "normal" diet:

	Ca	Mg	P
Vitamin D	increase	—	increase
Ca	increase	increase (?)	decrease
Mg	—	increase (decrease fraction)	—
P	increase	increase	increase (decrease fraction)
Lactose	increase	—	—
Protein	—	increase	—
Fat	decrease if high fat loss	increase (medium chain triglyceride)	—

significant role in Ca absorption; however, significantly increased Ca absorption may occur through the colon in patients with long-segment small-bowel resection.[25]

Variations in endogenous (intestinal secretory) losses of Ca can markedly affect measures of true percent Ca absorption.[26,27] Standard balance studies do not permit an estimate of such endogenous losses; these losses are included in fecal losses measured in balance studies. The resultant "balance" represents a "net" balance of intake minus all losses. With more recent [46]Ca stable isotope studies, **true Ca absorption appears to be as high as 90% of intake in preterm infants fed their own mothers' milk.**[28] Length of gestation and postnatal age of the infant appear to directly favor the amount of Ca absorbed, regardless of whether infants are fed full cream cow milk, modified cow milk or human milk.[29] The needs of the infant probably play an important role in stimulating the absorption of Ca.[1,2]

Vitamin D, either derived endogenously or from exogenous sources, is important in general for the active transport component of Ca absorption (see chapter 15). There is no uniform agreement on the effect of specific dietary items on Ca absorption. Dietary lactose[30,31] and phosphate[32,33] increase Ca absorption and retention. Extreme reduction in dietary P may impair Ca absorption, whereas large excesses of phosphorus and fat intake also may impair Ca absorption;[14,34] Mg also may depress Ca absorption to a modest extent in human adults.[35]

Magnesium absorption occurs throughout the small intestine, with absorption occurring in the jejunum at a rate similar to that in the ileum. In the usual range of intake, intestinal absorption of Mg is a linear function of intake in adults[35] and infants,[36] consistent with a *diffusion* process. However, decreased fractional absorption with increasing concentration is consistent with a facilitated diffusion or saturable component also.[35] It is not certain to what extent the endogenous fecal excretion of Mg influences the reports of studies of intestinal Mg absorption. The endogenous fecal excretion of Mg for adults appears small, with a small obligatory secretory loss of Mg of approximately 0.36 mg/kg/day.[37]

In the usual range of Mg intake, Mg absorption probably is higher in infants (46-73%) than in adults (25-60%).[3] Mg absorption does not appear to vary with gestational age in low birthweight infants between 29 and 34 weeks' gestation,[38] and there is no significant increase in Mg absorption with increasing postnatal age during the first month after birth.[39]

Vitamin D and its metabolites quantitatively have little effect on intestinal Mg absorption in humans.[4,40] Dietary items such as protein[41] and easily absorbed fat in the form of medium-chain triglyceride[40] may improve Mg absorption. In full-term breastfed infants, phosphate supplement to human milk improves Mg absorption and retention.[32] In the adult, dietary phosphorus intake has been reported to correlate with urinary Mg excretion but there is no net effect on Mg balance.[42] Ca intake usually is thought to have little or no influence on Mg absorption in human adults[35] or infants.[43,44] A more recent study showed that in the usual range of Ca intake, Mg absorption was increased by Ca.[42] However, urinary Mg excretion was positively correlated with dietary Ca, and there was no net effect on Mg balance.

Phosphorus absorption occurs throughout the small intestine but is greatest in the jejunum and least in the ileum.[45-48] It is absorbed from the intestinal lumen by *simple diffusion*[46,49] and by an *active transport* proccess dependent on Ca^{2+} and potassium ions,[50] Na^+-K^+-ATPase,[51] and vitamin D.[45,47,48] The active transport mechanisms may be rate-limiting for P absorption. The latter mechanism may not be important except perhaps in vitamin D deficient states;[4] in preterm infants, P absorption appears not to be significantly affected by vitamin D intake.[52]

The extent of P absorption varies with P needs. **Phosphorus absorption for preterm infants fed human milk with low P content frequently approaches 90% of intake,**[33,53] whereas adults on a normal intake of P have a P absorption of 60-70%.[54,55] In infants, the percent P absorption decreases and urinary P excretion increases as P intake (in milk) is increased.[56,57] However, the absolute amount of P retained with higher P content milk (such as cow milk formula) remains greater than in that of infants fed low P milk (such as breast milk).

In normal circumstances, most P is absorbed

separate from Ca. A large excess of either Ca or P may reduce the absorption of the other mineral because of precipitation of insoluble calcium phosphate.[54] Intestinal P absorption generally is more complete than Ca absorption when milk from human or cow sources is ingested, and the average P retention, expressed as percent of intake, is always higher than that of Ca.[33,36,52-58] Soluble dietary phosphates, such as those found in meat or milk, essentially are completely absorbed from the mid-jejunum, whereas insoluble or undigestible phosphate contained in certain vegetable fibers may not be absorbed. The phytate in soy formula is thought to be responsible for binding to P and reducing its absorption.[59]

The extent of intestinal P secretion is not well defined. It is assumed to be quantitatively small in the growing young infant, since P retention approaches 90% or more when young infants are fed low P milk.[3,53]

Urinary Excretion (Table 3)

Calcium transport occurs in most segments of the nephron, with the exception of the descending and ascending thin limbs of the loop of Henle. In the nephron, approximately 80% of the filtered Ca is reabsorbed in the proximal convoluted and straight tubules. An estimated 10 to 20% of the filtered Ca is reabsorbed in the thick ascending limb of loop Henle and the distal nephron. The fraction of filtered Ca that is excreted is approximately 1 to 2% in the adult.

In contrast to Ca reabsorption in the nephron, only 20-30% of filtered Mg is reabsorbed in the proximal tubule and most (50-60%) of the filtered Mg is reabsorbed in the loop of Henle, largely in the thick ascending limb. Approximately 10% of the filtered Mg is delivered into the distal nephron. The fraction of filtered Mg that is excreted is approximately 3 to 4% in the adult.

Approximately 75% of filtered P is reabsorbed in the proximal convoluted tubule. There is considerable uncertainty concerning the handling of phosphate by the remainder of

the nephron.[60] Comparison of distal puncture fluid with urine suggests that an additional 10% of the filtered load is reabsorbed either in the distal tubule or collecting duct.[61] Thus, under normal circumstances, 85 to 90% of filtered phosphate is reabsorbed by the kidney.

Some common factors of clinical importance that may increase urinary excretion of Ca, Mg and P include: increased loading of the respective minerals; increased sodium intake with resultant positive sodium balance and extracellular fluid expansion; and intravenous and oral glucose loading. Hypercalcemia inhibits Mg reabsorption in the loop of Henle, and Mg infusion inhibits Ca reabsorption in the loop of Henle. Phosphorus intake either orally or intravenously decreases urinary Ca and Mg excretion particularly in the phosphorus deficient state. **The kidney in the human infant adapts well to retaining P,** particularly under conditions of low P intake such as with human milk feeding, and during increased need such as for bone growth and mineralization.[1-4]

Total parenteral nutrition is well known to result in increased urinary excretion of Ca and possibly Mg. The mechanisms involved are complex and may include excessive fluid, sodium, amino acid (particularly sulfur amino acids), glucose and vitamin D intake.[1]

CALCIUM, MAGNESIUM AND PHOSPHORUS NEEDS IN INFANTS

As thou knowest not how the bones grow in the womb of her that is with child. (Solomon, writing in *Ecclesiastes*, Circa 900 B.C.)

Oral Requirements

The requirements for Ca, Mg and P in an infant vary with growth rate, and primarily concern the need to meet demands for bone mineralization and maintain serum (total and ionized) concentrations of these minerals within a defined range. **The recommended daily intake in early infancy for infants born at term may be based on those fed primarily on human milk.** However, since Ca absorption in term infants fed cow-milk-based formulas is generally lower than in those fed human milk, a higher Ca content in cow milk formula would be preferred. The recommended daily intake is about 60 mg of Ca/kg, up to a total daily intake of about 800 mg at one year of age; 8 mg of Mg/kg, up to a total daily intake of about 150 mg at one year; and 40 mg of P/kg, up to a

TABLE 3.   Renal Reabsorption of Ca, Mg and P

	Ca	Mg	P
Proximal convoluted tubule	80%	20-30%	75-80%
Loop of Henle		50-60%	—
	10-20%		
Distal Nephron		10%	10-15%

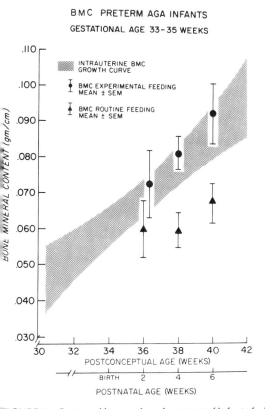

BMC PRETERM AGA INFANTS
GESTATIONAL AGE 33-35 WEEKS

INTRAUTERINE BMC GROWTH CURVE

BMC EXPERIMENTAL FEEDING MEAN ± SEM

BMC ROUTINE FEEDING MEAN ± SEM

BONE MINERAL CONTENT (gm/cm)

POSTCONCEPTUAL AGE (WEEKS)

BIRTH   2   4   6

POSTNATAL AGE (WEEKS)

FIGURE 2. Postnatal bone mineral content of infants fed an experimental formula fortified with calcium and phosphorus. Infants were of gestational ages 33-35 weeks. Experimental group was compared with infants fed routine cow milk formula, and with intrauterine bone mineralization curve. Bone mineral content in experimental group was not different from intrauterine bone mineral curve and was significantly higher than bone mineral content in routinely fed infants at 4-6 weeks' postnatal age. Values depicted are M ± SEM. (From Steichen JJ, Gratton TL, Tsang RC. Osteopenia of prematurity: the cause and possible treatment. J Pediatr 1980; 96:528-534, with permission.)

total daily intake of about 800 mg at one year.[62,63] **For preterm infants, the recommended daily intakes of Ca and P, per unit body weight, are higher[64] than those for term infants, and are usually based on intrauterine accretion rates.**[5-7,65]

The exact amount and duration of Ca and P supplement required for preterm infants still are not known. The amount varies with gestational age and infant weight. There are conflicting reports on success in increasing bone mineral content to match the in utero rate of development through the use of Ca and P supplementation.[66-69] The two reports that indicated success in matching postnatal changes in bone mineral content to "fetal" rates used large amounts of Ca and P supplement.[66,67] The total Ca intake in these two studies were

210-250 mg/kg/day and total P intakes were 112-125 mg/kg/day (Fig. 2). The duration of Ca and P supplementation required also may be important, since a "conventional" 6-week period of Ca and P supplementation has been reported to fail to prevent development of radiographic rickets in an extremely small preterm infant with a birth weight of 660 gm.[70] It would seem reasonable at the present time to recommend an intake of Ca and P that may match the intrauterine accretion of these minerals. Assuming an average Ca retention of 64% and a P retention of 71%,[3] *a maximum intake of approximately 200 mg Ca and 100-120 mg P/kg/day, over 8 to 10 weeks or until the infant achieves a postnatal weight of 2-2.5 kg* (i.e., near the time of discharge from hospital), should meet the Ca and P needs of the small preterm infant. Phosphorus intake may need to be slightly more than half the amount of Ca intake (see the section on Ca:P ratio).

Calcium- and phosphorus-fortified "preterm infant formulas" are commerically available for use in hospitalized infants. For infants receiving human milk feeding, Ca and P supplementation may be attained by using Ca- and P-fortified "preterm infant formulas" as a *complement*, powdered cow-milk-based fortifier for human milk (so-called "human milk fortifier") or lyophilized human milk powder as fortifier. The availability of lyophilized human milk powder in North America is limited and is being used currently on an experimental basis.[71]

It should be pointed out that the major problem of bone demineralization and rickets, associated with Ca and P deficiency in preterm infants, occurs predominantly in infants who are severely ill with multiple clinical complications.[1,72] In such infants, there are also practical difficulties in ingestion of intakes to match intrauterine mineral accretion rates.

For preterm infants tolerating adequate volumes of milk, the Mg intake from human milk is probably adequate to supply an amount comparable to the fetal accretion.[3] The intake of Mg from standard formulas ranges from 12-30 mg/kg/day and may be as much as threefold greater than the highest suggested daily intake.[64]

Parenteral Requirements

The goal of nutrient delivery to infants who cannot be fed enterally is to achieve growth rates of all tissues similar to those in infants fed normally. Current recommendations are de-

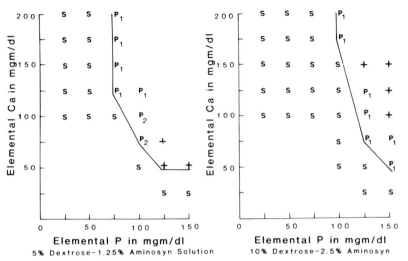

FIGURE 3. Ca and P contents achievable theoretically in parenteral nutrition fluid without precipitation. P indicates visible precipitation, S indicates soluble zone. (From Venkataraman PS, Brissie EO, Jr, Tsang RC. Stability of calcium and phosphorus in neonatal parenteral nutrition solution. J Pediatr Gastroenterol Nutr 1983; 2:640-643, with permission.)

Precipitation Observed in mixtures of Ca and P Solutions at 4°C

+   Immediate Precipitate Observed

P₁   Precipitate in 24 Hours

P₂   Precipitate in 48 Hours

S   No Visible Precipitate in 48 Hours at 4°C

rived from oral requirements and knowledge of enteric absorption. It is only recently that Ca and P can be consistently maintained in parenteral nutrition solutions in relatively large quantities (Fig 3).[73,74] The achievable quantities in theory range from those comparable to intrauterine accretion rates of Ca and P, to Ca and P retention rates of term and preterm infants fed human milk or various formulas.[1]

The optimal range of Ca and P to be delivered in parenteral nutrition for infants has not been defined. The reported quantity of Ca infused has varied from 10-200 mg/kg/day, and P infused has varied from approximately 9-109 mg/kg/day, with Ca:P ratios that have ranged from 4:1 to 1:8.[1,75] From very recent data,[76] a parenteral nutrition solution with a "high" content of 60 mg of Ca and 47 mg of P/dl can result in a stable metabolic milieu, as indicated by normal and stable serum concentrations of 1,25 dihydroxyvitamin D, and normal and stable renal tubular reabsorption of phosphorus, for large preterm (birth weight > 1500 gm) and term infants. These Ca and P contents were calculated to approximate the range of reported intake from human milk. In this study, the calciuria associated generally with the use of parenteral nutrition solutions was not increased with the relatively high Ca and P contents in the intravenous solutions. Preliminary data indicate that these Ca and P contents also may be suitable for use in very-low birthweight infants.[77]

The intravenous requirement for Mg in infancy has been estimated to be 10-25 mg/day.[64,78] In one report,[79] parenteral nutrition solutions containing 2.4 mg of Mg/dl resulted in hypomagnesemia in 11 of 42 infants. Serum Mg concentrations were normal in infants studied after the Mg content of the solution was increased to 4.8-7.2 mg/dl; the Mg delivered was 7.2-10.8 mg/kg/day. In another report,[76] parenteral nutrition solutions with 9.6 mg of Mg/dl delivering an average of 12 mg of Mg/kg/day resulted in a transient episode of hypermagnesemia in 5 of 18 infants studied. In neither of the reports was Mg loss from gastrointestinal fluid losses replaced separately. The exact requirement for Mg given intravenously is difficult to define, since it is not an usual practice for the clinician to replace Mg losses from gastrointestinal fluid losses, which may vary from 0.5-17 mg/dl; in addition, urinary Mg losses may be influenced by other nutrients delivered in parenteral nutrition (see the section on Urinary Excretion). However, it would appear that an intravenous intake of 7-10 mg/kg/day would be sufficient for most infants.

Calcium:Phosphorus Ratio

The Ca:P ratio varies widely in foods, from a high of 2.8:1(gm:gm) in green vegetables to a low of 0.06:1 in meat. The approximate ratio by weight for human milk is 2:1, for cow milk is

1.2:1, for commercial infant formula is 1.3-1.5:1 and for commercial preterm infant formula is 2:1.[63,80]

Studies of monkeys and adult humans fed large amounts of P have failed to show clear-cut adverse effects.[63] However, the high P content of cow milk ("evaporated") formula with its lower Ca:P ratio is one factor in the pathogenesis of *neonatal tetany,* a situation not encountered in the human milk fed infant[63,81] Hypocalcemic tetany and convulsions induced by cow milk is well known.[82,83]

The *Archives of Pediatrics* was the first American journal entirely devoted to Pediatrics. In the first paper published, in the first issue in 1884, practical hints were given on convulsions in children. The young physician was urged to evoke order from chaos when he made a house call to see a convulsing child. The secret was to keep everyone busy in preparing a warm bath, moving the patient to a larger bedroom, removing his clothing, wrapping him in a flannel blanket, and looking for mustard to put in the hot bathwater. By the time all these had been done the convulsion would probably have abated. (Cone TE Jr. History of American Pediatrics, Little, Brown & Co., Boston, 1979; 127.) One assumes that if the convulsions were due to cow milk ingestion, the condition would have been generally self-resolving and the management "appropriate"! (RCT).

It is likely there are much higher numbers of *asymptomatic hypocalcemic infants* related to cow milk formula feeding. The use of "humanized" cow milk formula recently has been reported to result in hypocalcemic tetany and convulsions, and (presumably compensatory) elevation of serum parathyroid hormone concentrations in otherwise healthy infants (Fig. 1).[84] The P load of such milks (Ca:P ratio 1.3 by weight), though lower than those of cow milk (Ca:P ratio 1.2:1), is still higher than that of human milk.

In general, infants are remarkably tolerant of a wide range of Ca:P ratios in their diet. A number of factors theoretically may influence the development of symptoms in infants receiving varying dietary intakes of Ca and P. First, the absolute quantity of Ca and P delivered in the diet: a grossly "imbalanced" Ca:P ratio in a single food item (e.g., green leafy vegetable or meat), ingested in limited quantities, will have little impact on Ca and P homeostasis. Second, the maturity of intestinal absorption and, in particular, the renal excretory system, since the more mature infant theoretically will have greater capacity to excrete excess minerals and thus minimize the disturbance to the body's homeostasis. Human milk with its low P content and a Ca:P ratio of approximately 2:1 by weight appears most appropriate for Ca and P homeostasis, at least for the term infant.

For the preterm infant, the ideal Ca:P ratio in the diet is not known. The preterm infant is generally thought to be deficient in both Ca and P and the extent of deficiency is inversely proportional to the gestational age and birth weight.[1] Intestinal absorption of Ca and P appears to be well developed even in the small preterm infant, but the renal excretory capacity appears to be limited, thus potentially decreasing the limit of tolerance for intakes of Ca and P.

In theory, the Ca:P ratio and the absolute quantity of each mineral in the diet should allow for normal bone mineralization and soft tissue growth. In utero bone Ca and P accretion occur in the ratio of 2:1 by weight. The relatively greater soft tissue accretion in the growing small preterm infant compared with term infants would result in a small but significantly increased P demand, since approximately 15% of total body P is found in soft tissue.[1,2] Thus a Ca:P ratio of slightly less than 2:1 may be more appropriate for the preterm infant, probably at least until the weight reaches 2-2.5 kg.

For infants requiring parenteral nutrition, widely varying Ca:P ratios of the infusate from 4:1-1:8 have been reported.[1,75] However, Ca and P needs and ratios will be affected by factors that influence urinary Ca and P excretion, and by intercompartmental shifts of P that may occur with injudicious use of intravenous nutrients. For example, excess glucose infusion, particularly after a period of "starvation," can result in severe hypophosphatemia because of a rapid shift (from fat) to glucose as the predominant fuel and the high demand for phosphate ion in the production of phosphorylated intermediates of glycolysis, and the intracellular "trapping" of phosphate.[1,2,4,85,86]

Using solutions in current use, it is possible to achieve high Ca and P contents. A parenteral nutrition infusate containing 60-80 mg of Ca and 47-62 mg of P/dl (Ca:P ratio of 1.3:1 by weight, or 1:1 by molar ratio) is being studied. From preliminary data it appears satisfactory for use in infants when used with caution. The lower total content of Ca and P probably can be used for larger preterm and term infants, and higher amounts for small preterm infants. Careful evaluation of serum Ca and P concentrations should be performed when these relatively high Ca and P content solutions are used. "Stepwise" increase in Ca and P content over the first few days of parenteral nutrition would minimize the potential risk of

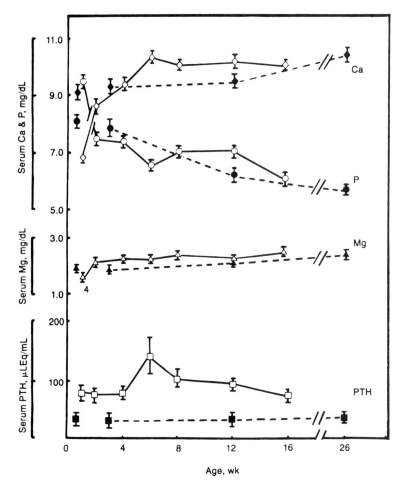

FIGURE 4. Evidence of secondary hyperparathyroidism in infants after hypocalcemia tetany. Sequential changes in serum Ca, P, Mg and parathyroid hormone (PTH) concentrations in tetanic infants versus 18 control infants fed human milk. All five infants were studied for the duration of the study but samples were not available from all time points. Serum Ca and Mg concentrations were initially corrected in tetanic infants but subsequently became higher relative to control infants. Serum phosphate concentration was initially high in tetanic infants vs. control infants but subsequently declined, with no significant difference between the two groups. Serum PTH concentrations were consistently high in tetanic infants vs control infants. Values depicted as mean ± SEM. (From Venkataraman PS, Tsang RC, Greer FR, et al. Late infantile tetany and secondary hyperparathyroidism in infants fed humanized cow milk formula. Am J Dis Child 1985; 139:664-668, with permission.)

hypercalcemia and hyperphosphatemia and their sequelae.[76]

DEFICIENCY

In 1803 Johnson stated, "Bonhomme found that chickens fed lime phosphate had harder bones. This had also been fed profitably to children with rickets and was claimed as a means of improving dentition and the healing of fractures. In mothers at the time of delivery of infants, the softness of bones was recognized and the failure of fractures to heal was appreciated." (Verzar F (ed). Clive M. McCay. *Notes on the History of Nutrition Research*. Berne, Hans Huber Publishers, 1973; page 173.)

There is a lack of an easily recognizable syndrome in infants associated with specific minor nutritional deficiency of Ca, Mg and P. This is in part because many of the symptoms and signs are nonspecific and can occur in the sick infant for other reasons.

Nutritional specific "deficiency" of Ca alone is rarely diagnosed. It may in part contribute to the cause of early neonatal hypocalcemia and to bone demineralization and rickets of small preterm infants.[1,2,4,87] Excessive urinary losses of Ca from diuretic usage in sick infants may predispose to osteopenia.[88] Deficiency of Ca *and* P presumably are the major contributors to rickets and fractures in very-low birth-weight infants.[1]

Unreplaced Mg losses from chronic gastrointestinal or biliary fistula and injudicious use of fluid and electolyte therapy probably are the major situations in which infants are predisposed to nutritional Mg deficiency. Congenital selective intestinal Mg malabsorption and congenital Mg-losing nephropathies are other conditions that predispose the infant to Mg deficiency.[1,4]

Nutritional deficiency of P specifically contributes to bone demineralization and rickets in small preterm infants, especially those who receive human milk feedings.[89] Rickets in association with chronic P deficiency, as occurs with inherited hypophosphatemic rickets, is thought to contribute to decreased stature.[90] Hypophosphatemia (serum P < 4 mg/dl) is relatively common in preterm infants, especially those who receive human milk feedings; extreme hypophosphatemia (serum < 1.5 mg/dl) is relatively uncommon in otherwise stable preterm infants tolerating full enteral feeding. Extreme hypophosphatemia may occur in infants receiving intravenous fluid or parenteral nutrition, usually associated with inadequate or no P administration, and is aggravated by injudicious use of fluid and electrolyte therapy, which increases urinary P loss and intercompartmental shifts of P. Rapid increase in nutrient delivery after a prolonged period of inadequate nutrition is responsible for a relative deficiency in P, and resultant hypophospha-temia, as a part of the "refeeding" syndrome.[86] Phosphorus deficiency is often only one facet of the typical "hypophosphatemic syndrome,"[55,91,92] since the condition usually occurs in the sick infant with complex disorders and multiple nutrient deficiencies.

TOXICITY

Under normal circumstances, toxicity associated with Ca, Mg and P is usually iatrogenic. Fortunately most of the potential toxicity associated with disturbed serum concentrations and tissue content of these elements is preventable by meticulous attention to details of fluid and electrolyte management, mechanical ventilatory efforts (to minimize acid-base disturbances), and diuretic therapy.

Excessive administration of Ca, Mg or P results in abnormally elevated circulating concentrations of these minerals and their clinical sequelae.[1,2,4] The intestinal tract and the physicochemical dietary interactions described earlier are to some extent effective barriers to excessive absorption of orally administrated Ca, Mg and P.

The major source of potential toxicity occurs with parenteral administration of these minerals. Alternate infusion of Ca and P as a means of avoiding Ca-P precipitation in intravenous fluid is an inefficient means of nutrient delivery; hyperphosphatemia, phosphaturia and hypocalcemia during P infusion, and hypercalcemia and hypercalciuria during Ca infusion have been reported with its use.[93] Phosphorus alone has been shown to reverse rickets in preterm infants. However, its use may result in biochemical complications as listed above; in addition, metastatic calcification may occur from excess P.[94] It is an inefficient means to maximize mineral retention in preterm infants.[95] It is therefore essential that serum concentrations of these minerals be measured regularly, especially if the goal is to deliver amounts of Ca and P comparable to the intrauterine accretion rate. Hypermagnesemia is a well-known complication of parenteral nutrition (see earlier comments).

Frequently, Ca, Mg and P toxicity result from therapeutic maneuvers unrelated directly to the administration of these minerals. For example, fluid restriction in association with Ca and P supplement apparently can cause intestinal milk curds and intestinal obstruction.[96] Chronic furosemide administration may result in Ca-containing nephrolithiasis,[97] cholelithiasis,[98] and bone demineralization in infants.[88] Chronic furosemide therapy has a growth-inhibitory effect associated with low bone mineral content in nursing young rat pups.[99] Thiazide diuretics are effective in reducing the calciuric effect of furosemide;[97] in adults, chronic thiazide usage is associated with higher bone mineral content when compared with adults not receiving diuretic therapy, matched for age and bone mass index.[100] However, use of a thiazide diuretic may be associated with hypokalemia, hypercalcemia and other metabolic disturbances,[101] and its efficiency and safety in the neonate require further study.

Toxins also may be given to infants incidental to the delivery of Ca, Mg and P. Aluminum, a toxin known to result in osteodystrophy, may contaminate intravenous products, particularly Ca and P salts.[102] The major route of aluminum excretion is through the kidney. In spite of an elevated urinary aluminum excretion in infants receiving parenteral nutrition, only approximately 40% of the aluminum load apparently is excreted via the urine. Presumably, a large proportion of aluminum load is retained, confirmed by histologic evidence of aluminum accumulation in bone of infants who received total parenteral nutrition.[103] Bone aluminum content may be increased in infants who receive total parenteral nutrition when compared with adult norms.[104]

Recently we reported that calcium gluconate contributes > 80% of the total aluminum contamination of the usual parenteral nutrition solution.[102] If a low aluminum containing Ca and P salt is used, markedly reduced aluminum loading is possible (Fig. 5). Brain aluminum content is elevated in uremic infants fed standard commercial cow milk formula when compared with adult norms.[105] High Ca and P formulas for preterm infants also have been reported to have an even greater extent of aluminum contamination than standard cow milk formula.[104-107] As with intravenous Ca and

ALUMINUM CONTAMINATION IN PARENTERAL NUTRITION

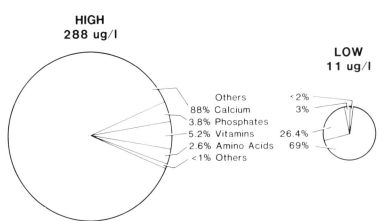

FIGURE 5. The extent of aluminum contamination in various components of parenteral nutrition solution, and the possible alternatives that may be used to lower the aluminum contamination. (Adapted from Koo WWK, Kaplan, LA, Horn J, Tsang RC, Steichen JJ. Aluminum in parenteral nutrition solution— sources and possible alternatives. J Parenter Enteral Nutr 1986; 10:591-595.)

P products, lowering of aluminum contamination in infant formula is potentially feasible, by lowering the aluminum contamination of raw materials, manufacturing processes and storage containers.[107]

RECOMMENDATIONS (Table 4)

Oral Intake

The Ca, Mg and P content and Ca:P ratio of human milk appear to be the optimal standard for term infants and probably for preterm infants who achieve a body weight of 2 kg or more. For infants fed cow milk formulas the Ca content should be higher by about 40% to correct for lower Ca absorption rates.

From current knowledge, a high Ca and P intake appears appropriate for small, growing preterm infants. Intakes to achieve in-utero accretion rates of these minerals would require a maximum daily intake of 200 mg of Ca and 100-120 mg of P/kg/day, assuming retention rates for Ca and P of 64% and 71%, respectively, until a body weight of at least 2 kg.

Intravenous Intake

Parenteral nutrition solutions containing Ca, Mg and P contents of, respectively, up to 60 mg, 7 mg and 45 mg/dl with a Ca:P ratio of 1.3:1 by weight and 1:1 by molar ratio, are suggested as suitable to maintain Ca, Mg and P homeostasis in large preterm and term infants requiring parenteral nutrition.

The Ca and P needs of the small preterm infant are higher, and these minerals may be given in total quantities at most about 25%

TABLE 4.   Suggested Daily Intakes of Ca, Mg and P for Young Infants

	Calcium		Magnesium		Phosphorus	
Oral intake	mg/kg[1]	mg[2]	mg/kg[1]	mg[2]	mg/kg[1]	mg[2]
Term[3]	60	800	8	150	30	800
Preterm[4]	< 200	—	8	—	< 120	—
Intravenous intakes[5]						
mg/dl	< 60-80		5-7		< 45-60	

[1]Suggested intake for young infants.
[2]Recommended intake for older infants (> 3 months)—see reference 64. For preterm infants > 3 months of age, the intake probably should be the same as that of infants born at term.
[3]Calculated from human milk intake. Cow milk formulas usually contain approximately 20-40% higher Ca to compensate for lower absorption, and higher P content (by approximately 100-280%) compared to human milk.
[4]Maximum intake until 2 kg body weight.
[5]Upper range for preterm and lower range for term infants. Ca and P content should be increased step-wise over 3 days, beginning from 70% of recommended intake.

higher than those for term infants. Since fluid intake usually is higher per unit body mass, the actual concentrations of Ca and P in parenteral fluids need not be increased much from those suggested for larger preterm and term infants. However, the margin of saftey in such infants probably is smaller. The Mg needs probably are comparable to those of term infants.

The recommended amounts of Ca, Mg and P could be more safely administered if their contents are increased stepwise over the first 3 days to reach the maximum, to allow for physiologic adaptation to the increased mineral loading. Daily monitoring of serum Ca, Mg and P concentration for the first 3 to 4 days, and thereafter at weekly intervals, is essential to monitor for disturbances in Ca, Mg and P.

CASE REPORT

A male infant was born at term weighing 4.6 kg, without birth asphyxia or maternal diabetes. Apgar scores were 9 and 10 at 1 and 5 minutes respectively. A family history of parathyroid adenoma was present in the maternal aunt. After a relatively benign immediate postnatal course, complicated only by hyperbilirubinemia and managed with phototherapy, the child was sent home on the sixth day of life, while receiving a standard cow milk formula.

On the seventh day of life the mother noted "twitching" of the left arm and leg. Bilateral jerking movements ensued intermittently and five of these episodes were noted. On the eighth day of life the pediatrician saw the infant and referred him to a pediatric neurologist. While an electroencephalogram was being done, the infant had a seizure and convulsion activities were recorded on electroencephalogram. The infant was then admitted to the Neonatal Intensive Care Unit.

On admission the infant's weight was 4.40 kg, head circumference was 36 cm, and length was 51 cm. Physical examination was essentially normal, except for some "jitteriness" while the infant was quiet without seizures.

Serum sodium was 136 mEg/L, potassium 4.8 mEq/L, chloride 102 mEq/L, glucose 63 mg/dl, blood urea nitrogen 5 mg/dl, calcium 7.3 mg/dl, magnesium 1.6 mg/dl, and phosphorus 9.2 mg/dl. Twelve hours after admission the serum calcium concentration was 6.2 mg/dl. The next day it was 6.1 mg/dl.

Questions and Answers

Q. What are the considerations for diagnosis?
A. Maternal hyperparathyroidism can be associated with neonatal *hypoparathyroidism* and tetany. Other forms of primary hypoparathyroidism can occur at this age; for example, DiGeorge's syndrome should also be considered and cardiac and thymic abnormalites should be sought. Magnesium deficiency can also lead to secondary hypoparathyroidism. Cow milk formulas have high phosphate contents relative to human milk, and neonatal tetany occurring at one week is a classic time for presentation.

Q. Is a serum calcium 7.3 mg/dl low enough to be considered as hypocalcemia?

A. Yes, in a term infant. Normal term infants *rarely* have serum calcium concentrations less than 8.5 mg/dl. Note also that the serum phosphorus concentrations are elevated, and magnesium concentrations are borderline low. This is a typical biochemical picture for cow milk formula related neonatal tetany, which should be considered as the first possibility. Other common causes of neonatal hypocalcemia are prematurity, birth asphyxia and maternal insulin-dependent diabetes, but these causes usually result in hypocalcemia prior to 48 hours of life ("early" hypocalcemia). These factors were not present in this infant.

Q. How would you treat this infant?
A. Acute correction with calcium salts intravenously may be needed if the seizures persist. Changing to a low-phosphate formula such as Similac PM60/40 theoretically might be of help, or to human milk if it is still available. Supplementation with calcium may be required for a short period. In general these infants appear to adapt to the phosphate load, and the disorder is transitory.

Acknowledgment

Supported in part by grants from NIH 1R01 HD 18505, NIH RR 00123, NIH HD 11725, and NIH Clinical Associate Physician Award 3M01 RR00123-21S1 (W.K.).

REFERENCES

1. Koo WWK, Tsang RC. Bone mineralization in infants. Prog Food Nutr Sci 1984;8:229-302.
2. Koo WWK, Tsang RC. Calcium, phosphorus and vitamin D needs of the high risk newborn. In Nowak AJ, Erenberg A (eds): Factors Influencing Orofacial Development in the Ill, Preterm Low Birth Weight, and Term Neonate. Publication Office of Maternal and Child Health, Bureau of Health Care Delivery, U.S. Department of Health and Human Services, 1985;30-41.
3. Greer FR, Tsang RC. Calcium, phosphorus, magnesium, and vitamin D requirements for the preterm infant. In Tsang RC (ed): Vitamin and Mineral Requirements in Preterm Infants. New York, Marcel Dekker Inc., 1985;99-136.
4. Koo WWK, Tsang RC. Calcium and magnesium metabolism in health and disease. In Werner M (ed): CRC Handbook of Clinical Chemistry, Vol. II, in press.
5. Widdowson EM, McCance RA. The metabolism of calcium, phosphorus, magnesium and strontium. Pediatr Clin North Am 1965;12:595-614.
6. Ziegler EE, O'Donnell AM, Nelson SE, Fomon SF. Body composition of the reference fetus. Growth 1976;40:320-341.
7. Sparks JW. Human intrauterine growth and nutrient accretion. Semin Perinatol 1984;8:74-93.
8. Trotter M, Hixon BB. Sequential changes in weight, density, and percentage ash weight of human skeletons from an early fetal period through old age. Anat Rec 1974;179:1-18.
9. Natelson S, Richelson MR, Sheid B, Bender SL. X-ray spectroscopy in the clinical laboratory. I. Calcium and potassium. Clin Chem 1959;5:519-531.
10. Moore EW. Ionized calcium in normal serum, ultrafiltrates, and whole blood determined by ion exchange electrodes. J Clin Invest 1970;49:318-334.
11. Carruthers BM, Copp DH, McIntosh HW. Diurnal variation in urinary excretion of calcium and phosphate and its relation to blood levels. J Lab Clin Med 1964;63:959-968.
12. Lowenstein FW, Stanton MF. Serum magnesium levels in the United States, J Am Coll Nutr 1986;5:399-414.
13. Walser M. Ion association. VI. Interactions between calcium, magnesium, inorganic phosphate, citrate and protein in normal human plasma. J Clin Invest 1961;40:723-730.

14. Parfitt AM, Kleerekoper M. The divalent ion homeostatic system—physiology and metabolism of calcium, phosphorus, magnesium and bone. In Maxwell MH, Kleeman CR (eds): Clinical Disorders of Fluid and Electrolyte Metabolism, 3rd ed. New York, McGraw Hill Book Co., 1980;269-398.

15. Stearns G, Warweg W. Studies of phosphorus of blood. I. The partition of phosphorus in whole blood and serum, the serum calcium and plasma phosphatase from birth to maturity. J Biol Chem 1933;102:749-765.

16. Hopkins T, Howard JE, Eisenberg H. Ultrafiltration studies on calcium and phosphorus in human serum. Bull Johns Hopkins Hosp 1952;91:1-21.

17. Van Leeuwen AM. Net cation equivalency (base binding power) of the plasma proteins. Acta Med Scand 1964; 422(Suppl):1-212.

18. Arnaud SB, Goldsmith RS, Stickler GB, et al. Serum parathyroid hormone and blood minerals: interrelationships in normal children. Pediatr Res 1973;7:485-493.

19. Meites S. Pediatric Clinical Chemistry. A survey of normals, methods, and instrumentation, with commentary. Washington, D.C., American Association for Clinical Chemistry. 1977;176-177.

20. Mostellar ME, Tuttle EP Jr. The effects of alkalosis on plasma concentration and urinary excretion of inorganic phosphate in man. J Clin Invest 1964;43:138-149.

21. Tsang RC, Oh W. Neonatal hypocalcemia in low birth weight infants. Pediatrics 1970;45:773-781.

22. Tsang RC, Donovan EF, Steichen JJ. Calcium physiology and pathology in the neonate. Pediatr Clin North Am 1976; 23:611-625.

23. Greer FR, Tsang RC, Levin RS, et al. Increasing serum calcium and magnesium concentrations in breast-fed infants: Longitudinal studies of minerals in human milk and in sera of nursing mothers and their infants. J Pediatr 1982;100:59-64.

24. Specker BL, Lichtenstein P, Mimouni F, et al. Calcium regulating hormones and minerals from birth to 18 months: a cross sectional study. II. Effects of sex, race, age, season and diet on serum minerals, parathyroid hormone, and calcitonin. Pediatrics 1986;77:891-896.

25. Hylander B, Ladefoged K, Jarnum S. The importance of the colon in calcium absorption following small-intestine resection. Scand J Gastrointestinal 1980;15:55-60.

26. Barltrop D, Mole RH, Sutton A. Absorption and endogenous fecal excretion of calcium by low birthweight infants on feeds with varying contents of calcium and phosphate. Arch Dis Child 1977;52:41-49.

27. Moore LJ, Machlan LA, Lim MO, et al. Dynamics of calcium metabolism in infancy and childhood. I. Methodology and quantification in the infant. Pediatr Res 1985;19:329-334.

28. Ehrenkranz RA, Ackerman BA, Nelli CM, Janghorbani M. Absorption of calcium in premature infants as measured with a stable isotope ^{46}Ca extrinsic tag. Pediatric Res 1985; 19:178-184.

29. Shaw JCL. Evidence for defective skeletal mineralization in low birth weight infants: the absorption of calcium and fat. Pediatrics 1976;57:16-25.

30. Ziegler EE, Fomon SJ. Lactose enhances mineral absorption in infancy. J Pediatr Gastroenterol Nutr 1983;2:288-294.

31. Cochet B, Jung A, Griessen M, et al. Effects of lactose on intestinal calcium absorption in normal and lactase-deficient subjects. Gastoenterol 1983;84:935-940.

32. Widdowson EM, McCance RA, Harrison GE, Sutton A. Effect of giving phosphate supplements to breast fed babies on absorption and excretion of calcium, strontium, magnesium and phosphorus. Lancet 1963;2:1250-1251.

33. Senterre J, Putet G, Salle B, Rigo J. Effects of vitamin D and phosphorus supplementation on calcium retention in preterm infants fed banked human milk. J Pediatr 1983; 103:305-307.

34. Southgate DAT, Widdowson EM, Smits BJ, et al. Absorption and excretion of calcium and fat by young infants. Lancet 1969;1:487-489.

35. Brannon PG, Vergne-Marini P, Pak CYC, et al. Magnesium absorption in human small intestine. Results in normal subjects, patients with chronic renal disease, and patients with absorptive hypercalciuria. J Clin Invest 1976;57:1412-1418.

36. Benjamin HR, Gordon HH, Marples E. Calcium and phosphorus requirements of premature infants. Am J Dis Child 1943;65:412-425.

37. Shils ME. Experimental human magnesium depletion. Medicine 1969;48:61-85.

38. Okamoto E, Muttart CR, Zucker CL, Heird WC. Use of medium-chain triglycerides in feeding the low-birth-weight infant. Am J Dis Child 1982;136:428-431.

39. Tantibhedhyangkul P, Hashim S. Medium-chain triglyceride feeding in premature infants: effects on calcium and magnesium absorption. Pediatrics 1978;61:537-545.

40. Wilz DR, Gray RW, Dominguez JH, Lemann J Jr. Plasma $1,25(OH)_2$ vitamin D concentrations and net intestinal calcium, phosphate, and magnesium absorption in humans. Am J Clin Nutr 1979;32:2052-2060.

41. McCance RA, Widdowson EM, Lehmann H. Effect of protein intake on absorption of calcium and magnesium. Biochem J 1942;36:686-691.

42. Laksmanan FL, Rao RB, Kim WW, Kelsay JL. Magnesium intakes, balances and blood levels of adults consuming self selected diets. Am J Clin Nutr 1984;40:1380-1389.

43. Moya M, Domenech E. Role of calcium-phosphate ratio of milk formulae on calcium balance in low birth weight infants during the first three days of life. Pediatr Res 1982;16:675-681.

44. DeVizia B, Fomon SJ, Nelson SE, et al. Effect of dietary Ca on metabolic balance of normal infants. Pediatr Res 1985; 19:800-806.

45. Chen TC, Costillo L, Korychka-Dahl M, DeLuca HF. Role of vitamin D metabolites in phosphate transport of rat intestine. J Nutr 1974;104:1056-1060.

46. Juan D, Liptak P, Gray TK. Absorption of inorganic phosphate in the human jejunum and its inhibition by serum calcitonin. J Clin Endocrinol Metab 1976;43:517-522.

47. Walling MW. Intestinal Ca and phosphate transport: differential responses to vitamin D_3 metabolites. Am J Physiol 1977; 233:E488-494.

48. Wasserman RH. Intestinal absorption of calcium and phosphorus. Fed Proc 1981;40:68-72.

49. McHardy GJR, Parsons DS. The absorption of inorganic phosphate from the small intestine of the rat. Q J Exp Physiol 1956;41:398-409.

50. Harrison HE, Harrison HC. Intestine transport of the phosphate: action of vitamin D, calcium and potassium. Am J Physiol 1961;201:1007-1012.

51. Taylor AN. In vitro phosphate transport in chick ileum: effect of cholecalciferol calcium, sodium and metabolic inhibitors. J Nutr 1974;104:489-494.

52. Senterre J, Salle B. Calcium and phosphorus economy of the preterm infants and its interaction with vitamin D and its metabolites. Acta Pediatr Scand (Suppl) 1982;296:85-92.

53. Rowe J, Rowe D, Horak E, et al. Hypophosphatemia and hypercalciuria in small premature infants fed human milk: evidence for inadequate dietary phosphorus. J Pediatr 1984; 104:112-117.

54. Wilkinson R. Absorption of calcium, phosphorus and magnesium. In Nordin BEC (ed): Calcium, Phosphate and Magnesium Metabolism. New York, Churchill Livingstone 1976:36-112.

55. Stoff JS. Phosphate homeostasis and hypophosphatemia. Am J Med 1982;72:489-495.

56. Shenai JP, Reynolds JW, Babson SG. Nutritional balance studies in very low birth weight infants: enhanced nutrient retention rates by an experimental formula. Pediatrics 1980; 66:233-238.

57. Huston RK, Reynolds JW, Jensen C, Buist NRM. Nutrient and mineral retention and vitamin D absorption in low birth weight infants: effect of medium chain triglycerides. Pediatrics 1983;72:44-48.

58. Fomon SJ, Owen GM, Jensen RL, Thomas LN. Calcium and phosphorus balance studies with normal full term infants fed pooled human milk or various formulas. Am J Clin Nutr 1963;12:346-357.

59. Shenai JP, Jhaveri BM, Reynolds JW, et al. Nutritional balance studies in very low birth weight infants. Role of soy

formula. Pediatrics 1981;67:631-637.

60. Knox FG, Osswald H, Marchand R, et al. Phosphate transport along the nephron. Am J Physiol 1977; 233:F261-F268.

61. Amiel C, Kuntziger H, Richet G. Micropuncture study of handling of phosphate by proximal and distal nephron in normal and parathyroidectomized rat: evidence for distal reabsorption. Pfluegers Arch 1970;317:93-109.

62. Committee on Dietary Allowances. Minerals, Food and Nutrition Board. Recommended dietary allowances. Washington, D.C., National Academy of Science, 1980;125-136.

63. Committee on Nutrition. American Academy of Pediatrics. Calcium, phosphorus, and magnesium. In Forbes GB, Woodruff CW (eds): Pediatric Nutrition Handbook, 2nd ed. Chicago, American Academy of Pediatrics 1985;111-122.

64. Committee on Nutrition. American Academy of Pediatrics. Nutritional needs of low birth weight infants. Pediatrics 1985; 75:976-986.

65. Ziegler EE, Biga RL, Fomon SJ. Nutritional requirements for the premature infants. In Suskind RM (ed): Textbook of Pediatric Nutrition. New York, Raven Press 1981;29-39.

66. Steichen JJ, Gratton TL, Tsang RC. Osteopenia of prematurity: the cause and possible treatment. J Pediatr 1980; 96:528-534.

67. Greer FR, Steichen JJ, Tsang RC. Effects of increased calcium, phosphorus, and vitamin D intake on bone mineralization in very low brith weight infants feed formula with polycose and medium-chain triglycerides. J Pediatr 1982; 100:951-955.

68. Modanlou H, Lim MO, Hansen JW. Growth, biochemical status and mineral metabolism in very low birth weight infants receiving fortified preterm human milk. J Pediatr Gastroenterol Nutr 1986;5:762-767.

69. Greer FR, McCormick A, Loker J. Improved bone mineral content without correction of urinary signs of "phosphate deficiency syndrome" in preterm infants fed own mother's fortified breast milk. Clin Res 1984;32:806A.

70. Koo WWK, Oestreich AE, Sherman, R, et al. Failure of high calcium and phosphorus fortification in the prevention of rickets of prematurity. Am J Dis Child 1986;140:857-858.

71. Schanler RJ, Garza C, O'Brien-Smith E. Fortified mother's milk for very low birth weight infants: results of macromineral balance studies. J Pediatr 1985;107:767-774.

72. Koo WWK, Gupta JM, Nayanar VV, et al. Skeletal changes in premature infants. Arch Dis Child 1982;57:447-452.

73. Eggert LD, Rusho WJ, MacKay MW, Chan GM. Calcium and phosphorus compatibility in parenteral nutrition solution for neonates. Am J Hosp Pharm 1982;39:49-53.

74. Venkataraman PS, Brissie EO, Jr, Tsang RC. Stability of calcium and phosphorus in neonatal parenteral nutrition solution. J Pediatr Gastroenterol Nutr 1983;2:640-643.

75. Adamkin DH. Nutrition in very low birth weight infants. Clin Perinatol 1986;13:419-443.

76. Koo WWK, Tsang RC, Steichan JJ, et al. Parenteral nutrition for infants: effects of high versus low calcium and phosphorus content. J Pediatr Gastroenterol Nutr 1987;6:96-104.

77. Koo WWK, Tsang RC. Minimal vitamin D, high calcium and phosphorus requirement of preterm infants receiving parenteral nutrition. Pediatr Res 1987;21:366A.

78. Committee on Nutrition. American Academy of Pediatrics. Commentary on parenteral nutrition. Pediatrics 1983; 71:547-552.

79. Koo WWK, Fong T, Gupta JM. Parenteral nutrition in infants. Aust Paediatr J 1980;16:169-174.

80. Leveille GA, Zabick ME, Morgan KJ. Nutrients in Foods. Massachusetts, The Nutrition Guild, 1983;2-283.

81. Anonymous. Dietary phosphorus and secondary hyperparathyroidism in infants receiving humanized cow's milk formula. Nutr Rev 1986;44:107-109.

82. Bakin H. Pathogenesis of tetany of the newborn. Am J Dis Child 1937;54:1211-1226.

83. Gittleman IJ, Pincus JB. Influence of diet on the occurrence of hyperphosphatemia and hypocalcemia in the newborn infant. Pediatrics 1951;8:778-787.

84. Venkatarman PS, Tsang RC, Greer FR, et al. Late infantile tetany and secondary hyperparathyroidism in infants fed humanized cow milk formula. Am J Dis Child 1985; 139:664-668.

85. Derr R, Zieve L. Intracellular distribution of phosphate in the underfed rat developing weakness and coma following total parenteral nutrition. J Nutr 1976;106:1398-1403.

86. Weinsler RL, Krumdieck CL. Death from overzealous total parenteral nutrition: the refeeding syndrome revisited. Am J Clin Nutr 1980;34:393-399.

87. Koo WWK, Tsang RC. Rickets in infants. In Nelson NM (ed): Current Therapy in Neonatal Perinatal Medicine. Toronto, B.C. Decker, 1985;299-304.

88. Venkataraman PS, Han BK, Tsang RC, Daugherty CC. Secondary hyperparathyroidism and bone disease in infants receiving long term furosemide therapy. Am J Dis Child 1983;137:1157-1161.

89. Koo WWK, Antony G, Stevens LHS. Continuous nasogastric phosphorus infusion in hypophosphatemic rickets of prematurity. Am J Dis Child 1984;138:172-175.

90. Herweijer TJ, Steendijk R. The relation between attained adult height and the metaphyseal lesions in hypophosphatemic vitamin D resistant rickets. Acta Pediatr Scand 1985; 74:196-200.

91. Fitzgerald F. Clinical hypophosphatemia. Ann Rev Med 1978;29:177-189.

92. Knochel JP. The clinical status of hypophosphatemia. N Engl J Med 1985;313:447-449.

93. Kimura S, Nose O, Seino Y, et al. Effects of alternate and simultaneous administration of calcium and phosphorus on calcium metabolism in children receiving total parenteral nutrition. J Parenter Enteral Nutr 1986;10:513-516.

94. Laflamme GH, Jowsey J. Bone and soft tissue changes with oral phosphate supplements. J Clin Invest 1972;51:2834-2840.

95. Carey DE, Goetz CA, Horak E, Rowe JC. Phosphorus wasting during phosphorus supplementation of human milk feedings in preterm infants. J Pediatr 1985;107:790-792.

96. Cleghorn GJ, Tudehope DI. Neonatal intestinal obstruction associated with oral calcium supplementation. Aust Paediatr J 1981;17:298-299.

97. Hufnagle KG, Khan SN, Penn D, et al. Renal calcifications: a complication of long term furosemide therapy in preterm infants. Pediatrics 1982;70:360-363.

98. Barth RA, Brasch RC, Filly RA. Abdominal pseudotumor in childhood: Distended gallbladder with parenteral hyperalimentation. Am J Roentgenol 1981;136:341-343.

99. Koo WWK, Guan ZP, Tsang RC, et al. Growth failure and decreased bone mineral of newborn rats with chronic furosemide therapy. Pediatr Res 1986;20:74-78.

100. Wasnich RD, Benfante RJ, Yano K, et al. Thiazide effect on the mineral content of bone. N Engl J Med 1983;309:344-347.

101. Reynolds JEF, Prasad AB (eds): Martindale: the Extra Pharmacopoeia, 28th ed. London, The Pharmaceutical Press 1982;600-602.

102. Koo WWK, Kaplan LA, Horn J, Tsang RC, Steichen JJ. Aluminum in parenteral nutrition solution—sources and possible alternatives. J Parenter Enteral Nutr 1986;10:591-595.

103. Koo WWK, Kaplan LA, Bendon R, et al. Response to aluminum in parenteral nutrition during infancy. J Pediatr 1986;109:877-883.

104. Sedman AB, Klein GL, Merritt RJ, et al. Evidence of aluminum loading in infants receiving intravenous therapy. N Engl J Med 1985;312:1337-1343.

105. Freundlich M, Faugere MC, Zilleruelo G, et al. Milk formula causes aluminum toxicity in uremic infants. Lancet 1985; 2:527-528.

106. Weintraub R, Hams G, Meerkin M, Rosenberg A. High aluminum content of infant milk formulas. Arch Dis Child 1986;61:914-916.

107. Koo WWK, Kaplan, LA, Krug Wispe SK. Aluminum contamination of infant formulas. JPEN, in press, 1988.

11

Trace Elements

CLARE E. CASEY, Ph.D.
PHILIP A. WALRAVENS, M.D.

ABSTRACT

This chapter addresses physiology, deficiency, and toxicity of the essential trace elements and provides recommendations for oral and intravenous intakes during
infancy.

Trace element. Constitutes less than 0.01% of body
mass. These elements were originally so called because
their levels in tissues were too low to quantify and their
presence was reported in "trace" amounts.

Essential trace element. One for which a deficient intake
consistently results in an impairment of function and for
which supplementation with physiological levels of the
element in question, but not of others, prevents or cures
the impairment.[4a,b]

Elements currently regarded as essential. (A) Well-
established: zinc, copper, selenium, chromium, manganese, molybdenum, iodine, fluorine, cobalt. (B) Newer:
arsenic, lithium, nickel, silicon, vanadium. (C) Probable:
bromium, cadmium, lead, tin.

INTRODUCTION

Although there are now 15 trace elements
regarded as essential in mammalian nutrition,
only 8 of these (zinc, copper, iodine, selenium,
fluorine, chromium, manganese, and molybdenum) are currently known to have any importance in human nutrition (Table 1). Indeed,
only the first 5 are of routine practical interest
in pediatrics. Deficiencies of several (manganese, chromium, molybdenum) may occur under specialized conditions, such as long-term
parenteral feeding, use of elemental formulas,
or genetic disorders. At the other end of the
spectrum, several elements (e.g., lead, alumi-
nium) are of concern in pediatric nutrition for
potential toxicity rather than potential deficiency.[1]

In spite of the increasing sophistication in
analytical measurements of trace elements
and our increased understanding of their biochemical functions, with the exception of
iodine and selenium, techniques for the description of nutritional status are still rudimen-
tary. The most commonly used measure of
nutritional status is the concentration of the
element in blood, but for metals other than
zinc and copper even such measurements are
rarely available on a routine basis. There is
currently not enough information about the
physiology of most elements, especially during
infancy, to adequately interpret blood concentrations. They do not necessarily reflect levels
in other tissues or functional availability. In
early infancy, in particular, blood concentrations of several elements (including zinc,
copper and manganese) appear to change
with age after birth regardless of the intake of
the element.

Even for an abundant and widely investigated element such as zinc, there are large
gaps in our understanding of its cellular functions and metabolic pathways. For elements
such as chromium and manganese, the essentiality of which has long been established, there
is very little information on which to discuss
nutritional requirements, especially in infancy,
so that many of the recommendations for
dietary intakes remain very tentative.[2,3]

COPPER

Copper, in medical circles, is most often
associated with the protean and frightening
manifestations of Wilson's disease. Recognition of presenting signs is a clinical challenge,
as they may reflect liver disease, behavioral or
neurologic changes or even hemolytic diseases. Copper chelation in this syndrome may
be life-saving and is even recommended for affected individuals prior to appearance of
symptoms.[5] This attention to the toxic effects
of copper distracts from the important role
copper plays in cell metabolism. Furthermore,
deficiency states do exist and are being reported in increasing numbers. **Clinical findings in copper deficiency correlate well with
biological or enzymatic functions of cuproenzymes.**

TABLE 1.   Essential Trace Elements of Practical Importance in Human Nutrition

Element	Discovery of Biological role	Functions	Human deficiency	Human toxicity
Zinc	1869	Enzymes in all classes; nucleic acid, protein synthesis; growth, immune function	✔	✔
Copper	1928	Ceruloplasmin; enzymes in synthesis of cartilage, bone, myelin	✔	✔
Selenium	1957	Glutathione peroxidase	✔	✔
Chromium	1959	Potentiation of insulin	✔	
Manganese	1931	Mucopolysaccharide synthesis; superoxide dismutase	?	✔
Molybdenum	1953	Metabolism of sulphur compounds, xanthine	✔	✔
Iodine	c.1840	Thyroid hormones	✔	✔
Fluorine	1800s	Structural component of bones and teeth	✔	✔

TABLE 2.   Copper Enzymes in Humans

Cuproprotein	Site	Function
Cytochrome oxidase	Mitochondria	Electron transport
Superoxide dismutase	Cytosol and mitochondria	Converts superoxide ions to oxygen and peroxide
Ceruloplasmin	Plasma	Amine oxidase, ferroxidase, copper transport
Ferroxidase II	Plasma	Ferroxidase
Lysyl oxidase	Connective tissue	Cross-linking of collagen and elastin
Tyrosinase	Skin, eye	Synthesis of melanin
Dopamine β-hydroxylase	Adrenal	Catecholamine synthesis

PHYSIOLOGY

Copper is a constituent of many enzymes, where it may be found alone or with iron, zinc or manganese. Some of the better known cuproenzymes and their most important functions are listed in Table 2. With its role in electron transport, copper enhances efficiency of energy production via oxidative phosphorylation. It is involved in protection of cell membranes against oxidative damage through the superoxide dismutase enzymes. In rats fed a milk diet low in iron and copper, a milk-induced anemia occurs that iron supplementation alone will not correct. This requirement for copper to correct apparent iron deficiency is explained by the ferroxidase function of ceruloplasmin. The latter oxidizes ferrous iron released from storage sites to the ferric state. Ferric iron binds to apotransferrin and is transported to the marrow for heme synthesis. Erythropoietin synthesis, furthermore, may be dependent on an adequate tissue copper supply; cerebral protein and myelin deposition are also copper-dependent functions.[1]

Some cuproproteins do not presently have known enzymatic functions. Examples include albocuprein I and II, which have been isolated from brain, and the metallothioneins, a group of cytoplasmic proteins with high sulfhydryl content that are capable of binding zinc, cadmium and copper. These proteins are found particularly in hepatocytes, intestinal cells and renal tubular cells.

Metallothionein-bound copper accumulates in the fetal liver during the last 3 months of gestation, giving the neonate a large hepatic reserve of copper. The liver of term infants contains 200–400 μg of copper per gram dry weight, or some 10- to 20-fold the adult hepatic copper concentration. In infants, this copper was previously thought to be associated with a special protein called neonatal hepatic mitochondrocuprein. Metabolic pathways of copper are summarized in Figure 1, which depicts the fate of dietary copper in a standard adult presumed to be in balance. **The importance of biliary excretion is evident, since it is some 30-fold higher than urinary losses.** Of recent interest is the discovery of a new cuproprotein, provisionally named transcuprein, which may be the predominant vehicle of copper transport to the liver in the portal circulation.[6] Identification of transcuprein re-

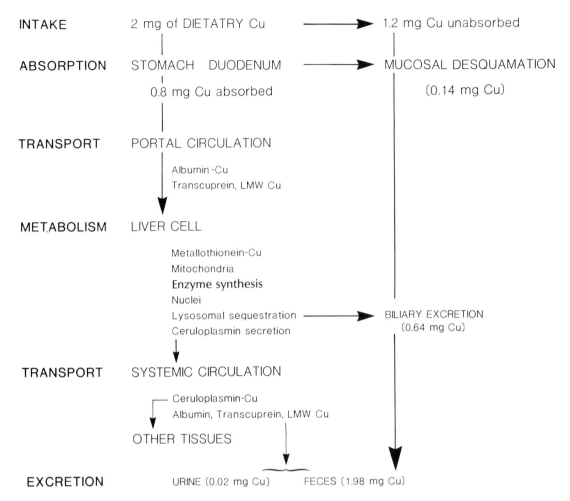

FIGURE 1.   Copper metabolism in a normal adult. Cu = copper; LMW = low molecular weight.

quired the use of high specific activity Cu[67] radioisotope, which has also provided new information on the transport functions of ceruloplasmin. Copper in plasma is found in four fractions, transcuprein and albumin carrying 15% each respectively; ceruloplasmin accounts for 60% of plasma copper, and the remaining 10% is in various low molecular weight components.[7] The affinity of transcuprein for copper is greater than that of albumin but both will freely exchange copper molecules. Albumin and transcuprein probably transport copper to kidney and liver. In the latter, ceruloplasmin synthesis and secretion occurs, with ceruloplasmin-bound copper presently considered the preferred transport form to other tissues such as brain, muscle and bones. The complex fate of copper in the liver may be schematized as follows. After uptake from the portal circulation, copper is bound to hepatic metallothionein from which it is re-

leased for enzyme synthesis in mitochondria and cytosol, transferred to the nuclei, and incorporated into ceruloplasmin, which is released into the plasma compartment. Copper breakdown products are normally sequestered in lysosomes and excreted in bile. In cases of copper overload, production of ceruloplasmin may also serve as a diversionary pathway for the excess intracellular hepatic copper. Urinary excretion of copper is normally minimal and presumably occurs as a result of filtration of low molecular weight components.

REQUIREMENTS

Term Infants

It has been estimated that term infants and growing children require a daily intake of 50–100 µg of copper per kg of body weight. The Food and Nutrition Board of the National

Academy of Sciences recommends a daily copper intake of 80 µg/kg.[8] Because copper is present in most foods, such levels of intake are easily achieved except when unmodified cow milk, the copper content of which rarely exceeds 180 µg/L, is the main source of nutrients. Salmenpera and colleagues from Finland have reported normal serum concentrations of copper and ceruloplasmin in infants breast-fed exclusively for up to 12 months.[9] The administration of copper supplements to the mothers did not increase breast-milk copper, and individual intakes of copper by the infants ranged from 3–40 µg/kg/day with a median value of 11 µg/kg/day at 9 months. Even on these low intakes, there was no evidence of copper deficiency and the infants' serum copper and ceruloplasmin concentrations achieved expected age-dependent increases. It is possible that Cu absorption from breast milk, like that of zinc and iron, is greater than that from cow milk or formula. At the same time liver copper reserves in the term infant should be sufficient, if no excess losses from diarrhea or other causes occur, to cover needs during most of the first year of life.

Parenteral needs for term infants have been calculated to be 20 µg/kg/day.[10] Balance studies by Zlotkin and Buchanan have confirmed that in term infants an intravenous intake of copper as little as 16 µg/kg/day will allow balance, and higher doses result in copper retention.[11]

Preterm Infants

Dauncey et al.[12] reported negative copper balances during the first month of postnatal life in preterm infants fed pasteurized human milk. More recently, however, Tyrala[15] was able to obtain positive balance by 34 weeks' postconception age (or 2–4 weeks postnatally) in five of ten infants receiving a formula enriched with medium-chain triglycerides. Intrauterine retention rates were achieved by three of the preterm infants, but such accumulation rates may not be an appropriate measure of adequacy of copper intake. During the third trimester very large amounts of copper are deposited in the fetal liver, so that by term it contains 50–70% of the total body burden. Such stores appear to be available after birth in term infants and are gradually depleted once ceruloplasmin synthesis and secretion begins. Copper deficiency does not occur prior to the time of depletion of hepatic copper stores, which

are used to meet extrahepatic needs. Without provision for hepatic accumulation, the estimated desirable rate for copper retention is about 20–40 µg/kg/day. It is presently unknown if the provision of additional copper to preterm infants will result in hepatic accumulation similar to that occurring during pregnancy.

Ehrenkranz, using stable isotope techniques, demonstrated a 53% absorption of copper in formula-fed preterm infants of 2 weeks of age.[16] The absorption increased to 72% when preterm human milk was provided to the infants. The estimated safe and adequate level of intake for term infants of 80 µg/kg/day should also be sufficient to cover the needs of preterm infants.[8] Plasma copper and ceruloplasmin concentrations are low at birth and remain low for several weeks in preterm infants (plasma Cu ranges around 30 µg/dL). **Plasma concentrations of copper start to rise as ceruloplasmin synthesis is initiated between 6 and 12 postnatal weeks, varying with the gestational age of the infant.** Concentrations and rates of increase are not affected by the levels of oral copper intakes.[13,14]

In parenteral nutrition, Zlotkin[16] recommends 63 µg/kg/day or a level that closely approximates intrauterine accretion rates, and an even higher level (95 µg/kg/day) is advocated by James and colleagues.[17] Sutton and colleagues from Glasgow[18] concur with the recommendation of 63 µg/kg/day. Again, however, such levels include provision for hepatic storage, and Halliday and colleagues in Ireland comment that they have not encountered copper deficiency in infants with parenteral intakes of 20 µg/kg/day,[19] a level that corresponds to the recommendations of the American Medical Association's (AMA) expert panel. **In view of the potential of copper for hepatotoxicity, the 20 µg/kg/day level seems most prudent until hepatic maturity has been achieved and the risk of cholestasis lessened.** Parenteral nutrition in premature infants induces higher plasma copper concentrations than oral nutrition. This may represent an early sign of hepatotoxicity and caution is warranted.[20]

DEFICIENCY

Copper deficiency was first reported in 1964 by Cordano and colleagues in Peruvian infants recuperating from protein energy malnutrition whose diets were based on cow milk.[21] Earlier in 1956 copper deficiency had been postulated in association with iron deficiency and hypoproteinemia in what would now be considered a malabsorption syndrome. Interest was further spurred in 1971 by reports of copper deficiency in formula-fed preterm infants,[22] which were soon followed by Karpel and Peden's description of copper deficiency induced by parenteral nutrition.[23]

At that time regular plasma infusions were considered adequate for provision of trace elements to infants or adults receiving parenteral nutrition. The protein hydrolysate solutions that were initially used probably contained fair amounts of trace metals as contaminants. When the hydrolysates were replaced by parenteral solutions made from crystalline amino acids, a period of nutritional experimentation ensued which demonstrated for the skeptics the essentiality of copper, and subsequently of zinc, chromium, selenium and molybdenum in humans.

Copper deficiency syndromes should be suspected in the presence of a combination of physical signs, abnormal laboratory measurements and radiologic changes (Table 3). Hematologic changes, mainly neutropenia in the presence of hypocupremia, and any combination of clinical or radiologic signs, are often indicative of the syndrome, which according to recent reports from Israel may be more widespread among infants fed cow milk than previously thought. Cow milk normally contains 40–180 µg/L of copper; hence, it is difficult to provide the minimal requirement to rapidly growing infants. Copper deficiency was initially described in infants who had prolonged diarrhea, so it is not surprising that it occurs in nutritional malabsorption,[24] and it has been reported with peritoneal dialysis.[25] Of interest are recent accounts of copper deficiency in conditions in which the pH of the stomach and proximal intestine were changed by the administration of buffer.[26] The accompanying changes in acidity of the stomach and duodenum decreased solubility of dietary copper and deficiency ensued.

Many of the symptoms and radiologic changes of copper deficiency are present in Menkes' steely hair syndrome, an X-linked inherited disease characterized by wiry hair, progressive neurologic deterioration and ultimately death.[27] It was the Australians' recognition of the similarities between hair changes in Menkes' syndrome and the wool of copper-deficient sheep that led to the discovery of the role of copper in this disease. In Menkes' disease, there is a perturbation of copper metabolism which leads to deficiency in liver and brain, whereas excess copper accumulates in intestine, kidney, spleen, fibroblasts and other tissues, presumably through defective regulation of metallothionein synthesis.

TOXICITY

With the ingestion of milligram amounts of copper, such as occurs from contaminated cocktail shakers and water heaters, gastrointestinal symptoms follow with epigastric pains, emesis of green-blue products and diarrhea. After accidental or intentional ingestion of larger doses, serious systematic toxicity occurs, which has been studied in India, where ingestion of 1–30 gm of copper sulfate is a common method of suicide. This causes ulcerations of the gastrointestinal tract followed by hemolysis and hepatic and renal failure, leading to coma and shock.[28] Use of copper-containing skin medications on large inflamed surfaces has also caused fatalities. Hemodialysis with solutions of high copper content can cause hemolysis or febrile reactions similar to metal fume fevers.

TABLE 3.   Diagnosis of Copper Deficiency

Clinical	Laboratory*	Radiological
Pallor	Anemia	Osteoporosis
Depigmented skin and hair	Leukopenia: WBC <5000/µL	Flaring of anterior ribs
Poor weight gain	Neutropenia: PMN <1500/µL	Fractures or periosteal reaction
Diarrhea		
Edema	Plasma Cu decreased	Metaphyseal spurs
Distended veins	Serum ceruloplasmin decreased	
Neurologic findings	Bone marrow: cytoplasmic vacuoles in erythroid	
Hypotonia	and myeloid series; maturation arrest	
Apnea		
Psychomotor delay		

*WBC = white blood cell; PMN = polymorphonuclear cells.

Chronic copper poisoning has been demonstrated in an infant who presented with pink disease, or acrodynia. The child's family had an idiosyncrasy of using hot water from copper pipings and heater for all cooking purposes.[29] Copper contamination of milk and foods furthermore has been postulated as an etiologic factor in Indian childhood cirrhosis.[30]

ZINC

A biological role for zinc was first postulated in 1869 when Raulin showed that it was essential for growth of *Aspergillus niger*. Todd and colleagues demonstrated a requirement for zinc in mammalian nutrition in the 1930s but it was only in 1955 that porcine parakeratosis was recognized as a zinc responsive syndrome.[31] The first human zinc responsive syndrome was reported in 1961 by Prasad and coworkers at the U.S. Naval Medical Research Unit in Cairo, when they showed that zinc would cause increases in growth and sexual maturation in patients with dwarfism and hypogonadism.[32] Prior to this time it was felt that because of the widespread distribution of zinc in foodstuffs, human zinc deficiency was unlikely to occur.

Since the 1960s, however, many zinc-responsive syndromes have been described that can affect growth rates, sexual maturation and function, integumental integrity, appetite and food intake, olfactory perception, immune response and even psychocognitive functions. Biochemical correlates to the multiple presentations of zinc deficiency are not evident much of the time, and even measurements of plasma, hair or urine zinc may be misleading when attempting to confirm a diagnosis of marginal deficiencies. One still awaits the advent of an assay that would allow accurate and reproducible measurements of zinc nutritional status.

PHYSIOLOGY

The importance of zinc in mammalian metabolism derives from the role that it exerts in protein metabolism and protein synthesis. Recognition of zinc metalloenzymes started with erythrocyte carbonic anhydrase, and a growing list has been added, including alcohol dehydrogenase, carboxypeptidases A and B, alkaline phosphatase, various dehy-

INTESTINAL ABSORPTION OF ZINC

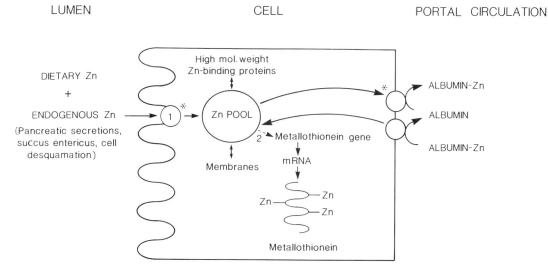

* Active transport site

1. Intestinal uptake increases in zinc deficiency
2. Metallothionein gene is activated in zinc sufficiency and excess zinc is stored in the cytosol

FIGURE 2.   Intestinal absorption of zinc.

drogenases and retinene reductase. Other enzymes use zinc as a cofactor, and at present some 100 systems are known to be either zinc dependent or zinc metalloproteins. Zinc is involved in nucleic acid metabolism as a component of various DNA and RNA polymerases. Amino acid utilization and polysome formation are also impaired in zinc-deficient animals, in which increased levels of ribonuclease may lead to excessive degradation of RNA. Host defense mechanisms are affected, and zinc also stabilizes cell membranes and may protect them from lipid peroxidation through its role in the superoxide dismutase enzyme systems. The effects of maternal zinc deficiency in experimental animals vary with the time of onset of the deficiency. Early in pregnancy zinc deficiency is highly teratogenic and affects principally the central nervous system. Deficiency of zinc later in pregnancy in rats causes intrauterine growth retardation and decreased fetal brain weight and DNA content.[33]

Dietary zinc is absorbed in the duodenum and proximal small intestine. In the intestinal lumen, dietary zinc mixes with zinc from pancreatic secretions and with the zinc-containing breakdown products from intestinal desquamation. After cellular uptake the metal may be transported to the serosal surface and actively secreted into the portal circulation where it binds to albumim. This mechanism is reversible, and uptake of portal zinc by intestinal cells also occurs. In cases of zinc sufficiency, an increasing zinc pool will trigger synthesis of intestinal cell metallothionein (Fig. 2), which can bind excess intracellular zinc. With desquamation this excess zinc will again become available for absorption, and zinc attached to low molecular weight protein fragments may adhere preferentially to the brush border. The luminal zinc binding site also has the capacity of increasing active transport of zinc in cases of zinc deficiency.[34]

Reported intestinal absorption levels in adults vary from 20 to 80% of ingested dietary zinc, with more recent estimates fluctuating between 20 and 40%.[32] Absorption also varies with the physical characteristics of the diet. Protein-bound zinc and breast milk zinc are readily absorbed. Some amino acids such as histidine and cysteine appear to facilitate absorption, whereas inhibitors include phytate and fiber. At alkaline pH, phytate, zinc and calcium form an insoluble complex in which the metal is unavailable for absorption. Excess

dietary copper or cadmium may also decrease zinc absorption by competing for cellular uptake and metallothionein binding. Inhibition of zinc absorption by high intakes of iron has been demonstrated in adults but is disputed in infants.[34]

Zinc is transported from the intestine mainly bound to albumin and taken up rapidly by the liver, pancreas, kidneys and spleen. Two-thirds of plasma zinc is albumin-bound, one-third appears in alpha-2-macroglobulin and a small portion is amino-acid bound.

Excretion occurs mainly through fecal losses. Urinary losses in adults range between 300 and 500 µg/day compared with a daily intake of approximately 10 mg. In infants, urinary zinc generally decreases from 30–50 µg/kg/day shortly after birth to levels of 10 µg/kg/day around 2–3 months of age.[35]

REQUIREMENTS

Term Infants
Oral. Very few balance studies of zinc have been performed on term infants. Cavell and Widdowson studied 10 neonates fed human milk at approximately one week of age and found 9 of 10 to be in negative zinc balance.[36] Ziegler and colleagues from Iowa performed balance studies with a variety of formulas on 55 normal healthy infants and children in whom an intake of 210 µg/kg/day of zinc resulted in apparent retention of zinc.[37] Depending on bioavailability of ingested zinc, calculated requirements vary from 1.0-3.1 mg/day of zinc for 2-month-old male infants when absorption is 60 and 20%, respectively. The 3.1-mg level corresponds to both the recommended dietary allowances (RDA) and the recommendations of the Committee of Nutrition of the American Academy of Pediatrics.[8]

Parenteral. Zinc requirements for term infants receiving parenteral nutrition have been estimated to be 100 µg/kg/day.[10] In presence of ongoing losses, such as intractable diarrhea or large stoma output, requirements can drastically increase, and infusion of 300-400 µg/kg/day has at times been necessary to compensate for stool losses.

Preterm Infants
Oral. Initial reports of zinc absorption and retention in premature infants fed pooled human breast milk were not encouraging, since negative balance persisted until the 60th day

of extrauterine life.[12] This negative balance was mainly due to marked losses of zinc in feces. In 1983, Voyer and colleagues from France reported positive balance in preterm infants of approximately 30-32 weeks' gestation, receiving a 70:30 whey-casein formula with a fat content that included 40% medium-chain triglycerides (MCT).[38] Apparent retention occurred at intakes of 200-270 µg/kg/day under those conditions, whereas comparable infants receiving human milk based formulas exhibited marked fecal zinc losses and were in negative balance. The principal difference between the two groups was in the absorption of fats, which averaged 90% for the MCT group but varied between 40-90% in the breast milk group. Confirmation of these observations was recently provided by Tyrala, who fed infants of 34 weeks' gestational age a whey-predominant MCT-containing formula with 12.5 mg of zinc per liter. Positive balance was achieved and generally exceeded the calculated intrauterine accretion rate of 432 µg/day.[15] Similarly Ehrenkranz and colleagues, using stable isotopes, found 32% absorption of zinc from cow milk formula and 53% absorption of added zinc in infants fed preterm human milk.[39] Calculations of intrauterine fetal zinc accretion range from 275-320 µg/kg/day between the 28th and 36th weeks of gestation. Assuming an average desirable retention value of 300 µg/kg/day, an absorption of 30% and an intake of 100-150 ml/kg/day, preterm formula should provide at a minimum 6 mg of Zn/L, and a level close to 9 mg/L is probably more realistic.

Parenteral. The AMA expert panel suggests an intake of zinc for infants on total parenteral nutrition (TPN) of 300 µg/kg/day. Higher levels of zinc infusion, 488 µg/kg/day, were recommended by James and colleagues,[17] who aimed at achieving intrauterine accretion rates. Zlotkin and Buchanan[11] estimated obligatory zinc urinary losses at 62 µg/kg/day in parenterally-fed infants, and recommended infusion of 438 µg/kg/day to duplicate intrauterine accretion rates. Appropriate levels of zinc for parenteral needs of preterm infants would thus range from 350-450 µg/kg/day.

DEFICIENCY (FIG. 3)

The original description of zinc deficiency by Prasad and colleagues in 1961 related to the

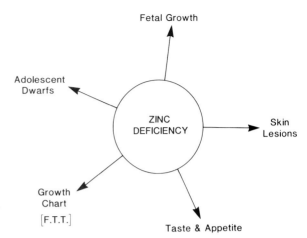

FIGURE 3.   Effects of zinc deficiency. FTT = failure to thrive.

adolescent dwarfism syndrome, which occurred frequently in the Middle East.

Concern about zinc in this country was mainly academic until Hambidge et al.[40] reported on a group of children with low zinc levels in hair, poor appetite, diminished taste acuity and short stature. Hair and plasma zinc concentrations of American infants were noted to be lower than those of infants from other countries, and subsequent research on the etiology of these findings led to a trial of supplementation of an infant formula with zinc.

Until 1975, the zinc content of American infant formulas was generally below 2 mg/L, which was less than that of cow milk. The addition of 4 mg of zinc to Similac formula (Ross Laboratories, Columbus, Ohio) was evaluated in a double-blind controlled study of healthy term infants and, surprisingly, a higher growth velocity was noted in the zinc-supplemented male infant group.[41] This suggested the existence of a mild zinc deficiency syndrome that could affect growth rates and appetite in infants and young children.

During this time, acrodermatitis enteropathica (AE) was recognized as a phenotypic manifestation of severe zinc deficiency in humans.[42] This disease has an autosomal recessive pattern of inheritance, and has long been of interest to dermatologists; the characteristic findings include weeping erythematous periorificial and acral skin lesions, diarrhea, mood changes and alopecia. Untreated, the disease often had a fatal outcome. In an important instance of misdiagnosis, hydroxyquinoline derivatives were prescribed to a patient with acrodermatitis to treat a suspected skin candidiasis, and this resulted in marked improvement of lesions and clearing of symptoms. Further research has shown that AE is caused by a block in intestinal zinc absorption, which fortunately can be easily overcome through the administration of zinc supplements. The protective role of hydroxyquinolines in this syndrome was probably a result of enhancement of zinc absorption and similar effects were derived from the provision of human breast milk, which was also recommended as treatment for AE.

A similar syndrome of acute, acquired zinc deficiency was reported in 1975 by Kay and Tasman-Jones[43] in adults receiving parenteral nutrition with solutions practically devoid of zinc. These observations have been confirmed in multiple reports of parenterally fed infants and adults and led to the recommendations of zinc supplementation of parenteral solutions. Since 1980, acute zinc deficiency has also been increasingly reported in preterm infants fed human milk,[44] which raises questions about the adequacy of preterm human milk as the sole source of nutrition for the rapidly growing preterm infant. Attempts at increasing zinc content of preterm human milk by giving supplements of 50-150 mg of zinc to lactating mothers were unsuccessful.[45] Transient zinc deficiency has also been reported in a full-term breast-fed infant.[46] Zinc absorption from breast milk is generally high but there is considerable variation in the zinc content of milk of individual mothers, which may in some instances lead to problems. The various signs and symptoms of mild, moderate and severe zinc deficiency in children and adolescents are summarized in Table 4.

TOXICITY

Zinc is relatively nontoxic and there exists a moderate margin of safety between physiologic requirements and toxic doses. However **supplementation with zinc at doses 10 times the RDA has resulted in copper deficiency.** This has occurred in adults receiving 150 mg of zinc daily and in one infant treated for symptomatic zinc deficiency with 30 mg daily.[47] If supplementation is maintained at levels 2-3 times the RDA, toxicity has not been observed. The inadvertent administration of 7.4 gm of zinc sulfate in a parenteral solution was followed by hepatic and kidney failure and death.[48]

SELENIUM

Although it is a relative newcomer to the list of essential trace elements, problems due to inadequate or excessive intakes of selenium are widely recognized, not only in specialized situations such as long-term parenteral nutrition but also in free-living populations.[49,50]

The biological significance of selenium was first recognized in 1934 when it was identified as the cause of lameness and death of livestock in parts of the Dakotas and Wyoming. These areas were subsequently shown to have high levels of selenium in soils and forage plants. Signs of what is now known as selenium toxicity were decribed in livestock in Tibet and western China by Marco Polo in 1295 and in Colombia in 1560 by early Spanish explorers.[47] In 1957, Schwartz and Foltz[50] gave a completely new direction to research on selenium in nutrition when they showed its essentiality as a nutrient for animals. An apparent interaction with vitamin E in several species suggested that selenium had an antioxidant function. The biochemical function of selenium was not elucidated until 1973, when it was discovered separately by Hoekstra's group in Wisconsin[51] and Flohe's group in West Germany[52] that glutathione peroxidase was a seleno-enzyme.

PHYSIOLOGY

Currently, the only known function of selenium in mammalian tissues is as an integral part of the enzyme glutathione peroxidase (GSHPx), one of the systems which, along with

TABLE 4.   Signs and Symptoms of Zinc Deficiency in Children and Adolescents

Mild	Moderate	Severe
Decreased growth velocity	Decreased growth velocity	Acral and peri-orificial skin lesions
Anorexia	Delayed sexual maturation	Failure to thrive
Hypogeusia	Rough skin	Diarrhea
Failure to thrive in infants	Pica	Mood changes
	Hepatosplenomegaly	Alopecia
		Photophobia

catalase, superoxide dismutase and vitamin E, protects cells from oxidative damage.[51] **While vitamin E mainly protects lipid membranes, GSHPx appears to act by destroying cytosolic hydrogen peroxide.[52]**

Selenium is generally well-absorbed, to more than 60% of the intake from a mixed diet.[53] Absorption from human milk has not been measured directly, but it is unlikely that it differs much from that of formulas. Two-year old infants absorbed 64% of selenium from a liquid formula based on cow milk, compared with 49% of the selenium in a soy-protein-based formula.[54] The primary route of excretion is in the urine, with 40-90% of the oral intake excreted in this way in adults. When intakes and plasma levels are low, the urinary excretion decreases, suggesting that some conservation occurs.

In both selenium-deficient and selenium-adequate areas, concentrations of selenium in cord blood reflect selenium levels in the adult population. However preterm values are lower than those of full-term infants. Levels tend to decline in early infancy, regardless of geographical area. In the United States, blood selenium concentrations in infants vary from region to region, but are generally higher than 80 ng/ml. In low selenium areas, blood levels in healthy adults approximate 60 ng/ml, and 45-60 ng/ml are typically found in infants, with no evidence that these are inadequate. Once mixed feeding is introduced, blood selenium concentrations start to increase again to the normal population range.[55-57]

It is important to note that blood concentrations of selenium are readily altered by changes in selenium intakes, so that a lower blood level in one group compared with another does not necessarily indicate a deficiency but may simply reflect differences in diet. Whole blood concentrations of selenium and GSHPx can be used as an index of selenium at lower levels of intake, however. Activity of GSHPx is correlated with selenium concentration up to about 100 ng of Se/ml.[49]

REQUIREMENTS

The metabolism and requirements of selenium have not been studied extensively during infancy. From isotope turnover and balance studies, a minimum requirement of 20 µg/day was calculated for healthy adults from New Zealand, a low selenium area.[58] Levander et al.[59] estimated a higher requirement of 70 µg/day for adults in the United States. Selenium requirements appear to be influenced by previous levels of intake, perhaps reflecting the level of tissue saturation. It is not known if such a variation in requirements may also apply to infants; however, concentrations of selenium in livers from New Zealand infants are about one-half levels in livers of infants from Canadian selenium-adequate areas.[60,61] For infants in the first year of life, a minimum dietary requirement of about 1 µg/kg/day may be estimated by extrapolation from adult needs. An intake greater than 1.5 µg/kg/day appears to be necessary to prevent the fall in blood selenium concentrations in the young infant[62] but there is no evidence that this fall is detrimental while levels remain greater than 40 ng/ml.[63] The current U.S. recommendation for an estimated safe and adequate intake is 10-40 µg/day up to 6 months, and 20-60 µg/day up to 1 year.[8]

Like blood levels, concentrations in human milk reflect selenium levels in the environment and can be increased in low selenium areas by maternal supplementation.[64-66] Concentrations in colostrum are higher than in mature milk which, in the U.S., contains about 15-20 ng of selenium/ml.[65,66] Smith et al.[66] found that the intake of selenium by fully breast-fed infants was about 10 µg/day, compared with 7 µg/day by formula-fed infants, and that this difference was reflected in higher serum selenium concentrations in the breast-fed infants. Cow milk based formulas in the United States contain about 5-8 ng/ml selenium, with similar levels in soy-based formulas. Levels may vary nationally according to the selenium content of cattle feeds and soils. Once mixed feeding is introduced, selenium intakes may increase markedly: Friel et al.[67] reported average daily intakes of about 40 µg of selenium by Canadian infants. Cereals contribute the greatest percentage to the total selenium intake.[67,68]

There is currently no evidence to suggest that the selenium intake of preterm infants should be different from that of full-term infants. On TPN, blood concentrations of selenium may fall rapidly, unless selenium intakes in the infusate are adequate. Blood selenium below about 30 ng/ml may be associated with biochemical abnormalities (see below). It is recommended that intravenous intakes be supplemented to give a total daily intake of about 1 µg/kg body weight.[62]

DEFICIENCY

A selenium responsive syndrome, Keshan disease, occurs in rural populations in several areas of China.[69] The syndrome is characterized by necrosis and fibrosis of the myocardium, resulting in acute or chronic heart failure, often fatal; some patients show a congestive cardiomyopathy.[70] Those most at risk include infants, young children and women of child-bearing age. Dietary intakes of selenium in affected populations are low, usually less than 3 µg/day, and blood concentrations in affected individuals are less than 20 ng/ml. Several trials showed that supplementation with selenite (1 mg of selenium daily) was effective in preventing new cases, but it is thought that the disease is not due to selenium deficiency alone.[49] Dietary intakes and blood concentrations of selenium as low as those in endemic Keshan areas have been measured in children in New Zealand and West Germany, but these subjects had no biochemical or clinical abnormalities that could be related to their low selenium status.[68,71]

Two different clinical deficiency syndromes have been reported in children and adults on TPN with inadequate selenium intakes. In a number of cases from New Zealand and the United States, the patients develop skeletal muscle pain and weakness, generally in the extremities, which may become incapacitating.[72,73] Blood selenium concentrations were very low (<10 ng/ml) and GSHPx activity was markedly decreased. Such cases have been effectively treated with 100-400 µg of selenium daily added to the infusate. This was equivalent to 3 µg/kg in the one pediatric case.[74]

Several probable cases of Keshan disease have also been reported in the United States, two of fatal cardiomyopathy in men on long-term TPN and another in a 2-year-old child whose diet was very low in both selenium and animal protein.[49] In the first case, the postmortem appearance of the heart was similar to that seen in Keshan disease, and selenium levels in the tissues were markedly decreased.

Biochemical disorders due to inadequate selenium intake may occur, in the absence of overt clinical symptoms, in association with low concentrations of selenium and GSHPx activity in the blood. The activity of the hexose monophosphate shunt, which is normally stimulated by the glutathione cycle, was reduced to 40% in erythrocytes and granulocytes from a patient on long-term TPN.[75] Gross[63] reported that blood selenium concentrations below 40 ng/ml were associated with increased erythrocyte fragility in orally-fed preterm infants. Very low blood levels of both selenium and GSHPx may occur in children with inborn errors of metabolism who are treated with special formulas of low selenium content.[68] However, no ill-effects due to selenium deficiency have yet been recorded in such patients.

A desirable goal in the treatment and prophylaxis of selenium deficiency in the United States should be to keep blood levels about 40 ng/ml, and probably above 60-70 ng/ml. Sodium selenite and selenate, selenious acid and selenomethionine have all been used as oral or intravenous sources of supplemental selenium, and all appear to be equally effective in increasing blood levels of GSHPx and selenium.

TOXICITY

Although selenium is an essential element in the diet, it is by no means harmless. It has a high inherent toxicity, and the level of toxcity varies according to the chemical state. Because there is a lack of specific data, a precise figure for the level of intake that would be harmful to humans is difficult to establish. A tentative maximum acceptable intake of selenium of 500 µg/day for adults (about 10 µg/kg) has been proposed[49] but this level is more than twice the upper limit of the estimated safe and adequate intake recommended by the National Research Council.

Very high environmental levels of selenium occur in various parts of the world including areas of Venezuela and the United States, most notably South Dakota. Dietary intakes of greater than 5 mg/day, with blood levels higher than 3200 ng/ml, were measured in an episode of human selenosis in China, which resulted from contamination of the soil by high-selenium coal dust. The effects of high intakes of selenium appear relatively mild and nonspecific—loss of hair, roughening of nails, nausea and fatigue. Abnormalities of the nervous system and skin were reported in the most severely affected Chinese villages.[76] Acute ingestion of more than 5 mg/kg of selenium as selenious acid resulted in death in a 3-year-old boy; conversely a 15-year-old girl who drank a solution providing 17 mg/kg of selenium as sodium selenite recovered fully. In animal studies, the lethal dose appears to be similar whether selenium is given orally or intravenously.

The recommended levels for oral and intravenous intake of selenium are much lower than the levels associated with toxicity. Blood levels can readily be monitored against excessive intakes; Jaffe et al.,[77] in Venezuela, suggested that a concentration of selenium in the blood of greater than 800 ng/ml was hazardous to children.

Selenium, iodine and fluorine occur mainly as small anions, and as such are rapidly and completely absorbed from the diet. This is in contrast to cationic elements such as copper, zinc and manganese, which are less well absorbed and are subject to dietary interactions and homeostatic control at the level of intestinal absorption.[4b] **The most important determinant of nutritional status with respect to the anionic elements is the level in the geochemical environment.** Large areas of the world are known to be naturally low in selenium, including Finland, New Zealand, and parts of China, but areas with near toxic concentrations also occur in China and the United States.[47]

IODINE

Problems with iodine nutrition, like those of selenium and fluorine, depend on geography rather than purely on diet. Recognition of the consequences of iodine deficiency, even if not an understanding of the causes, goes back millenia compared with only decades for the other two elements. It is unfortunate that in spite of our knowledge of the relatively simple measures, such as the use of iodized salt or injectable oils, which have all but eradicated iodine-deficiency diseases in some countries, endemic goiter and endemic cretinism remain severe public health problems in other areas.[74-76]

Goiter has been known to peoples in many parts of the world from ancient times; references to the disease can be found in Hindu and Chinese literature from 4000 years ago. Although iodine itself was unknown until 1811, effective remedial measures such as seaweed and preparations of animal thyroid were utilized empirically. Iodine was being prescribed to treat goiter by 1820, but subsequently fell into disrepute because of the toxic effects of the very large doses used. The prophylactic use of iodized salt to prevent goiter was first demonstrated in Ohio in 1920 and is now the most common mode of supplementing the iodine intake of populations in low iodine areas.[78,79]

PHYSIOLOGY

Iodine is an integral part of the thyroid hormones, which is its only known physiological function. Circulating iodine is avidly taken up by the thyroid gland where it is bound to thyroglobulin, an iodinated glycoprotein, from which the hormones thyroxine (T_4) and triiodothyronine (T_3) are formed. In iodine deficiency, the synthesis and release of thyroid hormones are decreased, resulting in low concentrations of T_4 and T_3 in the blood. These low concentrations stimulate the feedback mechanism involving the thyroid-hypothalamus-pituitary axis, causing an increased output of thyroid-stimulating hormone (TSH) by the pituitary. TSH acts to stimulate all steps of iodine metabolism, and to increase growth of the thyroid tissue, thus resulting in the enlarged gland of goiter.

Iodine status, therefore, generally is measured by assaying the thyroid hormones. In cord blood from a healthy, term infant, in an iodine-sufficient area, serum concentrations of T_4 are 90-130 ng/ml and TSH concentrations are in the range 12-15 µU/ml.[77,78] Shortly after birth, circulating concentrations of TSH increase and then fall again to birth levels by 72 hours. In response to this surge in TSH, concentrations of T_4 and T_3 increase in the first 24-72 hours after birth. Cord serum concentrations of T_4 in very preterm infants are lower, reflecting lower concentrations of circulating thyroid-binding globulin; cord T_4 concentrations increase with advancing gestational age. By 2 months, serum T_4 concentrations are similar to those in term cord blood and slightly higher than the adult level of 60-80 ng/ml, but TSH concentrations have fallen to 3-6 µU/ml, still higher than the adult norm of 2-3 µU/ml.[78]

Ingested iodine is very highly absorbed, with the main route of excretion being in the urine. Healthy infants with an adequate iodine intake will retain about 50% of the total intake.

REQUIREMENTS

The amount of iodine needed to replace that lost from the body by an adult is about 40-100 µg/day. Epidemiologic surveys have shown a very high prevalence of goiter when the average iodine intake in a population is less than 40 µg/day. When iodine intake reaches a critical level of 100 µg/day, prevalence of goiter is less than 10% and further increases in intake up to 500 µg/day make no further significant reductions.[8,78] From such data, the Food and Nutrition Board, National Academy of Sciences, calculated a minimum requirement of approximately 1 µg/kg/day, but, based on the intake from human milk, recommended a daily dietary intake for infants of 40 μg from birth to 6 months, increasing to 50 μg for 6 to 12 months. Levels of iodine in the U.S. national food supply are currently very high and this is reflected in breast milk concentrations. In recent surveys in the U.S., levels of 29-490 ng/ml were found, with a mean of 178 ng/ml.[79,80] The minimum intake by a fully breast-fed infant was 22 μg/day, well above the minimum requirement. Infant formulas are required by law to contain at least 5 μg of iodine per 100 kcal,[81] and most formulas on the market for both full-term and preterm infants supply 2-3 times this amount.

For infants of iodine-sufficient mothers, additional iodine does not appear to be necessary during short-term intravenous feeding.[82] Iodine/thyroid status of infants on long-term TPN should be monitored, and iodine supplements given at the minimum requirement of 1 μg/kg/day, if necessary. **Iodine is readily absorbed through the skin and is used extensively in products such as detergents and topical disinfectants.** Given its potential for toxicity, all such sources of iodine to the infant should be considered before supplementation is initiated.[60]

DEFICIENCY

Like selenium, the iodine status of human populations is greatly affected, in the absence of public health measures to increase iodine intakes, by iodine levels in local soils. **Iodine has been removed from soils by glaciation and weathering and deposited in the sea.** Thus, regions where iodine deficiency diseases are common (or were common until eradicated by population-based prophylaxis) are generally mountainous and distant from the oceans. These include countries of the Andean regions, the European Alps and central Africa, and mountainous regions of Asia and the Pacific, especially Nepal and New Guinea.[78] Figure 4 shows areas where iodine deficiency diseases are still common.

Although endemic goiter and its congenital corollary, endemic cretinism, are dramatic and highly visible diseases,[75] **iodine deficiency cannot be considered as a threshold phenomenon, but rather as a continuous spectrum of disorders.**[76,83] Iodine deficiency disorders will be present in almost all communities, with

OCCURRENCE OF ENDEMIC GOITER

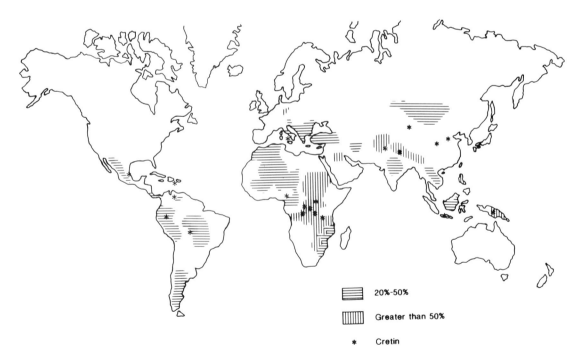

	20%-50%
	Greater than 50%
*	Cretin

FIGURE 4. Areas of iodine deficiency diseases. Countries in which the prevalence of endemic goiter is less than 20% (naturally or because of successful prophylaxis programs) are not included. The prevalence of endemic goiter as well as the presence of endemic cretinism are indicated. (Adapted from reference 78.)

the severity of manifestations and proportion of the population involved increasing as the average iodine intake decreases, until in some areas (such as Zaire), 100% of the population is affected.[74]

Because of the importance of thyroid hormones for normal development of the central nervous system, adequate iodine nutrition is most urgent during fetal and neonatal life.[84] Severe fetal iodine deficiency, resulting in endemic cretinism, still occurs in isolated areas of developing countries where environmental levels of iodine are low and there is a high prevalence of endemic goiter in the adult population. Results of supplementation trials with iodized oil in New Guinea suggested that **the effects of iodine deficiency on the developing brain occurred before 12 weeks' gestation.**[76] Later and milder degrees of iodine deficiency, both in utero and after birth, may have detrimental effects on growth and intellectual performance, even in the absence of more severe manifestations.[85]

In significant numbers of neonates (about 1 in 40,000 in the United States), the postnatal rise in serum T_4 and T_3 does not occur immediately after birth. About half of such cases have congenital hypothyroidism of varying etiologies and require replacement therapy with thyroid hormones. In the other 50%, hormone concentrations remain low for 4-6 weeks and then rise spontaneously. In healthy full-term infants, this transient neonatal hypothyroidism does not appear to have long-term consequences. In sick and preterm infants, the hypothyroidism may be more profound and longer lasting. However, there is still much debate as to whether these infants require hormone replacement.[86]

Although the transient neonatal hypothyroidism appears to be largely a problem of delayed maturation of the hypothalamic-pituitary-thyroid axis, there is also an influence of iodine nutrition. Beckers et al.[87] compared thyroid function in neonates from an iodine-sufficient part of Greece with infants from an area of mild endemic goiter. Serum concentrations of T_4 and T_3 were lower in preterm infants than in term infants, as expected, and both age groups had lower levels in the low-iodine area compared with infants of the same age in the iodine-adequate area. Delange and coworkers[88] found that infants born in Belgium (a low iodine area) excreted considerably less iodine in the urine and had lower iodine content in the thyroid gland than infants from

iodine-sufficient areas of North America. The incidence of transient neonatal hypothyroidism is higher in areas of endemic goiter.[89]

Neonatal hypothyroidism is normally a problem of glandular maturation or iodine deficiency but it may also be caused by excessive exposure of the fetal thyroid to iodine taken by the mother during pregnancy.[90]

TOXICITY

Thyrotoxic goiter has been recorded in several populations where iodine intake was very high from deliberate supplementation of bread or from high consumption of seaweed. Dietary intakes by adults in the United States generally are in the range of 64-677 µg/day. Such levels do not appear to be associated with ill effects.[78,79] Nonetheless, with the continued use of iodine-containing compounds in food processing and the dairy industry, the potential for chronic toxicity does exist in this country. Goiter in children is now likely to be associated with higher than normal urinary iodine excretion indicating high intake, rather than with low levels expected in iodine deficiency. Although there are no specific studies in infants, the American Medical Association concluded that there is currently no evidence for adverse physiological reactions associated with intakes of up to 1000 µg/day by healthy children. The highest concentration of iodine found in breast milk by Gushurst et al.[79] was 731 ng/ml, which would supply a daily intake to a breast-fed infant of about 600 µg/day. However, if the iodine content of the food supply continues to increase, it is possible that breast milk levels may reach toxic amounts, as levels of iodine in human milk correlate directly with maternal intake.

FLUORIDE

The role of fluoride in dental health was first recognized in the 1930s, when it was discovered that the primary cause of mottled enamel was a high level of fluoride in the domestic water supply. At the same time, it was noted that mottled teeth had a decreased susceptibility to decay. Some excellent epidemiological studies in the 1940s and 1950s, which included thousands of children, enlarged these observations to show the relationship between the content of the fluoride in the drinking water and indices of decayed-missing-filled teeth, over a wide range of fluoride concentrations.[96,97]

The recognition, supported by some of the best epidemiological studies in medicine, of the relationship between the level of fluoride in drinking water supplies and the incidence of dental caries in the corresponding population, has been termed "one of the greatest discoveries in the field of public health."[95]

Because of its very high ionization potential, fluorine forms exclusively anions, i.e., fluorides. Most fluorides are metabolized in the body and excreted in the ionic form, F^-.

It has frequently been debated as to whether fluorine should be regarded as an essential nutrient for humans. If the older definition is used, of an essential trace element being one that is required for life, then it is not. However, the definition now more commonly used is that given earlier, of an element essential for health and well-being; by this criterion, fluorine may be properly regarded as an essential element.

PHYSIOLOGY

Fluoride acts to strengthen dental enamel by substituting for hydroxyl ions (about 10% at normal fluoride intakes) in the hydroxyapatite crystalline mineral matrix of the enamel. The resulting fluorapatite is more resistant to both chemical and physical damage. Fluoride is incorporated into the enamel during the mineralization stages of tooth formation and also by surface interaction after the tooth has erupted.[97] Fluoride is similarly incorporated into bone mineral and theoretically may provide protection against osteoporosis later in life.

Absorption of dietary fluoride is about 80% from foods and fluids, and as high as 97% from soluble supplements such as sodium fluoride.[98] Fluoride is excreted mainly in the urine, with less than 10% of the intake appearing in the feces. Ingested fluoride is rapidly taken up into the bones and teeth of the growing infant and the excess is excreted in the urine, so that very low concentrations are maintained in the soft tissues and body fluids.[99] Plasma fluoride concentrations reflect the levels in drinking water; i.e., where the water contains 1 mg/L fluoride, mean plasma levels are about 20 ng/ml.[100]

REQUIREMENTS

Full-Term Infants

The large epidemiological studies that compared the health of teeth of children living in areas with different natural levels of fluoride in the water showed that the optimal intake of fluoride, that is, the level which provides excellent caries protection while minimizing the risk of enamel fluorosis, is that obtained from drinking water fluoridated to a level of 1.0 mg/L,[97] as illustrated in Figure 5.

At all ages, the major source of fluorine in the diet is water, and thus the levels of intake and desirable supplementation will depend on the exposure of the infant to the local water supply. In the formula-fed infant, the need for supplementation depends on the type of formula used (e.g., powder, liquid concentrate, ready-to-feed). Commercial formulas are now made with defluoridated water and contain varying but generally very low amounts of fluoride. Starting fluoride supplementation before 1 year of age does not appear to have any further benefit on prevention of caries in the permanent teeth. However, it does provide protection to the deciduous teeth. **The American Academy of Pediatrics now recommends that, in the absence of adequate fluoride in the water, infants be given supplemental fluoride, starting in the first 2 weeks after birth.**[101]

The recommended schedule for up to 2 years of age is:

Fluoride water content (mg/L)	<0.3	0.3 − 0.7	>0.7
Supplement dose (mg F/day)	0.25	0	0

An infant receiving only ready-to-feed formula should be given supplemental fluoride regardless of the level in the local water.

The fluoride content of human milk is low, 5-15 ng/ml, and intakes by fully breast-fed infants are about 4-15 µg/day in optimally fluoridated areas. The need to provide additional fluoride to the exclusively breast-fed infant is still a debated issue.[95] In a large study in Sweden, the frequency of caries was found to be identical in children who had been breast-fed compared with those who had received powdered cow milk diluted with water containing 1.2 mg/L fluoride.[102] The current recommendation for breast-fed infants is that they do not need additional fluoride if living in an area where the water is adequately fluoridated; otherwise they should receive the same supplement as formula-fed infants.[101]

Supplemental fluoride is easiest given to young infants in the form of drops containing fluoride alone or in combination with other prescribed vitamins or minerals. Fluoride drops (or a crushed portion of a tablet) may be

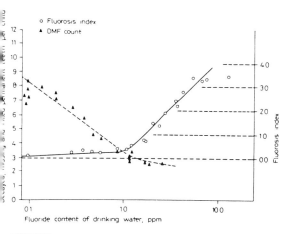

FIGURE 5. Relation between decayed-missing-filled teeth (DMF count), fluorosis index, and the concentration of fluoride in drinking water. (From Nikiforuk G. Understanding Dental Caries. II. Prevention, Basic and Clinical Aspects. Basel, Karger, 1985, with permission.)

mixed with the formula or other food, or drops can be given directly into the mouth.

Maternal Supplementation

Routine maternal supplementation with fluoride, above an optimal intake in the water supply, is not currently recommended during pregnancy or lactation. **The critical time for fluoride to exert the maximum cariostatic effects is during the mineralization of the surface of a crown.** Even for primary teeth, except for the anterior incisors, this process occurs mainly postnatally.[97] Consequently, there is no rationale for prescribing prenatal fluoride, and little benefit is to be expected.

The fluoride content of breast milk is relatively insensitive to maternal intake. In an area where water was fluoridated to 1 mg/L, breast milk fluoride levels were 11 ng/ml, compared with 7 ng/ml in milk from women living in an area with 0.2 mg/L in the water supply.[103] Even at much higher maternal fluoride intakes, which increased plasma levels 15-fold, there was only a very limited transfer of fluoride to the milk.

Preterm Infants

Defective primary dentition and hypoplasia in both deciduous and permanent teeth appear to be more common in children who were preterm or low birth weight than in those born at term. Histological examination of deciduous teeth from preterm infants showed that enamel made postnatally had improper mineralization and hypoplasia in the areas laid down shortly after birth. **Teeth erupt in the preterm infant at the same time postnatally as in the full-term infant, so that less time has been available for the proper degree of mineralization to occur before eruption.** The preterm infant is also at greater risk of generalized malnutrition, hypocalcemia and inadequate intake of vitamin D, all of which may contribute to the poor enamel formation. Mechanical trauma from respiratory or feeding tubes may exacerbate the effects of hypoplasia. Such injury to the deciduous teeth is also known to be an etiological factor for enamel hypoplasia in the permanent teeth.[104]

Given the wide variety of influences on the developing enamel, fluoride supplementation, beyond the levels indicated above, is unlikely to provide additional protection to the preterm infant and may entail toxicity. Attention to calcium nutrition, early introduction of adequate feeding, changes in the placement of orotracheal tubes, and institution of oral feeding as soon as clinically possible are likely to be more beneficial.

TOXICITY

Fluoride has a very narrow therapeutic range. The optimal dosage to prevent dental caries appears to be 0.05-0.07 mg/kg/day, and mild fluorisis begins to occur with intakes of 0.1 mg/kg/day.[101] **In areas where the water supply contains greater than 2.5 mg/L fluoride, there is a significant increase in dental fluorosis.** Since fluorosis or mottling of the enamel is due to an effect of the fluoride ion on the ameloblasts, it occurs only when elevated levels of fluoride (including excessive supplementation) are consumed during the first 8 years of life, when the crowns of the teeth are being formed.

Acute ingestion of very large amounts of fluoride causes cardiac and respiratory abnormalities and hypocalcemia. Death due to hyperkalemia and cardiac arrest may ensure.[105] The lethal dose in adults is in the order of 2.5-5 gm, or about 35 mg/kg. For this reason, it is generally advised that no more than 100 mg of fluoride be prescribed at once, so that even if the whole was accidentally swallowed by a small child, it would not be fatal.

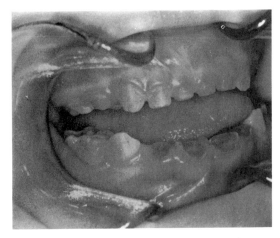

FIGURE 6. Nursing bottle caries, advanced stage. (Courtesy R.L. Braham, B.D., University of California, San Francisco.)

FLUORIDE AND DENTAL HEALTH

The aim in ensuring optimal fluoride intake is by and large directed toward protecting the permanent teeth, although when started in early infancy will also reduce the susceptibility to decay of the deciduous teeth. The formation of dental caries requires three factors—a susceptible tooth, cariogenic bacteria, and sugar. In a healthy, well-nourished infant, fluoride will reduce the susceptibility of tooth enamel to attack by cariogenic bacteria, but prevention of dental caries also requires good oral hygiene. New teeth should be cleaned by wiping with a soft cloth, until the infant is old enough for the teeth to be gently cleaned (by the parent!) with a soft brush. The child should not be left with a bottle in his mouth for extensive periods of time. The practice of putting an infant down to sleep with a bottle has led to rampant, "nursing bottle" caries in infants as young as 18 months. The prolonged contact of formula or juice (especially if it contains sucrose) provides an ideal environment for the growth of bacteria and formation of caries. Figure 6 demonstrates a case of such caries. A similar syndrome may occur occasionally in breast-fed infants who were never bottle-fed. In such cases the infant usually suckles from the breast for long periods while sleeping with the mother at night.[106]

MANGANESE

Manganese deficiency can be produced in several animal species, *with the most vulner-* *able period being during gestation and early* *infancy.* The main effects of deficiency are on neurologic function and cartilaginous structures.[1]

PHYSIOLOGY

Manganese is known to function in three main areas of metabolism: (1) glycosoaminoglycan synthesis, including the synthesis of the mucopolysaccharide matrix of cartilage; (2) carbohydrate metabolism, via the stabilization or activation of some gluconeogenic enzymes such as pyruvate carboxylase and isocitrate dehydrogenase; and (3) lipid metabolism.[107] Manganese is an integral component of the metalloenzyme mitochondrial superoxide dismutase, and alterations in the activity of this enzyme may account for the aberrations in membrane integrity observed in manganese deficiency. Manganese may also play a role in central nervous system function. Faulty metabolism of dopamine has been reported in animals with genetically disordered manganese metabolism. Supplementation with the element resulted in improvement of L-dopa metabolism and of the neurologic manifestations.[108]

Metabolism of manganese has not been studied extensively in infants. Full-term infants are in negative balance in the first week after birth, regardless of type of feeding (breast milk or cow milk). Sampson et al.[109] studied a group of full-term infants aged 1-248 days who had undergone cardiac surgery. They found negative balances when intakes from cow milk formulas were less than 8.5 µg/kg/day, and balance was generally negative in infants below 5 months of age. Absorption of manganese from cow milk is about 30%, with the absorbed manganese being mainly excreted in the bile and very little appearing in the urine.

REQUIREMENTS

The current recommendations by the U.S. National Academy of Sciences[8] for a safe and adequate intake of manganese are 0.5-0.7 mg for 0-6 months and 0.7-1.0 mg per day for 7-12 months. These levels are based on older data that may be inaccurate. More recent analyses show that the intake of manganese from human milk by an infant taking 750 ml milk per day is about 1-3 µg regardless of the age of the infant.[110] Bioavailability of manganese from breast milk and cow milk based formulas appears to be similar.[111] In the United

States, the lower limit for manganese in formulas is set by law at 5 µg/100 kcal.[85] Many of the cow milk based formulas available in the U.S. have added manganese and contain 5-25 µg/100 kcal, according to manufacturers' data, or from analysis, 70-1300 ng/ml.[112] Such levels would provide 56 µg to 1 mg to an infant consuming 800 ml of formula a day.

Once mixed feeding is introduced, daily intakes of manganese by breast-fed infants increase markedly. Gibson and colleagues[113] found that Canadian infants, receiving mixed foods along with breast milk or formula, obtained on average 0.5 mg of manganese daily at 3 months of age. By 6 months, the daily intake was 0.9 mg, and was 1.5 mg at 12 months. At 3 months, the major food sources for manganese were fruits and juices. In the older infants, cereals provided the greatest proportion of manganese, but fruit and juices were still a significant source.

There is currently no good measure of manganese status. The element is present in relatively low concentrations in most body fluids and is not routinely measured. Whole blood levels in the first 12 months are 14-17 ng/ml, with levels in erythrocytes being 25-fold greater than in serum. Changes in blood manganese concentrations during infancy are complex and do not unequivocally reflect dietary intakes. Hatano et al.[114] reported that erythrocyte manganese was higher (450 ng/gm Hb) at birth and fell during the first 4 months of postnatal life, before the introduction of solid foods, to adult levels of about 140 ng/gm Hb.

Concentrations in formula-fed infants were slightly higher than in breast-fed infants, presumably reflecting higher intakes from formula. Statsny et al.[112] reported serum manganese concentrations in healthy infants at 3 months of age averaged 4 ng/ml. They found that there was no difference in the mean serum level between fully breast-fed infants, with a manganese intake of 0.42 µg/kg/day, and formula-fed infants receiving 183 µg/kg/day. However, in the breast-fed group there was a strong correlation between manganese intakes and serum levels. Thus, the much higher levels of manganese consumed by formula-fed infants, or older infants receiving solids, do not seem to be associated with an increase in blood levels of manganese.

Intakes of manganese by preterm infants are of the same order as full-term infants receiving the same type of feeds.[115] The current recommendation by the American Medical Association[10] for manganese intakes in total parenteral nutrition is 2-10 µg/kg per day. There is no evidence to suggest that this level is excessive. A more extensive discussion of manganese nutrition in prematurity and TPN has been published.[62]

DEFICIENCY

Clinical deficiency of manganese has not been shown in man, although it has been suggested the high incidence of cartilaginous disorders in rural areas of South Africa may be related to low environmental levels of manganese.[116] Some workers but not others[117,118] have found lower blood concentrations of manganese in children with convulsive disorders as compared with those of healthy individuals.

TOXICITY

Manganese homeostasis is regulated by the liver, with excess being secreted in the bile. Large doses of manganese (20 mg/kg) caused mild intrahepatic cholestasis in experimental animals. When smaller doses of manganese were injected intravenously simultaneously with bilirubin, suppression of bile flow and more severe liver damage resulted. Blood levels of manganese are elevated in correlation with serum bilirubin in adults with various liver disorders, but no elevation was seen in either serum or liver manganese in infants dying of Indian childhood cirrhosis in whom liver copper was elevated.[119,120] Nonetheless, in view of its hepatotoxic potential, it is recommended that infants with biliary or liver disorders be given low manganese feedings. Exposure to very high levels of manganese in mining or industry may result in severe neurological disturbance similar to parkinsonism, but toxicity due to high dietary intakes of manganese has never been reported.

CHROMIUM

Chromium is important in maintaining proper glucose metabolism, possibly by potentiation of the action of insulin at the level of the cell membrane.[121] Chromium deficiency has been reported in two adult patients after long periods (1-3 years) of parenteral nutrition without added chromium and with glucose as main energy source.[122,123] The subjects

developed glucose intolerance and other dia-
betes-like symptoms, including a high requirement for exogenous insulin, peripheral neuropathy and weight loss in spite of high calorie
intakes. Several recent studies have found
some relationship between chromium status
and glucose utilization in healthy adults,[124,125]
and chromium supplementation has been
found to improve some cases of impaired
glucose tolerance in adults[126] and malnourished children.[127] However, there is currently
no good evidence to link inadequate chromium nutrition with either Type I or Type II
diabetes.

The healthy adult absorbs about 1% of ingested chromium, whether it is taken in a
mixed diet or as an inorganic supplement.[124]
Absorbed chromium is excreted mainly in the
urine. Normal plasma levels of chromium are
in the order of 0.1-0.2 ng/ml and are increased
by large supplemental intakes.

Few investigations have been made of chromium metabolism in infants. Intakes by the
fully breast-fed infant are very low, averaging
0.2 µg/day.[110] Formulas in the U.S. generally
contain more chromium (10-20 ng/ml)[128] than
human milk, which averages 0.1-0.8 ng/ml.
The current estimations for safe and adequate
intakes of chromium are 10-40 µg/day for an
infant from birth to 6 months, then 20-60
µg/day up to 12 months. These levels are
based on extrapolation from the adult intake.[8]
As in the case of manganese, however, there is
no evidence that this level of intake, compared
to that from human milk, is harmful. Because
the absorption of orally ingested chromium is
poor, it is relatively nontoxic and there have
been no reports of undesirable effects from
very high levels of intake.

A considerable amount of work has been done over the
past two decades on the biochemical function, *in vitro*
and *in vivo*, and on the human metabolism of chromium.
However, in 1979, it was realized that chromium suffers
from severe analytical problems: samples are very easily
contaminated during collection, storage and preparation
from the environment, glassware, water or chemicals;[128]
the normal levels in biological fluids are close to the
detection limits of many analytical techniques; in atomic
absorption spectrometry, the most commonly used technique, there is very high background absorption at the
chromium wavelength, and unless this is adequately com-
pensated for (not possible with older instruments), the
measured result may be orders of magnitude higher than
the true chromium concentration (Versieck J. Trace elements in human body fluids and tissues. CRC Crit Rev Clin
Lab Sci 1985;22:97-184; Guthrie BE, Wolf WR, Veillon C.
Background correction and related problems in the determination of chromium in urine by graphite furnace atom-

ic absorption. Anal Chem 1978:50;1900-1902.) Consequently, much of the earlier work on chromium (and
some more recent too) must be read very critically with respect to methodology. A good rule of thumb is that concentrations of chromium in plasma and urine from
healthy, unsupplemented individuals should be less than
0.5 ng/ml.

Friel and coworkers[67] reported chromium
intakes for full-term infants receiving mixed
diets, including human milk or formula and infant foods. Average intakes were 23 µg/day at
3 months, increasing to 57 µg/day by 12
months. At all ages, milk and formula provided
a high percentage (40-90%) of the total chromium, but by 12 months, fruits and juices were
the most important source. Intakes by preterm
infants were slightly higher than those of full-
term infants.

MOLYBDENUM

Deficiencies and toxicities involving molybdenum are important in animal husbandry in
various parts of the world,[1] but human problems with molybdenum nutrition are uncommon.[129]

An excessive intake of molybdenum may precipitate copper deficiency in animals even in conditions where copper intake appears adequate. The amount of sulphate in
the diet also affects the level of molybdenum at which
copper deficiency occurs. This is an example of *trace element interrelationships* whereby the dietary supply of one
element may affect the absorption or utilization of
another.[130] The practical importance of a molybdenum-
copper interaction in humans is not established, but an
excessive dietary intake (more than 1.5 mg/day) in adults
results in increased losses of copper in the urine. An interaction among high dietary levels of molybdenum and
fluorine and low intakes of copper may contribute to the
etiology of the crippling bone disorder, genu valgum,
which occurs in areas with very high natural levels of
molybdenum in India and Armenia. Other examples of
trace element interrelationships of practical importance in
human nutrition include interference of iron in zinc absorption, interference of zinc in copper absorption, resulting in clinical deficiency of copper, and the development
of anemia, due to lack of iron mobilization, in copper
deficiency.

Only three molybdoenzymes currently are
known to occur in mammals: sulphite oxidase,
xanthine oxidase/dehydrogenase, and aldehyde dehydrogenase. The most important is
sulphite oxidase, which catalyzes the oxidation
of sulphite to sulphate, the terminal step in
degradative sulphur metabolism.[130] Molybdenum in these enzymes is present as an active

form, synthesized in the liver and called the molybdenum co-factor, in which molybdate (MoO_4^{2-}) is complexed to a pterin through a disulphide linkage.[131] Dietary molybdenum is well absorbed—about 80% regardless of source.[129,132] The main route of excretion is via the kidneys. Current best estimates for molybdenum in plasma are less than 1 ng/ml, but levels may be increased by liver disease.[133]

Mature human milk contains 1-2 ng/ml of molybdenum (Casey, unpublished), so that intakes by the fully breast-fed infant will be 0.5-1.5 µg/day. The amount supplied by formulas is unknown but probably more than this as cow milk generally contains higher concentrations: 2-70 ng/ml. By 1 year of age, infants on mixed diets are receiving about 120 µg of molybdenum per day.[134]

Several inborn errors of molybdoenzyme metabolism have been described:[135-137] (1) In sulphite oxidase deficiency, the principal features are profound mental retardation and dislocated lenses. Biochemical features include abnormal sulphur compounds in urine. (2) Xanthine oxidase deficiency is usually mild or symptomless but it may cause kidney stones and myopathy. Biochemical features include decreased serum uric acid and increased urine xanthine compounds. (3) Combined deficiencies of sulphite and xanthine oxidases result in seizures, profound mental retardation and dislocated lenses; biochemical abnormalities include features of (1) and (2).

These inherited diseases are due to defective synthesis of the molybdenum cofactor.[137] Sulphite oxidase and the combined deficiencies are serious diseases with a bad prognosis for which there is as yet no effective treatment.

The requirements for molybdenum in TPN have not been extensively studied. It is recommended that infants on long-term parenteral nutrition receive supplemental molybdenum at a rate of 1-2 µg/kg/day.[62] There is one reported case of molybdenum deficiency in an adult after 12 months on unsupplemented TPN.[135] The clinical features included tachycardia, tachypnea and mental changes leading to coma. The patient had decreased serum uric acid and elevated urine levels of sulphur metabolites. The condition was corrected with supplemental intravenous molybdenum.

ALUMINUM

Although we are exposed to high amounts of aluminum in the natural environment and to additional intakes from antacids, cosmetics, beverage cans, cooking utensils and drinking water, historically aluminum has not been regarded as a significant toxicant for human populations. Normally the skin, lungs and gastrointestinal tract act as effective barriers against uptake of aluminum, and absorption of oral intake (about 2-3 mg/day in the adult) is less than 1%. Absorbed aluminum is excreted almost entirely in the urine.[138] Importantly, biliary excretion of aluminum is negligible, even when renal function is impaired, and patients with renal failure have an increased body burden of aluminum. Ultrafilterable aluminum readily crosses the blood-brain barrier and is deposited in the brain tissue. Aluminum is known to be neurotoxic in humans and in uremic patients excessive cerebral accumulation results in a dementing disease, dialysis encephalopathy.[139,140] There is increasing evidence also that aluminum toxicity may be responsible for the fracturing osteomalacia that often occurs in dialysis patients. The occurrence of dialysis encephalopathy at various centers was related to the level of aluminum in the water used in dialysis,[139] and high oral intakes of aluminum from other sources such as antacids and phosphate binding gels may have contributed.[141] Water supplies for dialysis are now routinely deionized so that the incidence of dementia and fracturing bone disease have declined dramatically. However a more insidious form of bone disease has been described that appears to be due to excessive oral intake of aluminum. Young children with compromised renal function are especially vulnerable.[142]

In 1985, it was reported that ill and preterm neonates are at risk of aluminum toxicity, even in the absence of overt renal disease. Such infants often have reduced renal function and aluminum absorption tends to be higher in neonates. Sedman and colleagues[143] found that preterm infants who had received intravenous therapy showed elevated levels of aluminum in bone and plasma (37 ng/ml compared with 5 ng/ml in plasma of healthy infants). They speculated that the high aluminum in bone may be a factor in the development of osteopenia frequently seen in such infants. Intravenous solutions may contain extremely high concentrations of aluminum (Table 5). These workers showed by analysis of autopsy tissues that intravenously fed preterm infants were subjected to aluminum loading. They were less certain however that oral feeding was a problem, in spite of measuring con-

TABLE 5.   Aluminum Content of Infant
Formulas, Human Milk and Intravenous Solutions*

Product	Aluminum content (ng/ml)
Enteral products	
Human milk	4–10
Cow milk based formulas: USA	200–400
Soy formula: USA	1500
Cow milk based formulas: UK	90–500
Soy formulas: UK	300
Water (Colorado)	4–12
Intravenous products	
15% KCl	6–225
10% Ca gluconate	3000–5000
10% Intralipid	9–100
Heparin	300–800
Albumin	1800
Water for injection (UK)	128

Formulas are ready to feed or made up with low aluminum water (less than 5 ng/ml)

*Data from references 143–145.

centrations of aluminum in formulas of 200-300 ng/ml. The daily intake of intravenously fed infants may be up to 100 μg of aluminum, of which 78% was retained, compared with an intake of 160-320 μg/day by a formula-fed infant, of which less than 0.05% is absorbed (A. Sedman, personal communication).

The concentration of aluminum in breast milk is generally very low, but formulas may have quite high levels regardless of whether purchased as ready-to-feed or in powder form. In the latter case, additional aluminum will be added by the water used to reconstitute. There are currently no recommended standards for aluminum in domestic water supplies and levels may vary widely according to geographical location. Soy formulas in particular appear to contain high amounts of aluminum. Table 5 gives levels of aluminum in milks and formulas and in commonly used intravenous solutions.[144] Aluminum concentrations may vary from lot to lot and it is likely that much of it is added during processing.

Although it is currently unclear exactly to what extent excessive aluminum accumulation may contribute to overt disease in preterm or sick neonates, it is advisable that formulas and solutions of low aluminum content be used for such infants, especially where there is impaired renal function or during intravenous feeding.[145]

OTHER ELEMENTS

The only known function of the essential trace element *cobalt* is as part of the vitamin B_{12} (cyanocobalamin) molecule. Very little B_{12} is manufactured by bacteria in the gastrointestinal tract of monogastric animals, as opposed to ruminants, so humans require a dietary source. A dietary intake of cobalt apart from this does not appear to be important. Vitamin B_{12} nutrition is discussed in Chapter 12.

Several other trace elements, including *nickel, vanadium,* and *silicon,* are regarded as essential for animals.[1] Little is known about their metabolism in humans and they are not at present thought to be of practical importance in human nutrition.

Other elements are of concern in pediatrics because of their potential for toxicity rather than potential for deficiency. Apart from aluminum, discussed above, excessive exposure to *lead* is of greatest concern.[146] Levels of lead in whole blood of 40-80 μg/ml may be associated with behavioral and learning disabilities in children, in the absence of other clinical symptoms of lead poisoning. The threshold of risk is now considered to be a whole blood level of 30 μg/ml of lead. The Food and Drug Administration has established a long range goal that lead intake from all sources should not exceed 100 μg/day in children from birth to 5 years.[147] Intakes of lead by infants fed exclusively human milk or formula are less than 20 μg/day.[148] Older infants, up to 1 year of age, on mixed feeding obtain on average less than 50 μg of lead daily from food. However, environmental factors may be of greater importance than diet. Excessive exposure to lead has been recorded in inner city environments from lead paint in old housing,[149] and from ingestion of high lead soils near major highways and other areas with high traffic density. As lead levels in gasoline are reduced, however, the average blood levels in the population of the U.S. are falling.[150] Folk remedies, such as azarcon, a powder containing 90% lead tetroxide and used to treat abdominal problems (empacho), also have caused lead poisoning in infants and children.[151]

Specific outbreaks of *cadmium* and *mercury* poisoning, due to environmental contamination, have occurred in several countries with devastating consequences to those people exposed.[152,153] The fetus and young infant are usually the worst affected in such situations. However, under normal circumstances, ex-

TABLE 6.   Recommended Daily Oral Intakes of Trace Elements

	Preterm	Birth–6 Months*	7–12 Months
Copper (µg/kg)	80	80	80
Zinc (mg)	0.3–0.6	3	5
Selenium (µg)	10–40	10–40	20–60
Iodine (µg)	40	40	50
Fluorine (mg) †	0.25	0.25	0.25
Manganese (µg/kg)	2–5	10	500–1000 (µg/day)
Chromium (µg/kg)	0.2–0.5	10	20
Molybdenum (µg/kg)	0.2–0.5	2	40–80 (µg/day)

*Does not include solely breast-fed infants below 4–6 months.
† In regions where the water supply contains less than 0.3 mg/L.

posure to these elements is low and neither should pose a problem in routine practice.

SUMMARY

The recommendations for oral and intravenous intakes of trace elements during infancy are given in Tables 6 and 7. It can be appreciated from the foregoing discussion that most of these figures must be regarded as tentative. For elements such as chromium and molybdenum, so little is known about the metabolism in infancy that the recommendations can be little more than guesswork based on the usual intakes from human milk or mixed diets. Even for better studied elements such as zinc or copper, there are still questions concerning absorption from different formulas, so that the recommendations should not be regarded as final.

CASE REPORTS

Case 1: Zinc. Lisa L, a 7-week-old female infant, was admitted to Denver General Hospital for treatment of diarrhea and failure to thrive. She was the third child of a single mother living on welfare. Her birthweight was 2.54

TABLE 7.   Recommended Daily Intravenous
Intakes of Trace Elements (µg/kg/day)

	Preterm	Birth–6 Months	7–12 Months
Copper	20	20	20
Zinc	400	100	100
Selenium		1–2	
Iodine		1	
Fluorine			
Manganese		2–10	
Molybdenum		1–2	
Chromium		0.2	

kg, the neonatal course was described as uneventful and the infant was fed Enfamil, of which she would only take 1-2 oz at a feeding. A few days prior to admission she was seen by a practitioner who diagnosed an upper respiratory infection with otitis, gave an intramuscular injection of lincomycin and wrote a prescription for amoxicillin by mouth. In the following days, increasing diarrhea led to evaluation at the community hospital and, on admission, the infant's weight was 2.0 kg. The examination revealed a marasmic infant with some edema of the inferior extremities. Pertinent laboratory assays included a hematocrit of 22%, total protein of 5 gm/dl, albumin 2.2 gm/dl, and plasma zinc 56 µg/dl. The infant was rehydrated, transfused and started on a slow regimen of parenteral nutrition and continuous intragastric drip of dilute Pregestimil. An extensive work-up for diarrhea failed to reveal an etiology for the malnutrition.

On the tenth hospital day, by which time the infant's weight had reached 2.7 kg, an erythematous rash was noted on the face, arms, perianal area, and buttocks, and was spreading down the legs. A visiting consultant diagnosed acquired zinc deficiency and recommended increasing the zinc intake from the previous 200 µg/kg/day to a level of 1000 µg/kg/day. This was accomplished by increasing the parenteral zinc concentration to provide 400 µg/kg/day and by adding another 500 µg/kg/day through the nasogastric tube. The skin lesions started to clear within 24 hours and the infant's subsequent hospital course was benign. She was discharged to foster care.

Questions and Answers

Q.   Wasn't the zinc intake adequate in this infant?
A.   Clinical manifestations of severe zinc deficiency may occur in infants who are receiving apparently adequate amounts of the element. However, during periods of catch-up growth, such amounts may be insufficient to meet the needs for deposition of new tissue. The diagnosis is easily confirmed by a trial of supplementation with zinc.

Q.   Does zinc have a nonspecific effect on growth, or is this effect only evident in zinc deficiency?
A.   Zinc does not have a nonspecific effect on growth, and improvements in growth rates after zinc supplementation are indicative of a preexisting deficiency.

Case 2: Copper. A 17-week-old infant was transferred to University Hospital in Denver for evaluation of an acrodermatitis syndrome. This child was born at 32 weeks' gestation and she weighed 1580 gm. There were mild problems of respiratory distress but they quickly resolved and she gained well on mother's milk. At nine weeks of age she developed the characteristic rash of acrodermatitis, and the diagnosis of zinc deficiency was confirmed by the demonstration of hypozincemia (21 μg/dl).

Treatment was started with 30 mg of zinc daily, which corresponded to a dose of 7 mg/kg. Lesions and symptoms cleared quickly, but upon arrival to our institution, the child who then weighed 4.5 kg was noted to be anemic and leukopenic. Further evaluation revealed hyperzincemia greater than 150 μg/dl and hyperzincuria approaching 1 mg/24 hours. The plasma copper was 33 μg/dl, lower than the 54 μg/dl obtained at 13 weeks of age, and spur formation was found on radiologic examination of the femurs. A diagnosis of copper deficiency was made and copper supplements provided, while the zinc supplement was temporarily withheld. The mother's milk was assayed for copper content, which was within the normal range of 600 μg/L.

Q.   Isn't it rare to have two trace element deficiencies?
A.   The occurrence of two trace element deficiencies in one infant was at the time both rare and a diagnostic challenge. Copper deficiency in this case, which had not previously been reported in breast-fed infants, was probably caused by interference of copper absorption by the large quantities of zinc given to treat the acrodermatitis syndrome. The response to withholding zinc and providing copper supplements was rapid.

Q.   Does overadministration of zinc interfere with other minerals?
A.   Theoretically it can also interfere with iron absorption but to date this has not been demonstrated in children.

REFERENCES

1. Underwood EJ. Trace Elements in Human and Animal Nutrition, 4th ed. New York, Academic Press, 1977.
2. Casey CE, Robinson MF. Some aspects of nutritional trace element research. In Siegel H (ed): Metal Ions in Biological Systems, Volume 16. New York, Marcel Dekker, 1983; 1–26.
3. Walravens PA, Hambidge KM. Trace elements in nutrition. In Kelley VC (ed): Practice of Pediatrics. Philadelphia, Harper and Row, 1982, vol. 6, ch. 8.
4a. Mertz W. The essential trace elements. Science 1981; 213:1332–1338.
4b. Mertz W. Metabolism and metabolic effects of trace elements. In Chandra RK (ed): Trace Elements in Nutrition of Children. New York, Raven Press, 1985; 107–119.
5. Walshe SM. Copper: its role in the pathogenesis of liver disease. Semin Liver Dis 1984;4:252–263.
6. Weiss KC, Linder MC. Copper transport in rats involving a new plasma protein. Am J Physiol 1985;249:E77–E88.
7. Wirth, PL, Linder MC. Distribution of copper among components of human serum. J Natl Cancer Inst 1985;75:277–284.
8. Recommended Dietary Allowances: Report of the Food and Nutrition Board, National Research Council, 9th ed. Washington, D.C., National Academy of Sciences, 1980.
9. Salmenpera L, Perheentupa J, Pakarinen P, Siimes MA. Copper nutrition in infants during prolonged exclusive breastfeeding: low intake but rising serum concentrations of copper and ceruloplasmin. Am J Clin Nutr 1986;43: 251–257.
10. American Medical Association. Guidelines for essential trace elements preparations for parenteral use. JAMA 1979;241:2051–2054.
11. Zlotkin SH, Buchanan BE. Meeting zinc and copper requirements in the parenterally fed preterm and full term infant. J Pediatr 1983; 103:441–446.
12. Dauncey MS, Shaw JLL, Urman J. The absorption and retention of magnesium. zinc and copper by low birth weight infants fed pasteurized human breast milk. Pediatr Res 1977;11:991–997.
13. Hillman LS. Serial serum copper concentrations in premature and SGA infants during the first 3 months of life. J Pediatr 1981;98:305–308.
14. Hillman LS, Martin L, Fiore B. Effect of oral copper supplementation or serum copper and ceruloplasmin concentrations in premature infants. J Pediatr 1981;98: 311–313.
15. Tyrala EE. Zinc and copper balances in preterm infants. Pediatrics 1986;77:513–517.
16. Ehrenkranz RA, Nelli CM, Gettner PA, et al. Determination of copper absorption in premature infants with 65 Cu as an extrinsic stable isotopic tracer. Pediatr Res 1986;20:409A.
17. James BE, Hendry PG, MacMahon RA. Total parenteral nutrition of premature infants. II. Requirements for micronutrient elements. Aust Paediatr J 1979;15:67–71.
18. Sutton AM, Harvie A, Cockburn F, et al. Copper deficiency in the preterm infant of very low birth weight. Arch Dis Child 1985;60:644–651.
19. Halliday HL, Lappin TRJ, McMaster D, Patterson CC. Copper and the preterm infant. Arch Dis Child 1985;60:1105–1106.
20. Tyrala EE, Manser JI, Brodsky NL, et al. Distribution of copper in the serum of the parenterally fed premature infant. J Pediatr 1985;106:295–298.
21. Cordano A, Baertl JM, Graham GG. Copper deficiency in infancy. Pediatrics 1964;34:324–336.
22. Al-Rashid RA, Spangler J. Neonatal copper deficiency. N Engl J Med 1971;285:841–843.
23. Karpel JT, Peden VH. Copper deficiency in long-term total parenteral nutrition. J Pediatr 1972;8:32–36.
24. Goyens P, Brasseur D, Cadranel S. Copper deficiency in infants with active celiac disease. J Pediatr Gastroenterol Nutr 1985;4:677–680.
25. Becton DL, Schultz WH, Kinney TR. Severe neutropenia caused by copper deficiency in a child receiving continued ambulatory peritoneal dialysis. J Pediatr 1986;108:735–737.
26. Nisni Y, Kittaua E, Fukuda K, et al. Copper deficiency associated with alkali therapy in a patient with renal tubular acidosis. J Pediatr 1981;98:81–83.
27. Danks DM, Campbell PE, Stevens BJ, et al. Menkes' kinky hair syndrome: an inherited defect in copper absorption with widespread effects. Pediatrics 1972;50:188–201.
28. Chuttani HK, Gupta PS, Gulati S, Gupta DH. Acute copper sulfate poisoning. Am J Med 1965;39:849–854.
29. Salmon MA, Wright T. Chronic copper poisoning presenting as pink disease. Arch Dis Child 1971;46:100–110.
30. Tanner MS, Bhave SA, Kantarjiaxc AM, Panait AM. Early introduction of copper-contaminated animal milk feeds as a possible cause of Indian childhood cirrhosis. Lancet 1983;2:992–95.
31. O'Dell BL. History and status of zinc nutrition. Fed Proc 1984;43:2821–2822.
32. Prasad AS, Halsted JA, Nadhimi M. Syndrome of iron deficiency anemia, hepatosplenomegaly, dwarfism, hypogonadism and geophagia. Am J Med 1961;31:532–546.
33. McKenzie JM, Fosmire GJ, Sandstead HH. Zinc deficiency during the latter third of pregnancy: Effects on fetal rat brain, liver and placenta. J Nutr 1975;105:1466–1475.
34. Solomons NW, Cousins RJ. Zinc. In Solomons NW, Rosenberg IH (eds): Absorption and Malabsorption of Mineral Nutrients. New York, Alan R. Liss, 1984;125–197.
35. Krebs NF, Hambidge KM. Zinc requirements and zinc intakes of breast-fed infants. Am J Clin Nutr 1986;43:288–292.
36. Cavell PA, Widdowson EM. Intakes and excretions of iron, copper and zinc in the neonatal period. Arch Dis Child 1964;39:496–502.
37. Zeigler EE, Edwards BB, Jensen RL, et al. Zinc balance studies in normal infants. In Kirchgessner M (ed): Trace Element Metabolism in Man and Animals-3. Universitat Munchen, Freising-Weihenstephan, 1978;292–295.

38. Voyer M, Davakis M, Antener I, Valleur D. Zinc balances in preterm infants. Biol Neonate 1982;42:87–92.

39. Ehrenkranz RA, Nelli CM, Gettner PA, et al. The influence of food zinc (Zn) absorption in premature infants. Pediatr Res 1986;20:409A.

40. Hambidge KM, Hambidge C, Jacobs M, Baum JD. Low levels of zinc in hair, poor growth and hypogeusia in children. Pediatr Res 1972;6:868–872.

41. Walravens PA, Hambidge KM. Growth of infants fed a zinc supplemented formula. Am J Clin Nutr 1976;29:1114–1121.

42. Moynahan EJ. Acrodermatitis enteropathica: A lethal, inherited human zinc deficiency disorder. Lancet 1974; 2:399.

43. Kay RG, Tasman-Jones C. Acute zinc deficiency in man during intravenous alimentation. Aust N Z J Surg 1975; 45:325–330.

44. Aggett PJ, Atherton DJ, More J, et al. Symptomatic zinc deficiency in a breast-fed, pre-term infant. Arch Dis Child 1980;55:547–550.

45. Courtney Moore ME, Moran JR, Greene HL. Zinc supplementation in lactating women: evidence for mammary control of zinc secretion. J Pediatr 1984;105:600–602.

46. Bye AME, Goodfellow A, Atherton DJ. Transient zinc deficiency in a full-term, breast-fed infant of normal birth weight. Pediatr Dermatol 1985;2:308–311.

47. Hambidge KM, Walravens PA, Neldner KH, Daugherty NA. Zinc, copper and fatty acids in acredermatitis enterpathica. In Kirchgessner M (ed): Trace Element Metabolism in Man and Animals-3. Universitat Munchen, Freising-Weihenstephan, 1978;413–417.

48. Brocks A, Reid H, Glazer H. Acute intravenous zinc poisoning. Br Med J 1977;1:1390–1391.

49. National Research Council. Selenium in Human Nutrition, revised edition. National Academy of Sciences, Washington D.C., 1983.

50. Schwartz K, Foltz CM. Selenium as an integral part of factor 3 against dietary necrotic liver degeneration. J Am Chem Soc 1957;79:3292–3293.

51. Rotruck JT, Pope AL, Ganther HE, et al. Selenium: biochemical role as a component of glutathione peroxidase. Science 1973;179:588–590.

52. Flohe L, Gunzler WA, Schock HH. Glutathione peroxidase: a selenoenzyme. FEBS Lett 1973;32:132–134.

53. Barbezat GO, Casey CE, Reasbeck P, et al. Selenium. In Solomons NW, Rosenberg IH (eds): Absorption and Malabsorption of Mineral Nutrients. New York, Alan R. Liss, 1984;231–258.

54. Solomons NW, Torun B, Janghorbani M, et al. Absorption of selenium from milk protein and isolated soy protein formulas in preschool children: studies using stable isotope tracer 74 Se. J Pediatr Gastroenterol Nutr 1986;5:122–126.

55. Lombeck I, Kasperek K, Feinendegen LE, Bremer HJ. Low selenium state in children. In Spallholz JE, Martin JE, Ganther HE (eds): Selenium in Biology and Medicine. Westport, CT, AVI, 1981;269–282.

56. McKenzie RL, Rea HM, Thomson CD, Robinson MF. Selenium concentration and glutathione peroxidase activity in blood of New Zealand infants and children. Am J Clin Nutr 1978;31:1413–1418.

57. Ward KP, Arthur JR, Russell G, Aggett PJ. Blood selenium content and glutathione peroxidase activity in children with cystic fibrosis, coeliac disease, asthma, and epilepsy. Eur J Pediatr 1984;142:21–24.

58. Stewart RDH, Griffiths NM, Thomson CD, Robinson MF. Quantitative selenium metabolism in normal New Zealand women. Br J Nutr 1978;40:45–54.

59. Levander OA, Morris VC. Dietary selenium levels needed to maintain balance in American adults consuming self-selected diets. Am J Clin Nutr 1984;39:809–815.

60. Casey CE, Guthrie BE, Friend GM, Robinson MF. Selenium in human tissues from New Zealand. Arch Environ Health 1982;37:133–135.

61. Bayliss PA, Buchanan BE, Hancock RGV, Zlotkin SH. Tissue selenium accretion in premature and full-term human infants and children. Biol TE Res 1985;7:55–61.

62. Casey CE, Hambidge KM. Trace minerals. In Tsang RC (ed): Vitamin and Mineral Requirements of Preterm Infants. New York, Marcel Dekker, 1985;153–184.

63. Gross S. Hemolytic anemia in premature infants: relationship to vitamin E, selenium, glutathione peroxidase and erythrocyte lipids. Semin Hematol 1976;13:187–199.

64. Kumpulainen J, Salmenpera L, Siimes MA, et al. Selenium status of exclusively breast-fed infants as influenced by maternal organic or inorganic selenium supplementation. Am J Clin Nutr 1985;42:829–835.

65. Robberecht H, Roekens E, Van Caille-Bertrand M, et al. Longitudinal study of the selenium content of human breast milk in Belgium. Acta Paediatr Scand 1985;74:254–258.

66. Smith AM, Picciano MF, Milner JA. Selenium intakes and status of human milk and formula fed infants. Am J Clin Nutr 1982;35:521–526.

67. Friel JK, Gibson RS, Balassa R, Watts JL. Selenium and chromium intakes of very low birthweight pre-term and normal birthweight full-term infants during the first twelve months. Nutr Res 1985;5:1175–1184.

68. Lombeck I, Ebert KH, Kasperek K, et al. Selenium intake of infants and young children, healthy children and dietetically treated patients with phenylketonuria. Eur J Pediatr 1984;143:99–102.

69. Yang GX, Chen J, Wen Z, et al. The role of selenium in Keshan disease. Adv Nutr Res 1984;6:203–231.

70. Li G, Wang F, Kang D, Li C. Keshan disease: An endemic cardiomyopathy in China. Hum Pathol 1985;16:602–609.

71. Robinson MF, Thomson CD. The role of selenium in the diet. Nutr Abs Rev 1983;53:3–26.

72. van Rij AM, Thomson CD, McKenzie JM, Robinson M. Selenium deficiency in total parenteral nutrition. Am J Clin Nutr 1979;32:2076–2085.

73. Brown MR, Cohen HJ, Lyons JM, et al. Proximal muscle weakness and selenium deficiency associated with long term parenteral nutrition. Am J Clin Nutr 1986;43:549–554.

74. Kein CL, Ganther HE. Manifestations of chronic selenium deficiency in a child receiving total parenteral nutrition. Am J Clin Nutr 1983;37:319–328.

75. Baker SS, Lerman RH, Krey SH, et al. Selenium deficiency with total parenteral nutrition: Reversal of biochemical and functional abnormalities by selenium supplementation: A case report. Am J Clin Nutr 1983;38:769–774.

76. Yang GX, Wang SX, Zhou RX, Sun S. Endemic selenium intoxication of humans in China. Am J Clin Nutr 1983;37:872–881.

77. Jaffe WG, Raphael MD, Mondragon MC, Cuevas MA. Clinical and biochemical studies on school children from a seleniferous area. Arch Latinoam Nutr 1972;22:595–611.

78. Matovinovic J. Endemic goiter and cretinism at the dawn of the third millenium. Ann Rev Nutr 1983;3:341–412.

79. Pharoah POD. Iodine deficiency: a study of endemic goitre and cretinism in a remote human population. In Mills CF, Bremner I, and Chesters JK (eds): Trace Element Metabolism and Animals-5. Slough, U.K., Commonwealth Agricultural Bureaux, 1985;929–932.

80. Hetzel BS, Maberly GF. Iodine. In Mertz W (ed): Trace Elements In Human and Animal Nutrition, Volume 2, 5th ed. Orlando, FL, Academic Press, 1986;139–208.

81. Klein AH, Oddie TH, Parslow M, et al. Developmental changes in pituitary-thyroid function in the human fetus and newborn. Early Human Devel 1982;6:321–330.

82. Delange F. Physiopathology of iodine nutrition. In Chandra RK (ed): Trace Elements in Nutrition of Children. Nestle Nutrition, New York, Vevey/Raven Press, 1985; 291–299.

83. Gushurst CA, Mueller JA, Green JA, Sedor F. Breast milk iodide: reassessment in the 1980s. Pediatrics 1984;73:354–357.

84. Bruhn JC, Franke AA. Iodine in human milk. J Dairy Sci 1983;66:1396–1398.

85. Infant Formula Act, 1980. Public Law 96-359 (United States of America).

86. Gough DCS, Laing I, Astley P. Thyroid function on short-term total parenteral nutrition without iodine supplements. JPEN 1982;6:439–440.

87. Warkany J. Teratogen update: iodine deficiency. Teratology 1985;31:309–311.
88. Hetzel BS, Hay ID. Thyroid function, iodine nutrition and fetal brain development. Clin Endocrinol 1979;11:445–460.
89. Bautista A, Barker PA, Dunn JT, et al. The effects of oral iodized oil on intelligence, thyroid status, and somatic growth in school-age children from an area of endemic goitre. Am J Clin Nutr 1982;35:127–134.
90. Erenberg A. Thyroid function in the preterm infant. Pediatr Clin North Am 1982;29:1205–1211.
91. Beckers C, Cornette C, Georgoulis A, et al. The effects of mild iodine deficiency on neonatal thyroid function. Clin Endocrinol 1981;14:295–299.
92. Delange F, Dalhem A, Bourdoux P, et al. Increased risk of primary hypothyroidism in preterm infants. J Pediatr 1984;105:462–469.
93. Sava L, Delange F, Belfiore A, et al. Transient impairment of thyroid function in newborn from an area of endemic goitre. J Clin Endocrinol Metab 1984;59:90–95.
94. Theodoropoulos T, Braverman LE, Vagenakis AG. Iodide-induced hypothyroidism: a potential hazard during perinatal life. Science 1974;205:502–503.
95. Committee on Nutrition. Pediatric Nutrition Handbook, 2nd ed. Elk Grove Village, Illinois, American Academy of Pediatrics, 1985.
96. Dean HT. Fluorine in the control of dental caries. Int Dent J 1954;4:311–337.
97. Nikiforuk G. Understanding Dental Caries. II. Prevention, Basic and Clinical Aspects. Basel, Karger, 1985.
98. Machle WF, Scott EW, Sargent EJ. The absorption and excretion of fluorides. I. The normal fluoride balance. J Ind Hyg Toxicol 1942;24:199–
99. Nizel AE. Nutritional aspects of pediatric dental-oral health problems: an overview. In Walker WA, Watkins JB (eds): Nutrition in Pediatrics. Boston, Little, Brown, 1985;727–739.
100. Guy WS, Taves DR. Relationship between (F⁻) in drinking water and human plasma. J Dent Res 1973;52:238.
101. American Academy of Pediatrics, Committee on Nutrition. Fluoride supplementation. Pediatrics 1986;77:758–761.
102. Ericsson Y, Ribelius U. Wide variations of fluoride supply to infants and their effect. Caries Res 1971;5:78–88.
103. Esala S, Vuori E, Helle A. Effect of maternal fluorine intake on breast milk fluorine content. Br J Nutr 1982;48:201–204.
104. Noren JG. The effects of perinatal disorders on the developing dentition. In Nowak AJ, Erenberg A (eds): Factors Influencing Orofacial Development in the Ill, Preterm Low-Birth Weight, and Term Neonate. Proceed. Conf., University of Iowa, Iowa City, 1984;42–50.
105. Yolken R, Konecny P, McCarthy P. Acute fluoride poisoning. Pediatrics 1976;58:90–93.
106. Brams M, Maloney J. "Nursing bottle caries" in breast-fed children. J Pediatr 1983;103:415–416.
107. Gershwin ME, Beach RS, Hurley LS. Nutrition and Immunity. Orlando, FL, Academic Press, 1985.
108. Cotzias GC, Tang LC, Miller ST, et al. A mutation influencing the transportation of manganese, L-dopa and L-tryptophan. Science 1972;176:410–412.
109. Sampson B, Barlow GB, Wilkinson AW. Manganese balance studies in infants after operations on the heart. Pediatr Res 1983;17:263–266.
110. Casey CE, Hambidge KM, Neville MC. Studies in human lactation: zinc, copper, manganese and chromium in human milk in the first month of lactation. Am J Clin Nutr 1985;41:1193–1200.
111. Raghib MH, Chan W-Y, Rennert OM. Comparative biological availability of manganese from extrinsically labelled milk diet using sucking rats as a model. Br J Nutr 1986;55:49–58.
112. Stastny D, Vogel R, Picciano MF. Manganese intake and serum manganese concentrations of human milk-fed and formula-fed infants. Am J Clin Nutr 1984;39:872–878.
113. Gibson RS. Dietary intakes of trace elements in infants during their first year. Food Nutr News 1985;57(1):1–3.
114. Hatano S, Aihara K, Nishi Y, Usui T. Trace elements (copper,

zinc, manganese, and selenium) in plasma and erythrocytes in relation to dietary intake during infancy. J Pediatr Gastroenterol Nutr 1985;4:87–92.
115. Friel JK, Gibson RS, Balassa R, Watts JL. A comparison of the zinc, copper and manganese status of very low birth weight pre-term and full-term infants during the first twelve months. Acta Paediatr Scand 1984;73:596–601.
116. Fincham JE, Van Rensburg SJ, Marasas WFO. Mseleni joint disease—a manganese deficiency? S Afr Med J 1981;60:445–447.
117. DuPont CL, Tanaka Y. Blood manganese levels in children with convulsive disorder. Biochem Med 1985;33:246–255.
118. Hoffmann H. Manganese serum levels in epileptics. Klin Wochenschr 1980;58:157–158.
119. Lustig S, Pitlik SD, Rosenfeld JB. Liver damage in acute self-induced hypermanganemia. Arch Intern Med 1982;142:405–406.
120. Sharda B, Bhandari B, Sharma KD. Study of manganese in Indian childhood cirrhosis. Indian Pediatr 1983;20:193–195.
121. Anderson RA. Nutritional role of chromium. Sci Total Environ 1981;17:13–29.
122. Jeejeebhoy KN, Chu RC, Marliss EB, et al. Chromium deficiency, glucose, and neuropathy reversed by chromium supplementation, in a patient receiving long-term parenteral nutrition. Am J Clin Nutr 1977;30:531–538.
123. Freund H, Atamain S, Fischer JE. Chromium deficiency during total parenteral nutrition. JAMA 1979;241:496–498.
124. Anderson RA, Polansky MM, Bryden NA, et al. Urinary chromium excretion of human subjects: effects of chromium supplementation and glucose loading. Am J Clin Nutr 1982;36:1184–1193.
125. Lui VJK, Abernathy RP. Chromium and insulin in young subjects with normal glucose tolerance. Am J Clin Nutr 1982;35:661–667.
126. Anderson RA, Polansky MM, Bryden NA, et al. Chromium supplementation of human subjects: effects on glucose, insulin, and lipid variables. Metabolism 1983;32:894–899.
127. Carter JP, Kattab A, Abd-El-Hadi K, et al. Chromium (III) in hypoglycemia and impaired glucose utilization in kwashiorkor. Am J Clin Nutr 1968;21:195–202.
128. Piccano MF. Trace elements in human milk and infant formulas. In Chandra RK (ed): Elements in Nutrition of Children. Nestle Nutrition, New York, Vevey/Raven Press, 1985, 157–174.
129. Chappell WR, Meglen RR, Moure-Eraso R, et al. Human Health Effects of Molybdenum in Drinking Water, EPA-600/1-79-006. U.S. Environmental Protection Agency, 1979.
130. O'Dell BL. Bioavailability of and interactions among trace elements. In Chandra RK (ed): Trace Elements in Nutrition of Children. Nestle Nutrition, New York, Vevey/Raven Press, 1985, 41–62.
131. Coughlin MP. The role of molybdenum in human biology. J Inherited Metab Dis 1983;6(Suppl 1):70–77.
132. Alexander FW, Clayton BE, Delves HT. Mineral and trace metal balance in children receiving normal and synthetic diets. Quart J Med 1974;43:89–111.
133. Versieck J, Hoste J, Vanballenberghe L, et al. Serum molybdenum in diseases of the liver and biliary system. J Lab Clin Med 1981;97:535–544.
134. Tsongas T, Meglen RR, Walravens PA, Chappell WR. Molybdenum in the diet: an estimate of average daily intake in the United States. Am J Clin Nutr 1980;33:1103–1107.
135. Abumrad NM. Molybdenum—is it an essential trace metal? Bull N Y Acad Sci 1984;60:163–171.
136. Roth A, Nogues C, Monnet JP, et al. Anatomo-pathological findings in a case of combined deficiency of sulphite oxidase and xanthine oxidase with a defect of molybdenum cofactor. Virchow Archiv (Pathol Anat) 1985;405:379–386.
137. Beemer FA, Duran M, Wadman SK, Cats BP. Absence of hepatic molybdenum cofactor. An inborn error of metabolism associated with lens dislocation. Ophthal Paed Genet 1985;5:191–195.

38. Alfrey AC. Aluminum. Adv Clin Chem 1983;23:69-91.
39. Alfrey AC, LeGrende GR, Kaehny WD. The dialysis encephalopathy syndrome: possible aluminum intoxication. N Engl J Med 1976;294:184-188.
40. Petit TL. Aluminum neurobehavioral toxicology. In Dreosti IE, Smith RM (eds): Neurobiology of the Trace Elements 2. Neurotoxicology and Neuropharmacology. Clifton, New Jersey, Humana Press, 1983; 237-274.
41. Andreoli SP, Bergstein JM, Sherrard DJ. Aluminum intoxication from aluminum-containing phosphate binders in children with azotemia not undergoing dialysis. N Engl J Med 1984;310:1079-1084.
42. Sedman AB, Miller NL, Warady BA, et al. Aluminum loading in children with chronic renal failure. Kidney Int 1984;26:201-204.
43. Sedman AB, Klein GL, Merritt RJ, et al. Evidence of aluminum loading in infants receiving intravenous therapy. N Engl J Med 1985;312:1337-1343.
44. McGraw M, Bishop N, Jameson R, et al. Aluminum content of milk formulae and intravenous fluids used in infants. Lancet 1986;1:157.
45. Freundlich M, Abitol C, Zilleruelo G, et al. Infant formula as a cause of aluminum toxicity in neonatal uraemia. Lancet 1985;2:527-529.
146. Rutter M. Raised lead levels and impaired cognitive/behavioral functioning: a review of the evidence. Dev Med Child Neurol 1980;22(Suppl 1).
147. Bander LK, Morgan KJ, Zabik ME. Dietary lead intake of preschool children. Am J Public Health 1983;73:789-794.
148. Ryu JE, Zeigler EE, Nelson SE, Fomon SJ. Dietary intake of lead and blood lead concentration in early infancy. Am J Dis Child 1983;137:886-891.
149. Mielke HW, Blake B, Burroughs S, Hassinger N. Urban lead levels in Minneapolis: the case of the Hmong children. Environ Res 1984;34:64-76.
150. Boeckx RL. Lead poisoning in children. Anal Chem 1986;58:274A-287A.
151. Bose A, Vashistha K, O'Loughlin BJ. Azarcon por empacho—another cause of lead toxicity. Pediatrics 1983;72:106-108.
152. Fassett DW. Cadmium. In Lee DHK (ed): Metallic Contaminants and Human Health. New York, Academic Press, 1972;98-124.
153. Goldwater LJ, Clarkson TW. Mercury. In Lee DHK (ed): Metallic Contaminants and Human Health. New York, Academic Press, 1972;17-55.

12

Nutritional Anemia of Infancy: Iron, Folic Acid, and Vitamin B$_{12}$

PETER R. DALLMAN, M.D.

ABSTRACT

Iron, folic acid, and vitamin B$_{12}$ are appropriately discussed in the same chapter because a deficiency of any of them will eventually lead to anemia. Most of the following discussion addresses iron deficiency because it is very common and easily prevented.

Menghini proved that iron was present in blood in 1747. He dried a sample of blood and then ground it to a fine powder. By applying a magnet he was able to lift out a portion of the powder. (De Ferreorum Particulerum sede in Sanguis. Commentar. Bononiens Bologna ii, p 475, 1747.)

INTRODUCTION

Iron, folic acid, and vitamin B$_{12}$ play an important role in the production of red blood cells. Iron is a constituent of hemoglobin, which accounts for about 75% of this element in the body. Folic acid and vitamin B$_{12}$ are essential for cell proliferation, which is active in the body as a whole during early development and in hematopoietic tissue throughout life. Deficiencies of vitamin B$_{12}$ and folic acid are relatively rare on a nutritional basis but may also result from certain inborn errors of metabolism. It is important that the latter are recognized in infancy, since they have serious neurological consequences and usually require lifelong treatment.

WHAT IS ANEMIA?

Because of the marked age-related changes that normally occur in hemoglobin concentration, it is essential to compare the patient's values to age-specific reference standards. The diagnosis of anemia in infancy requires a special awareness of the normal age-related changes in concentration of hemoglobin and related laboratory determinations.

Age-related changes in hemoglobin concentration were first recognized in the late nineteenth century. However, not until 1916 did Williamson report a large study that included infants and that employed quantitative spectrophotometric methods (Arch Intern Med 1916;18:505–28). More precise data with confidence limits were published in the thirties for both term and preterm infants (Merritt KK, Davidson LT. Am J Dis Child 1933;46:990–1010 and 1934;47:261–300). However, the general applicability of these values was somewhat hampered by technical limitations and the fact that they were derived mainly from lower socioeconomic groups in whom anemia is more common.

The current reference values shown in Figure 1 and Table 1 are based on nonindigent populations in whom laboratory studies and/or nutritional management excluded iron deficiency and other recognized causes of anemia. In a healthy term infant, the mean concentration of hemoglobin declines by about 30%, from about 17 to 11 gm/dl* within the first 6 to 8 postnatal weeks. These extremes represent highest and lowest values in any period of development. Anemia is usually defined as a hemoglobin concentration below the 95% range for healthy subjects of the same age (and sex, after 10 years of age). In order to avoid misdiagnosing anemia, a hemoglobin (or hematocrit) value must be interpreted in the context of the age- and birthweight-specific reference range[1-3] (Fig. 1 and Table 1).

The high hemoglobin value at birth results from a hypoxic intrauterine environment. Fetal red cell production is believed to be stimulated by elevated levels of erythropoietin, the humoral regulator of red cell production, which occur in response to tissue hypoxia.[4] The high rate of intrauterine red cell produc-

---

*To convert to the International System of Units, multiply by 10 to yield gm/L.

216

PRETERM INFANTS   TERM INFANTS

1000 to 1500g   1501 to 2000g   >3000g

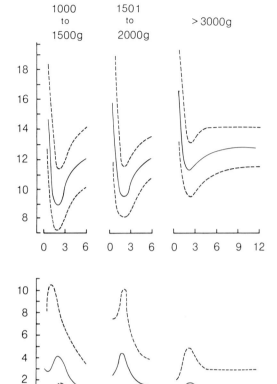

AGE, MONTHS

FIGURE 1. Hemoglobin concentration and reticulocyte count in preterm and term infants. Median values and 95% confidence limits are indicated for each of three birthweight categories. (Hemoglobin values are from Lundström et al: J Pediatr 1977;91:878; and Saarinen and Siimes: J Pediatr 1978;92:412; reticulocyte values are from unpublished data on the same infants from whom hemoglobin values were derived.)

TABLE 1.   Mean Hemoglobin (Hgb), Hematocrit (Hct), MCV and MCH with ± 2SD Ranges (95% Ranges) in Iron-supplemented Infants*

Age (months)	Hgb (g/dl)	Hct (%)	MCV (fl)	MCH (pg)
Term				
0.5	16.6 (13.4–19.8)	53 (41–67)	105 (88–122)	34 (30–38)
1	13.9 (10.7–17.1)	44 (33–55)	101 (91–111)	33 (29–37)
2	11.2 (9.4–13.0)	35 (28–42)	95 (84–106)	30 (27–33)
4	12.2 (10.3–14.1)	38 (32–44)	87 (76–98)	29 (25–33)
6	12.5 (11.0–14.0)	36 (32–40)	80 (70–88)	27 (24–30)
12	12.5 (11.0–14.0)	36 (32–40)	80 (70–88)	27 (24–30)
Preterm (1000–2000 gm)				
0.5	15.4 (10.7–20.0)	46 (31–62)	107 (91–123)	36 (30–42)
1	11.6 (8.1–15.1)	35 (23–46)	100 (87–112)	34 (29–38)
2	9.4 (7.2–11.7)	28 (21–36)	89 (75–102)	30 (26–34)
3	10.5 (8.6–12.3)	31 (25–37)	82 (72–92)	28 (24–32)
4	11.7 (9.7–13.8)	34 (29–39)	78 (68–88)	28 (24–32)
6	12.4 (11.0–13.8)	36 (31–40)	79 (68–90)	28 (24–32)

*Data are from Lundström et al., 1980 and Saarinen et al., 1978 and were rounded out in a few instances.

tion remains evident at birth from average reticulocyte counts of about 5% and 7 nucleated red cells/100 white cells in term infants. Values in preterm infants are often two to three times higher.

At birth, oxygen delivery to the tissues is suddenly facilitated as oxygen from the lungs virtually saturates the hemoglobin in arterial blood. The resulting improvement in tissue oxygenation results in diminished erythropoietin activity in the plasma and a decrease in the production of red cells.[5] In the peripheral blood, these changes are reflected in a precipitous fall in the reticulocyte count and the disappearance of nucleated red blood cells during the first few days after birth.

The marked depression in the rate of red blood cell production continues for 4 to 6 weeks. The resulting decline in hemoglobin concentration is independent of iron nutrition and occurs at a time when neonatal iron stores remain abundant. The fall in hemoglobin concentration is greatest in infants of lowest birth weight.[1,4,6] At about 2 months of age, infants with birth weights below 1500 gm have a mean hemoglobin concentration of about 9.0 gm/dl compared to 11.0 gm/dl in term infants; the corresponding value in infants with a birthweight between 1500 and 2000 gm is 9.5 gm/dl (Fig. 1).

After about 4–6 weeks of age, an increase in red cell production is signaled by a rise in the reticulocyte count (Fig. 1), and hemoglobin concentration in the term infant rises gradually after about 2 months of age. A mean hemoglobin value of 12.5 gm/dl is reached by 6 months and is then maintained through the remainder of the first 4 years of life. In the preterm infant, the rise in reticulocyte count after 2 months of age is even greater than in the term infant, but because of a more rapid rate of expansion of the blood volume, the hemoglobin values of preterm infant do not become equivalent to those of term infants until 4 to 6 months of age.[1]

In most respects, the breastfed infant serves as a model of optimal nutrition in infancy. However, the protein intake of very low birthweight (VLBW) infants fed human milk may be marginal, and their postnatal decline in hemoglobin concentration can be made slightly less pronounced if feedings of human milk contain added human milk protein.[8] This finding suggests that there may be a component of protein deficiency in the early anemia of the VLBW infant. Vitamin E deficiency as a possi-

ble basis for anemia in low birthweight infants is discussed elsewhere in this volume.

Although the reference values given in Figure 1 and Table 1 are applicable to most infants, an additional factor should be considered in respect to those infants requiring intensive care. During the first postnatal weeks, such infants often receive transfusions to replace blood removed for frequent laboratory studies. The transfused blood increases the percentage of adult hemoglobin and shifts the hemoglobin oxygen dissociation curve to the right, favoring oxygen delivery to the tissues.[4] Such infants, in whom there is an iatrogenic, preterm decline in percentage of fetal hemoglobin, may later stabilize at a hemoglobin concentration below the reference range.[7] Presumably, this is because the enhanced capacity for oxygen delivery of the adult hemoglobin depresses erythropoietin production and secondarily decreases red cell production.

The criteria for transfusing low birthweight infants for anemia have been discussed in two recent papers.[9,10] Increasing awareness of the risk of transmitting viral disease and reports on the transient nature of the post-transfusion rise in hemoglobin discourage the indiscriminate use of transfusion merely to correct a low hemoglobin value. This caution is reinforced by a recent study of randomly selected transfused and untransfused infants that showed that there was little or no benefit from transfusion.[10] On the other hand, in selected infants transfusion appears to reverse poor weight gain, poor feeding, and higher than expected pulse and respiratory rates.[9] Consequently, the decision to transfuse has to be based more on clinical than on laboratory criteria.

IRON DEFICIENCY

Term infants rarely develop iron deficiency anemia before 4 to 6 months of age. Preterm infants may become iron-deficient after 2 months of age. Effective prevention involves the use of iron-fortified formula for formula-fed infants and the use of ferrous sulfate in liquid form for breast-fed preterm infants.

The role of iron in the anemia of infancy became firmly established in 1928 when Helen Mackay reported a detailed longitudinal study of 541 infants from a low socioeconomic group in the East End of London (Arch Dis Child 1928;3:117–46). Her influential paper showed a clear distinction between the early and late anemia of infants; only the late anemia that occurred after 5 months of age re-

onded to iron treatment. The late anemia was shown to
e substantially milder in breast-fed infants than in infants
d a cow milk formula. She concluded that "the excellent
sults of treatment with iron preparations . . . point un-
istakably to iron deficiency as the factor of paramount
nportance" in the late anemia of infancy.

The major causes of iron deficiency in in-
ncy are a dilution of body iron by rapid
rowth and an iron-poor diet.[3,6] Blood loss is
ften an additional component[11] and oc-
asionally leads to more severe anemia than is
een with the other two causes alone.[12,13]
pecific causes of blood loss include prenatal
nd perinatal conditions such as fetal-maternal
ansfusion, placenta previa, rupture of umbili-
al vessels, and twin-to-twin transfusion; *dif-
fuse intestinal bleeding* related to ingestion of
esh cow milk in early infancy and celiac dis-
ase usually in later infancy; and *focal intes-
nal bleeding* associated with local anatomic
sions such as Meckel's diverticulum and pep-
c ulcer.

The *removal of blood for laboratory studies*
ften results in major iron losses in infants re-
uiring intensive care. For this reason, a care-
l log of blood removed for laboratory studies
ould be maintained for such infants.[14] **About
mg iron is lost with each 2 ml of blood.** To
rovide a frame of reference, total body iron in
e newborn averages 70 mg/kg.

HYSIOLOGY

Essential Iron and Storage Iron

1912, Ashby identified the liver as "the organ that has
e most to do with the storage . . . of iron." "When the
n is needed, it is given by the liver into the blood . . .
d used to make new hemoglobin and red blood cor-
scles." He also found that the concentration of liver
n was higher at birth than in the adult but that it
clined rapidly during early infancy (Lancet 1912;2:150–

Iron-containing compounds fall into two
tegories: the *essential compounds* that serve
etabolic or enzymatic functions and com-
ounds associated with iron storage.[3,15] The
st category functions in the transport and
ilization of oxygen for the production of
llular energy and includes hemoglobin, myo-
obin, the cytochromes, and iron-sulfur pro-
ins. The *storage compounds,* ferritin and
mosiderin, are involved in the maintenance
iron homeostasis. When the supply of

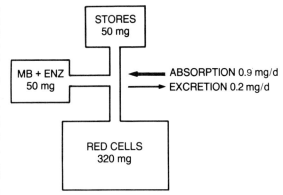

FIGURE 2.   Iron metabolism in the one year old infant. Iron absorption must exceed iron loss to allow for growth; however, daily iron absorption and loss, even in infancy, is normally a minute percentage of total body iron. MB + ENZ refers to myoglobin and enzyme iron.

dietary iron becomes inadequate, iron is mobilized from the storage compounds to maintain the production of hemoglobin and other essential iron compounds; not until the production of essential iron compounds becomes restricted is there known to be any impairment of body function.

The term iron deficiency is used here to refer to iron lack of sufficient severity to restrict the production of hemoglobin. Iron deficiency anemia occurs when the concentration of hemoglobin has fallen sufficiently due to iron lack to fulfill the laboratory definition of anemia, namely when it is below 95% reference range for age.

Iron Balance.   A distinctive feature of iron metabolism is the remarkable extent to which *the body conserves and reutilizes iron* once it has been absorbed (Fig. 2). The amount of body iron is regulated primarily through modulation of iron absorption over a more than 20-fold range.[16-18] **Iron absorption depends on the abundance of body iron stores, on the form and amount of iron in foods, and on the combination of foods in the diet.** It increases as storage iron becomes decreased. Iron excretion occurs mainly by loss with desquamation of the intestinal mucosa. The amount of iron lost in this manner varies only over a fourfold range, decreasing in iron deficiency and increasing in iron overload.[15] Consequently, the major determining factor in maintaining iron homeostasis is absorption.

A major difference in the iron balance of infants compared to adults is in the degree of dependence on dietary iron. In adult men,

ADULT

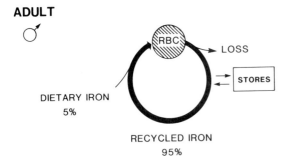

DIETARY IRON
5%

RECYCLED IRON
95%

**INFANT
1 YR.**

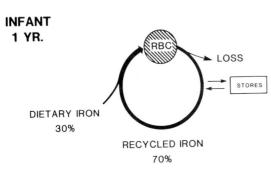

DIETARY IRON
30%

RECYCLED IRON
70%

FIGURE 3.   Greater dependence on dietary iron in the infant compared to the adult male. In adult men, about 95% of the iron required for the production of red blood cells is recycled from the breakdown of senescent red cells and only 5% comes from the diet. In contrast, one-year-old infants, due to their rapid growth, require about 30% from the diet.

about 95% of the iron required for the production of red blood cells is recycled from the breakdown of senescent red cells and only 5% comes from dietary sources (Fig. 3). The amount of iron absorbed approximates the small amount that is lost each day. In contrast, the average one-year-old infant derives less than 70% of red cell iron from senescent red cells and requires about 30% from the diet to meet the needs imposed by rapid growth. As a result, the amount of iron absorbed must be several times greater than iron losses. This difference helps to explain the high prevalence of iron deficiency in late infancy.

Absorption of Iron from Foods

Quantitative estimates of iron absorption began in the thirties and were based on balance studies in which the dietary intake of a nutrient was compared with fecal and urinary losses. This method was not only cumbersome and unpleasant but also particularly imprecise in respect to iron. Since most food iron is unabsorbed and appears primarily in the stool, small errors in stool collection and

iron analysis could lead to much larger discrepancies in estimating how much was retained by the body. Despite these handicaps, the balance studies of Sterns and Singer (J Nutr 1937;13:127–41) showed that iron-rich foods did not necessarily improve iron nutrition. Spinach and egg yolk had been widely recommended as good sources of iron, but iron from both was shown to be poorly retained by infants. On the other hand, iron-poor breast milk was associated with more positive iron balance than cow milk. These somewhat tentative conclusions were later confirmed when more precise measurements of iron absorption were performed in the seventies by isotopic methods.

There are two broad categories of iron in food. *Heme iron,* which is present in hemoglobin and myoglobin, is supplied mainly by meat and rarely accounts for more than a quarter of the iron ingested in most diets. Heme iron is relatively well-absorbed, and its absorption is little influenced by other constituents of the diet. Most of the remaining iron is present in the form of salts and is called *non-heme iron.* Since infant diets contain little meat, the vast preponderance of iron is in the non-heme form. The absorption of non-heme iron depends on how soluble it becomes in the intestine, and this, in turn, is determined by the composition of foods that are consumed in a meal.[16-18] Thus, the nature of the diet assumes greater importance than the absolute amount of iron ingested. **Absorption of the small amount of iron in breast milk is uniquely high,** 50% on the average, in contrast to 10% of iron from unfortified cow milk formula and 4% from iron-fortified cow milk formula.[21,23,24] Based on less direct evidence, it is estimated that also about 4% of the iron from iron-fortified dry infant cereals is absorbed[23] (Fig. 4).

Studies of iron absorption from various representative meals have been done primarily in adults,[16-18] but the results are also pertinent to the mixed diet of late infancy. Absorption of non-heme iron from a mixed meal is about four times greater when the major protein source is meat, fish, or chicken in comparison to the dairy products, milk, cheese or eggs. The beverage consumed with the meal plays an equally important role. Compared with water, orange juice will double the absorption of non-heme iron from the entire meal, whereas tea will decrease it by 75% and milk will decrease it to a lesser degree.

The most important enhancers of non-heme iron absorption are ascorbic acid and meat, fish, and poultry (Table 2). Major inhibitors are bran, polyphenols (including the tannates in

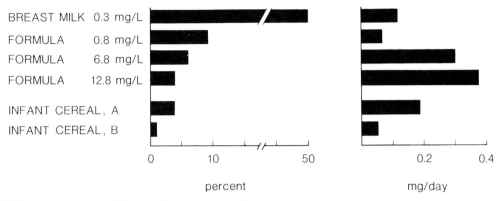

FIGURE 4. Iron absorption in infants. The percentage of iron absorbed from each food is shown on the left. The total amount of iron assimilation that would be predicted from the usual daily intake of these foods is shown on the right. The calculations are based on a daily intake of 750 ml of breast milk or formula and 10 gm of dry infant cereal. In the United States, fortified proprietary infant formulas currently contain about 12 mg/L of supplemental iron as ferrous sulfate; dry infant cereals contain 0.45 mg of fine particle reduced iron per gm of cereal. Infant cereal A is representative of products in current use in the United States; infant cereal B corresponds to products used prior to 1972 that were supplemented with less bioavailable forms of iron. (Calculations are based on the data of Rios E, et al: Pediatrics 1975;55:394; Saarinen UM, Siimes MA, et al: J Pediatr 1977;91:36; Saarinen UM, Siimes MA: Acta Paediatr Scand 1977;66:719.)

tea), and phosphate. The basis for the excellent absorption of iron from human milk is not known. The lower phosphate and protein content of human milk compared to cow milk, and the high concentration of the iron binding protein, lactoferrin, have been postulated to play a role but cannot explain this phenomenon entirely. There is some evidence that ingestion of human milk, per se, may influence the intestinal mucosa in a manner that facilitates iron absorption.[19]

IRON NEEDS DURING DEVELOPMENT

Many of the salient features of iron metabolism in newborn animals were described by Bunge in 1892 from measurements of food iron and body iron during early development. He found that "all of our most important foods have a much higher iron content than milk" and explained that the newborn "has already received its iron reserve for growth by birth." He wrote that "milk cannot be the predominant food after the suckling period has been completed." (Zeitschr Physiol Chemie 1892;16: 173–81.)

During pregnancy iron is efficiently transported from the maternal circulation to the fetus. This transport is scarcely impaired even when the mother has mild iron deficiency anemia.[3] At birth, the hemoglobin concentration is normally high and the liver reserves of storage iron are relatively generous. Conse-

TABLE 2. Enhancers and Inhibitors of Non-Heme Iron Absorption

Enhancers	Inhibitors
Ascorbic acid (orange juice)	Phosphates (cow milk, egg yolk)
Citric acid	Bran (whole grain cereals)
Meat (amino acids such as cysteine)	Oxalates (spinach)
Sugars	Polyphenols (tannates in tea)

quently most newborn infants are well supplied with iron.

In the term infant, there is little change in total body iron and little need for exogenous iron between birth and 4 months of age.[19] The usually abundant neonatal iron stores gradually decline during this period to provide for the synthesis of hemoglobin, myoglobin and enzyme iron (Fig. 5). Despite rapid growth and a substantial rise in blood volume, total hemoglobin iron scarcely increases because of the marked decline in concentration of hemoglobin. For this reason, iron deficiency is rare within the first few postnatal months unless there has been substantial loss of iron through perinatal or subsequent blood loss.

After about four months of age, there is a gradual shift from an abundance of iron to the marginal iron reserves that characterize the

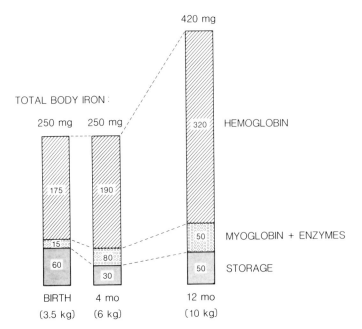

TOTAL BODY IRON :

FIGURE 5. Changes in body iron during infancy. Needs for exogenous iron are minimal between birth and about 4 months of age because there is little or no increase in total body iron during this period. In contrast, large amounts of iron must be assimilated during the remainder of infancy to allow for a rapid increase in total body iron. Estimates of body iron incorporate data from recent studies indicating higher values for myoglobin and enzyme iron than in earlier calculations. Storage iron at 12 months of age was assumed to be similar, on a body weight basis, to a mean of about 300 gm in women during the childbearing age. Hemoglobin iron calculations assume a hemoglobin concentration of 16.8 gm/dl and a blood volume of 90 ml/kg at birth and respective values of 12.5 gm/dl and 75 ml/kg at 4 and 12 months of age.

period of continued rapid growth during the remainder of infancy. This transition is primarily due to the large amount of iron required to maintain a constant hemoglobin concentration of about 12.5 gm/dl within a rapidly expanding body and blood volume. Between 4 and 12 months, an average of 0.9 mg of iron/day must be absorbed from the diet to provide 0.7 mg/day for growth and 0.2 mg/day to balance basal losses (Fig. 2). The rate and extent to which storage iron becomes depleted during this period depend on the magnitude of iron storage at birth and on the postnatal diet.

In term infants who receive unfortified cow milk formula, depletion of storage iron may occur as early as 4 months of age as indicated by a subnormal concentration of serum ferritin (< 10 µg/L).[18] In contrast, breastfed infants rarely exhaust their iron stores until after 6 months of age. The concentration of iron is similarly low in both forms of milk: well below 1.5 mg of iron/1000 kcal (or less than 1 mg/L), in contrast to roughly 6 mg/1000 kcal in a mixed infant diet. The reason that breast-fed infants deplete their iron stores more slowly is that the iron is much better absorbed from breast milk than from cow milk formula.[21,22] Nevertheless, in the absence of iron fortification or supplementation, iron stores eventually become marginal in breast-fed infants just at the age when solid foods begin to play an important role in the infant's diet.[20] The selection

of weaning foods, therefore, determines in large part whether an infant will progress from the harmless condition of low iron stores to the physiologic handicaps that are associated with iron deficiency anemia.

Low birthweight infants start out with a lower absolute amount of storage iron than term infants, since iron stores at birth are roughly proportional to body weight.[3,6] In addition, their postnatal iron needs are greater to allow for a more rapid rate of growth. As a result, low birthweight infants deplete their iron stores as early as 2 or 3 months of age, unless they receive iron-fortified formula or an iron supplement (if fed human milk).

PREVENTION OF IRON DEFICIENCY

There is now general agreement about most aspects of the prevention of iron deficiency (Tables 3 and 4). Only some relatively minor issues of timing remain controversial. Current recommendations will be summarized for term and preterm infants according to whether they are breastfed or formula-fed. In the following discussion, the term *fortification* refers to the addition of iron to a food, whereas *supplementation* signifies iron medication.

The iron needs of infants are more appropriately discussed in terms of the types of diet that prevent iron deficiency than in relation to milligrams of dietary iron required per day.[3,6,25] This is because of the marked variations in

TABLE 3.   Prevention of Iron Deficiency by Oral Ferrous Sulfate Drops and Iron-Fortified
                                    Cow Milk Formula

		Oral Ferrous Sulfate Drops	When to start iron-fortified formula
Term			
	Breast-fed	No	When weaned, if before 9 months
	Formula-fed	No	By 3 months
Preterm			
	Breast-fed	Between 2 and 8 weeks	When weaned, if before 9 months
	Formula-fed	Only in very low birthweight infants between 2 and 8 weeks	By 2 months

bioavailability of dietary iron from various kinds of infant foods. Furthermore, it is more practical to obtain a simple dietary history for infants than it is to attempt an estimate of their iron intake and absorption. However, it does become necessary to express iron requirements in quantitative terms when iron drops are administered.

Term Breast-fed Infants. Term breast-fed infants do not routinely require iron supplementation, since their iron stores rarely become depleted before 6 months of age (Fig. 6). Subsequently, an appropriate selection of solid foods will provide adequate dietary iron. Cereal and fruit juice are usually among the first non-milk foods given to infants. Iron-fortified dry infant cereal is generously fortified with iron (4.5 mg in a typical 10 gm serving) and the absorption of this iron can be enhanced by feeding an ascorbic-acid-rich food, such as orange juice or ascorbic-acid-fortified juice, at the same meal. Ready-to-serve cereals in jars are sometimes combined with fruit, but they are less heavily iron-fortified than dry infant cereals. Cream of wheat, though often fed to infants, contains little fortification iron. The absorption of iron from an entire meal can be enhanced by the inclusion of a small amount of meat. Egg yolk and spinach, though rich in iron, are now recognized to inhibit iron absorption. It also seems best *not* to feed solid foods near the time of breastfeeding, as this may reduce the excellent bioavailability of the small amount of iron in human milk.[26]

If breastfeeding is discontinued before 4 to 9 months, it is advisable to substitute iron-fortified infant formula rather than fresh cow milk. **Fresh cow milk commonly results in occult intestinal blood loss, especially before 6 months of age.**[11] Early use of fresh cow milk is the most common dietary characteristic shared by infants who are later found to have iron deficiency anemia when "screened" at about one year of age.

Term Formula-fed Infants. Cow milk formula is available in "unfortified" or iron-fortified forms. "Unfortified" formula has a minute amount of iron added to supply at least 1.5 mg of iron per reconstituted liter and iron-fortified formula has 12 mg of iron as ferrous sulfate added per reconstituted liter. Since infants who are fed "unfortified" formula may deplete their iron stores as early as 4 months of age, it is advisable to change to iron-fortified formula before about 3 months of age.

Whether iron-fortified formula is preferable right from birth is uncertain. On the one hand, it is more convenient to give a single formula throughout infancy. On the other hand, it can be argued that additional iron is not really needed before 3 or 4 months and that iron is poorly absorbed during the first few months of infancy when iron stores are still abundant (Fig. 7). Another argument against the initial use of iron-fortified formula involves a theo-

TABLE 4.   Ways to Improve Iron Nutrition
                 (and Overall Nutrition) in Infants

A. Unfortified foods:
   1. Maintain breastfeeding for at least 4 months
   2. No fresh cow milk until after about 9 months
   3. Use ascorbic-acid-rich foods and fruit juice and/or meat with meals of solid food after about 6 months
B. Iron- and ascorbic-acid-fortified foods:
   1. If cow milk formula is used, use a formula fortified with iron and ascorbic acid
   2. Use infant cereal or milk-cereal products that are fortified with iron or iron and ascorbic acid
   3. Use ascorbic-acid-fortified fruit juice with meals of solid foods
C. Iron supplementation (ferrous sulfate or similarly bioavailable compounds)
   1. In low-birthweight infants start iron at 2 to 8 weeks of age and continue at least through 6 months of age at the following amounts (from formula and/or drops) according to birthweight:
      1500–2500 gm   2 mg/kg/day
      1000–1500 gm   3 mg/kg/day
      < 1000 gm   4 mg/kg/day
   2. For established iron deficiency; 3 mg/kg/day

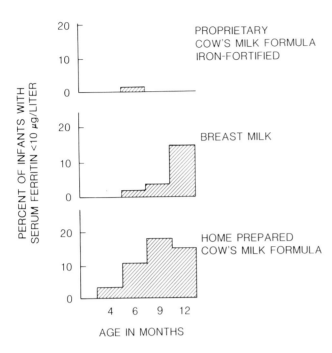

FIGURE 6. Depletion of iron stores as a function of milk feeding during infancy. The vertical axis shows the percentage of term infants with serum ferritin values below 10 µg/L. The percentage of infants with low serum ferritin values increased during the latter part of the first year of life in infants fed unfortified (home-prepared) formula and to a lesser degree in infants fed human milk (Saarinen, J Pediatr 1978;93: 177).

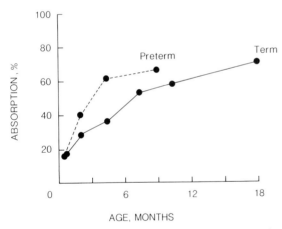

FIGURE 7. Age-related changes in absorption of iron in infancy. Studies were done by whole body counter after administration of 0.56 mg ^{59}Fe(II) with ascorbate under fasting conditions. Iron absorption increases with age as iron stores diminish. This change occurs earlier in the preterm than in the term infant. The data are from Götze et al. (Msch Kinderheilk 1970;118:210) and additional unpublished results from the same group.

retic risk of increased enteric infections. Transferrin and lactoferrin are iron-binding proteins present in milk. Both have bacteriostatic properties that disappear when they become saturated with iron. Despite animal and in vitro evidence that iron-fortified formula or oral iron medication might predispose to infections, epidemiologic support for this hypothesis in infants remains scant. This issue remains widely debated and is discussed in several reviews.[27,28]

Over two-thirds of the formula sold in the United States is iron-fortified.[29] The use of iron-fortified formula is a reliable way of preventing iron deficiency. The use of iron-fortified formula in the Federal Special Supplementary Food Program for Women, Infants and Children (WIC) has probably contributed to a decline in prevalence of iron deficiency among infants in the United States. The Committee on Nutrition of the American Academy of Pediatrics has recommended that the change from breast milk or formula to fresh cow milk can take place at any time between 6 and 12 months.[30] This author leans toward making the change closer to 12 months in order to provide a convenient and effective vehicle for fortification iron and to avoid the risk that parents will feed skim milk or low fat milk to infants; these are commonly used even though they provide an inadequate caloric density food for infants.

There is good evidence that fortifying cow milk formula with 12 mg iron/L as ferrous sulfate is effective in preventing iron deficiency. In much of Europe, cow milk formula is fortified with 6 mg iron/L. This lower amount probably is also adequate and results in almost as much iron assimilation because the percentage absorbed increases as the amount administered is decreased.[24] Thus, about 6% of the iron is absorbed from the formula fortified with 6 mg of iron/L compared with 4% from the 12 mg of iron/L formula.

Low Birthweight Infants. LBW infants fed human milk almost invariably develop iron deficiency anemia unless they are given iron supplements (Fig. 8).[31] The Committee on Nu-

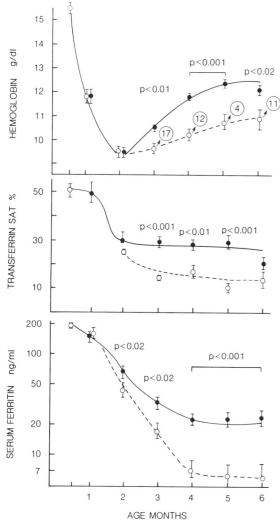

FIGURE 8. Iron supplementation in preterm infants. Serum ferritin, transferrin saturation, and hemoglobin concentrations are shown for infants who received no iron supplementation (—0—) or 2 mg iron/kg/day starting at 2 weeks of age (—•—). Means ± SEM are indicated. Serum ferritin concentration became significantly lower in the unsupplemented groups at 2 months of age, indicating the development of iron deficiency. The number of unsupplemented infants at each age who required initiation of iron supplementation because they developed anemia is shown within the circles. (From Lundström U, Siimes MA, et al. J Pediatr 1977;91:878, with permission.)

trition recommends 2 mg of iron/kg/day to a maximum of 15 mg iron/day for LBW infants.[32] This can be given as a single daily dose in the form of a liquid ferrous sulfate preparation starting at about one month of age. The iron is best absorbed when given before or between feedings. Intestinal intolerance to iron is rarely a problem in infants at these doses. A recent study showed no difference in prevalence of side effects between infants fed iron at a dose of 3 mg/kg/day and placebo-treated infants.[33] The dose should be increased for VLBW infants to accommodate their greater iron needs for growth.[6] A suggested dosage schedule is as follows:

Iron dose (as ferrous sulfate) mg/kg/day	Birth weight gm
4	< 1000
3	100–1500
2	1500–2500

Medication should be continued until at least 6 months of age and perhaps as long as 12 months, depending on the nature of the diet.

There are differences of opinion regarding the exact age at which iron medication should be started in preterm infants. There is no urgency to administer iron before iron stores become depleted at about 2 months of age. However, a starting age of 1 month seems equally appropriate, especially for infants in whom there has been substantial blood loss for laboratory studies or in association with the delivery. There is no value in earlier initiation of iron because iron stores actually become augmented in the first postnatal weeks as the fall in hemoglobin concentration releases more iron than can be recycled for the production of new red blood cells.

In *formula-fed preterm infants* it is reasonable to begin iron-fortified formula by about 1 or 2 months of age. Iron-fortified formula (containing 12 mg of iron/L) is adequate as the sole source of iron in infants with a birthweight > 1500 gm and supplies the equivalent of 2 mg of iron/kg. Infants of lower birthweight may need an additional 1 or 2 mg/kg as ferrous sulfate,[6] starting at about 1 month of age, to bring them up to a total of 3 mg/kg/day (birthweight 1000–1500gm) or 4 mg/kg/day (birthweight < 1000gm). As in the case of the human milk-fed preterm infant, the issue of exactly when to provide an additional source of iron is unresolved.

Evidence of vitamin E deficiency may still occur among < 1500 gm birthweight infants fed iron-fortified formula at 2 weeks of age.[33a] However, changes in formula composition, including decreased unsaturated fatty acids and increased vitamin E, have resulted in the partial resolution of this problem.[33b]

DIAGNOSIS

"Screening" for iron deficiency anemia is generally included as part of a routine health maintenance visit between about 9 and 12 months of age for term infants and between 3 and 6 months for preterm infants.[34] The prevalence of iron deficiency at these ages is probably well below 10% in the United States and substantially lower when nutritional counselling is emphasized.[35,36] **Acute infection is a frequent source of confusion because it is the most common cause of anemia other than iron deficiency,** and because laboratory abnormalities that mimic iron deficiency can persist for several weeks, even after recovery from a mild upper respiratory infection.[35] For this reason it is best to delay screening for anemia if there has been an illness in the previous few weeks.

The measurement of hemoglobin concentration is the most useful laboratory test in screening for iron deficiency anemia, since it directly reflects the quantity of the most abundant essential iron compound in the body. A micro-hematocrit may be more convenient in an office or clinic and is a close second choice. However, the hematocrit does not exactly parallel the hemoglobin concentration and is apt to be normal despite a subnormal hemoglobin value. This is because the microcytic, hypochromic cells of iron deficiency have slightly less hemoglobin than normal for any given packed cell volume. In addition, some degree of stiffness of the red cell membranes in iron deficiency probably results in more trapped plasma when red cells are packed by centrifugation.

The most helpful two values to remember in the screening for anemia in infants are:

Hemoglobin < 11.0 gm/dl
Hematocrit < 33%

These values apply from 6 months to 4 years of age, when iron deficiency anemia is most common. Values for the period between birth and 6 months of age differ so markedly according to age and birthweight that it is usually necessary to refer to tables or figures (Table 1, Fig. 1).

Since venipuncture is often difficult in infants, blood is more commonly obtained from skin puncture blood. While this is a justifiable sacrifice of accuracy for the sake of practicality, it is necessary to be aware of the *large sampling error* involved (a 1 SD sampling error of more than 1.0 gm/dl[14] compared to 0.3 gm/dl for venipuncture blood), even when appropriate care is taken to warm the extremity and avoid squeezing to obtain the sample. The practical implication of the large sampling error is that almost half of those infants whose hemoglobin is in the mild anemic range between 10.0 and 10.9 gm/dl prove not to be anemic when a repeat analysis is obtained on venipuncture blood.[31] Not surprisingly, there are differences of opinion about how to proceed when a skin puncture result suggests mild anemia in the following ranges:

Hemoglobin between 10.0 and 10.9 gm/dl or
Hematocrit between 30 and 33%

Some reasonable options are as follows:

1. A trial of iron therapy (see Iron Treatment) if the history is suggestive, i.e., low birthweight and/or prolonged use of fresh cow milk or unfortified formula.

2. A recheck of skin-puncture blood after one or more months if iron deficiency is thought to be unlikely on the basis of history or if there has been a recent infection.

3. A repeat hemoglobin analysis (and red cell indices) of venipuncture blood if the history is suggestive, with or without an additional laboratory testing.

The hemoglobin analysis is usually part of a routine of blood count done on an electronic counter. Such blood counts provide *red cell indices*, of which the mean red cell volume *(MCV)* and mean red cell hemoglobin *(MCH)* are the earliest to become abnormal in iron deficiency. If the indices are available, they should not be ignored. The following values between 6 months and 4 years of age support the diagnosis of iron deficiency if they accompany anemia or a low-normal hemoglobin:

MCV < 72 fl

MCH < 24 pg

Only a few causes of anemia are characterized by microcytosis, as indicated by a low MCV with or without low MCH; these include primarily iron deficiency and thalassemia minor.

Some electronic counters provide a quantitative measure of anisocytosis or the variation in red cell size, termed the *red cell distribution width* or RDW. Although the RDW appears on many laboratory reports, its usefulness remains uncertain. A few years ago, reports indicated that an elevated RDW was evidence of iron deficiency, whereas a normal RDW was typical of thalassemia minor and infection,[37] but this remains to be firmly established.

Confirmatory tests for iron deficiency include the serum ferritin, serum iron/iron binding capacity (transferrin saturation), and the erythrocyte protoporphyrin. Only rarely is it useful or cost effective to use more than one of these. The selection of a confirmatory test depends on availability, cost, and the most likely differential diagnosis in the particular clinical setting. However all three tests can be affected by infection.

The *serum ferritin* will probably prove to be the *most reliable test*, since it is depressed only in iron deficiency. It is most useful in infants who have been entirely well in the previous 2 weeks, since the result may be in the normal range despite iron deficiency if there has been a recent infection or inflammation; infection or inflammation raises serum ferritin concentrations. It requires a small amount of blood and can easily be done on a skin puncture sample.

The *erythrocyte protoporphyrin* can also be done on a skin puncture sample. Some clinics use an instrument that gives an immediate result on a drop of fresh blood. However the test is less well standardized than the other two confirmatory tests. Elevated values reflect depressed hemoglobin production and are characteristic not only of iron deficiency but also of concurrent or recent infection and lead toxicity.

The *serum iron/iron binding capacity* (transferrin saturation) is the most widely available of the three confirmatory tests but requires the largest volume of blood (venipuncture). Results fluctuate considerably with time of day, the nature of recent meals, and other factors. Typically the serum iron is depressed and the iron binding capacity elevated in iron deficiency, but the latter is not a consistent finding and its absence by no means excludes the diagnosis. A low transferrin saturation and serum iron are characteristics of both iron deficiency, or recent or concurrent infection.

The following values are consistent with iron deficiency in infancy:

> Serum ferritin < 10 ng/ml or µg/L
> Erythrocyte protoporphyrin > 2.5 µg/gm Hgb
> 30 µg/dl whole blood, or 70 µg/100 ml packed RBC
> Transferrin saturation < 10%

TREATMENT

In 1832, Blaud reported that tablets containing ferrous sulfate and potassium carbonate helped young women whose "coloring matter is lacking" in the blood (Rev Med Franc Etrang 1832;45:341–67). About 50 years later, Bunge, professor of medicine at Basel and one of the first to investigate mineral metabolism and nutrition, ridiculed Blaud's pills, which by then were in worldwide use. He pointed out that the iron ended up in the stool and insisted that only organic iron compounds could serve as precursors to hemoglobin. Inorganic forms of iron continued to be used but with less faith in their efficacy. Skepticism increased when Whipple and coworkers reported in 1920 that cooked liver was more effective than ferrous carbonate in promoting regeneration of blood in dogs made anemic by bleeding (Am J Physiol 1920;53:236). The failure to realize that iron in the intestine had to be in a *soluble* form to be absorbed was a major obstacle to research in iron nutrition for over a century. However, convincing evidence that inorganic iron compounds could be used for hemoglobin synthesis was finally presented in 1932 by Castle and coworkers who found that "the amount of iron given parenterally in hypochromic anemia corresponds closely to the amount of iron gained in the circulating hemoglobin" (J Clin Invest 1932;11:91–110).

Treatment of established iron deficiency anemia usually involves changes in the diet (see Prevention) as well as the administration of iron, usually as ferrous sulfate for infants. The most widely used preparations for infants are in liquid form and are administered by a dropper, marked to deliver 0.6 or 1.2 ml (15 and 30 mg of iron, respectively). A dose of 3 mg/kg/day represents about 30 mg/day for the average 1-year-old infant.[30] This dose is well tolerated as a single, before-breakfast dose.[33] If there are gastrointestinal symptoms, the dose can be divided or decreased. However, one dose per day has the advantage of favoring compliance.

Doses of iron in excess of 3 mg/kg/day unnecessarily risk side effects and do not result in a more rapid response. Indeed, even the lower amount of iron present in iron-fortified formula is rapidly effective in reversing severe iron deficiency anemia in preterm infants.[38] This is because iron absorption is markedly enhanced in iron deficiency, allowing small doses to be efficiently utilized. Parents should be alerted to the danger of toxicity due to accidental ingestion and reassured about the dark color of the stool with iron treatment.

Staining of teeth may occur, but this is not permanent and can be removed by gentle brushing.

The rate of response to iron treatment is rapid, with half correction of the anemia, on the average, after 2 weeks, and two-thirds correction after 4 weeks. A repeat hemoglobin (or hematocrit) determination to check for a therapeutic response can therefore be done after 2 to 4 weeks of treatment. Treatment should be maintained for 3 to 4 months to allow some accumulation of storage iron.

The most common cause for lack of a response is failure to administer the medication. Only rarely is there a failure to absorb iron; this can be detected by measuring a fasting serum iron concentration and repeating the determination 2–4 hours after a test dose of 3 mg iron as ferrous sulfate/kg.[39] The increase in serum iron should be greater than 30 µg/dl.

In some infants, iron deficiency anemia, presumed to have developed primarily on a nutritional basis, recurs after it has been corrected by treatment. If this happens, the possibility of occult blood loss should be investigated.

IRON EXCESS

Two important issues in regard to iron excess involve the predisposition to vitamin E deficiency that may result from administration of iron to preterm infants during the first postnatal month and iron poisoning as a result of accidental ingestion.

Preterm infants weighing less than 1500 gm at birth have marginal supplies of vitamin E due to low placental transfer of the vitamin, decreased tissue stores, and impaired absorption (Chapter 16). Their vitamin E needs generally can be satisfied either by breast milk or by the currently marketed infant formulas that are not iron-fortified. However, even a dose of 2 mg of iron/kg per day at 2 weeks of age (an amount that can be supplied by iron-fortified formula) can predispose to vitamin E deficiency.[33a] For this reason, it seems advisable to delay giving iron-fortified formula until 1 month of age to preterm infants weighing less than 1500 gm at birth.

Accidental ingestion of iron remains one of the most common causes of fatal poisoning in children. When prescribing iron for infants, it is important to caution parents to keep the medications out of reach, particularly of older siblings between the ages of 1 to 5 years. Patients who are found to have a serum iron concentration in excess of 300 µg/dl commonly have diarrhea, vomiting, leukocytosis, hyperglycemia, and radiographic evidence of iron ingestion (radiographic signs usually can be seen with tablets rather than with liquid preparations).[39a] Management involves prompt removal of iron by induction of emesis or by lavage with a 1 to 5% bicarbonate solution and chelation of absorbed iron by administration of deferoxamine.

MEGALOBLASTIC ANEMIAS

Megaloblastic anemias are relatively rare in infants.[40,41] The causes in order of frequency are folate deficiency, vitamin B_{12} deficiency and inborn errors of metabolism including hereditary orotic aciduria.

In 1879, Paul Ehrlich described a histologic staining technique that facilitated the identification of various types of blood cells (Arch Anat Physiol Phys Abth 1879;571). Shortly thereafter he described large nucleated red cells, which he called megaloblasts, in the peripheral blood of patients with pernicious anemia (Berlin Klin Wschr 1880;117:405). In 1907, Arneth provided a detailed report on the morphologic abnormalities of neutrophils in peripheral blood. Figure 9 shows one of his diagrams illustrating both the large neutrophil size and the increased number of nuclear lobulations in a patient with severe megaloblastic anemia.

Many of the laboratory manifestations of megaloblastic anemias are related to an impairment of DNA synthesis, particularly in rapidly proliferating hematopoietic cells. These characteristics will be described before discussing the individual disorders.

Hypersegmentation of the nucleus in circulating neutrophils is a useful aid to early diagnosis, since it is easy to detect on a routine blood smear (Fig. 10). Hypersegmentation should be suspected when a quick examination shows numerous neutrophils with four, five, or more distinct lobes. This impression can then be confirmed by a lobe count in 100 neutrophils; an average of more than 3.4 lobes per cell is considered abnormal. However, more frequently the subjective impression of hypersegmentation will lead to analyses of serum and red cell folate and serum vitamin B_{12} concentrations. About 1% of healthy individuals have hypersegmented neutrophils. Consequently, if hypersegmentation is used as a basis for diagnosis, its disappearance should be verified after treatment.

Increased red cell size is believed to result

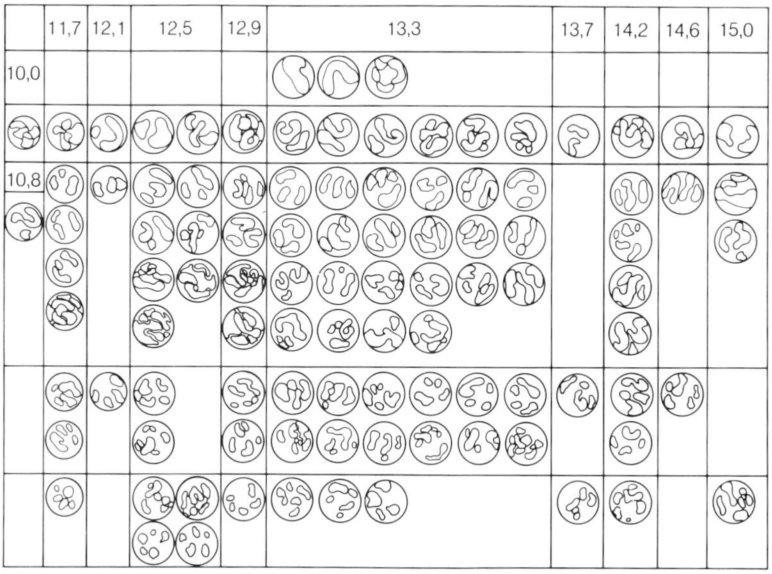

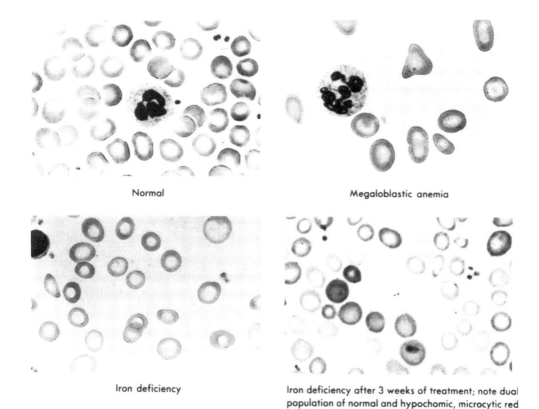

	11,7	12,1	12,5	12,9	13,3	13,7	14,2	14,6	15,0
10,0									

FIGURE 9. Nuclear hypersegmentation and enlargement of neutrophils in a patient with severe megaloblastic anemia. The diagram shows cells of increasing diameter in μm in the vertical columns from left to right and increasing numbers of nuclear lobules along the horizontal rows from top to bottom. (From Arneth J. Diagnose und Therapie der Anämien. Würzburger Abhandlungen aus dem Gesamtgebiet der praktischen Medizin. 1 Suppl Bd, 1907.)

Normal

Megaloblastic anemia

Iron deficiency

Iron deficiency after 3 weeks of treatment; note dual population of normal and hypochomic, microcytic red cells.

FIGURE 10.   Peripheral blood morphology.

TABLE 5. Causes of Folate and Vitamin B_{12} Deficiency

	Folate	Vitamin B_{12}
Inadequate intake	Evaporated milk formulas, goat milk, prolonged heating of formula	Breast milk of vegetarians who consume no eggs or dairy products
Inadequate absorption	Chronic diarrhea, broad spectrum antibiotics, congenital malabsorption, inflammatory bowel disease, sprue, gluten enteropathy	Pernicious anemia, disease or absence of terminal ileum
Inadequate transport or utilization	Drugs	Congenital deficiencies of transcobalamin I or II
Increased requirement	Hemolytic disease of very low birthweight newborn infants. Deficiencies in enzymes of folate metabolism	Deficiencies in enzymes of vitamin B_{12} metabolism

from a skipped cell division due to impaired DNA synthesis during red cell maturation. It is not as early a finding as hypersegmentation. In clinical practice, an elevated MCV for age (Table 1) is often the first evidence of a megaloblastic disorder, because it is part of a routine blood count by electronic counter. However, *blood loss* and *hemolytic anemia* are far more common causes of an elevated MCV; these two conditions are associated with polychromatophilia and reticulocytosis attributable to the *large cell volume of young erythrocytes* from increased red cell production. The elevated MCV of increased red cell production can be easily distinguished from that of megaloblastic disorders, since only the latter is associated with hypersegmented neutrophils and macro-ovalocytes (large oval red cells). The great variation in size of red cells (anisocytosis) is also evident on the blood smear and is reflected by an elevated RDW. Megaloblastic, nucleated red blood cells are noted in the peripheral blood in severe or advanced cases. Megaloblasts are nucleated red blood cells that are larger than normal and in which the nucleus appears immature for the stage of cytoplasmic development. The megaloblastic disorders may also be associated with mild neutropenia and/or thrombocytopenia. Megaloblastic changes of the bone marrow are obvious only with relatively severe and chronic deficiencies.

Other laboratory abnormalities common to megaloblastic anemias are an elevated lactate dehydrogenase and occasionally a mild increase in unconjugated bilirubin, both reflecting ineffective erythropoiesis (destruction of immature red cells before release from the bone marrow).

FOLATE DEFICIENCY

In 1937, Lucy Wills and coworkers inferred the existence of a new nutritional factor in crude liver, which was subsequently shown to be folic acid. She found that crude liver cured megaloblastic anemia in a group of pregnant women in India who had had no response to a partially purified, aqueous extract of liver that was known to be effective in treating pernicious anemia (Biochem J 1937;31:2136–47). Folic acid was first isolated in pure form from four tons of spinach and given its name by Mitchell and associates in 1941 (Am Chem Soc J 1941;63:2284). Only a few years later, Zuelzer and Ogden reported 25 infants with megaloblastic anemia who were successfully treated with folic acid (Am J Dis Child 1946;71:211–243).

Folate deficiency may result from a low dietary intake or malabsorption of folate, or vitamin-drug interactions (Table 5).[40,41] It can develop rapidly within a few weeks of birth, because there is scant storage of folate in the newborn (in contrast to large stores of vitamin B_{12}).

Dietary Lack of Folate

A dietary lack of folate is most common under circumstances that increase its requirement, such as rapid body or cell growth in the preterm infant and in severe hemolytic disease of the newborn. There is a group of rare inborn errors of folate metabolism that may present with megaloblastic anemia in infancy. Some of the various mechanisms involved have been reviewed.[41a]

Infants require about 10 times as much folate as adults on the basis of body weight. The recommended intake of folate for infants varies between 30 and 65 µg/day. Folate is abundant in green vegetables and liver. Breast milk and fresh pasteurized cow milk contain about 50 µg/L. Heat treatment lowers the folate content of milk. Thus, heat sterilizing a home-prepared formula can decrease its folate content by about half. Evaporated milk has less than 20 µg of folate/reconstituted liter. The widespread use of heat-sterilized, evaporated milk formulas in the 1940s and 1950s probably accounted for folate deficiency being common at that time. Goat milk is an even poorer source of folate than evaporated milk, with less than 6 µg/L, and severe megaloblastic anemia may result if it is the main source of calories.

Among otherwise healthy infants, folate deficiency has been reported primarily in low birthweight infants who were fed formulas based on heated or boiled evaporated milk[42,43] or pasteurized milk.[44] In proprietary infant formulas, the presence of ascorbic acid decreases the loss of folic acid with heating, but evaporated milk and pasteurized milk contain relatively little ascorbic acid.

It is doubtful whether infants fed human milk or proprietary cow milk formulas are at risk of nutritional folate deficiency. Breast-fed term infants have far higher serum and red cell folate values throughout infancy than adults.[45] Term infants fed proprietary formulas usually have elevated folate levels, probably because of the very high level of folate fortification now used in the United States. Proprietary cow milk formulas contain about 160 µg of folate/L compared to about 50 µg/L in human milk.[45] The current folate content of U.S. formulas should therefore provide generously even for low birthweight infants once their formula consumption reaches about 300 mg/day. However, at least some European formulas may be marginal in this respect, e.g., a formula containing 20 µg of folate/L resulted in much lower serum folate levels in preterm than in term, breastfed infants.[46]

Very low birth weight infants probably should be given supplemental folate, as well as a supplement that includes other vitamins, to support their very rapid growth, especially until their human milk or formula intake increases sufficiently to provide adequate folate (about 300 ml/day, or at a body weight of 2000 gm). Before that time, supplemental folic acid at a dose of about 0.1 mg/day seems reasonable. The same dose for a period of 2 or 3 months also seems appropriate for infants with hemolytic disease of the newborn, whose folate requirements are greater than normal.[47]

Malabsorption of Folate

Folate deficiency due to malabsorption may occur with chronic diarrhea. At least two mechanisms are likely to be responsible. First, diarrhea may result in a deficiency in intestinal conjugase. Consequently, the conjugated polyglutamate forms of folate that predominate in the diet may not be broken down to the monoglutamate form that can be absorbed. Thus, a small dose of unconjugated folate (the usual therapeutic form) can produce a prompt therapeutic response, whereas large amounts of dietary polyglutamic folate might have no effect. Second, diarrhea may interfere with the normal enterohepatic circulation of folate by resulting in excessive losses due to rapid intestinal passage. There are also rare cases of congenital malabsorption of folate that have been recognized in infants who developed severe megaloblastic anemia at 2 to 3 months of age.[48]

Intestinal bacteria normally may supplement the dietary folate supply. Partial elimination of intestinal bacteria by prolonged use of broad-spectrum antibiotics may be associated with folate deficiency.

Drug Interactions

Folate analogues such as methotrexate and certain antibiotics such as trimethoprim (Septra, Bactrim) inhibit dihydrofolate reductase, an enzyme required for the production of the active form of the vitamin. Megaloblastic changes in bone marrow and peripheral blood are common with methotrexate therapy. A different mechanism is responsible for the folate deficiency associated with the use of phenytoin and other anticonvulsants. These drugs interact with polyglutamates in the intestinal lumen and interfere with their digestion to the absorbable monoglutamate form. Administration of pterolyglutamic acid, the usual therapeutic form of folate that is unconjugated, reverses the folate deficiency.

Diagnosis[33,34,41]

The manifestations of dietary folate deficiency in infants include hypersegmentation of neutrophils,[42,43] megaloblastic changes on the blood smear,[43] generally noted between 6 and 12 weeks of age, and poor growth.[44] Anemia and neurologic manifestations such as hypotonia are only evident in severe or advanced cases. As a deficiency of folate progresses, abnormalities develop in the following sequence: low serum folate, hypersegmentation of neutrophil nuclei, low red cell folate, megaloblastic bone marrow, and macrocytic anemia. Most cases are mild and do not progress through this entire sequence.

Folate deficiency may first be suspected when hypersegmented neutrophils and/or elevation of the MCV are noted. Confirmation of the diagnosis is then obtained by a determination of serum and red cell folate, and serum vitamin B_{12} concentration. Although serum folate reflects recent dietary changes, it may be too sensitive to dietary fluctuations to be an ideal test of chronic folate status. The red cell folate level is a more stable and reliable index of folate status. A serum folate below 3 ng/ml is subnormal; the lower limit for red cell folate is 140 ng/ml. Serum vitamin B_{12} levels are normal in folic acid deficiency. However, **a potential source of confusion is the low red cell folate that can occur in vitamin B_{12} deficiency** (see p. 233).

Folate deficiency is likely to coexist with iron deficiency in infants fed only an evaporated milk formula or goat milk. With this combination of deficiencies, the MCV and some of the other laboratory tests give unpredictable results. However, hypersegmentation of the neutrophil nuclei is still likely to be a helpful test, unless the folate supply from the diet or from medication was increased during the few days prior to the test.

Treatment

A therapeutic dose of folate, 0.5-1.0 mg/day of pteroylglutamic acid (10 or more times the daily allowance), may be given when the diagnosis of folate deficiency is firmly established. Large doses of folate mistakenly given to a patient with vitamin B_{12} deficiency can *worsen* the clinical manifestations. A safe maintenance dose to prevent deficiency or to correct it slowly is 0.1 mg/day.

Folic acid is available in 0.1, 0.4, 0.8, and 1.0-mg scored tablets. Folate in liquid multivitamin preparations for oral use is not available commercially because of its lability under the pH conditions used in such formulations. However, a pharmacist can use vials of injectable folate to formulate a liquid preparation that can be stored under refrigeration for about 1 month. If anemia is present, treatment can be monitored by the reticulocyte response and by the rate of rise in hemoglobin and hematocrit, which are similar to the response during the iron treatment of iron deficiency anemia.

VITAMIN B_{12} DEFICIENCY

The term *pernicious anemia* originated in the late 19th century to describe a syndrome that was invariably fatal. In 1926, Minot and Murphy reported on the dramatic response of 45 patients with pernicious anemia after they were fed 120 to 240 gm of cooked liver per day (JAMA 1926;87:470). This observation led to their being awarded the Nobel Prize in 1934. Crystalline vitamin B_{12} was isolated and named in 1948 (Rickes et al. Science 1948; 107:396). Within months, West showed that the injection of minute amounts of the pure vitamin was highly effective in reversing pernicious anemia (Science 1948; 107:398).

Vitamin B_{12} deficiency is important despite its rarity because of the danger of *irreversible neurologic damage* unless it is diagnosed and treated early, and because most causes of the deficiency require continuing therapy throughout life.[40,41] Most cases are due to a *defect in absorption*.

Dietary vitamin B_{12} is usually present in considerable excess over requirements. **The vitamin is unique in that it enters the food chain entirely through synthesis by microorganisms.** The vitamin is absent in plants (except for the bacteria in the root nodules of certain legumes and through contamination by microorganisms). Exclusively breast-fed infants ingest about 0.3 µg/day of vitamin B_{12}, an amount that is considered more than adequate. **An exception is breast milk from vegetarian mothers** who regularly consume no eggs or dairy products. Prolonged consumption of such a diet will lead to a markedly subnormal concentration of vitamin B_{12} in maternal milk and eventually to megaloblastic anemia with neurologic changes in the nursing infant.

The absorption of a physiologic amount of vitamin B_{12} is dependent upon the formation of a complex between the vitamin and a mucoprotein (intrinsic factor) produced by the parietal cells of the stomach. The complex is taken up by the distal ileum. Vitamin B_{12} is then freed from the complex and released into the circulation. In the plasma, vitamin B_{12} is bound to a specific serum transport protein (transcobalamin II). The vitamin is stored in the liver. These stores are large in the newborn, averaging about 25 µg, and are rarely depleted before 1 year of age.

Pathogenesis of Vitamin B_{12} Deficiency

The types of conditions that can lead to vitamin B_{12} deficiency are summarized in Table 4. With the exception of dietary deficiency, most vitamin B_{12} deficiency results from the absence of intrinsic factor or from a failure to absorb the vitamin-intrinsic factor complex.

The term *pernicious anemia*[50] is reserved for those conditions in which there is a deficiency of intrinsic factor. Two types of pernicious anemia are distinguished in children; in both of them, malabsorption of vitamin B_{12} can be corrected if intrinsic factor is supplied. *Juvenile pernicious anemia* occurs in older children and is similar to pernicious anemia in the adult.[51] Gastric atrophy and decreased secretion of acid and pepsin commonly are associated with antibodies to intrinsic factor or to parietal cells. Concurrent endocrinopathies and manifestations of immune deficiency also may be present. In contrast, *congenital pernicious anemia* usually is evident during late infancy.[52] Although secretion of normally active intrinsic factor is lacking, the morphology and secretory function of the gastric mucosa are normal. There are no demonstrable antibodies or associated endocrinopathies, and long-term follow-up examination does not show progression to the typical adult form of pernicious anemia. An autosomal recessive inheritance pattern is suggested by a high incidence of consanguinity and the occurrence in siblings.[53]

Other causes of deficiency are not properly called pernicious anemia, since there is no lack of intrinsic factor. These include removal of the vitamin from the intestinal lumen by parasites or bacteria, as with heavy infestations of fish tapeworm *(Diphyllobothrium latum)*. Bacterial consumption of vitamin B_{12} in intestinal diverticuli or blind loops also can result in removal of the vitamin before it is absorbed.

Since vitamin B_{12} is selectively absorbed by the distal half of the ileum,[45] surgical removal of this area of bowel for treatment of intussusception, regional enteritis, or congenital malformation results in a lifelong deficiency.[54] Chronic disease of the ileum, most commonly regional enteritis, can also produce a deficiency of vitamin B_{12} but usually one that is

mild and manifested primarily by a low serum concentration of the vitamin. Vitamin B_{12} absorption and transport are also decreased in a rare inherited deficiency or abnormality of transcobalamin II.[55] Presumably the transport protein is necessary as an acceptor in the transport of the vitamin across the ileal mucosa.

Diagnosis

Most forms of vitamin B_{12} deficiency do not become evident until late infancy, since neonatal liver stores normally are so abundant. Exceptions are the development of megaloblastic anemia in the breastfed infant of a mother with vitamin B_{12} deficiency and in the inherited deficiency of transcobalamin II. Depression of serum vitamin B_{12} below 100 pg/ml and the appearance of hypersegmented neutrophils are the earliest manifestations.[37] Late findings of vitamin B_{12} deficiency include megaloblastic anemia, megaloblastic changes in the bone marrow, leukopenia, thrombocytopenia, and mild jaundice, similar to the findings of folate deficiency. However, neurologic manifestations generally are quite distinct from those of folate lack. They include posterior and lateral column demyelinization in the spinal cord and associated paresthesias, sensory deficits, loss of deep tendon reflexes, slowing of mental processes, confusion, and memory defects. Neurologic changes may precede anemia. **Inappropriate administration of large doses of folate (well in excess of 0.1 mg/day in an adult) to vitamin B_{12}-deficient individuals can aggravate the neurologic manifestations.**

The serum folate concentration is usually normal or elevated in vitamin B_{12} deficiency, but the red cell folate can be a source of confusion since it is often decreased. Consequently, all three tests, *serum B_{12}, serum folate,* and *red cell folate,* are helpful in the differential diagnosis of vitamin B_{12} and folate deficiency. If the dietary history is unremarkable, absorption of [57]Co-vitamin B_{12} may be determined by the Schilling test. A standard dose of the labeled vitamin is given orally after a fast; 2 hours later a flushing dose of vitamin B_{12} is given parenterally. This allows the excretion of labeled vitamin B_{12} into the urine in readily detectable amounts. Less than 7% of the administered label is recovered in the urine in 24 hours if there is a lack of intrinsic factor or a defective absorption of vitamin B_{12} for other reasons. If absorption is impaired, the Schilling test is repeated with oral intrinsic factor. Enhancement of urinary excretion of the radiolabel with intrinsic factor confirms the diagnosis of intrinsic factor deficiency. The availability of assays for intrinsic factor in gastric juice provides an alternative diagnostic tool.

Treatment

Most cases of vitamin B_{12} deficiency that are not of dietary origin require treatment throughout life. Optimal doses for infants and children are not as well defined as those for adults. If the diagnosis is firmly established, an intramuscular dose of 50 to 100 μg may be used to initiate therapy. Maintenance therapy then consists of monthly intramuscular injections in the same dosage range.

Hereditary Orotic Aciduria

Megaloblastic anemias related to deficiencies of folic acid or vitamin B_{12} should be distinguished from the rare disorder of pyrimidine biosynthesis, hereditary orotic aciduria.[56] This defect may result in megaloblastic anemia, leukopenia, retarded growth and development, and excessive urinary excretion of orotic acid. It appears to be inherited as an autosomal recessive trait. The heterozygotes are detectable by enzyme assays but are hematologically normal and are asymptomatic.

CASE REPORT

A 3-month-old infant was seen at a follow-up office visit and was found to have a hemoglobin concentration of 8.0 gm/dl. The infant weighed 1650 gm at birth and was discharged from the nursery after an uneventful course at 4 weeks of age. The infant has been fed pumped breast milk since shortly after birth and was continued on breast-feeding after discharge. Weight gain was satisfactory. The infant had had a hemoglobin concentration of 9.0 gm/dl at 2 months of age.

Questions and Answers

Q.   Should the infant have been treated with iron drops previously? If so, starting when?
A.   Iron in the form of ferrous sulfate (with multivitamins) should have been started at the time of discharge at a dose of 2 mg elemental iron/kg/day.

Q.   Was the infant anemic at the 2 month visit?
A.   No (see Table 1).

Q.   Was the infant anemic at 3 months of age?

A.   Yes (see Table 1). Furthermore, any significant fall in hemoglobin concentration between 2 and 3 months is unusual and should suggest iron deficiency.

Q.   The mother had been advised to give iron and vitamin drops on discharge but disregarded the advice, believing that breast milk was a "complete food." If the mother now agrees to administer the iron-vitamin preparation, will this be adequate or is a higher dose of iron necessary?
A.   The iron-vitamin preparation (or iron alone, at 2 mg/kg/day) will be adequate to allow for treatment of the anemia.

Q.   When should the hemoglobin concentration be checked again?
A.   In 3 to 4 weeks at which time the concentration should have risen to a value near or within the normal range.

REFERENCES

1. Lundström V, Siimes MA. Red blood cells values in low birth weight infants: ages at which values become equivalent to those of term infants. J Pediatr 1980;86:1040–1042.
2. Saarinen VM, Siimes MA. Developmental changes in red blood cell counts and indices of infants after exclusion of iron deficiency by laboratory criteria and continuous iron supplementation. Pediatrics 1978;92:412–416.
3. Dallman PR, Siimes MA, Stekel A. Iron deficiency in infancy and childhood. Am J Clin Nutr 1980;33:86–118.
4. Dallman PR. Anemia of prematurity. Ann Rev Med 1981;32:143–60.
5. Brown MS, Phibbs RH, Garcia JF, Dallman PR. Postnatal changes in erythropoietin levels in untransfused premature infants. J Pediatr 1983;103:612–617.
6. Siimes MA. Iron nutrition in low-birth-weight infants. In Stekel A (ed): Iron Nutrition in Infancy and Childhood. New York, Raven Press, 1984;75–91.
7. Stockman JA III, Garcia JF, Oski FA. The anemia of prematurity. Factors governing the erythropoietin reponse. N Engl J Med 1977;296:647–650.
8. Rönnholm KAR, Siimes MA. Haemoglobin concentration depends on protein intake in small preterm infants fed human milk. Arch Dis Child 1985;60:99–104.
9. Stockman JA, Clark DA. Weight gain: a response to transfusion in selected preterm infants. Am J Dis Child 1984;138:828–830.
10. Blank JP, Sheagren TG, Vajaria J, et al. The role of RBC transfusion in the premature infant. Am J Dis Child 1984;138:831–833.
11. Fomon SJ, Ziegler EE, Nelson SE, Edwards BB. Cow's milk feeding in infancy: gastrointestinal blood loss and iron nutritional status. J Pediatr 1981;98:540–545.
12. Woodruff CW, Clark JL. The role of fresh cow's milk in iron deficiency. I. Albumin turnover in infants with iron deficiency anemia. Am J Dis Child 1972;124:18–23.
13. Wilson JF, Lahey ME, Heiner DC. Studies on iron metabolism: V. Further observation on cow's milk-induced gastrointestinal bleeding in infants with iron-deficiency anemia. J Pediatr 1974;84:335–344.
14. Blanchette VS, Zipursky A. Assessment of anemia in newborn infants. Clin Perinatol 1984;11:489–510.
15. Bothwell TH, Charlton RW, Cook JD, Finch CA. Iron Metabolism in Man. Oxford, Blackwell Scientific Publications, 1979.
16. Hallberg L. Bioavailability of dietary iron in man. Ann Rev Nutr 1981;1:123–147.
17. Charlton RW, Bothwell TH. Iron absorption. Ann Rev Med 1983;34:55–68.
18. Cook JD, Bothwell TH. Availability of iron from infant food. In Stekel A (ed): Nutrition in Infancy and Childhood. New York, Raven Press, 1984;119–143.

19. Dallman PR. Iron deficiency in the weanling: a nutritional problem on the way to resolution. Acta Paediatr Scand 1986;323:59-67.
20. Saarinen UM. Need for iron supplementation in infants on prolonged breast feeding. J Pediatr 1978;93:177-180.
21. Saarinen UM, Siimes MA, Dallman PR. Iron absorption in infants: High bioavailability of breast milk iron as indicated by the extrinsic tag method of iron absorption and by the concentration of serum ferritin. J Pediatr 1977;91:36-39.
22. McMillan JA, Landaw SA, Oski FA. Iron sufficiency in breast-fed infants and the availability of iron from human milk. Pediatrics 1976;58:686-691
23. Rios E, Hunter RE, Cook JD, et al. The absorption of iron as supplements in infant cereal and infant formulas. Pediatrics 1975;55:686-693.
24. Saarinen UM, Siimes MA. Iron absorption from infant formula and the optimal level of iron suppplementation. Acta Paediatr Scand 1977;66:719-722.
25. Committee on Nutrition. Pediatric Nutrition Handbook. Elk Grove, Illinois, American Academy of Pediatrics, 1985.
26. Oski FA, Landaw SA. Inhibition of iron absorption from human milk by baby food. Am J Dis Child 1980;134:459-460.
27. Committee on Nutrition. Relationship between iron status and incidence of infection in infancy. Pediatrics 1978; 62:246-250.
28. Weinberg ED. Iron withholding: a defense against infection and neoplasm. Phys Rev 1984;64:65-102.
29. Martinez GA, Krieger FW. 1984 milk feeding patterns in the United States. Pediatrics, 1985;76:1004-1008.
30. Committee on Nutrition, American Academy of Pediatrics. The use of whole cow's milk in infancy. Pediatrics 1983, 72:253-255.
31. Lundström U, Siimes MA, Dallman PR. At what age does iron supplementation become necessary in low-birth-weight infants? J Pediatr 1977;91:878-883.
32. Committee on Nutrition, American Academy of Pediatrics. Iron balance and requirements in infancy. Pediatrics 1969; 43:134-142.
33. Reeves JD, Yip R. Lack of adverse side effects of oral ferrous sulfate therapy in 1-year-old infants. Pediatrics 1985;75: 352-355.
33a Gross SJ, Gabriel E. Vitamin E status in preterm infants fed human milk or infant formula. J Pediatr 1985;106:635-640.
33b Zipurski A. Vitamin E deficiency anemia in newborn infants. Clin Perinatol 1984;11:393-402.
34. Dallman PR, Reeves JD. Laboratory diagnosis of iron deficiency. In Steckel A (ed): Nutrition in Infancy and Childhood. New York, Raven Press, 1984;11-44.
35. Dallman PR, Yip R, Johnson C. Prevalence and causes of anemia in the United States, 1976-80. Am J Clin Nutr 1984;39:437-445.
36. Reeves JD, Yip R, Kiley VA, Dallman PR. Iron deficiency in infants: The influence of milk antecedent infection J Pediatr 1984;105:874-879.
37. Bessman JD, Gilmer PR Jr, Gardner FH. Improved classification of anemias by MCV and RDW. Am J Clin Path 1983;

80:322-326.
38. Gorten MK, Cross ER. Iron metabolism in premature infants. II. Prevention of iron deficiency. J Pediatr 1964;64:509-520.
39. Massa E, MacLean WC Jr, Lopez de Romaña G, et al. Oral iron absorption in infantile protein-energy malnutrition. J Pediatr 1978;93:1045-49.
39a Lacouture PG, Wason S, Temple AR, et al. Emergency assessment of severity in iron overdose by clinical and laboratory methods. J Pediatr 1981;39:89-91.
40. Meyers PA, Miller DR. Megaloblastic anemias. In Miller DR, Baehner RL, McMillan CW (eds): Blood Diseases of Infancy and Childhood. St. Louis, C.V. Mosby Co., 1984; 147-170
41. Shojania AM. Folic acid and vitamin B_{12} deficiency in pregnancy. Clin Perinatol 1984;11:433-459.
41a Erbe RW. Inborn errors of folate metabolism. N Engl J Med 1975;293:753-57, 807-812.
42. Burland WL, Simpson K, Lord J. Response of low birth-weight infants to treatment with folic acid. Arch Dis Child 1971;46:189-194.
43. Strelling MK, Blackledge DG, Goodall HB. Diagnosis and management of folate deficiency in low birthweight infants. Arch Dis Child 1979;54:271-277.
44. Matoth Y, Zehavi I, Topper E, Klein T. Folate nutrition and growth in infancy. Arch Dis Child 1979;54:699-702.
45. Smith AM, Picciano MF, Deering RH. Folate intake and blood concentrations of term infants. Am J Clin Nutr 1985;41:590-598.
46. Ek J, Behnke L, Halvorsen KS, Magnus E. Plasma and red cell folate values and folate requirements in formula-fed premature infants. Eur J Pediatr 1984;142:78-82.
47. Gandy G, Jacobson W. Influence of folic acid on birthweight and growth of the erythroblastic infant. Arch Dis Child 1977;52:1-6, 7-15, 16-21.
48. Poncz M, Colman N, Herbert V, et al. Therapy of congenital folate malabsorption. J Pediatr 1981;98:76-79.
49. Lindenbaum J. Status of laboratory testing in the diagnosis of megaloblastic anemia. Blood 1983;61:624.
50. Kass L. Pernicious Anemia. Philadelphia, W.B. Saunders, 1976,247.
51. Spurling CL, Sacks MS, Jiji RM. Juvenile pernicious anemia. N Engl J Med 1964;271:995-1003.
52. Heisel MA, Siegel SE, Falk RE, et al. Congenital pernicious anemia: Report of seven patients, with studies of the extended family. J Pediatr 1984;105:564-568.
53. Furuhjelm V, Nevanlinna HR. Inheritance of selective malabsorption of vitamin B_{12}. Scand J Haematol 1973;11:27-34.
54. Valman HB, Roberts PD. Vitamin B_{12} absorption after resection of ileum in childhood. Arch Dis Child 1974;49:932-935.
55. Hitzig WH, Dohmann V, Pluss HJ, Vischer D. Hereditary transcobalamin II deficiency: clinical findings in a family. J Pediatr 1974;85:622-628
56. Rogers LE, Warford LR, Patterson RB, Porter FS. Hereditary orotic aciduria. A case with family studies. Pediatrics 1968;42:415-422.

13

Water-Soluble Vitamins: C, B$_1$, B$_2$, B$_6$, Niacin, Biotin, and Pantothenic Acid

RICHARD J. SCHANLER M.D.

ABSTRACT

The recommended intakes of seven water-soluble vitamins (ascorbic acid, thiamin, riboflavin, niacin, pyridoxine, biotin, and pantothenic acid) are evaluated for term and preterm infants fed either enterally or parenterally. The estimated vitamin needs for the term infant are satisfied by feeding either human milk or commercial formula. The ascorbic acid intake from evaporated milk is inadequate. The preterm infant does not receive sufficient water-soluble vitamins from human milk. The vitamin needs during total parenteral nutrition (TPN) for term and preterm infants are unknown. Recent data are included that suggest that the intake of these water-soluble vitamins from TPN is adequate for term infants, whereas preterm infants receive an excessive intake of ascorbic acid and biotin.

INTRODUCTION

"No animal can live on a mixture of pure protein, fat, and carbohydrate . . . even when the inorganic material is carefully adjusted . . . other unknown substances are essential to life."[1]

This was the belief echoed in 1906 by Gowland Hopkins of Cambridge when he realized that his rats failed to grow when fed a mixture of known nutrients derived from milk.[1] He was able to induce normal growth when small amounts of untreated milk were added to their diet. Casimir Funk coined the term "vitamine" in 1912 to illustrate that these "unknown substances" were vital to life. Soon after, J.C. Drummond modernized the spelling and suggested that the consecutive alphabetical nomenclature be adopted since so many of these vital nutrients were being discovered.[1]

It must be noted that the concept of vitamin-deficiency disease was novel in the early 1900s. The clinical symptoms of vitamin-deficient patients were attributed to undiscovered infectious agents. The early discoverers of vitamins had to fight the prevailing opinion that positive factors, such as infectious agents, were responsible for what we now call deficiency ("negative factors") diseases.[2]

In 1988 a need still exists for information concerning vitamin needs for the infant born either at term or prematurely. The recommended intakes of ascorbic acid, thiamin, riboflavin, pyridoxine, niacin, biotin, and pantothenic acid for term and preterm infants do not address minimal intakes or intakes required during periods of stress. **The current, best estimate of the vitamin needs is based on the term infant who is breast-fed ad libitum.**[3] This model, unfortunately, does not apply to the very low birthweight, preterm infant.

In the first six months of life the breast-fed term infant achieves a satisfactory intake of these water-soluble vitamins, provided the maternal diet is adequate.[4] The commercial formula-fed term infant also achieves an optimal intake of these vitamins.[4] Recent studies that document the milk consumption of breast-fed infants during the first four months of life conclude that, although normal growth patterns are achieved, the milk intakes of these normal infants are significantly lower than intakes previously reported for formula-fed infants.[5,6] Our knowledge of optimal intakes of water-soluble vitamins, therefore, may be inaccurate. Because there are no reports of water-soluble vitamin deficiency states in breast-fed infants of well-nourished mothers, actual water-soluble vitamin needs may be less than previously suggested. In addition, several investigators recently have re-evaluated the water-soluble vitamin composition of human milk. These data, for certain vitamins, differ from values reported earlier. For these reasons, the recommended intakes of water-soluble vitamins may need reevaluation.

The maintenance vitamin needs of the preterm infant are unknown. Such infants may be at increased risk of deficiency for these vitamins because of limited intake and absorption.[3,4,7] In addition, problems peculiar to the preterm infant, such as high protein intakes, use of whey vs casein-dominant formulas, exposure to hyperoxic environments, lack of early nutritional intervention, and use of multiple medications, may affect their needs for vitamins.

Water-soluble vitamins are not stored in the body.[7] Because of favorable transplacental transport mechanisms, however, these vitamins accumulate in the fetus and neonate. In general the fetomaternal gradients for these vitamins are 2–5:1.[8] In the first day of life the newborn infant is saturated with vitamins but this condition is transient. Increased urinary losses and diminished intake in the first week of life provide a setting for vitamin deficiency.[7,9]

The status of the seven water-soluble vitamins in the preterm infant has been summarized previously.[10,11] This chapter will expand the available information to include the needs of the term infant and the infant receiving total parenteral nutrition (TPN).

ASCORBIC ACID

Scurvy, or ascorbic acid deficiency, was the first dietary deficiency disease to be recognized. The history of ascorbic acid and scurvy dates back to the ancient Egyptians, Greeks, and Romans. Before scurvy was recognized as a disease of dietary deficiency, it was thought to be a venereal disease and was treated as such![12]

In 1535, the Newfoundland Indians advised Jacques Cartier to feed his crew extracts from the needles of spruce trees to stop an epidemic. Two hundred years later there were only "case reports" suggesting cures for scurvy. Backstrom reported a dramatic tale in 1734: A sailor, so overrun and disabled with scurvy was sent ashore to perish. He had lost the use of his limbs and could only crawl on the ground and "graze" on the grasses. In a short time he was restored completely to health. The grass was the herb scurvy-grass, *Cochlearia officinalis*, which has a high antiscorbutic value.[1]

In 1747, James Lind performed a human experiment to determine the etiology of scurvy. He took several men suffering from scurvy on board ship and administered different diets to each. Only those men who ate oranges and limes recovered! It took over 50 years for his results to be recognized. In 1804 the British Navy ordered lemon juice (then, often called "lime juice") for all crew members and the term "limeys" for British sailors was introduced.[1,12]

The isolation of ascorbic acid from paprika, its characterization, and its name are attributed to Szent-Gyorgy and Haworth, both of whom shared the Nobel Prize for this work in 1937.[1,12]

Scurvy did not become a matter of concern for infants until the end of the nineteenth century when the use of pasteurized milk and artificial formula became prevalent. Infantile scurvy was observed in well-to-do families who had the means to purchase commercial artificial formulas.[2] Ingalls, in 1938, described three cases in which scurvy was identified in preterm infants who died between 26 and 57 days of life.[13] These infants were fed pooled, pasteurized human milk exclusively. He suggested that the daily dose of ascorbic acid for small (preterm) infants should approximate the amount of this vitamin contained in unpasteurized human milk. Preterm infants also may be more vulnerable to ascorbic acid deficiency than term infants because of a defect in their metabolism of tyrosine.[10]

PHYSIOLOGY

The two principal forms of ascorbic acid are L-ascorbic acid and the oxidized form, dehydroascorbic acid. L-ascorbic acid appears to be the biologically active form of the vitamin.

Ascorbic acid accelerates hydroxylation reactions in many biosynthetic reactions. It may provide electrons to enzymes that require prosthetic metal ions in a reduced form to achieve full activity, such as the hydroxylation of proline and lysine in collagen synthesis.[14] **Many examples can be found of hydroxylase activity enhanced by ascorbic acid:** the hydroxylation of lysine and methionine in carnitine biosynthesis, the metabolism of tyrosine, and the synthesis of norepinephrine from dopamine. Ascorbic acid is of particular importance to the preterm infant because it enhances the activity of the immature hepatic enzyme, p-hydroxyphenylpyruvic acid oxidase, which increases the metabolism of tyrosine.[10,14] Twenty to thirty years ago, transient tyrosinemia as a result of possible ascorbic acid deficiency or high tyrosine and/or protein intakes was a common problem for preterm infants.[10,15,16]

Ascorbic acid is involved in the synthesis of neurotransmitters. A relationship may exist between this function and the observation that **the human fetal brain contains 4 to 11 times the amount of ascorbic acid found in the adult brain.**[17] These brain ascorbate contents decline with increasing gestational age, but the content remains threefold greater than that in adults even after four weeks of age. The significance of the brain ascorbate level is unclear but may be an important rationale for the provision of adequate ascorbic acid to the preterm infant. The rise in serum ascorbic acid levels reported following intraventricular hemorrhage in preterm infants may be a marker of the disruption of the blood-brain barrier.[10,18]

A potential role for the antioxidant properties of ascorbic acid also is emerging.[14,19] Ascorbic acid as an antioxidant, theoretically, may be of importance to the high-risk preterm infant who is exposed to hyperoxic environments and mechanical ventilation.[10]

Placental transfer results in a greater concentration of ascorbic acid in the fetus and in cord blood than in the mother.[20] With optimal nutrition the maternal/cord ascorbic acid ratio is 0.5. The fetus appears to be protected from maternal ascorbic acid deficiency.[10]

Ascorbic acid is absorbed in the upper small intestine. When the renal threshold is reached the vitamin appears unchanged in the urine. At moderate intakes, urinary excretion is the main source of elimination. At intakes above 3 gm/day, fecal excretion of the vitamin rises and protects the infant against excessive intakes.[12]

The availability of ascorbic acid is influenced by its physical characteristics. **The ascorbic acid content of human milk is reduced 90% by pasteurization.**[13] Storage time, temperature, and oxidation affect ascorbic acid levels.[10] **The ascorbate content of pooled human milk is 50% lower than that of fresh milk.**[13] Exposure to copper, iron, and oxygen also will reduce ascorbic acid levels. The plasma ascorbic acid concentration is reported to decline during febrile and gastrointestinal illnesses.[10,20]

AVAILABILITY AND NEEDS

The ascorbic acid needs of full-term infants are obtained from estimates of the availability of this vitamin from human milk. The ascorbic acid concentration of human milk remains generally stable during lactation, averaging 8 mg/100 kcal (range 5-13 mg/100 kcal, Table 1).[21-28] A slight decline, 9.7-7.6 mg/100 kcal, is observed between milks obtained from less than six months' lactation and those from 6-25 months of lactation.[26,29] When the lactating mother's diet is supplemented with ascorbic acid an increase in milk concentration of the vitamin occurs only if her diet has been deficient in ascorbic acid.[21,30] No effect of routine supplementation is reported for American women.[24,25,27,28]

Cow milk contains a low concentration of ascorbic acid, 0.1-1.4 mg/dl (0.1-2.0 mg/100 kcal), probably because the cow is able to synthesize this vitamin.[13,14,20] Undiluted evaporated milk contains 0.9 mg/100 kcal.[23] Commercially available infant formulas derived from cow milk are fortified to a level of 5.5 mg/dl (8 mg/100 kcal, Table 1). Formulas adapted specifically for preterm infants contain a range of ascorbic acid concentrations from 7-30 mg/dl (9-37 mg/100 kcal, Table 1).

Neonatal serum ascorbic acid concentrations decline during the first week and by five days are similar to maternal serum values at delivery.[20] This low level is maintained in infants fed unsupplemented cow milk. Based on studies of urinary excretion and body saturation, formula-fed term infants require a mini-

TABLE 1.   Vitamin Content of Human Milk, Commercial Formulas, and Evaporated Milk (per 100 kcal)

| Vitamin | Mature Human Milk | Commercial Formula | | Evaporated Milk ‡ |
		Term*	Preterm †	
Ascorbic acid (mg)	8 (5–13)‡	8	9–37	0.9
Thiamin (μg)	31 (21–36)	78–100	100–250	30
Riboflavin (μg)	49 (36–72)	147–156	160–617	250
Niacin (mg)	0.29 (0.27–0.34)	0.8–1.2	0.8–4.9	0.14
Biotin (μg)	0.9 (0.7–1.2)	1.5–2.3	2–37	2–5
Pantothenic acid (mg)	0.38 (0.37–1.00)	0.30–0.47	0.45–1.85	0.5

*Formulas routinely used for full-term infants, Enfamil (Mead Johnson & Co, Evansville, IN 47721), Similac (Ross Laboratories, Columbus, OH 43216), SMA (Wyeth Laboratories, Philadelphia, PA 19101).
† Formulas designed for use in preterm infants, Enfamil Premature Formula (Mead Johnson), Similac Special Care (Ross), Preemie SMA (Wyeth).
‡Average of published values (range), see text for details.
Note: For vitamin B_6 data see Table 6.

mum ascorbic acid supplement of approximately 10 mg/day to prevent scurvy. If supplemented with 20 mg/day, these infants demonstrate serum concentrations similar to those of breast-fed infants.[20] Breast-fed full-term infants probably have saturated ascorbic acid levels with respect to their need.[20,26]

The ascorbic acid needs of the preterm infant may be greater than those of the full-term infant. Transient tyrosinemia and high protein intakes ($\geqslant$5 gm/kg/day) are two conditions that may occur in preterm infants. To prevent hypertyrosinemia a daily intake of 75-100 mg of ascorbic acid was suggested for preterm infants who maintained high protein intakes.[10,16,20] There is disagreement, however, as to the long-term effects of mild transient tyrosinemia in the preterm infant.[10,20] This problem may be of less significance today, because protein intakes of 5-6 gm/kg/day are no longer recommended.[31] Furthermore, **serum tyrosine concentrations in preterm infants fed human milk and whey-dominant formulas are lower when compared with those in similar infants fed casein-dominant formulas.[10]** This finding suggests that preterm infant's ascorbic acid needs may not be significantly greater than those of the full-term infant, provided that human milk or whey-predominant formulas are used.

When clinical conditions in preterm infants prevent early initiation of enteral nutrition, the delay of vitamin supplementation may lead to ascorbic acid deficiency. Ascorbic acid intakes of less than 5 mg/kg/day result in a marked decline of plasma values, from 1.56-0.48 mg/dl during the first 14 days of life.[32] Normal plasma levels are maintained in preterm infants, however, when enteral feedings are begun and supplemented with ascorbic acid (5-10 mg/kg/day) by five days of life.[32]

The recommendations of the Committee on Nutrition (CON), American Academy of Pediatrics (Table 2), for the minimum ascorbic acid intake of term and preterm infants is 8 mg/100 kcal.[31] If protein intakes are in an appropriate range, the recommended dietary allowances (RDA) of 35 mg/day ascorbic acid for all infants in the first six months of life would be sufficient to prevent scurvy and establish tissue saturation.[33] An additional allowance of ascorbic acid for preterm infants is unnecessary.

Plasma ascorbate concentrations in term and preterm infants receiving total parenteral nutrition (TPN) have been reported recently;[34] term infants received 80 mg/day and preterm infants 52 mg/day of ascorbic acid (MVI Pediatric, Armour Pharmaceutical Co., Kankakee, IL). In term infants plasma ascorbate concentrations, evaluated for 21 days, rose to a maximum of 35% above baseline cord blood values. In preterm infants, evaluated for 28 days, plasma concentrations rose 135% above control values. Those infants with birthweights below 1000 gm had even higher plasma levels. Other investigators report that while preterm infants received 50 mg/kg/day of ascorbic acid in TPN, cord blood ascorbic acid values were regained in preterm infants at 7 days and were doubled by 14 days of life.[32] Intravenous needs in adults may be greater than the enteral needs because 50% of an intravenous dose of ascorbic acid is excreted in the urine.[35] The American Medical Association guidelines for multivitamin preparations suggest a dose of 80 mg/day for all infants but even 50 mg/day may be too high for preterm infants (Table 3).[36] Further studies are needed to evaluate lesser intravenous doses in this population.

DEFICIENCY

A deficiency of ascorbic acid results in the clinical presentation of scurvy (Table 4, Fig. 1). Petechial hemorrhages, which indicate increased capillary fragility, are the earliest clinical manifestations in adults. Infantile scurvy presents with the findings of irritability, tenderness, swelling, and *pseudoparalysis of the lower extremities.* Characteristic radiologic abnormalities, hyperkeratosis of hair follicles, and mental status changes characterize the

TABLE 2.   Recommended Vitamin Intakes for Term and Preterm Infants

Vitamin	CON* (per 100 kcal)	RDA† (units/day)
Ascorbic acid (mg)	8	35
Thiamin (μg)	40	300
Riboflavin (μg)	60	400
Niacin (mg)	0.25 (0.8‡)	6‡
B$_6$ (μg)	35§	300
Biotin (μg)	1.5	35
Pantothenic acid (mg)	0.3	2–3

Adapted from reference 10.
*Committee on Nutrition, American Academy of Pediatrics.[31]
†Recommended Dietary Allowances, birth to 6 months.[33]
‡As niacin equivalents
§Assumes B$_6$/protein: 15 μg/gm

TABLE 3.   Water-Soluble Vitamins for Term and Preterm Infants Receiving TPN

Vitamin	Term* (mg/day)	Preterm* (mg/day)	Comments	
Ascorbic acid	80	52	Term†	Preterm‡
Thiamin	1.2	0.78		
Riboflavin	1.4	0.90		
Niacin	17	11		
Pyridoxine	1.0	0.65		
Biotin	0.020	0.013	Preterm‡	
Pantothenic acid	5	3.2		

Modified from reference 34. Term infants (N = 26) received an average of 912 kcal/day. Preterm infants received an average of 76 kcal/day. Protein intakes varied from 1.5–4.0 gm/kg/day.
*American Medical Association Guidelines. Reference 36. Preterm infants given ⅔ of term infant dose.
†Plasma values in term infants significantly above baseline but not above reference controls.
‡Plasma values in preterm infants significantly above baseline and controls.

PRESENTATION

"SKIN" INVOLVEMENT

DERMATITIS ➜ NIACIN, BIOTIN, and RIBOFLAVIN

MUCOUS MEMBRANES

  ■ ERYTHEMA ➜ NIACIN

  ■ STOMATITIS ➜ RIBOFLAVIN

  ■ CHEILOSIS ➜ RIBOFLAVIN

  ■ GLOSSITIS ➜ RIBOFLAVIN and BIOTIN

  ■ FILIFORM ATROPHY ➜ RIBOFLAVIN and NIACIN

  ■ HEMORRHAGE ➜ ASCORBIC ACID

PETECHIAE ➜ ASCORBIC ACID

PALLOR (ANEMIA) ➜ ASCORBIC ACID and PYRIDOXINE

HAIR

  ■ ALOPECIA ➜ BIOTIN

  ■ FOLLICLE HYPERKERATOSIS ➜ ASCORBIC ACID

EDEMA ➜ THIAMIN

EYE

  ■ CORNEAL VASCULARIZATION ➜ RIBOFLAVIN

  ■ CATARACT ➜ RIBOFLAVIN

  ■ PHOTOPHOBIA ➜ RIBOFLAVIN

  ■ REDUCED TEARING ➜ RIBOFLAVIN

"NEUROLOGIC" INVOLVEMENT

SEIZURES ➜ THIAMIN and PYRIDOXINE

MENTAL STATUS CHANGES

  ■ MARKED ➜ THIAMIN and NIACIN

  ■ IRRITABILITY ➜ PYRIDOXINE, BIOTIN
                          and ASCORBIC AC

  ■ APATHY ➜ PANTOTHENIC ACID and
                  THIAMIN

PARESTHESIA ➜ PANTOTHENIC ACID and
                      THIAMIN

PSEUDOPARALYSIS ➜ ASCORBIC ACID

APHONIA ➜ THIAMIN

FIGURE 1.   Simplified differentiation of water-soluble vitamin deficiency states in infancy.

progression of the illness. Hemorrhagic manifestations in children may present with bleeding at the site of tooth eruption, bloody diarrhea, epistaxis, ocular bleeding, and petechiae at pressure points. Anemia, secondary to decreased iron absorption or abnormal folate metabolism, is a common finding.[14] Sepsis and failure to thrive are characteristics of preterm infants reported with scurvy.[13]

Serum ascorbic acid concentrations reflect recent ingestion of this vitamin.[20] Acceptable plasma ascorbic acid values are > 0.6 mg/dl. Values below 0.2 mg/dl are observed in scurvy.

TOXICITY

Problems encountered with the ingestion of high doses of ascorbic acid have been summarized previously.[10] Potential problems with acidosis may be encountered. The increased oxalic acid excretion would be detrimental in conditions such as congenital oxalosis/oxaluria, hyperuricemia, and cystinuria. Large doses of ascorbic acid decrease the absorption of vitamin B_{12}. Cases of a conditioned need for ascorbic acid have been reported in which the cessation of high ascorbic acid doses resulted in rapid onset of clinical scurvy.[12,14] The development of scurvy in offspring of a mother who took high doses of ascorbic acid routinely during pregnancy also has been reported.[15] Large doses also may result in excessive iron absorption, depression of copper status, and exacerbation of glucose-6-phosphate dehydrogenase (G-6-PD) deficiency.[15]

THIAMIN

In 1896, Christian Eijkman, a Dutch medical officer living in Java, described a water-soluble dietary factor that cured pigeons of the neuritis produced by feeding them only polished rice.[1] His discovery of the "antiberiberi factor" led the way to the present concept of vitamins, as nutritional and not infectious factors.[1,37]

In 1907 Braddon, in what is now Malaysia, made the observation that although rice-eating was related to beriberi, the preparation of the rice was of equal importance. When the rice was "parboiled" before milling, the Indian population did not develop the severe disease seen in the Chinese population who did not "parboil" the rice. He concluded, however, that some poison was destroyed by the boiling process! It was many years later when the real conclusion was described: the boiling process caused the water soluble vitamin to become dispersed into the innermost portion of the endosperm.[1]

TABLE 4.　Key Considerations in the History of the Infant with Water-Soluble Vitamin Deficiency

1. Feeding History
    a. maternal dietary deficiencies
        (1) current:　thiamin, pyridoxine
        (2) during pregnancy:　thiamin, pyridoxine
    b. breast feeding:　thiamin, pyridoxine
    c. "processed" milk:　ascorbic acid
    d. raw eggs:　biotin
    e. malnutrition:　thiamin, riboflavin, niacin, pantothenic acid
2. Gastrointestinal Disturbances (Vomiting, Diarrhea)
    thiamin, pyridoxine, niacin, pantothenic acid
3. Associated Medications/Therapies
    a. phototherapy:　riboflavin
    b. isoniazid:　pyridoxine
    c. antibiotics:　biotin
4. Possible Vitamin-Responsive Inborn Errors of Metabolism and Vitamin-Dependency States
    thiamin, pyridoxine, niacin, biotin

PHYSIOLOGY

Thiamin, vitamin B_1, functions as a coenzyme in biochemical reactions related to carbohydrate metabolism, i.e., the oxidative decarboxylation of alpha keto acids and pyruvate and transketolase reactions of the pentose pathway. Thiamin also is involved in the decarboxylation of branched-chain amino acids and may be involved in neuronal membrane excitability. Large doses of thiamin have proven successful in the treatment of certain metabolic disorders including a variant of maple syrup urine disease, Leigh's encephalopathy, thiamin-responsive anemia, and a condition characterized by severe lactic acidosis.[38]

Thiamin is phosphorylated in the intestinal mucosa to form thiamin pyrophosphate and adenylic acid. Thiamin is absorbed from the small intestine by both passive diffusion and active transport.[38] The absorption of thiamin is rate-limited and is slower during pregnancy.[8]

Although thiamin deficiency during pregnancy has been reported, no correlation is observed between maternal thiamin status and pregnancy outcome.[39] The fetomaternal gradient for thiamin favors the fetus and may protect against maternal deficiency. At delivery, cord blood thiamin concentrations are greater than maternal levels.[8,10]

Urinary excretion of thiamin parallels dietary intake except at low dietary intake levels.[39] Thiamin in excess of tissue needs is excreted in the urine.[37] Conditions involving heavy diureses, such as those accompanying diuretic therapy, may increase the urinary excretion of thiamin.[37,40]

Thiamin is destroyed or inactivated by heat, alkaline solutions, and ionizing radiation. Loss of vitamin occurs during milk pasteurization and sterilization.[10,37,40]

AVAILABILITY AND NEEDS

The thiamin content of human milk increases from 3 µg/100 kcal during the first five days of lactation to an average of 31 µg/100 kcal (range 21-36 µg/100 kcal) in mature milk (Table 1).[22,27,40-45] The thiamin concentration in milk is related to dietary intake in malnourished but not in well-nourished women.[30,41,45] The thiamin content of commercial formulas for full-term and preterm infants is 78-100 and 100-250 µg/100 kcal, respectively (Table 1). The average content of thiamin in cow milk and undiluted evaporated milk is 45 and 30 µg/100 kcal, respectively.[23]

The need for thiamin is related to the energy content of the diet. The thiamin intake of full-term breast-fed infants appears satisfactory.[33,41,42] Thiamin deficiency in breast-fed infants of well-nourished mothers has not been reported. The Committee on Nutrition's recommendation of 40 µg of thiamin/100 kcal of milk is higher than the average thiamin content of human milk (21-36 µg/100 kcal). Because thiamin deficiency in breast-fed infants has not been demonstrated, the recommended intake for this group should be re-evaluated. Formula-fed infants receive sufficient thiamin to meet these recommended intakes.

Thiamin intake from human milk for preterm infants is below minimum recommendations (Tables 2 and 5). A satisfactory content of thiamin is available from commercial formula (Table 5).

The thiamin needs of infants receiving TPN have not been described fully. When term and preterm infants received TPN which included 1.2 and 0.78 mg of thiamin per day, respectively, the red blood cell transketolase activity was normal.[34] The vitamin preparation was administered daily in doses which were unrelated to energy intake. When calculated based on their energy intake, the term infants received an average of 133 µg/100 kcal (based on an average intake of 912 kcal/day) and the preterm infants received 975 µg/100 kcal (based on 76 kcal/day)! Although the measurement of transketolase enzyme activity does not identify excessive intakes, no infant was deficient.[34] TPN patients theoretically may be more susceptible to thiamin deficiency, because of the associated stress, trauma, and sepsis that accompany its use.[46] Further studies are needed in this area.

DEFICIENCY

A deficiency of thiamin results in beriberi (Table 4, Fig. 1). The signs of this disease relate to the chronicity of the depletion, its severity, and associated stresses.[47] Early signs, in adults, of **"dry" beriberi** include wasting, peripheral neuropathy, paresthesias, and weakness. In addition to neurologic manifestations, severe deficiency will result in cardiovascular symptoms and signs. In **"wet" beriberi**, edema is

TABLE 5.   Comparison of Recommended Vitamin Intakes for Preterm Infants with Calculated Daily Vitamin Intakes from Human Milk, Formula, and Vitamin Supplement*

Vitamin	CON†	RDA‡	Human Milk (units/day)	Formulas	Supplement
Ascorbic acid (mg)	14	35	14	16–67	35
Thiamin (µg)	72	300	56§	180–450	500
Riboflavin (µg)	108	400	88§	288–1111	600
Niacin (mg)	0.45	6	0.52	1–9	8
B6 (µg)	63	300	77‖	112–450	400
Biotin (µg)	2.7	35	1.6§	4–67	0
Pantothenic acid (mg)	0.54	2–3	0.68	1–3	0

Modified from reference 10.
*Assume a growing preterm infant weighing 1.5 kg fed 120 kcal/kg/day. Average vitamin content of mature human milk and formulas designed for preterm infants derived from Tables 1 and 6. Vitamin supplement refers to 1 ml., Poly-Vi-Sol (Mead Johnson) or Vi-Daylin (Ross).
†From Committee on Nutrition,[31] value calculated for this hypothetical infant.
‡Recommended Dietary Allowance.[33]
§Vitamin intake inadequate.
‖Vitamin intake adequate providing maternal diet supplemented with pyridoxine.

prominent and may progress to fulminant cardiac failure ("cardiac beriberi").[40]

"Infantile" beriberi may occur between one and four months of life in breast-fed infants whose mothers have an intake deficient in thiamin. The nursing mother, however, may not have obvious signs of the deficiency. Although thiamin deficiency may be either acute or chronic, the acute cardiac symptoms and signs predominate.[40] Anorexia, apathy, vomiting, restlessness, and pallor progress to dyspnea and cyanosis from cardiomegaly and congestive heart failure with death in 24 to 48 hours. The infant with beriberi may have a striking characteristic cry; the infant is *aphonic*, he appears to be crying but no sound is uttered. A pseudomeningitic phase characterized by bulging fontanelle, seizures, and coma also has been reported.[38,48] Infantile beriberi has been reported in association with celiac disease.[48]

Wernicke's encephalopathy and Korsakoff's syndrome result from severe, acute thiamin deficiency often observed in alcoholics and in pregnancies associated with severe vomiting. The high intake of "empty" calories coupled with decreased intake of nutritionally adequate foods is thought to lead to the array of neurologic manifestations, including confusion, coma, ophthalmoplegia, nystagmus, ataxia, psychosis, and emotional disturbances. This form of thiamin deficiency is observed rarely in infants. When present, the symptoms of generalized encephalopathy predominate.

The most reliable measure of functional thiamin activity is the activity of *erythrocyte transketolase*. The "TPP-effect" (thiamin pyrophosphate) is the ratio of transketolase activity before and after the addition of thiamin diphosphate. Severe thiamin deficiency exists when this activity increases by more than 25%, mild deficiency by a ratio of 15-25%, and adequate status is suggested by a ratio of <15%.[37]

TOXICITY

No toxic effects have been observed for high oral doses of the vitamin. Extremely large intravenous doses may result in respiratory depression.[47]

RIBOFLAVIN

Riboflavin, initially isolated as "the yellow pigment" from milk, yeast, and animal organs, is required for all cellular growth.

This "growth-promoting" function originally was observed in rats. The responsible factor was initially thought to be similar to that which prevented pellagra, and its history is intertwined with that of vitamin H, biotin.[49] In 1932 the biological significance of the "yellow enzyme" was made apparent.

PHYSIOLOGY

Riboflavin is a constituent of two coenzymes, riboflavin-5-phosphate (FMN, flavin mononucleotide) and flavin adenine dinucleotide (FAD). These coenzymes are essential components of several enzymes (glutathione reductase, xanthine oxidase) involved in electron transport. **A deficiency of riboflavin affects glucose, fatty acid, and amino acid metabolism.** Riboflavin deficiency results in a reduction of liver and plasma essential fatty acids, linoleic and linolenic.[49] It also impairs the conversion of tryptophan to niacin because the conversion of the cofactor, pyridoxine, to the active pyridoxal form is impaired.

After phosphorylation, riboflavin is absorbed readily from the proximal small intestine. Absorption is reduced in biliary obstruction and in conditions which decrease intestinal transit time.[10] Urinary excretion of riboflavin depends upon dietary intake and saturation of tissue stores.[40]

A significant relationship has been reported to exist between diminished riboflavin intake and antenatal fetal mortality, prematurity, hyperemesis in pregnancy, and lactation failure.[50] The placenta is permeable only to riboflavin and not its coenzymes. FAD is converted by the placenta to free riboflavin. In the neonate, therefore, riboflavin is the predominant form of the vitamin.[8] As early as 20 weeks of gestation, fetal liver is able to convert riboflavin to FAD.[51] Cord blood concentrations of riboflavin are greater than maternal values at delivery.[8,51]

Riboflavin and its phosphate are decomposed by exposure to light and in strong alkaline solutions.[52] Phototherapy treatment for hyperbilirubinemia is reported to produce biochemical riboflavin deficiency in breast-fed newborn infants, as measured by activation of erythrocyte glutathione reductase.[52-55] Riboflavin, however, is resistant to heat, acid, and oxidation. The processes of pasteurization, evaporation, and condensation of milk do *not* destroy riboflavin.[49]

AVAILABILITY AND NEEDS

Based on the relationships between riboflavin and protein metabolism, riboflavin needs had been expressed in terms of protein utilized. This designation has been changed in recent years to relate to caloric intake, because of the close relationships between protein and calories and for practical considerations, such as the similarity to estimation of thiamin needs.[40]

The riboflavin concentration in human milk remains uniform throughout lactation and averages 49 μg/100 kcal (range 36-72 μg/100 kcal, Table 1).[22,27,42,43,45,56,57] Vitamin supplementation is reflected in a greater milk riboflavin concentration if maternal riboflavin intake is in a range below the recommended dietary allowance of 1.7 mg/day or, conversely, if mothers receive almost 3 times the RDA during the first six weeks of lactation.[30,33,45,57] The riboflavin content of cow milk and undiluted evaporated milk is 260 and 250 μg/100 kcal, respectively.[23]

Although evidence for biochemical riboflavin deficiency is reported in a survey of breast-fed full-term infants during *phototherapy,* the content of riboflavin in human milk generally satisfies the minimum recommendation for full-term infants (Table 2).[3,31,42,53] The possible intake of riboflavin from standard infant formulations, which contain 147-156 μg/100 kcal, is significantly greater than from human milk, 36-72 μg/100 kcal (Table 1). The content of riboflavin in human milk differs from the content specified in the CON recommendations, 60 μg/100 kcal, when the lower end of the possible range in values is considered. This difference depends upon the riboflavin value quantitated in human milk. Further study in full-term infants, especially those who receive prolonged phototherapy, is suggested to assess the precise need for this vitamin.

The preterm infant may have greater riboflavin needs due to the common and, possibly, prolonged use of phototherapy. If fed human milk, the riboflavin intake for a preterm infant would be inadequate (Table 5).[54-55] Commercial formulas, however, will provide the riboflavin needs of the preterm infant (Table 5).

For infants receiving conventional TPN, measurements of riboflavin status indicate no deficiencies, using daily intravenous riboflavin doses of 1.4 and 0.9 mg, in term and preterm infants respectively (Table 3).[34] The methods for assessing deficiency, however, do not detect excessive riboflavin intake. Term infants in this study received an average of 153 μg of riboflavin/100 kcal and preterm infants received 1180 μg/100 kcal! Further studies of the riboflavin needs during TPN are indicated.

DEFICIENCY

Ariboflavinosis is characterized by angular stomatitis, glossitis, cheilosis, seborrheic dermatitis around the nose and mouth, and eye changes which include reduced tearing, *photophobia,* corneal vascularization, and cataracts (Table 4, Fig. 1). Overt signs of deficiency are rare in inhabitants of developed countries. However, the Ten State Nutritional Survey revealed biochemical evidence of subclinical riboflavin deficiency in the following situations: women taking oral contraceptive agents, diabetic subjects, children from low socioeconomic families, children with chronic cardiac disease, the elderly, and infants undergoing phototherapy for hyperbilirubinemia.[48]

The urinary excretion of riboflavin falls in the early stages of deficiency, but the best correlation with a deficiency state is the activity of the enzyme erythrocyte glutathione reductase (EGR) before and after riboflavin administration.

TOXICITY

No toxic effects of overdosage are known.

NIACIN

Niacin is the term that describes the compounds nicotinic acid and nicotinamide (niacinamide).

In 1937, Elvehjem described niacinamide as the active component in liver extracts that cured "black-tongue" in dogs. At the same time other laboratories attributed a deficiency of this vitamin as the cause of *pellagra,* a condition in humans that parallels the canine disorder.[58]

PHYSIOLOGY

Nicotinamide, the amide of nicotinic acid, is the chief form of the vitamin. It functions as a component of the coenzymes nicotinamide adenine dinucleotide (NAD) and nicotinamide adenine dinucleotide phosphate (NADP). Niacin participates in multiple metabolic processes, including fat synthesis, intracellular respiratory metabolism, and glycolysis.

When describing the needs for niacin, the content of tryptophan in the diet must be ad-

dressed because dietary tryptophan is converted to niacin. Tryptophan pyrrolase converts tryptophan eventually to kynurenine and after multiple additional conversions to niacin. The conversion is catalyzed by riboflavin and vitamin B_6. Approximately 3% of administered tryptophan is converted to niacin in adults,[40] in whom one niacin equivalent (NE) equals 60 mg tryptophan or 1 mg niacin. The conversion of tryptophan to niacin is more efficient during pregnancy. There are no data available to determine the appropriate conversion factor for infants. Tryptophan accounts for 1.5% of the amino acids in proteins of animal origin.[47]

Niacin is *stable* in foods and can withstand heating and prolonged storage.

AVAILABILITY AND NEEDS

The concentration of niacin itself in human milk remains stable throughout lactation, and averages 0.29 mg/100 kcal (range 0.27-0.34 mg/100 kcal; Table 1).[22,42,43,59] If the mother is malnourished, niacin supplementation will increase the concentration in the milk.[30] Approximately 70% of the total niacin equivalents (NE) in human milk are derived from tryptophan. The tryptophan content of human milk, 22 mg/dL (33 mg/100 kcal), provides 0.37 NE/dl (0.55 NE/100 kcal). The content of NE in human milk, therefore, represents the sum of preformed niacin and niacin equivalents derived from tryptophan, or, a total of 0.8 NE/100 kcal.[33] Approximately 90% of NE in cow milk is derived from tryptophan.[47] The niacin content of cow milk is 0.12 mg/100 kcal, and the total NE are 1.2-1.6 NE/100 kcal. Undiluted evaporated milk contains 0.2 mg/dl of niacin (0.14 mg/100 kcal) and 1.6 NE/dl (1.2 NE/100 kcal.)[23]

The allowances for niacin are related to energy expenditure, because the coenzymes NAD and NADP function in the respiratory chain. In infants fed 6 NE per day, but not 4 NE, the urinary excretion of niacin metabolites remains normal, suggesting a normal status.[60] The recommended allowance for full-term infants is based on the niacin equivalents in human milk, 0.8 mg NE/100 kcal. Infants fed routine commercial formula would receive 0.8 to 1.2 mg preformed niacin/100 kcal (Table 1). Differences in needs of niacin related to intake of preformed niacin compared with niacin equivalents have not been evaluated and should be considered.

No data exist to support a specific recommendation for the preterm infant. The CON recommendations state that the minimum milk content should be 0.25 mg preformed niacin per 100 kcal. If the recommended protein intake is assumed to be approximately 2.5 gm/100 kcal, then the tryptophan content in formula would contribute 0.63 NE/100 kcal. Thus, provided there is 0.25 mg preformed niacin per 100 kcal of milk, the preterm infant would receive a milk with 0.88 of total NE/100 kcal, similar to the recommended milk content for full-term infants (Table 2).[33] Since the degree of conversion of tryptophan to niacin in infants is unknown, the recommendation probably should be given in terms of preformed niacin.

There are limited data available to assess the niacin needs of infants during TPN. Plasma "niacin" concentrations are similar to normal controls in term and preterm infants receiving TPN with niacin intakes of 17 and 11 mg/day, respectively.[34] The term infants received an average of 1.9 mg niacin/100 kcal and the preterm infants received 14 mg/100 kcal. The protein and tryptophan intakes were not specified in this evaluation (Table 3). Although deficiencies were not identified, without the protein and tryptophan intake data, it is difficult to determine whether the niacin requirements were met.

DEFICIENCY

A deficiency of niacin results in the clinical syndrome of pellagra, a disease endemic to corn-eating areas.

The first description of pellagra was given in 1730 by Casal who used the term "mal de la rosa" to describe the cutaneous inflammation observed before the dermatitis.[1] In 1771, Frapoli, in Italy, described a similar condition and the name pellagra was given: "pella" for skin, "agra" for unsightly or rough. At that time it was considered that this condition was related to diet.[40]

The significance of these descriptions and their relationship to diet were lost for hundreds of years. It was not until 1914 that the cause of pellagra was identified, by Joseph Goldberger, as a dietary deficiency and not due to an infectious agent.[1,40]

Pellagra is characterized by weakness, lassitude, dermatitis, inflammation of mucous membranes, diarrhea, vomiting, dysphagia, and in severe cases, dementia (Fig. 1, Table 4). **Cutaneous inflammation looks like a sunburn because, initially, only areas exposed to light are affected.** A familial disorder of tryptophan-niacin metabolism is Hartnup's disease, an impaired absorption of mono-amino/monocarboxylic acids including trypto-phan.[15]

The urinary excretion of niacin metabolites, chiefly N^1-methylniacinamide and N^1-methyl-6-pyridone-3-carboxamide, "pyridone," can be measured and is considered a good method in diagnosing niacin deficiency. Although the excretion of the pyridone falls earliest in niacin deficiency, it is the most difficult to assay. The N^1-methylniacinamide/creatinine ratio in random urine samples may be employed conveniently; values below 0.5 mg/gm creatinine suggests deficiency in adults.[40] Serum N^1-metabolites and nicotinamide can be assayed fluorimetrically.[58]

TOXICITY

Excess nicotinic acid produces cutaneous vasodilation. Niacin in large doses has been observed to reduce serum cholesterol levels and to protect against the recurrence of myocardial infarction.[10] The associated risks of arrhythmias, abnormal liver function tests, jaundice, increased gastric acid secretion, and gastrointestinal hypermotility warrant caution in such usage.[10,15,40]

VITAMIN B$_6$

A "pellagra-preventive" factor for rats, initially studied by Goldberger in 1926, was evaluated by Gyorgy in 1934. He named this substance vitamin B$_6$. Investigators then found that this substance did *not* cure pellagra in humans, but cured a "pellagra-like" condition in rats. This was the first acknowledgment of vitamin B$_6$ and the effects of its deficiency.

PHYSIOLOGY

B$_6$ refers collectively to three naturally occurring pyridines—pyridoxine (pyridoxol), pyridoxal, and pyridoxamine—and the phosphates of the latter two which are metabolically and functionally interrelated. Pyridoxal-5-phosphate and to a lesser degree pyridoxamine-5-phosphate are the major forms of B$_6$ in blood.[61,62] Pyridoxic acid is the chief excretory product of the B$_6$ vitamers.[62] The metabolic functions of vitamin B$_6$ include participation in interconversion reactions of amino acids, conversion of tryptophan to niacin and serotonin, metabolic reactions in the brain, carbohydrate metabolism, immune development, and the

biosynthesis of heme and prostaglandins. **Because of the relationship between B$_6$ and protein metabolism, it is customary to consider the ratio of these factors when assessing needs.**

Cord blood contains pyridoxal phosphate, pyridoxamine phosphate, and pyridoxic acid in greatest quantities.[62] The intake of vitamin B$_6$ during the last trimester of pregnancy determines the nutritional state of the infant with respect to this vitamin.[61,62] B$_6$ concentrations are greater in cord blood when compared with those in maternal blood.[63] Transport of the vitamin appears to become more active during the last trimester as assessed by increased cord blood:maternal blood ratios.

Absorption occurs in the upper small intestine. **High dietary protein intakes and destruction of vitamin B$_6$ by light are two factors that increase its needs.** Heat destruction may occur with the pyridoxal and pyridoxamine forms of the vitamin and such destruction was responsible for B$_6$ deficiency and seizures in infants fed improperly processed formulas.[6] For this reason, the heat-stable vitamer, pyridoxine, is used for the fortification of milk.

AVAILABILITY AND NEEDS

The content of B$_6$ in human milk reflects the mother's nutritional status with respect to this vitamin.[25,30,64-67] A marked difference in B$_6$ content is observed between milks obtained from mothers consuming the approximate RDA for B$_6$ (2.5 mg/day) and mothers whose intake of B$_6$ is greater than 2.5 mg/day (Table 6). The concentration of B$_6$ in milk obtained from mothers whose intake is at the RDA or is unspecified is 18 µg/100 kcal (range 9-2 µg/100 kcal).[22,42,43,64,65,67] Mothers who consume greater than 2.5 mg/day of B$_6$ have milk concentrations that average 43 µg/100 kcal (range 28-79 µg/100 kcal).[24,25,27,64-67] The B$_6$ content of human milk may decline with extended lactation.[29]

The milk B$_6$/protein ratio, generally used to assess B$_6$ status, reflects maternal intake of the vitamin, and its content may decline to levels as low as 7 µg/gm in milk obtained from unsupplemented mothers (Table 6). When maternal B$_6$ intake is at the RDA or unspecified the average ratio is 15 µg/gm (range 7-2 µg/gm).[22,64-67] With intakes greater than the RDA, the average ratio is 27 µg/gm (range 14-37 µg/gm).[64,65,67] The ratio derived from fo

TABLE 6.   Vitamin B_6 Content of Human Milk, Commercial Formulas, and Evaporated Milk (per 100 kcal)

| Vitamin | Mature Human Milk | Commercial Formula | | Evaporated Milk ‡ |
		Term*	Preterm †	
$_6$ (µg)	18 (9–27)‡ §	59–62	62–250	55
$_6$ (µg/g protein)	15 (7–25)§	27–28	25–91	16
$_6$ (µg)	43 (28–79)∥	—	—	—
$_6$ (µg/g protein)	27 (14–37)∥	—	—	—

Formulas routinely used for full-term infants, Enfamil (Mead Johnson & Co, Evansville, IN 47721), Similac (Ross Laboratories, Columbus, OH 43216), SMA (Wyeth Laboratories, Philadelphia, PA 19101).
Formulas designed for use in preterm infants, Enfamil Premature Formula (Mead Johnson), Similac Special Care (Ross), Preemie SMA (Wyeth).
Average of published values (range), see text for details.
Mature milk obtained from women whose B_6 intake was unspecified or ⩽ 2.5 mg/day.
Mature milk obtained from women whose B_6 intake was ⩾ 2.5 mg/day.

ula received by six-month-old infants fed *ad bitum* is 20 µg/gm.[68]

The range of vitamin B_6 concentrations in ow milk-based formulas routinely used for ull-term infants, 59-62 µg/100 kcal, satisfies ie recommended allowances (Tables 2 and). Cow milk and undiluted evaporated milk ontain 50-90, and 55 µg/100 kcal, respec- vely.[23] **Goat's milk is deficient in vitamin
$_6$.**[69]

Full-term infants become B_6-deficient when 2d mother's milk containing a low content of ie vitamin, 9-12 µg/100 kcal. B_6 deficiency as been reported in formula-fed infants:[70]

---

uring 1952-1953 a peculiar phenomenon occurred mong infants (between 2 and 4 months of age) charac- rized by epileptiform convulsions unassociated with her signs of illness ... infants presented a strikingly uni- orm picture: normal birth history, normal growth and evelopment, a continuous good state of health un- ... convulsions occurred ... all of these infants had een artificially fed ... liquid SMA ... when fed another ilk formula ... were free from convulsions. No cases ere reported among infants receiving powdered SMA. ictors ... which may have been responsible were a dif- rent mode of sterilization in the can which may have estroyed pyridoxine.[71]

A dose of B_6, 0.3 mg/day, prevented the eizures.[70] A greater B_6 intake, however, was equired to normalize biochemical measure- nents of deficiency.[70] Recent reports of ealthy breast-fed infants receiving a low vita- nin B_6 intake of 0.1 mg/day, however, have ot indicated detrimental effects.[64,65]

Low plasma pyridoxal phosphate (PLP) alues were observed in preterm infants on the rst day of life, but plasma PLP rose to greater

levels with the provision of a whey-dominant cow milk formula.[72]

It seems most prudent to recommend vita- min B_6 supplementation to lactating women. Inadequately supplemented women produce milk with B_6 contents that are below the CON recommendations. There is insufficient evi- dence to suggest that deficiency states exist in full-term breast-fed infants. Commercially available infant formulas contain sufficient B_6 to meet estimated needs of term and preterm infants (Tables 2, 5, and 6). The human milk- fed preterm infant would not receive adequate B_6. Further studies are needed to define the B_6 needs of infants.

The data also are limited regarding the B_6 needs of infants receiving TPN. Assays of plasma activity of glutamic-oxaloacetic trans- aminase, in term and preterm infants receiving TPN with B_6 doses of 1.0 and 0.65 mg/day, respectively, have been interpreted as reflect- ing a normal vitamin B_6 status (Table 3).[34] These assays, however, do not differentiate be- tween normal and excessive intakes. When computed on the basis of caloric intake, the vitamin intake appears excessive in both groups.

DEFICIENCY

Quantitative assays for vitamin B_6 generally employ the microbiological assay of *Saccharo- myces* sp.[24,64,67] Methods for the assessment of vitamin B_6 nutritional status include the tryp- tophan loading test, the measurement of py- ridoxic acid in the urine, the PLP assay, and the measurement of transaminase activity in the blood. These methods have been reviewed.[62]

The transaminase measurement is sensitive and used by several investigators to assess B_6 inadequacy.[24,62] The erythrocyte glutamic pyruvic transaminase index (EGPT) measures the enzyme activity before and after the addition of PLP. Normal individuals have an index of less than 1.25.[62]

In infants, dietary deprivation or malabsorption of vitamin B_6 results in hypochromic microcytic anemia, vomiting, diarrhea, failure to thrive, listlessness, hyperirritability, and seizures (Fig. 1, Table 4). In adults, vitamin B_6 deficiency may result in depression, confusion, peripheral neuritis, electroencephalographic abnormalities, and seizures. In chronic liver or renal disease there is an increased rate of PLP degradation.[61]

Several conditions are associated with abnormalities in B_6 metabolism that require pharmacologic doses of the vitamin for adequate function. These B_6-dependency syndromes include the following conditions: pyridoxine-dependent seizures in the neonate, pyridoxine-responsive hypochromic microcytic anemia, xanthurenic aciduria, cystathioninuria, and homocystinuria. Infants receiving isoniazid may require additional B_6 because the drug binds to the vitamin.[38]

TOXICITY

Doses up to 1 mg/kg/day were tolerated without ill effects in animals. Although most investigators agree that high doses of pyridoxine in humans do not pose a risk, a recent report describes sensory neuropathy in adults ingesting megadoses of pyridoxine.[73]

BIOTIN

Biotin, or, vitamin H (haut is the word for skin in German) as named by Gyorgy in 1931, was originally investigated in rats made deficient by feeding raw egg white. "Egg white injury" was produced by the heat labile protein, avidin, which bound and, therefore, inactivated biotin.

PHYSIOLOGY

Biotin has coenzyme functions in the metabolism of fat and carbohydrate, specifically as a component of several carboxylase enzymes. **Biotin is synthesized by intestinal bacteria, which explains why a deficiency state is less likely to occur.** A deficiency state is observed, however, when gastrointestinal flora is suppressed or when biotin absorption is diminished, such as occurs in diets which consist of raw eggs.

Various biotin-dependent carboxylase deficiency states have been described. The multiple carboxylase defect (pyruvate, propionyl coenzyme-A, and methylcrotonyl CoA carboxylase) has been shown to be biotin responsive.[15]

Biotin is absorbed by passive diffusion in the intestine. It is transported bound to plasma proteins. Urinary excretion reflects dietary intake; fecal excretion, generally unaffected by intake, indicates enteric synthesis.[33,74]

AVAILABILITY AND NEEDS

The biotin content of human milk **increases** with the duration of lactation.[22,43,59,75] The average biotin concentration in mature human milk is 0.9 μg/100 kcal (range 0.7-1.2 μg/100 kcal, Table 1).[22,42,43,59,75] In milk produced during the first week after delivery, the average biotin content is 0.07 μg/100 kcal.[22,43,59,7] Dietary supplementation of malnourished women will result in a rise in the biotin content of the milk.[30] Cow milk is a rich source of biotin, 2-5 μg/100 kcal.[74] Commercial formula contains 1.5-2.3 μg/100 kcal (Table 1).

Recommended intakes for biotin have not been established. Urinary biotin excretion in infants increases in the first days of life and then declines until six months when, possibly related to diet, rises gradually to adult values.[5] The diets of growing infants after weaning contain as much as 1 mg/100 kcal biotin.[7] Biotin deficiency has not been reported for infants fed either human milk or formulas despite a wide range of intakes.

Recent measurements of biotin in human milk utilizing improved methodologies have shown that the biotin content is less than considered previously. Since the CON recommendations of 1.5 μg of biotin/100 kcal were based on previous measurements these recommendations probably should be re-evaluated. No deficiencies of biotin have been reported for enterally-fed term and preterm infants.

Biotin deficiencies have been reported, however, when it was omitted from TPN solutions.[76,77] Plasma biotin concentrations are reported for term and preterm infants receiving TPN with biotin doses of 20 and 13 μg/day, respectively.[34] At these doses, blood levels remain stable for term infants but rise to more than ten times baseline values for preterm infants during four weeks of study. Since these values are several fold greater than aver age adult values, the B_6 doses for the preterm infant probably are excessive (Table 3).

DEFICIENCY

Biotin deficiency develops in adult volunteers after one month on a biotin-deficient diet which includes a large proportion of raw egg white. Symptoms of biotin deficiency include anorexia, nausea, glossitis, pallor, mental changes, alopecia, and a fine maculosquamous dermatitis which becomes exfoliative (Fig. 1, Table 4).[9,15] Biotin deficiency has been reported in patients with short gut syndromes when the vitamin was omitted from TPN solutions.[76,77] A young girl receiving TPN for six months reportedly developed a scaly dermatitis, alopecia, pallor, irritability, lethargy, and markedly reduced urinary excretion and plasma concentration of biotin.[76] Administration of biotin corrected these abnormalities. Biotin may enhance the treatment of seborrheic dermatitis, Leiner's disease, propionic acidemia, and B-methylcrotonylglycinuria.[15,77] Antibiotics reportedly may affect biotin status by decreasing enteric synthesis of the vitamin.[77]

Biotin is assayed commonly by microbiological methods.

TOXICITY

There are no reports of overdosage from biotin.

PANTOTHENIC ACID

Pantothenic acid (pantos is the Greek word for everywhere) was described and named in 1933 by Williams. The name is appropriate, because pantothenic acid is found in a variety of biological materials.[78]

PHYSIOLOGY

Pantothenic acid is the amide formed from pantoic acid and B-alanine. Its primary role in metabolism is its incorporation into coenzyme A. Pantothenic acid is a factor in acyl group transfers in the synthesis of fatty acids, cholesterol, steroids, the oxidation of fatty acids, pyruvate, and alpha-ketoglutarate, and in other acetylation reactions.[11,15,33,78] There is endogenous synthesis of the vitamin from pantoic acid and B-alanine.[11] The plasma concentration of pantothenic acid in the neonate is several-fold greater than that in the mother.[11]

AVAILABILITY AND NEEDS

The concentration of pantothenic acid in mature human milk is approximately 0.38 mg/100 kcal (range 0.37-0.39 mg/100 kcal, Table 1).[22,42,43,59,79] Supplementation of malnourished women or consumption of extreme amounts results in increases in the milk content of pantothenic acid.[30,79,80] A recent study, using a double enzyme method to release the bound vitamin, suggests that the level in mature milk is as high as 0.7-1.0 mg/100 kcal.[80] In cow milk, 30-35% of the vitamin is lost in processing.[79] The content of pantothenic acid is 0.5 mg/100 kcal in cow milk and undiluted evaporated milk.[23]

The CON recommendation for pantothenic acid appears adequate. The safe and adequate intake from human milk or formula of 2-3 mg/day appears achievable for infants during the first year of life (Table 2).[33,79]

Pantothenic acid needs during TPN are unknown. When term infants received 5 mg/day in TPN, their plasma concentrations during three weeks of study were stable.[34] Preterm infants receiving 3.2 mg/day, however, had plasma pantothenic acid levels that rose to more than two standard deviations above baseline values.[34] Since these values in preterm infants were much higher than usual adult values it appears that intravenous administration of this daily amount to preterm infants is excessive (Table 3). Further studies are necessary to define these vitamin needs.

DEFICIENCY

Deficiency of pantothenic acid is observed in many animal species but only under extraordinary circumstances in man. Pantothenic acid deficiency is considered to have caused the *"burning feet syndrome"* described in World War II prisoners in the Far East.[78] Under rather extraordinary conditions, experimental deficiency has been produced in volunteers fed the antagonist omega-methylpantothenic acid as part of a pantothenic acid-deficient diet.[11,78] Subjects developed burning feet, gastrointestinal disturbances, headache, insomnia, fatigue, and muscle weakness.[78] A deficiency of pantothenic acid is also observed in severe malnutrition (Table 4, Fig. 1).

There are two steps in the assay of pantothenic acid. Because the vitamin is 85 to 90% protein bound, it must first be released by enzymatic hydrolysis. After this step, the vitamin is assayed either by microbiological or radioimmunological methods.[78-80]

TOXICITY

Pantothenic acid is relatively nontoxic. High doses have been reported to produce water retention and diarrhea.[33]

SUMMARY

Overt clinical deficiency of the seven water-soluble vitamins (ascorbic acid, thiamin, riboflavin, niacin, pyridoxine, biotin, and pantothenic acid) is not observed in full-term infants who are either breast-fed from adequately nourished mothers or fed commercial formula, although infants fed evaporated milk preparations receive an inadequate amount of ascorbic acid. Precise recommendations for the intake of water-soluble vitamins, however, are unavailable. The consensus approach, to derive vitamin needs from estimates of the amount of milk consumed by breast-fed full-term infants, is limited in at least three ways: (1) there is significant variability in the methodologies used to determine the concentrations of these vitamins in human milk (e.g., pantothenic acid), (2) the milk consumption of breast-fed infants is lower than that of formula-fed infants,[5,6] and (3) the bioavailability of vitamins from human milk and formula may differ. Until these potential limitations are evaluated fully, clinical observation and experience will determine appropriate vitamin needs for this population.

The vitamin needs for the infant born prematurely are unknown. In addition to the limitations described for infants born at term, the preterm infant may experience a delay in nutritional intervention, a limitation in fluid intake, and also may suffer associated conditions which impose additional needs for vitamins. As calculated in Table 5 from CON recommendations and the RDA, the human milk-fed preterm infant may receive an inadequate supply of thiamin, riboflavin, biotin, and possibly, pyridoxine. Commercial formulas designed for preterm infants, in accordance with minimum CON recommendations and the RDA, supply sufficient amounts of the seven water-soluble vitamins. Supplemental water-soluble vitamins probably should be given to preterm infants who are fed human milk. If milk intake is restricted severely, the formula-fed preterm infant also should receive water-soluble vitamin supplementation. This vitamin supplement should be continued until the infant's intake exceeds 300 kcal/day or he achieves a body weight of 2.5 kg.[4]

The data derived from term and preterm infants receiving TPN are insufficient to determine precise vitamin needs. The American Medical Association guidelines for TPN-vitamin administration, however, may be too generous for ascorbic acid and biotin in preterm infants (Table 3). Although toxicities reportedly are uncommon for water-soluble vitamins, a conditioned need for ascorbic acid is observed.[12,14,15] Further evaluations of vitamin status and the interaction of vitamin status with vitamin, energy, and protein intakes are required before any precise recommendations can be provided.

Acknowledgments. I thank E. R. Klein for editorial advice and N. Hayley for secretarial assistance. This work is a publication of the USDA/ARS Children's Nutrition Research Center, Department of Pediatrics, Baylor College of Medicine and Texas Children's Hospital. This project has been funded in part with federal funds from the U.S. Department of Agriculture, Agricultural Research Service under Cooperative Agreement #58-7MNI-6-100. The contents of this publication do not necessarily reflect the views or policies of the U.S. Department of Agriculture, nor does mention of trade names, commercial products, or organizations imply endorsement by the U.S. Government.

REFERENCES

1. Chick H. The discovery of vitamins. Progr Food Nutr Sci 1975;1:1-20.
2. Faber HK, McIntosh R, eds. History of the American Pediatric Society. New York, McGraw-Hill Book Co., 1900.
3. Committee on Nutrition, American Academy of Pediatrics. Commentary on breast-feeding and infant formulas, including proposed standards for formulas. Pediatrics 1976;57: 278-285.
4. Committee on Nutrition, American Academy of Pediatrics. Vitamin and mineral supplement needs in normal children in the United States. Pediatrics 1980;66:1015-1021.
5. Butte NF, Garza C, Smith EO, Nichols BL. Human milk intake and growth of exclusively breast-fed infants. J Pediatr 1984;104:187-195.
6. Fomon SJ. Infant Nutrition, 2nd ed. Philadelphia, W.B. Saunders, 1974;24-25,231-233.
7. Greene HL. Water soluble vitamins. In Lebenthal E (ed): Textbook of Gastroenterology and Nutrition in Infancy, vol. 1. New York, Raven Press, 1981;585-594.
8. Baker H, Frank O, Thomson AD, et al. Vitamin profiles of 174 mothers and newborns at parturition. Am J Clin Nutr 1975;28:56-65.
9. Hamil BM, Coryell M, Roderuck C, et al. Thiamine, riboflavin, nicotinic acid, pantothenic acid and biotin in the urine of newborn infants. Am J Dis Child 1947;74:434-446.
10. Schanler RJ, Nichols BL. The water soluble vitamins C, B_1, B_2, B_6, and niacin. In Tsang RC (ed): Vitamin and Mineral Requirements in Preterm Infants. New York, Marcel Dekker Inc, 1985;39-62.
11. Gross SJ. Choline, pantothenic acid, and biotin. In Tsang RC (ed): Vitamin and Mineral Requirements in Preterm Infants. New York, Marcel Dekker, Inc, 1985:191-201.
12. Jaffe GM. Vitamin C. In Machlin LJ (ed): Handbook of Vitamins. New York, Marcel Dekker, Inc., 1984: 199-244.

3. Ingalls TH. Ascorbic acid requirements in early infancy. N Engl J Med 1938;218:872-875.

4. Levine M. New concepts in the biology and biochemistry of ascorbic acid. N Engl J Med 1986;314:892-902.

5. Moran JR, Greene HL. The B vitamins and vitamin C in human nutrition. II. "Conditional" B vitamins and vitamin C. Am J Dis Child 1979;133:308-314.

6. Light IJ, Berry HK, Sutherland JM. Aminoacidemia of prematurity. Am J Dis Child 1966;112:229-236.

7. Adlard BPF, De Souza SW, Moon S. Ascorbic acid in the fetal human brain. Arch Dis Child 1974;49: 278-282.

8. Arad ID, Eyal FG. High plasma ascorbic acid levels in preterm neonates with intraventricular hemorrhage. Am J Dis Child 1983;137:949-951.

9. Fisher AB, Bassett DJP, Forman HJ. Oxygen toxicity of the lung: biochemical aspects. In Fishman AP, Renkin EM (eds): Pulmonary Edema. Bethesda, American Physiological Society, 1979:207-216.

0. Irwin MI, Hutchins BK. A conspectus of research on vitamin requirements of man. J Nutr 1976;106:823-879.

1. Selleg I, King CG. The vitamin C content of human milk and its variation with diet. J Nutr 1936;11:599-606.

2. Macy IG. Composition of human colostrum and milk. Am J Dis Child 1949;78:589-603.

3. Adams CF. Nutritive value of American foods. Agricultural Research Service, United States Department of Agriculture, Washington, D.C., 1975.

4. Thomas MR, Kawamoto J, Sneed SM, Eakin R. The effects of vitamin C, vitamin B_6, and vitamin B_{12} supplementation on the breast milk and maternal status of well-nourished women. Am J Clin Nutr 1979;32:1679-1685.

5. Sneed SM, Zane C, Thomas MR. The effects of ascorbic acid, vitamin B_6, vitamin B_{12}, and folic acid supplementation on the breast milk and maternal nutritional status of low socioeconomic lactating women. Am J Clin Nutr 1981;34: 1338-1346.

6. Salmenpera L. Vitamin C nutrition during prolonged lactation: optimal in infants while marginal in some mothers. Am J Clin 1984;40:1050-1056.

7. Thomas MR, Sneed SM, Wei C, et al. The effects of vitamin C, vitamin B_6, vitamin B_{12}, folic acid, riboflavin, and thiamin on the breast milk and maternal status of well-nourished women at 6 months postpartum. Am J Clin Nutr 1980; 33:2151-2156.

8. Byerley LO, Kirksey A. Effects of different levels of vitamin C intake on the vitamin C concentration in human milk and the vitamin C intakes of breast-fed infants. Am J Clin Nutr 1985;41:665-671.

9. Karra MV, Udipi SA, Kirksey A, Roepke JLB. Changes in specific nutrients in breast milk during extended lactation. Am J Clin Nutr 1986;43:495-503.

0. Deodhar AD, Rajalakshmi R, Ramakrishnan CV. Studies on human lactation. III. Effect of dietary vitamin supplementation on vitamin contents of breast milk. Acta Paediatr (Stockholm) 1964;53:42-48.

1. Committee on Nutrition, American Academy of Pediatrics. Nutritional needs of low-birth-weight infants. Pediatrics 1985;75:976-986.

2. Arad ID, Sagi E, Eyal FG. Plasma ascorbic acid levels in preterm infants. Int J Vit Nutr Res 1982;52:50-54.

3. Committee on Dietary Allowances, Food and Nutrition Board. Recommended Dietary Allowances, 9th ed. Washington, D.C., National Academy of Sciences, 1980.

4. Moore MC, Greene HL, Phillips B, et al. Evaluation of a pediatric multiple vitamin preparation for total parenteral nutrition in infants and children. Pediatrics 1986;77:530-538.

5. Slonka D. The clinical use of vitamins in total parenteral nutrition. Curr Concepts Hosp Pharm Manage 1979;1:4-9.

6. Nutritional Advisory Group, Department of Foods and Nutrition. Guidelines for multivitamin preparations for parenteral use. Chicago, American Medical Association, 1975.

7. Gubler CJ. Thiamin. In Machlin LJ (ed): Handbook of vitamins. New York, Marcel Dekker, Inc., 1984:245-297.

8. Moran JR, Greene HL. The B vitamins and vitamin C in human nutrition I. General considerations and "obligatory" B vitamins. Am J Dis Child 1979;133:192-199.

9. Heller S, Salkeld RM, Korner WF. Vitamin B_1 status in pregnancy. Am J Clin Nutr 1974;27:1221-1224.

40. Goldsmith GA. Vitamin B complex. Thiamine, riboflavin, niacin, folic acid (folacin), vitamin B_{12}, biotin. Progr Food Nutr Sci 1975;1:559-609.

41. Knott EM, Kleiger SC, Torres-Bracamonte F. Factors affecting the thiamine content of breast milk. J Nutr 1943;25:49-58.

42. Bates CJ. Normal vitamin requirements in neonates and infants. J Inherit Metab Dis 1985;1(Suppl):8-12.

43. Ford JE, Zechalko A, Murphy J, Brooke OG. Comparison of the B vitamin composition of milk from mothers of preterm and term babies. Arch Dis Child 1983;58:367-372.

44. Roderuck CE, Williams HH, Macy IG. Human milk studies. XXIII. Free and total thiamine contents of colostrum and mature human milk. Am J Dis Child 1945;70:162-170.

45. Nail PA, Thomas MR, Eakin R. The effect of thiamin and riboflavin supplementation on the level of those vitamins in human breast milk and urine. Am J Clin Nutr 1980;33:198-204.

46. Cadorniga R. Vitamins in parenteral nutrition. Acta Vitaminol Enzymol 1982;4:141-151.

47. Goodhart RS, Shils ME (eds): Modern Nutrition in Health and Disease, 6th ed. Philadelphia, Lea & Febiger, 1980.

48. Van Gelder DW, Darby, FU. Congenital and infantile beriberi. J Pediatr 1944;25:226-235.

49. Cooperman JM, Lopez R. Riboflavin. In Machlin LJ (ed): Handbook of Vitamins. New York, Marcel Dekker, Inc., 1984:299-327.

50. Brzezinski A, Bromberg YM, Braun K. Riboflavin deficiency in pregnancy. J Obstet Gynecol 1947;54:182-186.

51. Lust JE, Hagerman DD, Villee CA. The transport of riboflavin by the human placenta. J Clin Invest 1954;33:38-40.

52. Bates CJ, Liu DS, Fuller NJ, Lucas A. Susceptibility of riboflavin and vitamin A in breast milk to photodegradation and its implications for the use of banked breast milk in infant feeding. Acta Paediatr Scand 1985;74:40-44.

53. Hovi L, Hekali R, Siimes MA. Evidence of riboflavin depletion in breast-fed newborns and its further acceleration during treatment of hyperbilirubinemia by phototherapy. Acta Paediatr Scand 1979;68:567-570.

54. Ronnholm KAR. Need for riboflavin supplementation in small preterms fed with human milk. Am J Clin Nutr 1986;43:1-6.

55. Lucas A, Bates C. Transient riboflavin depletion in preterm infants. Arch Dis Child 1984;59:837-841.

56. Roderuck CE, Coryell MN, Williams HH. Human milk studies. XXIV. Free and total riboflavin contents of colostrum and mature milk. Am J Dis Child 1945;70:171-175.

57. Hughes J, Sanders TAB. Riboflavin levels in the diet and breast milk of vegans and omnivores. Proc Nutr Soc 1979;38:95A.

58. Hankes LV. Nicotinic acid and nicotinamide. In Machlin LJ (ed): Handbook of Vitamins. New York, Marcel Dekker, Inc., 1984:329-377.

59. Coryell MN, Harris ME, Miller S, et al. Human milk studies. XXII. Nicotinic acid, pantothenic acid and biotin contents of colostrum and mature human milk. Am J Dis Child 1945; 70:150-161.

60. Holt LE Jr. The adolescence of nutrition. Arch Dis Child 1956;31:427-438.

61. Committee on Dietary Allowances, Food and Nutrition Board. Human vitamin B_6 requirements. Washington, D.C., National Academy of Sciences, 1978.

62. Driskell JA. Vitamin B_6. In Machlin LJ (ed): Handbook of Vitamins. New York, Marcel Dekker, Inc., 1984:379-401.

63. Brin M. Abnormal tryptophan metabolism in pregnancy and with the oral contraceptive pill. II. Relative levels of vitamin B_6-vitamers in cord and maternal blood. Am J Clin Nutr 1971;24:704-708.

64. Styslinger L, Kirksey A. Effects of different levels of vitamin B_6 supplementation on vitamin B_6 concentrations in human milk and vitamin B_6 intakes of breastfed infants. Am J Clin Nutr 1985;41:21-31.

65. Borschel MW, Kirksey A, Hannemann RE. Effects of vitamin B_6 intake on nutriture and growth of young infants. Am J Clin Nutr 1986;43:7-15.

66. Andon MB, Howard MP, Moser PB, Reynolds RD. Nutritionally relevant supplementation of vitamin B_6 in lactating women: effects on plasma prolactin. Pediatrics 1985;76:

769–773.

67. West KD, Kirksey A. Influence of vitamin B_6 intake on the content of the vitamin in human milk. Am J Clin Nutr 1976; 29:961–969.

68. Filer LJ, Martinez GA. Intake of selected nutrients by infants in the United States. Clin Pediatr 1964;3:633–645.

69. Johnson GM. Powdered goat's milk. Clin Pediatr 1982;21: 494–95.

70. Bessey OA, Adam DJD, Hansen AE. Intake of vitamin B_6 and infantile convulsions: A first approximation of requirements of pyridoxine in infants. Pediatrics 1957;20:33–44.

71. Molony CJ, Parmelee AH. Convulsions in young infants as a result of pyridoxine (vitamin B_6) deficiency. JAMA 1954; 154:405–406.

72. Reinken L, Mangold B. Pyridoxal phosphate values in preterm infants. Int J Vitam Nutr Res 1973;43:472–478.

73. Schaumburg H, Kaplan J, Windebank A, et al. Sensory neuropathy from pyridoxine abuse—A new megavitamin syndrome. N Engl J Med 1983;309:445–448.

74. Roth KS. Biotin in clinical medicine—a review. Am J Clin Nut 1981;34:1967–1974.

75. Goldsmith SJ, Eitenmiller RR, Feeley RM, et al. Biotin conten of human milk during early lactational stages. Nutr Re 1982;2:579–583.

76. Mock DM, DeLorimer AA, Liebman WM, Sweetman L, Bake H. Biotin deficiency: an unusual complication of parentera alimentation. N Engl J Med 1981;304:820–823.

77. Bonjour JP. Biotin in man's nutrition and therapy—a review Int J Vitam Nutr Res 1977;47:107–118.

78. Fox HM. Pantothenic acid, In Machlin LJ (ed): Handbook o Vitamins. New York, Marcel Dekker, Inc., 1984:437–458

79. Song WO, Chan GM, Wyse BW, Hansen RG. Effect of pan tothenic acid status on the content of the vitamin in huma milk. Am J Clin Nutr 1984;40:317–324.

80. Johnston L, Vaughn L, Fox HM. Pantothenic acid content o human milk. Am J Clin Nutr 1981;34:2205–2209.

14

Vitamin A

RICHARD D. ZACHMAN, Ph.D., M.D.

ABSTRACT

Although vitamin A was the first of the fat-soluble vitamins discovered, the full extent of its mechanism of action is still unknown. Likewise, although vitamin A deficiency is a worldwide problem, easily recognized in its severe form, the sequelae of borderline sufficiency, or possibly a functional deficiency in certain classes of infants, are not recognized or well studied.

The preterm infant is at risk for vitamin A (retinol) deficiency. Liver stores increase during gestation, and plasma levels are lower than term infants. Intravenous supplementation has often been inadequate in the past. The stress and tissue injury accompanying certain diseases and the potential for retinol interacting with other nutrients are other factors that impact on the determination of the retinol status of such patients and are considerations in meeting their retinol nutritional requirements.

INTRODUCTION

In the early 1900s the field of nutrition was in crisis because chemical analysis alone failed to accurately predict the nutritional value of foodstuffs.[1] E.V. McCollum, an organic chemist in the Department of Agricultural Chemistry at the University of Wisconsin, noted in 1907 that purely wheat-fed cows were stunted and blind, oat-fed cows fared somewhat better, while the corn-fed cows did well. All cows had been fed rations of the same chemical (i.e., total nitrogen, etc.) composition, so what was the basis of the difference?

After buying a dozen albino rats from a pet dealer in Chicago, McCollum started one of the first rat colonies ever used for experimental nutrition purposes. In 1913, McCollum and Davis published a milestone paper clearly showing that all fats were not nutritionally equal for young rats.[2] Butterfat and the ether extract of egg yolk provided growth, but lard or olive oil did not. The growth-promoting lipid was present in the small "non-saponifiable fraction" of fat, and this fraction could be transferred to olive oil, which then would support growth.[3] This ether-soluble growth-promoting "lipin" was later named vitamin A.

Although in 1913 vitamin A was the first of the fat soluble vitamins discovered, the full extent of its mechanism of action is still unknown. Deficiency and toxicity from vitamin A have been noted worldwide in man—but most of these data are on young children and adults,

with few observations on neonates in either the human or experimental animal. Neonates, especially preterm infants, have limited tissue reserves of vitamin A and therefore are potentially at risk for deficiency.

Many reviews covering the chemistry, metabolism and mechanism of action of vitamin A, and considerations of the global nature of vitamin A deficiency in children, have been published recently.[4-8] The present discussion therefore will only give a limited overview of those aspects of vitamin A, and the chapter will focus on the perinatal and infant aspects of vitamin A nutrition.

PHYSIOLOGY

CHEMISTRY AND NOMENCLATURE

The structure of vitamin A was deduced in 1931. Now the term vitamin A is used generically for closely related derivatives of β-ionone that possess biological activity described to the vitamin (Fig. 1). The basic constituent of the vitamin A group is called all *trans* retinol.[4,5] The structure of retinol consists of a β-ionone ring, the highly conjugated double-bond system on the hydrocarbon side chain and the potentially active alcohol group that can be oxidized (to retinal [retinaldehyde], then retinoic acid) or esterified by reacting with acyl CoA fatty acids. This structure accounts for retinol's physiochemical properties of lipid solubility, spectral absorption at near-ultraviolet wavelengths (328 nm), ease of *cis-trans* isomerization, sensitivity to oxidation and epoxide formation, and a potential for metabolic reactivity.

METABOLISM

Ingested plant carotene (a precursor of retinol) or animal-tissue retinyl esters release retinol in the proximal small intestine after the action of hydrolases of the pancreas and intestinal brush border (Fig. 2). Free retinol is then absorbed into the intestinal mucosal cells, re-

STRUCTURE OF VITAMIN A

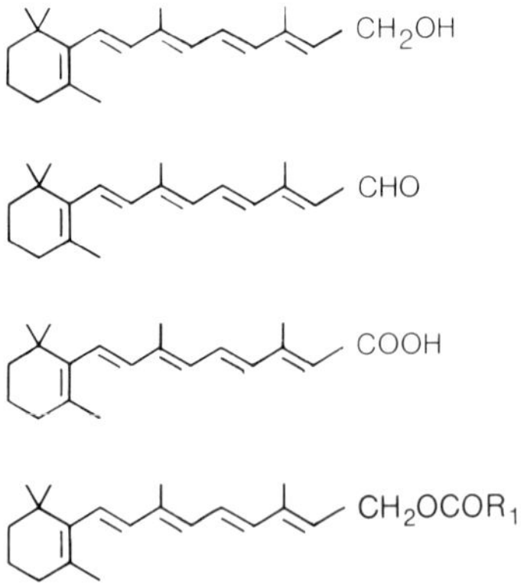

all trans Retinol

Retinal (Retinaldehyde)

Retinoic Acid

Retinyl Ester
R_1 = fatty acid

β -ionone ring   → Hydrophobicity (lipid soluble)
Hydrocarbon chain

Conjugated double   → UV absorption at 328 nm
    bond system

                                                  → Ease of peroxidation, epoxy formation,
                                                    and cis/trans isomerization

Reactive alcohol   → Oxidation and conjugation
    terminal group

FIGURE 1.   Structure and properties of vitamin A.

esterified, and incorporated into chylomicrons. This process is apparently facilitated by a newly discovered cellular binding protein type II (CRBP-II) found almost exclusively in the absorptive cells of the small intestine,[9] and distinctly different from the well-known cellular retinol binding protein (CRBP) found in nearly all tissues.[10]

Chylomicrons and lipoprotein-bound retinyl esters are predominantly taken up by the liver for deposition and storage, mostly as retinyl palmitate. Subsequently, a highly regulated hydrolysis process liberates free retinol for its delivery to target tissues.

Retinol is mobilized from liver as a specific complex of retinol-binding protein (RBP). In plasma, the RBP-retinol complex (holo-protein) combines with transthyretin (TTR) for circulation. RBP is a small protein of a molecular weight of about 21,000 and possesses a single-binding site for retinol. The turnover of the RBP (holo-protein) complex in plasma is about 11–16 hours, and the turnover of the free RBP apoprotein (without retinol) is even more rapid.[5] After the circulating complex delivers retinol to the target tissues, the free RBP is excreted by the kidney. Diseases of the kidney diminish the catabolism of RBP, thus elevating plasma RBP, whereas liver parenchymal disease will lower plasma RBP. Infections and glucocorticoids are some examples of other factors associated with a rise in the level of plasma retinol and RBP.[6]

Many metabolites of retinol have been discovered in blood and urine.[5] Retinol can be reversibly oxidized to retinaldehyde and further oxidation yields retinoic acid. The oxidation of retinaldehyde to retinoic acid is not reversible and accounts for the observation made over 25 years ago by Dowling and Wald that **retinoic acid can support growth but not the visual function of retinol.**[11]

RETINOL METABOLISM

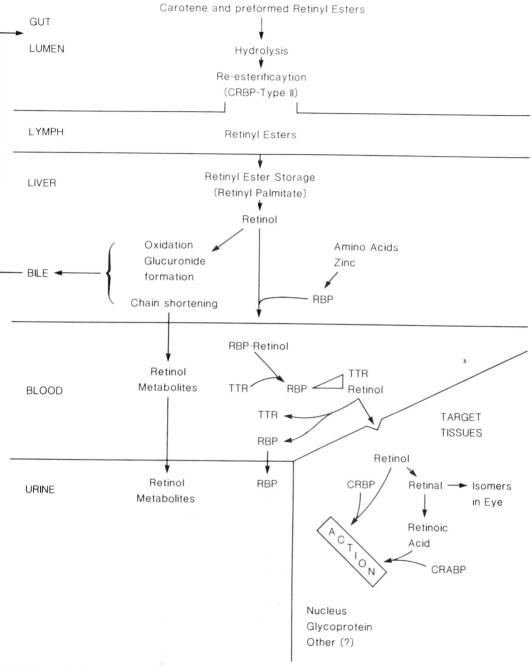

FIGURE 2.   Retinol metabolism. The anatomic and physiological compartments are separated by the heavy solid lines and retinol metabolism indicated by the arrows. Abbreviations are: CRBP-Type II—cellular retinol binding protein Type ; RBP—retinol binding protein; TTR—transthyretin; CRBP—cellular retinol binding protein; CRABP—cellular retinoic cid binding protein. Note: in plasma, the RBP retinol complex combines with TTR for circulation.

"The rat seems unable to reduce vitamin A acid to vitamin A; ... hence this substance might *not* be able to serve as precursor of the visual pigments, which need for their synthesis the alcohol and aldehyde."

The experiment for proof of this hypothesis consisted of three groups of weanling rats: Group 1, vitamin A (retinol) alcohol supplement; Group 2, vitamin A acid (retinoic acid) supplement; and Group 3, vitamin A deficient. Results of the experiment are seen in the accompanying table:

Supplement	Growth	Liver vitamin A	Visual thresholds
1. Retinol	Normal	300 µg/g	Normal
2. Retinoic acid	Normal	<10	Abnormal
3. Deficient	Weight loss at 6 weeks	<10	Abnormal

"The general tissue functions of vitamin A that support growth and maintenance in the rat are served also by vitamin A acid, but since this substance is not reduced, it forms neither the alcohol, the form in which vitamin A is stored, nor the aldehyde needed for the synthesis of visual pigments."[11]

Epoxy derivatives and β-glucuronidation of retinoic acid occur in liver, and these metabolites are excreted in bile. A portion of the retinoic-acid glucuronide undergoes enterohepatic circulation, and further oxidation, including chain-shortening by decarboxylation, occurs in the intestine and other organs; most of these biological metabolites appear in the urine.[5]

Olson has recently summarized[5] quantitative aspects of the disposition of the ingested vitamin. Of the 80% absorbed, some 20–50% is excreted in the feces and urine in about a week. The remainder is stored and metabolized much more slowly.

MECHANISMS OF ACTION

The uptake and utilization of retinol by target tissues are in some way facilitated by specific cellular-binding proteins. In the rod outer-segment of the eye, retinol undergoes oxidation to retinaldehyde, subsequent isomerization, and combination with opsin, forming *rhodopsin*. Subsequently, the action of light on rhodopsin leads to potential changes that facilitate the visual process.[4]

Retinol also has a role in reproduction and a general somatic function influencing growth and differentiation of epithelium. The molecular mechanism of these biological phenomena of retinol have not been completely elucidated but are the subject of intensive investigation.[6,12] Interaction with the nucleus, causing changes in nucleic acid formation and metabolism similar to the action of steroid hormones, has been proposed. Another possible mechanism of action is that retinol or one of its derivatives serves as a cofactor in specific glycoprotein synthesis.[12] Most tissues also contain cellular retinoic-acid-binding protein (CRABP). Retinoic acid can substitute for retinol in all functions except maintaining reproduction and vision.[12]

NEEDS OF TERM AND PRETERM INFANTS

GENERAL NEED RECOMMENDATIONS

At this writing, the 10th edition of the National Research Council's Recommended Dietary Allowance (RDA), reporting the amount of ingested retinol that should meet the needs of most individuals, has not yet been released. However, since 1984, several extensive reviews outlining the needs and recommendations for animal and humans have been published.[4,5,7,8]

The definition of the nutritional requirement for retinol is made complex because the requirement for a given organism depends on many criteria, including age and storage reserves, rate of growth and activity, intake of other nutrients, disease states, and stress, to name a few.[5,7] An exhaustive review of the literature has pointed out that there was limited information on the dietary level necessary to provide for liver storage in infants.[13]

Experimental data from which to derive the RDA for humans are limited to two small studies recently reviewed by Olson.[5] In the study of 1974,[14] in which 8 adult male volunteers were depleted of vitamin A, a dose of 600 µg/day was necessary to *restore normal dark adaptation*, as measured by electroretinograms, and to restore their plasma retinol to 20 µg/dl. Although it varies in certain countries,[4] most adult daily recommended intakes are 750–1000 µg of retinol* to maintain plasma levels and accumulate liver stores (Table 1). The recommendation is around 400 µg of retinol for infants.

---

*1 µg retinol = 1 retinol equivalent = 6 µg β-carotene = 3.33 International Units (IU)

TABLE 1.   Recommended Daily Allowance Expressed as Retinol Equivalents (RE)[5,8]

Population	Age (yr)	NRC–U.S., 1980*	WHO–FAO, 1974*	Canada*
Adult	⩾ 20	800–1000	750	—
Children	1–3	400	250	—
Infants	0.5–1.0	400	—	400
	0.0–0.5	420	300	400

1 RE = 1 μg retinol = 6 μg β-carotene = 3.33 International Units (IU)
*NRC–U.S. = Food and Nutrition Board of the National Research Council of the United States.[5] WHO–FAD = World Health Organization and the Food and Agricultural Organization of the United Nations.[5] Canada.[8]

PERINATAL ASPECTS POTENTIALLY AFFECTING NEEDS OF THE TERM AND PRETERM NEWBORN (Fig. 3)

Placental Transfer

Moore[15] speculated from his data in 1971 that the transfer of retinol from mother to fetus was probably controlled by something like liver RBP transport.

In mice and rats on a liberal supply of retinol, Moore found that the proportion of the vitamin passed to the fetus prenatally was small. When the maternal supply of retinol was restricted, the amounts of retinol passed to the offspring were only slightly less than with a liberal supply, i.e., the proportion of the maternal supply was much higher. "Probably the mechanism controlling the passage of retinol to the offspring, at least before parturition, is closely connected with that known to control the release of retinol from liver into the blood stream, which allows a constant blood level to be maintained until the liver reserves are almost exhausted."[15]

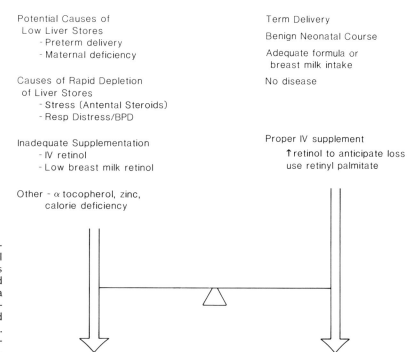

Some Theoretical Considerations of
Neonatal Retinol Balance Needs

Potential Causes of
Low Liver Stores
 - Preterm delivery
 - Maternal deficiency

Causes of Rapid Depletion
of Liver Stores
 - Stress (Antental Steroids)
 - Resp Distress/BPD

Inadequate Supplementation
 - IV retinol
 - Low breast milk retinol

Other - α tocopherol, zinc,
  calorie deficiency

Term Delivery

Benign Neonatal Course

Adequate formula or
breast milk intake

No disease

Proper IV supplement
 ↑ retinol to anticipate loss
 use retinyl palmitate

DEFICIENT   SUFFICIENT

FIGURE 3. Some theoretical considerations of neonatal retinol balance needs. Items on the left of the figure would increase the potential for a neonatal deficiency. Circumstances on the right should assure adequate retinol status. Abbreviations are: BPD—bronchopulmonary dysplasia; IV—intravenous.

After the development of sophisticated assays for RBP, this speculation was confirmed. Studies in pregnant rats demonstrated three phases of retinol accumulation in the fetus during development.[16] First (7–9 days of gestation), retinol accumulated in fetal tissues but RBP was low and at a constant level. Second (11–14 days of gestation), both retinol and RBP accumulated coincident with growth of the fetus. Finally (days 16–20 of gestation), there was a marked increase in fetal liver retinol with another rise in RBP as well. Fetuses and placentas of retinol-deficient mothers had low levels of RBP during these last days, but study of repletion of the dam suggested that the maternal RBP-retinol complex crossed the placenta. These various studies support the hypothesis that **retinol was transported from the mother to the fetus during the latter half of gestation (starting day 11) mainly by transplacental transport of maternal RBP bound retinol.**

Human placental transport of retinol is less completely understood. One study found a correlation between maternal and cord blood RBP levels,[17] but others demonstrated a lack of correlation between maternal and neonatal RBP levels in preterm[18] and term gestations.[19] Also, there is a relatively poor correlation between maternal and neonatal levels of retinol,[19] and cord retinol levels in concordant sex twins were as variable as values of other neonates born to different mothers.[18] These findings suggest that, at least in the last trimester, **the human fetus participates in the regulation of retinol transport across the placenta.**

Low Hepatic Retinol Stores

Animal studies support the notion that **liver stores of 20 µg/gm liver weight is the minimal acceptable reserve for retinol.**[20] This has also been proposed as the standard for human adults. If this value is used as a guideline for a minimal acceptable reserve for retinol, many term and preterm neonates are retinol-deficient.

Since 1972, several studies have demonstrated that frequently the mean liver retinol of newborns is ≤ 20 µg/gm, well below the concentration of most older age groups.[21] Preterm infants frequently have even lower means. In their study of assessing the age-dependent vitamin A status of children in the U.S., Olson et al.[22] analyzed the liver concentrations of several groups of infants dying from various

causes and noted that of 92 infants analyzed at ≤ 30 days, 43–100% had liver retinol of ≤ 20 µg/gm. In preterm (< 2.5 kg) and term infants, the mean value appeared independent of birthweight.

However, preterm infants in that study described as having "failure to thrive" had very low levels at the time of death (3.3 µg/gm). Using approximate liver weights to calculate the total body reserves of retinol, the total retinol reserves of 38-40 week gestation newborns is 1800 ± 516 µg (mean ± SEM), approximately twice the amount available to smaller, 25–32 week gestation, preterm infants. This is to be expected, since fetal rat liver retinol concentrations and amounts double in the last quarter of gestation.[23,24] Therefore, a preterm human neonate born at 30 weeks' gestation has both a low concentration of retinol in liver, frequently under suggested values described as adequate, and a *total reserve of retinol of only about one-half that of term infants.*

In the absence of direct routine analysis of the liver, low plasma retinol concentrations have been used as an indicator of vitamin A deficiency in humans. **A concentration of <10 µg/dl is generally accepted to be strongly indicative of vitamin A deficiency,**[25,26] although unless liver retinol concentrations are <5 µg/gm, there is no assurance of a direct correlation between serum and liver retinol values.[5]

Using this approach, several investigators have estimated the retinol status of the preterm infant by analyzing plasma retinol. Although there is no apparent direct relationship between plasma retinol and gestational age, most studies find that preterm infants of less than 36 weeks' gestation have lower plasma retinol values than term infants.[21]

Neonatal Disease

Neonates with bronchopulmonary dysplasia (BPD) have biochemical evidence of retinol deficiency.[18,27] This evidence is not based on actual tissue analysis of liver or lung but is based on the association of plasma retinol and liver retinol stores mentioned above. In one study, the 28-postnatal-day plasma concentration of retinol in BPD patients was significantly less than in matched controls.[27]

In another study[18] preterm infants who developed BPD had lower cord plasma retinol than those that did not develop BPD and also were lower at day 21 of life. Thirty to 40 percent of these BPD patients had plasma retinol concentrations <10 µg/dl. It is possible that the low plasma retinol levels in these patients were related to the route and amount of administration of retinol and calories, and this is in need of further study.

It also will be very important to learn the actual tissue amounts of retinol in neonatal disease. Tissue retinol contents may reflect specific tissue or overall body needs. In animals with a relative deficiency state, a greater percent of the total body retinol is present in lung tissue, lung and kidney.[28] Tissue retinol stores and levels of the binding proteins change with birth.[24,29] The extensive necrotizing bronchiolitis and squamous metaplasia in lung that occurs in BPD could cause a rapid exhaustion of lung retinol stores and the liver storage depot, but proof awaits investigation.

Type of Nutritional Intake
Breast Milk. Human milk content of retinol is approximately 50 µg/dl in the U.S. and possibly lower in other populations.[5,6] Assuming an intake of 600-750 ml per day, the mean intake of retinol by a well-feeding neonate, from day 3 to 7 of life, would be 300 to 375 µg of retinol. There is no evidence that this intake causes any problems of deficiency, so it is assumed that this intake is meeting the needs of well neonates.

A recent study suggests that the amount of milk retinol from mothers delivering term infants initially is higher than those delivering preterm infants; by the third post-partum week, the retinol content of both milk sources declines to similar levels.[30] β-carotene occurs in breast milk and this could supply some retinol.[31] However, only about 12% of fed carotene is absorbed by humans[4] and this is not all converted to retinol. It is assumed, in the recommendations for dietary intakes, that infants 0–6 months old obtain the majority of retinol as retinol and not carotene.

Proprietary Formulas. Proprietary formulas generally provide retinol in the range of 100–200 µg per 100 kcal,[32] which corresponds to a minimum daily intake of about 420–840 µg of retinol per day for a 3.5 kg neonate ingesting 120 kcal of feedings/kg/day. Again, this intake meets the apparent needs of the neonate.

Intravenous Supplementation. Recommendations for intravenous administration of retinol have been from 70–100 µg retinol/kg/day.[33] In a 3.5-kg infant that would directly provide 245–350 µg of retinol/day, intravenously, roughly equivalent to the RDA. However, two aspects of intravenous alimentation might well alter this need. First, the infants are probably ill and under stress and possibly mobilizing their retinol stores more rapidly. The patient might be a preterm infant with very low liver stores, who has an increase in peripheral target-tissue demand, as suggested in the studies with BPD. Second, intravenous administration of retinol is notoriously unreliable. Several studies have shown that **50-75% of the original retinol in the intravenous supply bottle is lost onto the supply tubing by the time it reaches the neonate.**[21] Hence, supplementation of the sick preterm infant over several days or weeks with intravenous fluids might well be different from the full-term infant feeding well on proprietary formula.

Relationship to Other Nutrients. The retinol needs of a neonate, especially the preterm infant, might very well be affected by the status of other nutrients such as vitamin E, zinc, protein and, calories.[5]

A relationship between vitamin E and vitamin A has been proposed for some time.[5] A recent study concluded that high dietary vitamin A (1500 µg/kg) decreases tocopherol (vitamin E) concentrations in plasma by acting only at the level of absorption of vitamin E from the gut.[34] This action is unlikely to be a problem in neonatal care, since most neonates would not be fed that much retinol.

An α-tocopherol-deficient diet affected the concentration of retinol and retinyl esters in several organs of the rat.[35] In liver, there was an increase in free retinol concentration but a decrease in total vitamin A (free retinol plus retinyl esters). In lung, there was a decrease in both free retinol and retinyl esters. Liver changes were possibly related to the in vitro inhibitory effects of α-tocopherol on liver retinyl hydrolase. Lung retinyl hydrolase, on the other hand, was stimulated by α-tocopherol in vitro.[35] The reason for the different responses by the hydrolase enzyme is unknown. Since there is evidence that many preterm infants have very low serum tocopherol concentrations compared to adults,[36] it is theoretically possible that retinol needs of preterm infants could be altered.

In general, zinc deficiency is associated with decreased serum vitamin A concentrations and tissue vitamin A stores. It is unclear whether zinc deficiency directly affects retinol nutrition and metabolism or merely lowers serum vitamin A concentrations and tissue stores as a result of reduced food intake accompanying zinc deficiency.[6] Zinc may well be essential for the synthesis of RBP in liver.[37] Zinc is the metal element involved in a family of metalloenzymes known as alcohol dehyrogenases; retinol dehydrogenase (retinal reductase) is an alcohol dehydrogenase that is responsible for interconversion of retinol to retinal and the reverse reaction.[37] In the past, a zinc-deficiency-like dermatosis was seen in some infants on intravenous parenteral nutrition;[38] reports have increased the recommendations for zinc in infant parenteral nutrition.[39] In our own institution, enterally fed preterm infants supplemented with additional daily zinc had statistically higher serum retinol concentratons in the first 7 days of life than in a non-supplemented group.[40] Serum RBP concentration was not affected in this or another previously reported study.[41] Thus, there is the theoretical potential that retinol needs of a neonate might be altered by zinc needs.

Dietary restriction of protein and energy cause a decrease in serum RBP concentrations; RBP is sensitive to dietary alterations because of its short biological half-life.[42,43] Preterm infants have lower plasma RBP concentrations than term neonates; lower concentrations might be related to low protein and caloric intake in some preterm infants.[44] Many sick preterm infants who are receiving nutrients only by intravenous alimentation have nutrient restrictions because of accompanying problems such as fluid overload or cholestatic jaundice. Under these circumstances then, if RBP synthesis was reduced, peripheral target tissues might not receive adequate retinol because of lack of mobilization of liver stores of retinol.

DEFICIENCY

Vitamin A deficiency remains a severe worldwide problem. The most affected population is children.[7] The predominantly recognized clinical signs and symptoms specific to vitamin A deficiency in humans are ocular. These signs have been grouped and termed *xerophthalmia*. The earliest of these symptoms is night blindness, followed by manifestations in the conjunctiva and cornea as a result of the loss of normal differentiation of epithelial tissue.[4,5,7] Conjunctival xerosis and corneal xerosis lead to ulceration, necrosis,

keratomalacia, and finally a corneal scar that can partially impair vision and is frequently irreversible. Retinol deficiency in weanling rats leads to disruption of the photoreceptor outer segments, decreased retinal rhodopsin content, and decreased electroretinogram (ERG) activity. Abnormalities of the ERG due to retinol deficiency accompanying cystic fibrosis have been demonstrated.[45] It is not known what effect the retinol status of preterm or term infants has on neonatal ERG, although recently interest in the ERG in small infants has emerged.

Frequent symptoms and signs of deficiency reported have been anorexia, slowed growth, increased susceptibility to infections, disturbances in the reproductive system, and increased cerebrospinal fluid pressure.[4,5,7] In animals, deficiency affects nearly every tissue of the body, especially, but not exclusively, those of primarily epithelial lining and origin, such as the digestive tract, urinary tract, and respiratory tract.[5]

Overt clinical signs of deficiency in the neonate apparently have not been reported. Even neonates dying with vitamin A content as low as 3 μg/gm liver were not described as having classical signs of vitamin A deficiency.[22] It is unlikely that their eyes were extensively examined premortem or postmortem, however.

Although an association between low plasma retinol concentrations and BPD in preterm infants has been shown,[18,27] further work needs to be done to determine if there is a casual relationship between low retinol stores and BPD, or whether insufficient supplementation of retinol occurs in these infants. Another neonatal illness with extensive involvement of epithelium, necrotizing enterocolitis, also has been suspected of being associated with vitamin A deficiency,[46] but this likewise is unproven.

TOXICITY

A moderate excess of vitamin A can be consumed and no harm occurs because most of the compound is merely stored. However, hypervitaminosis A does occur and has serious sequelae.

Moore and others[47] have described the observation of vitamin A poisoning of humans and dogs by the consumption of *polar bear liver*—first reported by arctic explorers in 1596. Typically, a few hours after the meal of polar bear liver, symptoms of drowsiness, headache, irritability and vomiting occur. Since polar bear liver contains 3,900–5,400 µg vitamin A/gm,[45] the consumption of 8 oz of liver would provide about 1.23 grams of vitamin A, about 10 times the total reserves of a typical adult male.

Since the introduction and availability of synthetic retinol compounds, toxicity all too commonly occurs because of overdosing.[4] The literature has recently been extensively reviewed.[4,5,7] Acute toxicity has occurred from single massive doses of 100,000 IU (30,000 µg) or more given to infants. Bulging cranial fontanelles are common, accompanied by nausea, vomiting, fever and neurologic symptoms. Chronic toxicity in children can occur when large doses of vitamin A, frequently being used for treatment of skin conditions, are purposely or accidentally abused by using too often. Symptoms include dry skin, alopecia and headaches. Usually, symptoms and signs disappear after cessation of ingestion of the vitamin, but continued abuse can lead to hepatotoxicity, bone fracture and death.[5,7]

Vitamin A is also very teratogenic. Recently, there have been reports of a high incidence of embryopathy in offspring of mothers who had received isotretinoin (13-cis-retinoic acid) for acne or dermatoses while pregnant.[48] It is hoped that the exact risk of this problem soon will be known so that such retinoic acid embryopathy can be avoided in the future.

SUMMARY OF NEEDS

The latest available recommendations of retinol needs for neonates and infants less than 6 months are around 420 µg of retinol/day.[5,6] This appears slightly higher than what would be the daily intake (375 µg) of a breast-fed term infant receiving 750 ml per day of breast milk containing 50 µg of retinol/dl. This range of intake seems both adequate and safe. In a term infant receiving 750 ml of standard proprietary formula (90 µg of retinol/dl), the vitamin A intake would be 675 µg, which would be higher than the RDA. Two concerns remain to be clarified: (1) the recommendations in part are based on turnover studies in a small group of human adults, and (2) there is some evidence that no signs of deficiency or reduced growth rate occurred in children receiving only 100-200 µg/day.[49,50]

The preterm infant might have problems in reaching the recommendation given above. Assuming a tolerance of enteral feedings of a proprietary formula containing 90 µg of reti-

nol/dl, a 1.5 kg neonate receiving 150 ml/kg/day would receive 135 µg of retinol/kg/day and a total of 203 µg of retinol per day.

$$(150 \text{ ml/kg} \times 90 \text{ µg of retinol}/100 \text{ ml} = 135 \text{ µg of retinol/kg})$$

In comparison, a 3.5-kg counterpart term neonate with a similar intake on a per kg basis (135 µg/kg) would receive a vitamin A intake of 473 µg, exceeding slightly the RDA. It is possible that turnover, utilization, and absorption efficiency rates of retinol are different between the term and preterm infant, especially in the first few weeks of life. However, as yet there are no data on the question of whether retinol supplements should be based on gestational age, or weight in the first 6 months of life. Until there are specific data, it seems reasonable to start with the recommended formulations.

In sick preterm infants receiving retinol by the intravenous route, much of the retinol is adsorbed onto the supply tubing.[21] Recommendations for intravenous retinol previously have been 70-100 µg of retinol/kg/day, lower than enteric recommendations, probably based on the assumption of attaining delivery above that by the enteral route. However, one should account for anticipated losses of about 60-75% and increase accordingly the concentration of retinol in the intravenous solution. Alternatively, intravenous *retinyl palmitate* might be used at a dose of 100 µg/kg/day since relatively little of the palmitate is adsorbed to tubing.[51]

Deficiency of vitamin A is most easily induced experimentally, and most frequently described clinically in a growing and malnourished population. It is likely that various tissues may have different specific requirements for vitamin A. It seems possible that a *"conditional deficiency,"* or one where an increased amount of exogenous retinol would be necessary in specific conditions of "stress" could arise in the sick term infant. The present RDAs for 0-6 month infants for retinol already are high when compared to an adult on a per kg basis, which may help cover the situation of the neonate born with low liver stores and anticipated growth. Whether these recommendations cover a "conditional deficiency" or increased needs for retinol that occur possibly with prematurity associated illnesses will require further research and observation to answer.

CASE REPORT

A 7.0-kg female infant was admitted to the hospital at 4½ months of age with hyperirritability and a recent onset of anorexia. The physical examination revealed a tense, bulging anterior cranial fontanelle, spread sutures, and a head circumference of 44 cm. The skin was generally dry and there was desquamation of the palms and soles. There was no jaundice or hepatosplenomegaly. No definite skin tenderness was apparent.

Past history revealed that the term infant was 3.6 kg at birth with no neonatal problems, and she went home breastfeeding. At the one-month examination, the physician told the mother that the infant was not gaining weight very well and said something about being sure she gave the vitamin supplement. This discussion was misinterpreted by the parents, and they started giving the supplemental vitamin dose with every feeding instead of one dose daily. In addition, they had recently gone into the chicken-raising business, and beginning at 2½ months the infant was given chicken liver daily in the form of a thick soup or slurry. This was started because the parents remembered their grandparents talking about liver as a good source for some vitamin.

The total serum vitamin A concentration (retinol plus retinyl ester) was 150 µg/dl. The child was treated with a regular diet and the tense fontanelle treated with three spinal taps over a 10-day period. Both the chicken liver soup and supplemental vitamin were discontinued, and she was discharged in 2 weeks. At 3 weeks after discharge, the skin had improved, the fontanelle was flat, and the serum vitamin A was 50 µg/dl.

Questions and Answers

Q. What is an estimate of the vitamin A that might be ingested with this approach for 2 months?
A. Estimation of excess vitamin A given to infant:
  (a) Vi-Daylin (1500 I.U. vitamin A/ml)
    5/ml/day × 1500 I.U./ml × 0.3 µg retinol/
    I.U. × 60 days = 135 mg
  (b) liver (250 µg/g) and assume one ounce consumption per day:

    250 µg/gm × 30 gm/oz × 60 days = 450 mg
    _____
    Total: 585 mg extra retinol
    given over the 2 months

REFERENCES

1. Schneider HA. Rats, fats, and history. Perspect Biol Med 1986;29:392-406.
2. McCollum EV, Davis M. The necessity of certain lipins during growth, J Biol Chem 1913;15:167-175.
3. McCollum EV, Davis M. Observations on the isolation of the substance in butterfat which exerts a stimulating influence on growth. J Biol Chem 1914;19:245-250.
4. Pitt AJ. Vitamin A. In Diplock AT (ed): Fat Soluble Vitamins, London, William Heinemann, Ltd., 1985;1-75.
5. Olson JA. Vitamin A. In Maclin LJ (ed): Handbook of Vitamins: Nutritional, Biochemical, and Clinical Aspects. New York, Marcel Dekker, Inc., 1984;1-43.
6. Goodman DeW S. Vitamin A and retinoids in health and disease. N Engl J Med 1984;310:1023-1031.
7. Underwood BA. Vitamin A in animal and human nutrition. In Sporn MB, Roberts AB, Goodman DS (eds): The Retinoids, Vol I, Orlando, FL, Academic Press, Inc., 1984;281-392.

8. Beaton GH. Nutritional needs during the first year of life: Some concepts and perspectives, Pediatr Clin North Am 1985;32:275-288.
9. Crow JA, Ong DE. Cell-specific immunohistochemical localization of a cellular retinol-binding protein (type two) in the small intestine of rat. Proc Natl Acad Sci USA 1985;82:4707-4711.
10. Ong DE, Crow JA, Chytil F. Radioimmunochemical determination of cellular retinol and cellular retinoic acid binding protein in cytosols of rat tissue. J Biol Chem 1982;257:13385-13389.
11. Dowling JE, Wald G. The biological function of vitamin A acid. Proc Natl Acad Sci USA 1960;46:587-608.
12. Zile MH, Cullum ME. The function of vitamin A: current concepts. Proc Soc Exp Biol Med 1983;172:139-152.
13. Rodriquez ME, Irwin MI. A conspectus of research on vitamin A requirements in man. J Nutr 1972;102:909-968.
14. Sauberlich HE, Hodges RE, Wallace DL, et al. Vitamin A metabolism and requirements in the human studied with the use of labelled retinol. Vitam Horm 1974;32:251-275.
15. Moore T. Vitamin A transfer from mother to offspring in mice and rats. Int J Vitam Nutr Res 1971;41:301-306.
16. Takahashi YI, Smith JE, Goodman DS. Vitamin A and retinol binding protein metabolism during fetal development in the rat. Am J Physiol 1977;233:E263-E272.
17. Dostalova L. Correlation of the vitamin status between mother and newborn at delivery. Dev Pharmacol Ther 1982;4:45-47.
18. Hustead VA, Gutcher GR, Anderson SA, Zachman RD. Relationship of vitamin A (retinol) status to lung disease in the preterm infant. J Pediat 1984;105:610-615.
19. Vobecky JS, Vobecky J, Shapcott D, et al. Biochemical indices of nutritional status in maternal, cord, and early neonatal blood. Am J Clin Nutr 1982;36:630-642.
20. Olson JA. New approaches to methods for assessment of nutritional status of the individual. Am J Clin Nutr 1982;35:1166-1168.
21. Zachman RD. Vitamin A. In Farrell PM, Taussig LM (eds): Bronchopulmonary Dysplasia and Related Chronic Respiratory Disorders. 90th Ross Conference on Pediatric Research. Columbus, Ross Laboratories, 1986;86-92.
22. Olson JA, Gunning DB, Tilton RA. Liver concentrations of vitamin A and carotenoids, as a function of age and other parameters of American children who died of various causes. Amer J Clin Nutr 1984;39:903-910.
23. Ismadi SD, Olson JA. Dynamics of the fetal distribution and transfer of vitamin A between rat fetuses and their mother. Int J Vitam Nutr Res 1982;52:111-116.
24. Zachman RD, Kakkad B, Chytil F. Perinatal rat lung retinol (vitamin A) and retinyl palmitate. Pediatr Res 1984;18:1297-1299.
25. Pitt GAJ. The assessment of vitamin A status. Proc Nutr Soc 1981;40:173-178.
26. Underwood BA. The determination of vitamin A and some aspects of its distribution, mobilization, and transport in health and disease. World Rev Nutr Diet 1974;19:123-172.
27. Shenai JP, Chytil F, Stahlman MT. Vitamin A status of neonates with chronic lung disease. Pediatr Res 1985;19:185-189.
28. Moore T (ed). Vitamin A. Amsterdam, Elsevier Publishing Co., 1975;208-210, 508.
29. Ong DE, Chytil F. Changes in levels of cellular retinol and retinoic acid-binding proteins of liver and lung during perinatal development of the rat. Proc Natl Acad Sci USA 1976;73:3976-3978.
30. Vaisman N, Mogilner BM, Sklan D. Vitamin A and E content of preterm and term milk. Nutr Res 1985;5:931-935.
31. Ostrea EM, Balun JE. Winkler R, Porter T. Serum antioxidant levels of vitamin E and beta carotene in newborn infants: Effects of gestational age, maternal serum concentration, and breast feeding. Am J Obstet Gynecol 1986;154:1014-1017.
32. Hay WW Jr. Nutrition of the fetus and premature infant. Perinatol-Neonatol 1985;4:19-29.
33. American Academy of Pediatrics. Pediatric Nutrition Handbook. Washington, D.C., 1979;395; and Nutrition Advances Group of the Department of Food and Nutrition of the AMA. JPEN 1979;3:258-261.

34. Frigg M, Broz J. Relationships between vitamin A and vitamin E in the chick. Int J Vit Nutr Res 1984;54:125–134.

35. Napoli JL, McCormick AM, O'Meara B, Dratz EA. Vitamin A metabolism: α-Tocopherol modulates tissue retinol levels *in vivo*, and retinyl palmitate hydrolase *in vitro*. Arch Biochem Biophys 1984;230:194–202.

36. Gutcher GR, Raynor WJ, Farrell PM. An evaluation of vitamin E status in premature infants. Am J Clin Nutr 1984;40:1078–1089.

37. Solomons NW, Russell RM. The interaction of vitamin A and zinc: implications for human nutrition. Am J Clin Nutr 1980;33:2031–2040.

38. Arlette JP, Johnson MM. Zinc deficiency dermatosis in preterm infants receiving prolonged parenteral alimentation. Am Acad Dermatol 1981;5:37.

39. Expert Panel for Nutrition Advising Group, AMA. Guidelines for essential trace element preparations for parenteral use. JAMA 1979;241:2051–2054.

40. Hustead VA, Greger J, Gutcher GR. The effect of zinc supplementation in the vitamin A status of preterm infants. Pediatr Res 1985;19:223A.

41. Lockitch G, Godolphin W, Pendray MR, et al. Serum zinc, copper, retinol, binding protein, pre-albumin, and ceruloplasmin concentrations in infants receiving intravenous zinc and copper supplementation. J Pediatr 1983;102:304–308.

42. Shetty PS, Jung RT, Watrasierwicy KE, James WPT. Rapid turnover transport proteins: An index of subclinical protein-energy malnutrition. Lancet 1979;2:230–232.

43. Smith FR, Suskind R, Thanangkul O, et al. Plasma vitamin A, retinol binding protein and prealbumin concentrations in protein calorie malnutrition. Am J Clin Nutr 1975;28:732–738.

44. Moskowitz R, Pereira GR, Heaf L, et al. Retinol binding protein (RBP) levels in premature infants: Effects of nutrient intake. Pediatr Res 1982;16:301A.

45. Fulton AB, Hansen RM, Underwood BA, et al. Scotopic thresholds and plasma retinol in cystic fibrosis. Invest Ophthalmol Vis Sci 1982;23:364–370.

46. Brandt RB, Mueller DG, Schroeder JR, et al. Serum vitamin A in premature and term neonates. J Pediatr 1978;92:101–104.

47. Moore T. Pharmacology and toxicology of vitamin A. In Sebrell WH Jr, Harris RS (eds): The Vitamins: Chemistry, Physiology, Pathology, Methods, Vol. I. New York, Academic Press, 1967;280–294.

48. Lammer EJ, Chen DT, Hoar RM, et al. Retinoic acid embryopathy. N Engl J Med 1985;313:837–841.

49. Batista M. Considerations about the problem of vitamin A in northeastern Brazil. Hospital 1969;75:817–832.

50. Patwardhan VN. Hypovitaminosis A and epidemiology of xerophthalmia. Am J Clin Nutr 1969;22:1106–1118.

51. Gutcher GR, Lax AA, Farrell PM. Vitamin A losses to plastic intravenous infusion devices and an improved method of delivery. Am J Clin Nutr 1984;40:8–13.

15

Vitamin D

BONNY L. SPECKER, Ph.D.
FRANK GREER, M.D.
REGINALD C. TSANG, M.D.

"Rickets is indeed a price paid by man for his abandonment of a life out-of-doors and a natural diet for a life in houses and a diet of denatured food stuffs; it is a sign of the operation of the immutable law of nature that *nothing out of accord with her shall flourish.*" Edward A. Parks, 1923

ABSTRACT

Vitamin D is not present in significant amounts in naturally occurring food items except oily fish. It is produced endogenously in skin upon exposure to ultraviolet radiation and is transported throughout the body bound to a specific vitamin D binding protein. Vitamin D undergoes hydroxylation in the liver to 25-hydroxyvitamin D which is often used as a serum indicator of vitamin D status. The 25-hydroxyvitamin D metabolite is further converted to 1,25-dihydroxyvitamin D in the kidney, a process that is regulated by parathyroid hormone (PTH), and decreased calcium and phosphorus. The 1,25-dihydroxyvitamin D metabolite is the biologically active form of vitamin D which acts on intestine, bone and kidney to ensure calcium and phosphorus homeostasis. Deficiency of vitamin D in infancy results in rickets and supplementation of 400 IU of vitamin D/day is recommended for infants not exposed to adequate amounts of ultraviolet radiation.

INTRODUCTION

A clearer understanding of vitamin D physiology has been gained in recent years with the development of laboratory assays for the determination of vitamin D metabolite concentrations in serum. Various factors have been noted to have an influence on vitamin D metabolism during infancy, including maternal and environmental influences as well as the infant's age, race and diet.

PHYSIOLOGY

GENERAL PHYSIOLOGY

Vitamin D is derived either exogenously from dietary sources or is produced endogenously in the epidermis of skin upon exposure to ultraviolet (UV) radiation (290 to 320 nm wavelength). **Unlike other vitamins, vitamin D is not present in significant amounts in naturally occurring food items except oily fish.**

Two chemical forms of vitamin D exist: vitamin D_2 (ergocalciferol), which is of plant

FIGURE 1. Two chemical forms of vitamin D exist: vitamin D_2 (ergocalciferol), which is of plant origin, and vitamin D_3 (cholecalciferol), which is of animal origin.

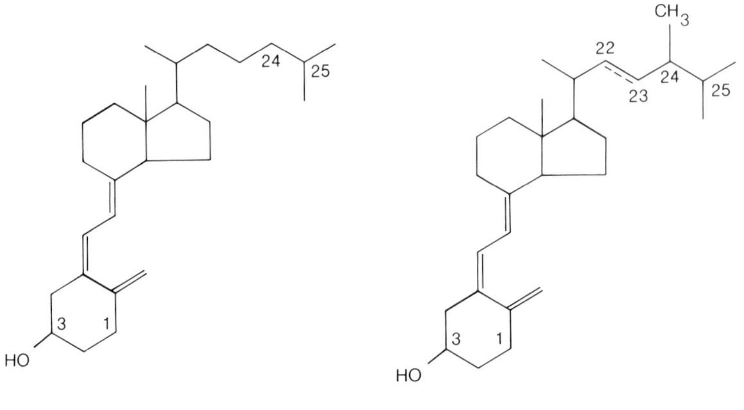

CHOLECALCIFEROL (D_3)

ERGOCALCIFEROL (D_2)

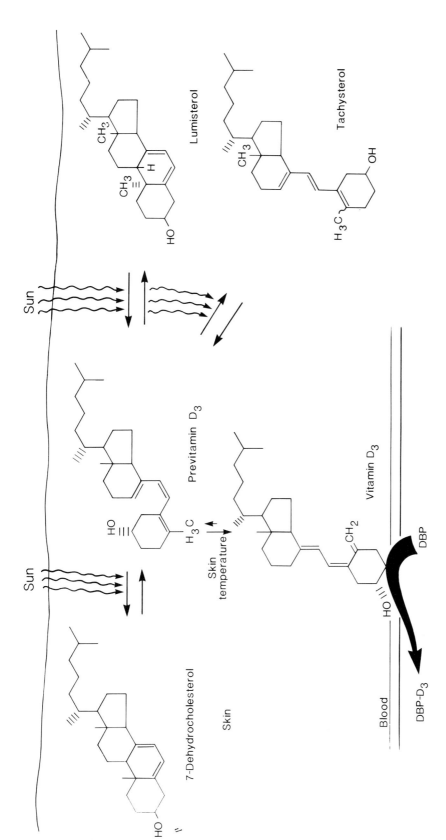

FIGURE 2.   Formation of vitamin D_3 in skin. 7-Dehydrocholesterol is converted to pre-vitamin D_3, which undergoes thermal isomerization to vitamin D_3, which is carried in the blood bound to vitamin D binding protein. During continual exposure to the sun, pre-vitamin D_3 also photoisomerizes to lumisterol$_3$ and tachysterol$_3$, which are biologically inert photoproducts; that is, they do not stimulate intestinal calcium absorption. As soon as pre-vitamin D_3 stores are depleted (because of thermal isomerization to D_3), exposure of lumisterol and tachysterol to ultraviolet radiation will promote the photoisomerization of these isomers to pre-vitamin D_3. (From Holick et al. Science 1981;211:590–593, with permission.)

origin, and vitamin D_3 (cholecalciferol), which is of animal origin (Fig. 1). In general terms, both forms of vitamin D appear to be metabolized similarly and further discussion will refer to both the D_2 and D_3 forms and their metabolites, unless otherwise specified.

Hess and Weinstock in 1925 irradiated excised human skin with a mercury-vapor lamp, fed it to rats, and were able to prevent rickets. They concluded therefore that the anti-rachitic factor was formed from the human skin.[1]

In the skin, 7-dehydrocholesterol (7-DHC), an intermediate in cholesterol biosynthesis, is converted to previtamin D_3 by UV radiation;[2] previtamin D_3 is isomerized to vitamin D_3; vitamin D is released into the circulation bound to vitamin D binding protein. Excessive amounts of previtamin D_3 in the skin can be further converted to either lumisterol or tachysterol (Fig. 2), which are stored in skin and are in equilibrium with previtamin D_3.[3] In addition, these metabolites have a low affinity for vitamin D binding protein and therefore do not enter the circulation; thus lumisterol may provide a storage site for vitamin D and possibly a *protective mechanism* against vitamin D toxicity resulting from UV exposure.

The diet is another source of vitamin D in countries where fortification of foodstuffs with vitamin D is practiced, or where fish oil is routinely consumed. In general, the absorption rate of vitamin D is linearly related to the dose, suggesting that absorption takes place by simple passive diffusion, presumably after stabilization by bile salts.[4] The role of bile salts is confirmed by findings of decreased vitamin D absorption in adult subjects with fat malabsorption due to bile salt deficiency.[5] In normal adults, an absorption of vitamin D between 62 and 91% (mean 78%) has been reported,[6] but in adults with T-tube biliary drainage after elective cholecystectomy[7] the absorption rate of vitamin D_3 is only 3.9%.

In full-term infants (3-21 days) with inoperable brain deformities, Kodicek reported that between 77 and 87% of an oral dose of labeled vitamin D was absorbed within three days.[8] Vitamin D and its metabolites may be excreted in the bile into the intestine and undergo intestinal reabsorption; the physiologic significance of this enterohepatic circulation is unclear.[7,9,10]

Vitamin D is more properly considered a steroid hormone than a vitamin in the classic sense; D_3 itself may be regarded as a prohormone or precursor.[11]

Since the late 1960s it has been known that vitamin D undergoes 25-hydroxylation to 25-hydroxyvitamin D (25OHD) in the liver and 1α-hydroxylation in the kidney to 1,25-dihydroxyvitamin D (1,25-$(OH)_2D$). The concentration of the former compound in serum is often used as an indicator of vitamin D status. $1,25(OH)_2$ D is essentially a hormone and plays a major factor in calcium metabolism; its concentration is used as an indicator of calcium and phosphorus needs; **elevated concentrations occur when there is increased need for calcium and phosphorus.** The primary role of $1,25(OH)_2D$ is to stimulate absorption of calcium and phosphorus from the small intestine; it also appears to promote reabsorption of calcium and phosphorus in the kidney, and, in concert with parathyroid hormone (PTH), the mobilization of calcium and phosphorus from bone.

The synthesis of 25-OHD by the liver generally is not tightly controlled and is dependent on the availability of vitamin D. However, **the synthesis of $1,25(OH)_2D$ is under strict endocrine control** through regulation of 1α-hydroxylase in the kidney.[12] The major stimulus for this enzyme appears to be PTH, whose secretion is increased by a decrease in extracellular calcium concentration. The enzyme also is stimulated directly by reduced serum calcium and phosphorus concentrations (Fig. 3).

Cellular receptors for $1,25(OH)_2D$ have been identified in many different tissues.[13] In the intestinal mucosa, the $1,25(OH)_2D$ receptor complex stimulates nuclear transcription of genetic information which codes for calcium binding protein (CaBP). In some species, calcium absorption from the intestinal mucosa begins before the appearance of CaBP in the cytoplasm, suggesting an alternative mechanism for the effect of $1,25(OH)_2D$ on intestinal calcium transport,[14] possibly due to $1,25(OH)_2D$ altering mucosal membrane lipid composition.[15,16]

PHYSIOLOGY IN THE INFANT

For the human infant there are three potential sources of vitamin D and its metabolites. The first source is from maternal transfer of vitamin D or its metabolites across the placenta to the fetus. The second source is dietary intake of vitamin D and its metabolites from human milk, formula, vitamin D fortified milk or direct oral supplements of the vitamin. The third source is the photosynthesis of endo-

25 liver
1 kidney.

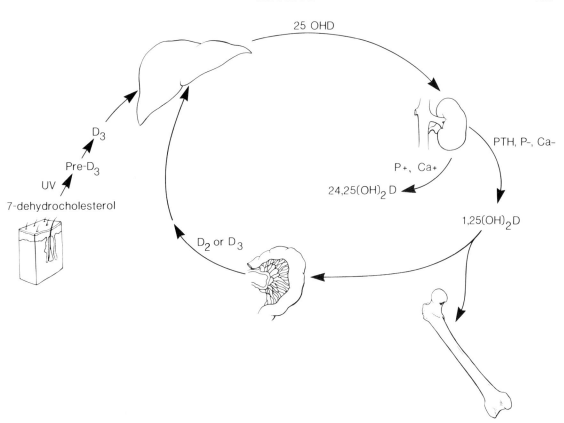

FIGURE 3. Vitamin D₃, which is normally produced in the skin, is converted to 25-hydroxylation in the liver. 25-Hydroxyvitamin D is the major vitamin D metabolite and is often used as an indicator of vitamin D status. 25-Hydroxyvitamin D is further converted to either 24,25-dihydroxyvitamin D or 1,25-dihydroxyvitamin D. The renal conversion of 1,25-dihydroxyvitamin D is stimulated by calcium lack, phosphate lack and parathyroid hormone (PTH). 1,25-Dihydroxyvitamin D₃ results in stimulation of intestinal calcium and phosphate absorption and mobilization of calcium from bone. (From Tsang et al. Clin Perinatol 1981;8:287–306, with permission.)

genous vitamin D in the skin of infants following sunshine exposure.

Vitamin D and some of its metabolites cross the placenta but the relative importance of placental transfer, or fetal synthesis of vitamin D metabolites in the fetus is unknown. Vitamin D crosses the placenta from mother to fetus in the rat[31] and sheep[18], but not in the cow.[19] In man, from indirect evidence, it has been suggested that very little vitamin D itself normally crosses the placenta to the fetus;[20] when very large amounts of vitamin D₂ (100,000 IU/day) are given, some placental crossover of vitamin D₂ occurs.

In rat, sheep, cow, and human, 25-OHD crosses the placenta from mother to fetus.[18,19,21] In humans, cord blood 25-OHD concentrations are generally lower than maternal levels with a significant correlation between the two;[22-28] in two studies cord blood values were similar to maternal values.[29,30] Cord blood 25-OHD concentration at term also reflects the seasonal variation of maternal 25-OHD concentration.[25,26] From studies in Asian immigrants in Great Britain it has been suggested that the **fetal–neonatal 25-OHD status is significantly dependent on maternal 25-OHD status.**[17] These data are consistent with maternal-fetal transfer of 25-OHD in the human.

1,25(OH)₂D, synthesized by the maternal kidney from 25-OHD, probably does not cross the placenta from mother to fetus in rat[31] and cows,[19] though it may do so in sheep[18] and monkey.[32] Transfer of 1,25(OH)₂D across the perfused human placenta in vitro has been reported,[33] and in a single pregnant mother receiving very large oral doses of 1,25(OH)₂D.[34] In human studies, cord blood concentrations of 1,25(OH)₂D are lower than maternal serum concentrations, and a correlation has been found in some[11,23-25] but not all studies.[27-30]

The role of the fetal kidney in the synthesis

of 1,25(OH)$_2$D is not clear. In the pregnant rat, maternal nephrectomy does not prevent 1,25 (OH)$_2$D synthesis from labeled 25-OHD, and labeled 1,25(OH)$_2$D is found on both the maternal and fetal sides of the placenta,[35-37] implying a site for synthesis of 1,25(OH)$_2$D in pregnancy that is not exclusively in the maternal kidney. In sheep, fetal kidney may be important in the synthesis of 1,25(OH)$_2$D[38]. In the human fetus, the role of fetal kidney in 1,25(OH)$_2$D synthesis is not known. The term human placenta can synthesize 1,25(OH)$_2$D in vitro,[39,40] though whether the synthesis is occurring on the maternal or fetal side of the placenta remains controversial.[41,42]

It is unknown to what extent the fetus is able to store vitamin D or its metabolites for utilization after birth. Vitamin D is stored in fat in the rat[43] and may be stored in muscle and other tissues in the adult human.[44] It appears that 25-OHD is rapidly released after its formation in the rat liver and not stored in tissues.[45]

The diet is the second source of vitamin D for the infant. Commercial infant formulas in the United States are fortified with 400 IU of vitamin D per liter. Human milk often contains less than 40 IU of vitamin D/L and this has stimulated research on the adequacy of human milk for the vitamin D needs of breast-fed infants.[46] Almost all of the vitamin D activity in human milk can be accounted for by *vitamin D* (parent compound, concentration 39-380 pg/ml) *and 25-OHD* (concentration 150-375 pg/ml); the concentration of 1,25(OH)$_2$D in human milk is negligible.[47-49] In spite of original claims to the contrary[50] the contribution of vitamin D sulfate, a water-soluble metabolite of vitamin D, to the biological activity of vitamin D in human milk is insignificant.[51]

It is not known exactly how vitamin D and 25-OHD gain access to human milk. Vitamin D binding protein (DBP) may play a role as it is found in human milk and appears to be of plasma origin. Vitamin D and its metabolites bind to DBP with varying affinities, 25-OHD being more tightly bound than vitamin D.[52]

Because of the weaker interaction between vitamin D and the plasma carrier as compared to 25-OHD, one could speculate that vitamin D, as a free molecule, is more easily diffusible into human milk. This is supported by the effect of maternal ultraviolet B light on the vitamin D content of human milk. In a recent study, lactating mothers receiving 1.5 minimal erythemal doses (MED) of total body ultraviolet-B light (about 90 seconds of irradiation), had a ten-fold increase in milk vitamin D$_3$ concentration with little change in milk 25-OHD concentration.[53]

In addition to UV-B light, maternal supplements of vitamin D may also affect the vitamin D concentration of human milk. In lactating mothers given an oral dose of vitamin D of 2500 IU/day for two weeks, breast milk concentration increased from <20 to 140 IU/L, all of the increase being accounted for by vitamin D and 25-OHD in the milk.[52] In a more dramatic case, a mother taking 100,000 IU/day of vitamin D$_2$ achieved a breast milk concentration of 7000 IU/L, which was almost exclusively vitamin D$_2$ and 25-OHD$_2$.[54] Recently in a cross-sectional study, breast milk vitamin D concentrations also have been found to be correlated with vitamin D intakes in ranges normally consumed (0-700 IU/day).[55]

The third source of vitamin D in infants is from the photosynthesis of vitamin D$_3$ in skin. Seasonal variations have been observed in older children[56,57] and during infancy.[58,59] In a recent study in Cincinnati, Ohio it has been estimated that throughout the year a conservative estimate of **2 hours a week of sunshine exposure in fully clothed (hands and head exposed), white, breast-fed infants will maintain serum 25-OHD concentrations above 11 ng/ml,** the lower limit of the normal range.[59] This estimate has been confirmed in a study in Beijing, China, where infants were randomly assigned to experimental sunshine (taken outside 2 hours per day) compared with conventional sunshine exposure.[60] Thus, a minimum amount of time in sunshine in temperate climates appears sufficient to maintain adequate vitamin D status for a large proportion of the population.

Serum Vitamin D Metabolite Concentrations in Infancy

Table 1 summarizes the normative data from a recent large cross sectional study of 198 infants less than 18 months of age and the factors found to be related to vitamin D metabolites.[61,62] The normative ranges are based on the mean ± 2 standard deviations. The range for serum 25-OHD is large and includes serum concentrations that may be associated with vitamin D deficiency. Based on observed serum 25-OHD concentrations during vitamin D deficiency rickets and values observed in adults, the lower limit of the normal range is considered to be approximately 11 ng/ml.

TABLE 1.   Normal Ranges Birth to 18 Months of Life

	n	x	Normal Range (± 2SD)	Important Variables*
iCa (mg/dl)	196	5.26	4.84–5.68	↓ with age, ↓ in formula-fed
Ca (mg/dl)	193	9.73	8.55–10.91	↓ in summer
Mg (mg/dl)	194	2.10	1.72–2.48	↓ in summer
P (mg/dl)	194	6.56	4.88–8.24	↓ in winter months, ↓ with age, ↓ with blacks, ↓ in human milk-fed
cPTH (ng/ml)	145	1.2	0.9–1.6	↓ in winter
DBP (µg/ml)	163	358	212–504	↑ with age, ↓ in summer, ↓ in human milk-fed
25-OHD (ng/ml)	199	46	4–88	↓ in winter, ↓ in human milk-fed
1,25(OH)$_2$D (pg/ml)	189	61	13–109	↓ in white infants ↓ in summer

*Race, age, season and diet investigated. No sex differences in any variable.

Serum 25-OHD concentrations are decreased during winter months compared to summer and in breast-fed infants compared to formula-fed infants. No change in serum 25-OHD with age was observed.

Serum 1,25(OH)$_2$D concentrations increase in full term infants during the first 24 hours of life,[30] presumably reflecting the ability of the neonatal kidneys to actively synthesize 1,25 (OH)$_2$D. **In the first 18 months of life, serum 1,25-(OH)$_2$D concentrations have been found to be higher in black infants compared to white infants; 1,25(OH)$_2$D concentrations are also higher during winter months compared to summer months.**[61] These findings are interpreted to imply active synthesis of 1,25(OH)$_2$D in situations where low vitamin D status potentially could occur.

ASSESSMENT OF VITAMIN D NEEDS

The current recommended daily allowance for vitamin D for infants in the United States is 400 IU/day and is based on studies completed during the 1930s.[63] These studies were completed in a group of infants fed cow milk: term infants fed milk containing 60-135 units of biological vitamin D activity per quart did not develop rickets and had growth rates comparable to other infants reported in the literature of the period.[64] Infants given 340-400 units of vitamin D per day (1 teaspoon of cod liver oil) were found to grow at more rapid rates.[65]

Based on studies on the prevention of rickets, the promotion of linear growth, and on theoretic promotion of intestinal absorption of calcium, the vitamin D requirement was thought to range from 100 to approximately 400 units/day.

Doses higher than 400 units/day did not result in a greater degree of protection against rickets, a greater promotion of linear growth, or an increase in the retention of calcium. Although these early studies have been questioned, doses of 300-500 IU of vitamin D/day have been found to result in rapid healing of severe vitamin D deficiency rickets, supporting the effectiveness of this dose of vitamin D.

The American Academy of Pediatrics Committee on Nutrition, in their 1963 report, supported the view that full-term infants fed cow milk formulas or human milk should receive a total of 400 IU of vitamin D/day from all dietary sources and that this amount would prevent rickets and promote optimal calcium and phosphorus metabolism.[65] These values represent the total recommended daily intake from all ingested sources, and assume adequate amounts of calcium and phosphorus in the diet and *no sunlight exposure*. This value also incorporates a safety factor beyond a minimum daily requirement of the normal infant.

Standard infant formula contains 400 IU/L of vitamin D which is sufficient to maintain adequate vitamin D status. However human milk usually contains low amounts of vitamin D (<40 IU/L) and the infant fed human milk may need supplemental vitamin D. "Triple vitamin" (A, C and D) preparations were developed prior to the modern infant formulas, during a period when "evaporated" milk was used. Due to the low amount of vitamins A, C and D in evaporated milk, these vitamin preparations were often given to infants. Today the triple vitamin preparation can be readily used for the infant fed human milk.

Greer and coworkers in 1981 completed a double blind prospective study to determine whether or not supplemental vitamin D affected vitamin D status and bone mineralization in full-term, breast-fed infants.[66] Nine infants were randomly assigned to a vitamin D supplement of 400 IU per day and 9 infants to a placebo. By 12 weeks of age, infants receiving placebo had a significant decrease in bone mineralization and serum 25-OHD concentration compared to the vitamin D supplemented group (Fig. 4). However, differences in bone mineral content (BMC) were not significant between groups at 26 or 52 weeks of age.[66]

In Greer's study, serum 25-OHD concentrations declined progressively in the first 6 months of life in the placebo group but did not decline in the supplemented group. The decline in serum 25-OHD concentrations may have been a result of decreased sunlight exposure; by study design, 16 of the 18 infants were born during the summer months and thus the first 6 months theoretically were associated with progressive decrease in sun exposure. Roberts and coworkers, in a non-randomized study, also found differences by 4 months of age in mean 25-OHD concentrations between vitamin D–supplemented and non-supplemented breast-fed infants.[67] However, no difference in bone mineral content between the vitamin D supplemented and non-supplemented infants was observed.

Investigators have found that even though maternal vitamin D status may be adequate, some infants fed human milk alone may be at a risk of vitamin D deficiency.[68,69] Recently the specific relationship between sun exposure and 25-OHD has been quantitated in infants; Specker and coworkers determined the relationship between serum 25-OHD concentrations and sunshine exposure in full-term exclusively breast-fed infants.[59] Sunshine exposure in infants was quantitated using an ultraviolet dosimeter and a sunshine and clothing diary to estimate surface area exposed to sunshine. There was a direct correlation between serum 25-OHD concentrations and sunshine exposure in these infants.

In an additional longitudinal study quantitating sunshine exposure during the first year of life, in winter- or summer-born breast-fed infants, Specker et al. found a **cyclical seasonal pattern in serum 25-OHD concentrations.[70]** High 25-OHD concentrations were found in summer-born infants dropping to low concentrations in winter; low serum 25-OHD concentrations were present in winter-born infants, which rose in summer; the changes in the two groups of infants mirrored each other, and in each group closely paralleled the extent of sunshine exposure (Fig. 5).[70] In a study in Scandinavia it was noted also that adequate vitamin D status can be obtained during summer months in infants fed human milk; during winter months supplementation of 400 IU/day vitamin D appeared to be necessary and adequate.[68]

As to the vitamin D needs of preterm infants, speculations have been made that the ability to hydroxylate vitamin D is a maturational change and that preterm infants have a decreased ability to produce 25-OHD.[71] However, several studies recently have not supported this hypothesis,[72,73] and the preterm infant appears to have adequate 25-hydroxylase activity. Many excellent reviews on the vitamin D requirements of preterm infants have been published.[74,75] In general, the vitamin D needs of preterm infants appear similar to those of full-term infants.

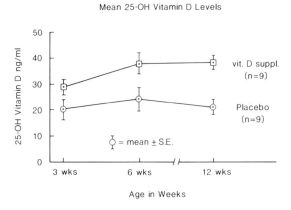

Mean 25-OH Vitamin D Levels

FIGURE 4. Effect of 400 IU of vitamin D/day on serum 25-hydroxyvitamin D concentrations. By 12 weeks of age, infants receiving placebo had a significant decrease in serum 25-hydroxyvitamin D concentration compared to the vitamin D supplemented group. (From Greer et al. J Pediatr 1982;100:919–922, with permission.)

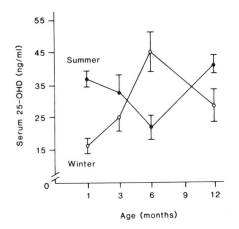

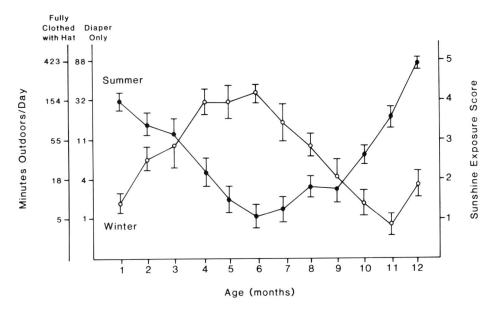

FIGURE 5. Significant changes in sunshine exposure occurs throughout the year and correlate with changes in serum 25-hydroxyvitamin D concentrations. These changes are significantly different for infants born during winter months (o) when compared to infants born during summer months (●). (From Specker BL, Tsang RC. J Pediatr, J Pediatr 1987;110:744-747, with permission.)

VITAMIN D DEFICIENCY AND TOXICITY

DEFICIENCY

Glisson in 1660 had established rickets as a clinical entity and believed it was the result of overeating.[76]

The derivation of the word "rickets" is obscure. One possibility is the Greek word for spine, "rhachis," converted into the word "rachitis" and then rickets. Another view is that the word arose from the Dorset dialect, to "rucket" (breathe with difficulty). Rucket in turn is possibly a derivation of the Scandinavian word "ruckle" (make a rattling noise in the throat). It may also be an eponym from the name of one Rickets who, in 1620, was active treating the disease in Dorset.[77] Another possibility is the early English "wrick" or "wrikken" (twist or sprain). By 1634 however the word was generally used as if it was general knowledge, although the medical profession called it "rachitis."[1]

The original description of rickets, as well as the first hint that it was a disease of urban dwellers, is due to Soranus of Ephesus (about A.D. 100), who ascribed the crooked legs of Roman toddlers both to maternal neglect and to the hardness of the street pavement which bent their soft bones.[78] It was Claudius Galenus (A.D. 130-210), in his De morborum-causis, who noticed thoracic deformities as well as *genu varus* or *valgus* in overfed children.

The first description of the modern age is the medical thesis, written in 1645, by Daniel Whistler.[79] The classical treatise "De Rachitide" of Francis Glisson appeared in 1650.[80] It was he who coined the word rachitis.

Rickets was common in industrialized cities in the nineteenth century and its incidence reported to be as high as 90% in British infants and children up to 4 to 5 years of age.[81] The Civil War also brought its rachitic toll. Already in 1870, as a consequence of the flight of former slaves to cities of the North, in Philadelphia 25% of all black children of less than five years of age had rickets.[82] As early as 1884, it was noted that there was a cyclical pattern to the incidence of rickets and tetany with increases during the winter months and decreases during the summer and autumn.[83] In 1885, Pommer established the pathology of rickets through histological studies.[84]

Possibly the most brilliant investigation into the cause of rickets was made by Theobald A. Palm, an English medical missionary in Japan who was "struck with the absence of rickets among the Janpanese." He studied the geographic distribution of rickets in 1890 and reported that "rickets came about as a result of lack of sunlight" and that its incidence was inversely related to the amount of sunshine at a given latitude. He even stated that "the important factor in the sunshine was the chemical activity of the sun's rays rather than its heat" and proposed a systematic use of sun baths as a preventive and therapeutic measure in rickets. Palm was astute enough also to point out that rickets was related to air pollution.[1]

In the early 1900s several hypotheses regarding the etiology of rickets were developed. Siegert had a theory of inheritance[85,86] which was supported by Sambon, who noted that pigmented skin increased the susceptibility to rickets and that a predisposition in that sense may be inherited.[87] In the late 1800s and early 1900s rickets also was thought to be a result of infectious disease. Koch felt he was able to produce rickets by means of inoculation with bacteria[88] and Edlefsen thought that the enlarged spleen in rickets was significant and regarded fever as an early manifestation of this infectious disease.[89] The occurrence of rickets in certain houses further suggested that it was related to an infectious agent.[88] **In 1909 Schmorl demonstrated seasonal variations in rickets in pathological studies and found the highest incidence of early manifestations of the disease to be between November and May.[90]**

Despite Funk's observation that rickets was a result of a substance missing in the diet, the credit for establishing the relationship between the development of rickets and a deficiency of vitamin D belongs to Mellanby, who in 1918 announced the production of rickets by means of a diet lacking in "an accessory factor."[92] In 1919 the British Medical Research Committee publicly stated that rickets was a deficiency disease due to a lack in the diet of an "antirachitic factor."[93]

Clinical signs of rickets include craniotabes, frontal skull bossing, rachitic rosary (enlarged costochondral junctions), widened ribs, bowed legs, and muscle weakness. Serum 25-OHD concentrations less than 15 ng/ml are often observed in cases with severe rickets.[94] In the early stage of rickets serum calcium concentration is low with normal serum phosphorus concentration (Fig. 6). Increases in parathyroid hormone, stimulated by the low serum calcium, result in an increase in serum 1,25 $(OH)_2D$, a normalization of serum calcium, and a decrease in serum phosphorus due to hyperphosphaturia. It is at this stage that typical rachitic bone features are present; serum 25-OHD concentrations are decreased but serum $1,25(OH)_2D$ concentrations may be normal or elevated.[95,96] Although concentrations of 1,25 $(OH)_2D$ may be elevated above the normal ranges, they still may be too low to maintain adequate mineral homeostasis.[97]

It is likely that the 1α-hydroxylase enzyme in the kidney is highly active in rickets, presumably stimulated by increased parathyroid hormone concentration and calcium and phosphorus deficiency. This suggestion is supported by consistent findings of increases in serum $1,25(OH)_2D$ to supranormal concentrations following the initiation of vitamin D therapy, even when vitamin D therapy is only 400 IU/day.[97] Presumably, supply of the substrate 25-OHD to a highly active 1α-hydroxylase produces marked elevation of serum 1,25 $(OH)_2D$ concentrations.

In 1914, Funk published the following: "it is very probable that rickets occurs only when certain substances in the diet essential for normal metabolism are lacking or supplied in insufficient amount. Substances occur in *good* breast milk, also in good cod liver oil, but are lacking in sterilized milk and in cereals."[91]

The first report of ultraviolet irradiation in the cure of rickets was made by Kurt Huldschinsky in 1919, a Berlin pediatrician who used a mercury-vapor quartz lamp, which includes ultraviolet irradiation, on four cases of advanced rickets, resulting in cures within two months. He even anticipated the current emphasis on vitamin D as a hormone by irradiating one arm of a rachitic child with ultraviolet light. X-rays showed that the calcium salts were deposited not only in the irradiated arm but in the other arm as well.[1]

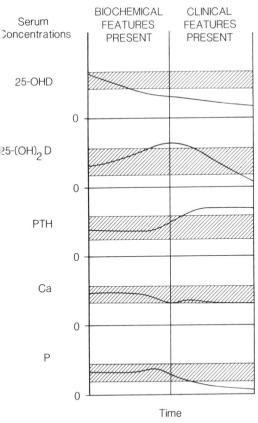

Serum Concentrations | BIOCHEMICAL FEATURES PRESENT | CLINICAL FEATURES PRESENT

25-OHD

0

25-(OH)$_2$ D

0

PTH

0

Ca

0

P

0

Time

FIGURE 6. Hypothetical time frame for development of vitamin D deficiency rickets.

TOXICITY

The clinical symptoms of vitamin D toxicity include nausea, anorexia, headache, growth retardation in children, diarrhea, polyuria, fatigue and restlessness. Kidney and cardiovascular damage may result from cellular and interstitial calcification, which also may occur in the lungs and intestine. Ironically, excessive amounts of vitamin D promote bone resorption.

In 1938 Jeans and Stearns suggested that daily intakes of vitamin D in the range of 1600 IU inhibited linear growth of normal infants and was therefore not desirable.[98] These data have come under criticism due to the small number of infants, the considerable variability in the growth patterns that were observed, and the inability to be confirmed by other workers. However, during the early 1950s in Great Britain and Switzerland there was a general emphasis on a high degree of maternal and infant dietary vitamin D supplementation such that an infant might routinely ingest 4000 IU of

vitamin D per day.[65] During this period of high vitamin D supplementation an "epidemic" of infantile hypercalcemia was discovered. Although no systematic study was done examining the relationship of vitamin D intake and infantile hypercalcemia, the incidence of hypercalcemia decreased dramatically when all sources of dietary vitamin D were withheld, supporting the thesis that high dietary vitamin D might indeed have been etiologically related to the incidence of infantile hypercalcemia.

RECOMMENDATIONS

Vitamin D intake is recommended at 400 IU/day for infants receiving limited sunshine exposure, in agreement with the American Academy of Pediatrics Committee on Nutrition recommendations.[65] This intake is recommended for term and preterm infants.

CASE REPORT

A one-year-old black male was noted to be "falling off" the growth curve at 6 to 7 months of age. Height, weight and head circumference measures at birth were between the 40th and 50th percentile. His development was normal except that he was not walking on his own. He had frequent upper respiratory tract infections. The child had been *exclusively breast-fed since birth.*

At presentation he was less than the 5th percentile in head circumference, height, and weight. Complete blood count and serum electrolytes, albumin, and total protein were determined and were normal. X-rays showed a 3-month bone age, "fraying" and cupping of the metaphyses of the long bones (Fig. 7), and peribronchial thickening. He had a serum calcium concentration of 7.9 mg/dl

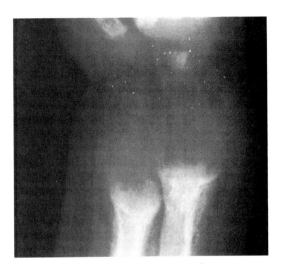

FIGURE 7. Radiograph of the wrist of a child showing classical signs of vitamin D deficiency rickets. "Fraying" and cupping of the metaphyses of the long bones are present.

(infant normal 8.6-10.9 mg/dl), serum phosphorus 3.6 mg/dl (infant normal 4.9-8.2 mg/dl), and alkaline phosphatase 792 IU/l.

His 25-hydroxyvitamin D (25-OHD) concentrations were undetectable (infant [breast-fed] normal 9-49 ng/ml). Serum 1,25-dihydroxyvitamin D (1,25-$(OH)_2$D) concentration was 97 pg/ml (infant normal 13-109 pg/ml), and intact PTH concentration was high (121 μl Eq/ml; adult normal 33-117 μl Eg/ml). The mother's serum 25-OHD concentration was 8 ng/ml (adult normal 11-68 ng/ml) and analysis of her milk revealed undetectable amounts of vitamin D and 25-OHD.

The infant was considered to have vitamin D deficiency rickets and was started on 400 IU of vitamin D/day in the form of Tri-Vi-Sol (Mead-Johnson, IN). Two weeks following the beginning of treatment, his serum 25-hydroxyvitamin D rose to 13 ng/ml, 1,25$(OH)_2$D was further elevated at 198 pg/ml, and intact PTH remained high at 113 μl Eg/ml. Five weeks following treatment his 25-OHD had risen to 26 ng/ml, 1,25$(OH)_2$D concentration had fallen to 76 pg/ml, PTH was 80 μl Eq/ml, and alkaline phosphatase had fallen to 180 IU/L.

Questions and Answers

Q.   Could the infant have vitamin D resistant rickets?
A.   Infants of vitamin D resistant rickets generally have *normal* serum 25-OHD concentrations. Vitamin D "resistant" rickets is a general term for rickets associated with hypophosphatemia, requiring very large doses of vitamin D. The largest number of subjects with vitamin D–resistant rickets involve a renal tubular disorder of phosphate metabolism: urinary losses of phosphate result in hypophosphatemia and hypophosphatemic rickets. Disturbance in vitamin D metabolism is not a primary feature although the production of 1,25$(OH)_2$D may be inappropriate; 1,25$(OH)_2$D production should be increased in the presence of hypophosphatemia; however in these subjects, 1,25$(OH)_2$D concentrations may be normal or low.

Two most interesting rare subtypes of "hypophosphatemic rickets" are now separated as: (1) a deficiency of renal 1-hydroxylase (vitamin D "dependency" rickets); and (2) target organ resistance to 1,25$(OH)_2$D (vitamin D dependent rickets type II, with alopecia). In both these instances, serum 25-OHD concentrations also would be normal. In 1-hydroxylase deficiency, the 1,25$(OH)_2$D concentrations would be extremely low, whereas in resistance to 1,25$(OH)_2$D, the 1,25$(OH)_2$D would be high. In both these conditions, serum PTH concentrations are elevated and hypocalcemia is a prominent feature. Therefore these conditions indeed can be clinically confused with nutritional vitamin D deficiency.

Q.   Why was only 400 IU/day given to treat rickets and not more?
A.   Most textbooks recommend large doses of vitamin D as treatment, often as a single intramuscular injection. This historical mode of treatment has not been evaluated by measurements of vitamin D metabolites, and the risks of vitamin D intoxication and hypercalcemia have not been determined.

We elected to treat with a dose of vitamin D that is thought to be close to the "physiologic" dose, on the assumption that it would be logical that a physiologic dose would be both appropriate and sufficient for a condition of presumed vitamin D deficiency. We speculated that a highly active renal 1-alpha-hydroxylase activity, stimulated by hypocalcemia, hypophosphatemia, and high serum PTH concentrations would allow for maximal production of 1,25$(OH)_2$D, provided sufficient 25-OHD substrate was available.

By giving a physiologic dose of vitamin D of 400 units day, supraphysiologic serum concentrations of 1,2 $(OH)_2$D would be produced. The normalized serum 25 OHD and the elevated 1,25$(OH)_2$D concentrations would maximize intestinal calcium and phosphorus absorption and rickets should be resolved. This dose of vitamin D also serves as a test to rule out rickets due to deficiency of renal 1-hydroxylase and target organ unresponsiveness to 1,25$(OH)_2$D; in both these instances, there would be no response to 400 IU of vitamin D.

Q.   Was the infant's race contributory to the etiology of rickets?
A.   In the United States at the present time, most of the cases of vitamin D deficient rickets in breast-fed infants occur in black infants or in groups with unusual dietary practices. It has been suggested that dark skin pigmentation blocks UV-B light necessary for vitamin D photosynthesis. The mother's marginal vitamin D status with undetectable low levels of vitamin D in the milk theoretically may have contributed to the development of rickets. A recent study has shown lower vitamin D concentrations in breast milk from black mothers than white mothers. At present, however, there is no clear evidence that black breast-fed infants are substantially at risk for development of rickets, provided infants are taken outdoors or receive vitamin D supplements.

REFERENCES

1. Cone TE. 200 Years of Feeding Infants in America. Columbus Ohio, Ross Laboratories, 1976.
2. Holick MF, Richtand NM, McNeill SC, et al. Isolation and identification of previtamin D_3 from the skin of rats exposed to ultraviolet irradiation. Biochemistry 1979;48:1003-1008.
3. Holick MF, MacLaughlin JA, Dopplelt SH. Regulation of cutaneous previtamin D_3 photosynthesis in man: skin pigment is not an essential regulator. Science 1981;211:590-593.
4. Hollander D. Intestinal absorption of vitamin A, E, D, and K. J Lab Clin Invest 1981;97:449-462.
5. Lo CW, Paris PW, Clemens TL, et al. Vitamin D absorption in healthy subjects and in patients with intestinal malabsorption syndromes. Am J Clin Nutr 1985;42:644-649.
6. Thompson GR, Lewis B, Booth CC. Absorption of vitamin D_{3-} 3_H in control subjects and patients with intestinal malabsorption. J Clin Invest 1960;45:94-102.
7. Clements MR, Chalers TM, Fraser DR. Enterohepatic circulation of vitamin D: a reappraisal of the hypothesis. Lancet 1984;1:1376-1379.
8. Kodicek E. The fate of ^{14}C-labeled vitamin D_2 in rats and infants. In Garattini S, Paoletti G (eds): Drugs Affecting Lipid Metabolism. Amsterdam, Elsevier, 1961;515-519.
9. Goldsmith RS. Enterohepatic cycling of vitamin D and its metabolites. Mineral Electrolyte Metab 1982;8:289-292.
10. The enterohepatic circulation of vitamin D is negligible. Nutr Rev 1985;43:76-78.
11. Henry HL, Norman AW. Vitamin D: metabolism and biological actions. Ann Rev Nutr 1984;4: 493-520.
12. Fraser DR. Regulation of the metabolism of vitamin D. Physiol Rev 1980;60:551-613.
13. Norman AW, Roth J, Orici L. The vitamin D endocrine system steroid metabolism, hormone receptors and biological response (calcium binding proteins). Endocr Rec 1982;3 331-366.
14. Bishop CW, Kendrick NC, DeLuca HF. Induction of calcium binding protein before 1,25-dihydroxyvitamin D_3 stimulation of duodenal calcium uptake. J Biol Chem 1983;258 1305-1310.
15. Rasmussen H, Matsumoto T, Fontaine O, Goodman DBP

Role of changes in membrane lipid structure in the action of 1,25-dihydroxyvitamin D_3. Fed Proc 1982;41:72–77.

16. Wasserman RH, Brindak ME, Meter SA, Fullmer CS. Evidence for multiple effects of vitamin D_3 on calcium absorption: response of rachitic chicks with or without partial vitamin D_3 repletion to 1,25-dihydroxyvitamin D_3. Proc Natl Acad Sci USA 1982;79:7939–7943.

17. Brooke OG, Brown IRF, Cleeve HJW. Observations on the vitamin D state of pregnant Asian women in London. Br J Obstet Gynecol 1981;88:18–26.

18. Ross R, Care AD, Taylor CM, et al. The transplacental movement of metabolites of vitamin D in the sheep. In Norman AW, Shaefer KV, Herrath D, et al (eds): Vitamin D Bone Research and Its Clinical Application. Berlin, de Gruyter, 1979;341–344.

19. Goff JP, Horst RL, Littledike ET. Effect of the maternal vitamin D status at parturition on the vitamin D status of the neonatal calf. J Nutr 1982;112:1387–1393.

20. Hollis BW, Pittard WB. Evaluation of the total fetomaternal vitamin D relationships at term: evidence for racial differences. J Clin Endocrinol Metab 1984;59:652–657.

21. Weisman Y, Sapir R, Harell A, Edelstein S. Maternal-perinatal interrelationships of vitamin D metabolism in rats. Biochem Biophys Acta 1976;428:388–395.

22. Weisman Y, Occhipinti M, Knox G, et al. Concentrations of 24,25-dihydroxyvitamin D and 25-hydroxyvitamin D in paired maternal-cord sera. Am J Obstet Gynecol 1978;130:704–707.

23. Gertner JM, Glassman MS, Coustan DR, Goodman DBP. Fetomaternal vitamin D relationships at term. J Pediatr 1980;97:637–640.

24. Wieland P, Fischer JA, Trechsel U, et al. Perinatal parathyroid hormone, vitamin D metabolites, and calcitonin in man. Am J Physiol 1980;239:E385–E390.

25. Bouillon R, Van Assche FA, Van Baelen H, et al. Influence of the vitamin D-binding protein on the serum concentration of 1,25-dihydroxyvitamin D_3. Significance of the free 1,25-dihydroxyvitamin D_3 concentration. J Clin Invest 1981;67:589–596.

26. Verity CM, Burman D, Beadle PC, et al. Seasonal changes in perinatal vitamin D metabolism maternal and cord blood biochemistry in normal pregnancies. Arch Dis Child 1981;56:943–948.

27. Seino Y, Ishida M, Yamaoka K, et al. Serum calcium regulating hormones in the perinatal period. Calcif Tissue Int 1982;34:131–135.

28. Markestad T, Aksnes T, Magnar U, Aarskog D. 25-Hydroxyvitamin D and 1,25-dihydroxyvitamin D of D_2 and D_3 origin in maternal and umbilical cord serum after vitamin D_2 supplementation in human pregnancy. Am J Clin Nutr 1984;40:1057–1063.

29. Fleischman AR, Rosen JF, Cole J, et al. Maternal and fetal serum 1,25-dihydroxyvitamin D levels at term. J Pediatr 1980;97:640–642.

30. Steichen JJ, Tsang RC, Gratton TL, et al. Vitamin D homeostasis in the perinatal period. 1,25-Dihydroxyvitamin D in maternal, cord, and neonatal blood. N Engl J Med 1980;302:315–319.

31. Noff D, Edelstein S. Vitamin D and its hydroxylated metabolites in the rat placental and lacteal transport, subsequent metabolic pathways and tissue distribution. Hormone Res 1978;9:292–300.

32. Schedewie H, Slikker W, Hill D, et al. Transplacental transfer of 1,25(OH)$_2$ vitamin D in subhuman primates. Clin Res 1979;27:813A.

33. Ron M, Levitz M, Chuba J, Dancis J. Transfer of 25-hydroxyvitamin D_3 and 1,25-dihydroxyvitamin D_3 across the perfused human placenta. Am J Obstet Gynecol 1984;148:370–374.

34. Marx SJ, Swart EG, Hamstra AJ, DeLuca HF. Normal intrauterine development of the fetus of a woman receiving extraordinary high doses of 1,25-dihydroxyvitamin D_3. J Clin Endocrinol Metab 1980;51:1138–1142.

35. Weisman Y, Vargas A, Duckett G, et al. Synthesis of 1,25-dihydroxyvitamin D in the nephrectomized pregnant rat. Endocrinology 1978;103:1992–1996.

36. Lester GE, Gray TK, Lorenc RS. Evidence for maternal and fetal differences in vitamin D metabolism. Proc Soc Exp Biol Med 1978;159:303–307.

37. Gray TK, Lester GE, Lorenc RS. Evidence for extrarenal 1 hydroxylation of 25-hydroxyvitamin D_3 in pregnancy. Science 1979;204:1311–1313.

38. Ross R, Chen M, Halbert K, Tsang RC. High in vivo fetal production rates of calcitriol in ovine pregnancy. Pediatr Res 1986;20:334A.

39. Weisman Y, Harell A, Edelstein S, et al. 1,25-Dihydromin D_3 and 24,25-dihydroxyvitamin D_3 in vitro synthesis by human decidua and placenta in vitro. J Clin Endocrinol Metab 1981;53:484–488.

40. Whitsett JA, Ho M, Tsang RC, et al. Synthesis of 1,25-dihydroxyvitamin D_3 by human placenta in vitro. J Clin Endocrinol Metab 1981;53:484–488.

41. Delvin EE, Arabian A, Glorieux FH, Mamer OA. In vitro metabolism of 25-hydroxycholecalciferol by isolated cells from human decidua. J Clin Endocrinol Metab 1985;60:880–885.

42. Zerwekh JE, Breslar NA. Human placental production of 1,25-dihydroxyvitamin D_3: Biochemical characterization and production in normal subjects and patients with pseudohypoparathyroidism. J Clin Endocrinol Metab 1986;62:192–196.

43. Rosenstreich SJ, Rich C, Volwiler W. Deposition in and release of vitamin D_3 from body fat. Evidence for a storage site in the rat. J Clin Invest 1971;50:679–687.

44. Mawer EB, Schaefer K. The distribution of vitamin D_3 metabolites in human serum and tissue. Biochem J 1969;114:74P–75P.

45. Dueland S, Helgerud P, Pederson JI, et al. Plasma clearance, transfer, and tissue distribution of vitamin D_3 from rat intestinal lymph. Am J Physiol 1983;245:E326–E331.

46. Greer FR, Tsang RC. Vitamin D in human milk: Is there enough? J Pediatr Gastroenterol Nutr 1983;2 (Suppl 1):S277–S281.

47. Hollis BW, Roos BA, Draper HH, Lamber PW. Vitamin D and its metabolites in human and bovine milk. J Nutr 1981;111:1240–1248.

48. Greer FR, Ho M, Dodson D, Tsang R. Lack of 25-hydroxyvitamin D and 1,25-dihydroxyvitamin D in human milk. J Pediatr 1981;99:233–235.

49. Reeve LE, Chesney RW, DeLuca HF. Vitamin D of human milk: identification of biologically active forms. Am J Clin Nutr 1982;36:122–126.

50. Lakdawala DR, Widdowson EM. Vitamin D in human milk. Lancet 1977;1:167–168.

51. Greer FR, Reeve LE, Chesney RW, DeLuca HF. Commentary—water soluble vitamin D in human milk—a myth. Pediatrics 1982;69:238.

52. Hollis BW, Lambert PW, Horst RL. Factors affecting the antiarchitic sterol content of native milk. In Holick MF, Gray JK, Anast CS (eds): Perinatal Calcium and Phosphorus Metabolism. New York, Elsevier, 1983;157–182.

53. Greer FR, Hollis BW, Cripps DJ, Tsang RC. Effects of maternal ultraviolet B irradiation on vitamin D content of human milk. J Pediatr 1984;105:431–433.

54. Greer FR, Hollis BW, Napoli JL. High concentrations of vitamin D_2 in human milk associated with pharmacologic doses of vitamin D_2. J Pediatr 1984;105:61–64.

55. Specker BL, Tsang RC, Hollis BW. Effect of race and diet on human milk vitamin D and 25-hydroxyvitamin D. Am J Dis Child 1985;139:1134–1137.

56. Chesney RW, Rosen JF, Hamstra AJ, et al. Absence of seasonal variation in serum concentrations of 1,25-dihydroxyvitamin D despite a rise in 25-hydroxyvitamin D in summer. J Clin Endocrinol Metab 1981;53:139–142.

57. Taylor AF, Norman ME. Vitamin D metabolite levels in normal children. Pediatr Res 1984;18:886–890.

58. Markestad T. Plasma concentrations of vitamin D metabolites in unsupplemented breast-fed infants. Eur J Pediatr 1983;141:77–80.

59. Specker BL, Valanis B, Hertzberg V, et al. Sunshine exposure and serum 25-hydroxyvitamin D concentrations in exclusively breast-fed infants. J Pediatr 1985;107:372–376.

60. Ho ML, Yen HC, Tsang RC, et al. Randomized study of sunshine exposure and serum 25-OHD in breast fed infants in Beijing, China. J Pediatr 1985;107:928–931.

61. Lichtenstein P, Specker BL, Tsang RC, et al. Calcium-regu-

lating hormones and minerals from birth to 18 months of age: A cross-sectional study I. Effects of sex, race, age, season and diet on vitamin D status. Pediatrics 1986;77: 883–890.

62. Specker BL, Lichtenstein P, Mimouni F, et al. Calcium-regulating hormones and minerals from birth to 18 months of age: A cross-sectional study. II. Effects of sex, race, age, season and diet on serum minerals, parathyroid hormone, and calcitonin. Pediatrics 1986;77:891–896.

63. Jeans PC, Stearns G. The human requirement of vitamin D. JAMA 1938;111:703–711.

64. Stearns G, Jeans PC, Vandecar V. The effect of vitamin D on linear growth in infancy. J Pediatr 1936;9:1–10.

65. American Academy of Pediatrics, Committee on Nutrition. The prophylactic requirements and the toxicity of vitamin D. Pediatrics 1963;31:512.

66. Greer FR, Searcy JE, Levin RS, et al. Bone mineral content and serum 25-hydroxyvitamin D concentration in breast-fed infants with and without supplemental vitamin D: one-year follow-up. J Pediatr 1982;100:919–922.

67. Roberts CC, Chan GM, Folland D, et al. Adequate bone mineralization in breast-fed infants. J Pediatr 1981;99: 192–196.

68. Ala-Houhala M. 25-Hydroxyvitamin D levels during breast-feeding with or without maternal or infantile supplementation of vitamin D. J Pediatr Gastroenterol Nutr 1985;4:220–226.

69. Rothberg AD, Pettifor JM, Cohen DF, et al. Maternal-infant vitamin D relationships during breast-feeding. J Pediatr 1982;101:500–503.

70. Specker BL, Tsang RC. Cyclical serum 25-hydroxyvitamin D paralleling sunshine exposure in exclusively breast-fed infants: mirror image in summer vs winter born. J Pediatr, 1987;110:744-747.

71. Hillman LS, Haddad JG. Perinatal vitamin D metabolism II: serial 25-hydroxyvitamin D concentrations in sera of term and premature infants. J Pediatr 1975;86:928–935.

72. Glorieux F, Salle B, Delvin E, David L. Vitamin D metabolism in preterm infants: Serum calcitriol values during the first five days of life. J Pediatr 1981;99:640–643.

73. Markestad T, Aksnes L, Finne P, Aarskog D. Plasma concentrations of vitamin D metabolites in premature infants. Pediatr Res 1984;18:269–272.

74. Greer F, Tsang RC. Calcium, phosphorus, magnesium and vitamin D requirements in the preterm infant. In Tsang RC (ed): Vitamin and Mineral Requirements in Preterm Infants. New York, Marcel Dekker, Inc., 1985;99–136.

75. Wolf H, Graff V, Offermann G. The vitamin D requirements for prematue infants. In Norman A, Schaefer K, Herrath D, Grigoleit H (eds): Vitamin D Bone Research and Its Clinical Application. Berlin, Walter de Gruyter, 1979;349–352.

76. Glisson F, et al. De rachitide, sive morbo puerili qui vulgo "The rickets" dicitur, tractatus. 2nd ed. London, 1660.

77. Ell B. Rickets and rachitis. Lancet 1977;1:113–114.

78. Peiper A. Quellen zur Geschichte der Kinderheilkunde. Bern, Verlag Hans Huber 1966,104.

79. Whistler D. Morbo puerili anglorum, quem patrio idiomate indigenae vocant the rickets. Lugduni Batavorum, 1645.

80. Glisson F. De rachitide sive morbo puerili qui vulgo the rickets dicitur. Londinium, 1650.

81. Parks EA. The etiology of rickets. Physiol Rev 1923;3:106–163.

82. Weick MT. A history of rickets in the United States. Am J Clin Nutr 1967;20:1234–1241.

83. Kassowitz M. Tetanie and Autointoxication im Kindersalter. Wien Med Presse 1887;38:97;139. Also in: Kassowitz M. Gesammelte Abhandlungen. Berling, 1914;192.

84. Pommer G. Untersuchungen ueber Osteomalacie and Rachitis, etc. Leipzig, 1885.

85. Siegert F. Beitrag zur Lehr von der Rachitis. Jahrb Kinderh 1903;58:929.

86. Siegert F. Die Aetiologie der Rachitis auf Grund neuerer Untersuchungen. Munchen Med Wochenschr 1905;52:622.

87. Sambon LW. Tropical clothing. J Trop Med 1907;10:67.

88. Koch J. Untersuchungen ueber die Lokalisation der Bakterien, das Verhalten des Knochenmarkes und die Veranderungen der Knochen, insbesondere der Epiphysen, bei Infektionskrankheiten. Mit Bemerkungen zur Theorie der Rachitis. Zeitschr Hyg Infetionskrankh 1911;69:436.

89. Edlefsen G. Ueber die Entstehungsursachen der Rachitis und ihre Verwandschaft mit gewissen Infektionskrankheiten Deutsch AerzteZeitg 1902;169:200.

90. Schmorl G. Die pathologische Anatomie der rachitischer Knochenerkrankung mit besonderer Berucksichtigung ihrer Histologie und Pathogenese. Ergebn Med Kinderh 1909 4:403.

91. Funk C. Die Vitamine, ihre Bedeutung fur die Physiologie und Pathologic, etc. Wiesbaden, 1914.

92. Mellanby E. The part played by an "accessory factor" in the production of experimental rickets (Proc Physiol Soc, Jan 26, 1918). J Physiol 1918;52:xi.

93. Report on the present state of knowledge concerning accessory food factors (vitamins). Compiled by a committee appointed jointly by the Lister Institute and the Medical Research Committee. London, 1919, H.M. Stat Off Med Research Comm, Spec Rep No. 38.

94. Arnaud SB, Stickler GB, Haworth JC: Serum 25-hydroxy vitamin D in infantile rickets. Pediatrics, 1976;57:221.

95. Markestad T, Halvorsen S, Halvorsen KS, et al. Plasma concentrations of vitamin D metabolites before and during treatment of vitamin D deficiency rickets in children. Acta Paediatr Scand 1984;73:225–231.

96. Garabedian M, Vainsel M, Mallet E, et al. Circulating vitamin D metabolite concentrations in children with nutritional rickets. J Pediatrics 1983;103:381–386.

97. Venkataraman PS, Tsang RC, Greer FR, et al. Late infantile tetany and secondary hyperparathyroidism in infants fed humanized cow milk formula. Am J Dis Child 1985;139 664–668.

98. Jeans PC, Stearns G. The effect of vitamin D on linear growth in infancy. I. The effect of intakes above 1,800 U.S.A. unit daily. J Pediatr 1938;13:730.

99. Tsang RC, Greer F, Steichen JJ. Perinatal metabolism of vitamin D: Transition from fetal to neonatal life. Clin Perinatol 1981;8:287–306.

16
Vitamin E

TERRI A. SLAGLE, M.D.
STEVEN J. GROSS, M.D.

ABSTRACT

Vitamin E is a fat soluble vitamin that functions as a biological antioxidant protecting polyunsaturated fatty acids of cell membranes from peroxidation. Infants are relatively vitamin E deificient at birth because of limited placental transfer of the vitamin. Healthy term infants achieve vitamin E sufficiency shortly after birth. However, the preterm infant is at risk for continued vitamin E deficiency because of greater requirements for vitamin E secondary to intestinal malabsorption and rapid postnatal growth. Colostrum contains relatively high concentrations of tocopherol and human milk is a good dietary source of vitamin E for both term and preterm infants. In the past, infant formulas contained low concentrations of α-tocopherol and large amounts of polyunsaturated fatty acids and were responsible for a syndrome of vitamin E deficiency marked by hemolytic anemia. While currently utilized formulas are manufactured to meet the vitamin E needs of infants, parenterally nourished infants remain at risk for the manifestations of vitamin E deficiency. Pharmacologic uses of vitamin E for the prevention of oxidant-induced injury to tissues such as retina and lung have been investigated. Since the efficacy of this usage of vitamin E has not been established and a wide range of toxicity has been reported, pharmacologic usage of vitamin E cannot be recommended.

INTRODUCTION

Vitamin E was discovered in 1922 when Evans and Bishop found that reproduction failed in rats fed a diet of rancid lard.[1]

Such animals are sterile. They are chiefly so in the first generation and wholly so in the succeeding one. The sterility of dietary origin yields a highly characteristic picture. Animals suffering from it do not differ so profoundly from normal ones in their ovarian function as they do in placental behavior. Approximately the same number of Graafian follicles mature and rupture per ovulation and the ova are fertilized and implanted. The placentae are normal. They may persist almost throughout gestation but show as early as the second day of establishment beginning blood extravasations which increase in extent. Resorption invariably overtakes the products of conception.[1]

They termed their "hitherto unrecognized dietary factor essential for reproduction" substance X. In 1924, Barnett Stone "asked for the abandonment of the term 'X' and the legitamacy of the letter E, next in order."[2] A pure form of vitamin E was isolated from wheat-germ oil in 1936 and Evans was soon called upon to offer a proper name for this purified substance.[2]

I promptly invited George M. Calhoun, our professor of Greek, to luncheon in Berkeley in our small faculty club. "Most scientists, medical men especially," said Calhoun, "have been guilty of coining Greek-Latin terms, bastards, of course, and we might have to do this." "What does the substance do?" he asked. "It permits an animal to bear offspring," I replied. "Well, 'childbirth' in Greek is tocos, and if it confers or brings childbirth, we will next employ the Greek verb phero. You have also said that the term must have an ending consonant with its chemical—'ol', it being an alcohol; your substance is 'tocopherol,' and the pleasant task assigned me quickly solved and not worth the delightful four-course dinner you have arranged."[2]

Animal models exist to support the role of vitamin E in maintaining the health of a wide variety of organ systems. Disorders as diverse as encephalomalacia in chicks and necrotizing myopathy in monkeys and mink result from vitamin E deficiency. Attempts to find human correlates of these animal disorders have met with limited success. Nevertheless, vitamin E has been advocated to combat many of the maladies of neonatal intensive care including kernicterus,[3] anemia,[4-7] retinopathy of prematurity,[8-11] and bronchopulmonary dysplasia.[12,13] Is it surprising that this "shady lady of nutrition" has come to be dubbed "a vitamin in search of a disease"?

PHYSIOLOGY

Vitamin E, discovered more than 50 years ago, has remained for half a century one of the great enigmas of nutritional science. Milton Scott, 1978[14]

Chemistry and Nomenclature

The chemistry of vitamin E is more complex than that of the other fat-soluble vitamins because there are eight naturally occurring compounds with characteristic antioxidant activity. The most active of these compounds is alpha tocopherol, which accounts for greater than 90% of vitamin E present in human tissues (Fig. 1).[15] While the d stereoisomer of α-tocopherol is the only naturally occuring form, the most commonly used pharmacologic forms of α-tocopherol contain both the d and l stereoisomers. This pharmacologic form has considerably less activity (approximately 75%) than the pure d form. The only other vitamers of importance in infant nutrition are beta and gamma tocopherol; these compounds respectively possess 33% and 10% of the acitivity of α-tocopherol.[16] Once extracted, the naturally occurring free alcohol form of α-tocopherol has a limited shelf-life due to its interaction with oxygen. Therefore, **commercially available forms of vitamin E are esterified to the acetate or succinate forms.** Since each of these forms of vitamin E has different biologic activity, preparations have been standardized to International Units (IU) where one IU is equivalent to the activity of one milligram of d,l α-tocopherol acetate. Table 1 compares the activities of the different tocopherol compounds.

Mechanism of Action

In humans, the primary (perhaps only) role of vitamin E is as a biologic antioxidant. Vitamin E acts by inhibiting the naturally occurring peroxidation of polyunsaturated fatty acids (PUFA) present in the lipid layers of cell membranes. Vitamin E is suited for this function by its ability to scavenge free radicals that are generated by the reduction of molecular oxygen and as normal by-products of oxidativ enzymes.[17] **This auto-oxidation is demonstrated in the kitchen when foods with high PUFA content become rancid after exposure to air.** Peroxidation begins when a hydrogen atom escapes from one of the carbons of a double bond, "unmasking" a highly reactive intermediate that can interact with free oxygen (Fig. 2). The lipid free radical formed interacts with another PUFA side chain and creates stable lipid hydroperoxides and more lipid free radicals. This process can repeat as potentially endless chain reaction.[18] Tappel identified vitamin E as a *chain-breaking antioxidant* because of its ability to readily substitute for oxygen in this reaction by donating stabilizing hydrogen ion to the "lipid free radical."[18] In the process of stopping fatty acid peroxidation, the α-tocopherol is oxidized to α-tocopherol quinone, which is excreted in the urine (Fig. 2).

Absorption

Free tocopherols are absorbed from the midportion of the small intestine and taken via chylomicrons into the gastrointestinal lymphatics. Bile and pancreatic juices are essential for normal absorption (Fig. 3). If an esterified form of vitamin E is given, complete *hydrolysis* must

TABLE 1.   Biologic Activity of Vitamin E Compounds

		IU/mg
d,l	α-tocopherol acetate	1.00
d,l	α-tocopherol	1.10
d	α-tocopherol acetate	1.36
d	α-tocopherol	1.49
d,l	α-tocopherol succinate	0.89
d	α-tocopherol succinate	1.21

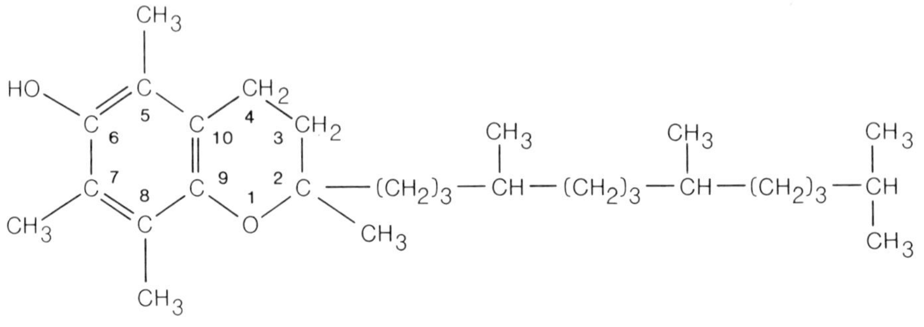

FIGURE 1.   The structure of α-tocopherol.

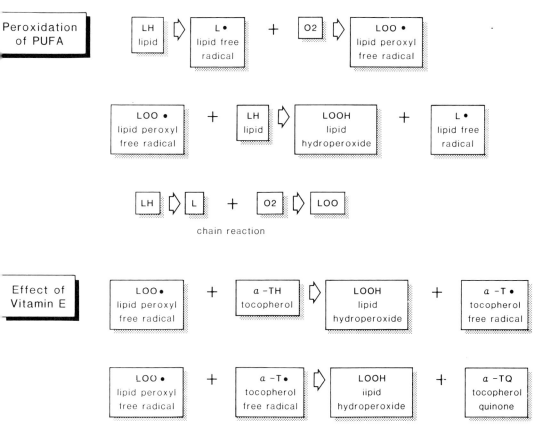

FIGURE 2. Suggested antioxidant theory of vitamin E. During the process of breaking the chain reaction of polyunsaturated fatty acid (PUFA) peroxidation, the α-tocopherol donates a *stabilizing hydrogen ion* to the lipid free radical and itself oxidized to tocopherol quinone.

cur in the intestinal lumen prior to absorption. Vitamin E then enters the venous circulation and is carried by nonspecific low density lipoproteins to all body tissues, where it is incorporated into cell membranes. At the tissue level, vitamin E isomers are concentrated where there is an abundance of fatty acids and, thus, tissue concentrations of the vitamin are related to the lipid content of specific organs. Adipose tissue, liver and skeletal muscle represent the major storage depots.[19] Despite high levels of vitamin E in adipose tissue and muscle, these stores are not readily mobilized during times of deficiency.[19]

Intestinal absorption of vitamin E by the neonate is variable and influenced by multiple factors (Table 2). Most important among these factors are the infant's gestational age, the components of the diet, and the preparation of vitamin E given. Human milk has a lower content of α-tocopherol and a lower ratio of vitamin E to PUFA than do currently utilized formulas.[24,25] Nevertheless, term and preterm infants attain vitamin E sufficiency sooner and have higher serum tocopherol levels when fed human milk.[24,25] These data suggest that absorption of vitamin E from human milk is significantly greater than that from cow-milk-based formula.

Nutritional Interactions

Feeding of diets with varying concentrations of polyunsaturated fatty acids results in corresponding changes in the PUFA content of cell membranes.[28,29] The increase in erythrocyte membrane PUFA resulting from an increased intake of dietary linoleic acid is associated with greater fatty acid peroxidation, more hydrogen peroxide–induced red cell hemolysis and increased requirements for vitamin E.[30,31]

The peroxidation of cell membranes may be catalyzed by iron, a potent generator of free radicals. For this reason, as well as its pos-

Tocopherol Transport

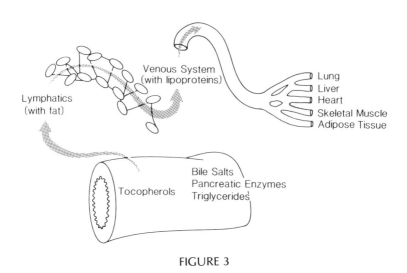

FIGURE 3

TABLE 2.   Factors Affecting Tocopherol
Absorption In Neonates

Factor	Effect on Absorption
1. Gestational age	Absorption decreased in infants less than 32 weeks' gestational age[20]
2. Fat absorption	Fat malabsorption states (e.g., cystic fibrosis and cholestasis) are associated with evidence of vitamin E deficiency[21,22]
3. Presence of lipoproteins	Abetalipoproteinemia associated with low serum vitamin E levels[23]
4. Nutritional source	Greater tocopherol absorption from human milk than from formula[24,25]
5. Amount ingested	Percent absorption decreases as amount ingested increases[16,26]
6. Preparation given	Absorption better with water miscible than fat-soluble forms[27]

sible direct inhibition of tocopherol absorption,[32] the addition of iron to the diet further increases the vitamin E requirement.

Williams et al.[31] have described the interaction of these three factors (vitamin E, polyunsaturated fatty acids and iron) in determining the vitamin E status in preterm infants. In their study, infants fed a formula high in PUFA (32% linoleic acid) demonstrated a greater degree of red cell hemolysis and a lower serum tocopherol concentration than did infants who received a low PUFA formula (13% linolei? acid). Additionally, infants who received sup plemental iron (approximately 2 mg/kg/day in the formula rich in linoleic acid had signifi? cantly lower hemoglobin levels and highe? reticulocyte counts than did infants in the other dietary groups.[31]

An interrelationship between vitamin E an? selenium-dependent glutathione peroxidas? has been found in animal species. Administra? tion of one antioxidant (vitamin E or selenium? may protect against deficiency of the othe? nutrient. A similar interaction between toco? pherol and selenium in infant nutrition is un? certain.[16]

REQUIREMENTS

... And it came to pass, as they were eating of the pot? tage, that they cried out, and said: "O man of God, there i? death in the pot." And they could not eat thereof. But h? said: "Then bring meal." And he cast it into the pot; an? he said: "Pour out for the people, that they may eat." An? there was no harm in the pot. Second Kings 40-42

The above passage may demonstrate th? earliest usage of the high vitamin E content o? grain ("meal") to prevent rancidity ("harm") i? foodstuffs. In modern times, although we con? tinue to modify the "meal," we do not alway? know the exact needs to prevent the "harm."

Perinatal Factors Affecting Needs

The total body content of tocopherol in the human fetus increases from about 1 mg at 5 months' gestation to approximately 20 mg at term.[33] This increase in tocopherol during gestation is paralleled by an increase in total body fat.[33] Blood concentrations of tocopherol in preterm and term infants at birth average less than half the value for normal adults of 1.05 ± 0.27 mg/dl and are only 20–30% of corresponding maternal levels.[34–37] **This suggests that placental transfer of vitamin E is limited.** Furthermore, increasing maternal blood tocopherol levels by administration of large doses of vitamin E (100–900 mg/day) to women during the last weeks of pregnancy results in minimal increase in cord blood levels.[38,39]

Additionally, Hägä and Lunde[40] found a significant correlation between plasma concentrations of β-lipoprotein, the principal carrier of tocopherol in plasma, and the vitamin E level in both cord and maternal blood at the time of delivery. The corresponding low concentrations of tocopherol and β-lipoprotein in cord blood suggests that differences in transport capacity rather than impermeability of the placenta for tocopherol alternatively can explain the low levels of the vitamin in newborn infants.

Assessment of Status

The assessment of vitamin E status in neonates depends upon the biochemical analysis of tocopherol in blood. Until recently, determinations of total tocopherols were performed by colorimetric procedures. These procedures were technically difficult, required large amounts of blood, and were imprecise because of interference by carotene.[14,19] High-performance liquid chromatography has eliminated these problems and allows the separation and quantitation of the α, β, and γ isomers of tocopherol.

The marked influence of circulating lipids on tocopherol concentrations makes it preferable to express plasma α-tocopherol concentrations as a ratio to β-lipoprotein, cholesterol or total lipid.[41] Additionally, a functional measure of tissue antioxidant activity such as the degree of erythrocyte hemolysis in dilute hydrogen peroxide, although nonspecific, is useful. **Vitamin E deficiency is most appropriately defined by a ratio of serum α-tocopherol to total lipid that is less than 0.8 mg/gm and erythrocyte hemolysis in hydrogen peroxide that is greater than 10%.**

Advisable Intakes for Term Infants

It has long been recognized that colostrum contains high concentrations of vitamin E,[42,43] and term infants who are breast-fed demonstrate dramatic increases in blood tocopherol levels from 0.38 ± 0.18 mg/dl to 1.46 ± 0.63 mg/dl within a few days after birth.[25] Blood tocopherol concentrations remain in the normal adult range until weaning.[25]

In contrast, term infants who are fed proprietary formula low in vitamin E maintain deficient blood levels of tocopherol (<0.8 mg/dl) for many months.[25] Therefore, the American Academy of Pediatrics Committee on Nutrition recommends that **formula designed for term infants contain a minimum of 0.3 IU of vitamin E per 100 kcal and at least 0.7 IU of vitamin E per gram of linoleic acid.**[44]

Table 3 summarizes the concentrations of vitamin E and ratios of vitamin E to linoleic acid in human milk and currently utilized infant formulas. All these formulas meet the above recommendations and, therefore, administration of additional vitamin E to term infants is not necessary.

Advisable Intakes for Preterm Infants

Because of limited tissue stores of tocopherol at birth, poor absorption of dietary fats, and rapid postnatal growth, the preterm infant has a greater requirement for vitamin E than does the term infant.

Milk produced by mothers of preterm infants ("preterm milk") is particularly suited to meet the vitamin E needs of the low birthweight infant. The concentration of α-tocopherol and ratio of α-tocopherol to lineolic acid in preterm milk decrease with progressing lactational stage but remain *higher* than those of mature human milk through at least the first 6 weeks postpartum (Table 4).[24,42]

In a recent study, Gross et al.[24] compared the vitamin E status of 36 very low birthweight infants fed one of three diets from birth to 6 weeks; all infants received routine multivitamin supplementation providing 4.1 mg of d α-tocopherol succinate per day. The results of this study are summarized in Table 5. After 6 weeks, infants fed *preterm milk* had a higher mean serum concentration of vitamin E (1.80

TABLE 3.   Tocopherol Content and E:PUFA Ratio of Milks Fed to Term Infants

Type of Milk	α-tocopherol content*		E:PUFA†
	mg/100 kcal	IU/100 kcal	
Human milks[24,42]			
Postpartum days 0–4	1.50 ± 0.80	2.20 ± 1.2	5.5 ± 2.2
Postpartum weeks 2–5	0.46 ± 0.17	0.68 ± 0.2	0.7 ± 0.5
Postpartum months 3–12	0.35	0.52	0.3
Enfamil, 67 kcal/dl (Mead-Johnson)	3.1	3.1	1.9
Similac, 67 kcal/dl (Ross)	3.0	3.0	1.5
SMA, 67 kcal/dl (Wyeth)	1.4	1.4	1.9

*Human milk contains d α-tocopherol (1 mg = 1.49 I.U.); proprietary formulas contain d, 1 α-tocopherol acetate (1 mg = 1 I.U.).
†E:PUFA ratios calculated as mg d α-tocopherol per gm linoleic acid.

Colostrum is rich in tocopherol and has a high vitamin E to PUFA ratio. Consequently, vitamin E sufficiency is readily attained in the breastfed infant. Commonly used infant formulas for term infants are manufactured to provide concentrations of α-tocopherol and ratios of α-tocopherol to PUFA in excess of estimated requirements.

TABLE 4.   Tocopherol Content and E:PUFA Ratio of Milks Fed to Preterm Infants

Type of Milk	α-tocopherol content*		E:PUFA†
	mg/100 kcal	IU/100 kcal	
Human milk**[24]			
Postpartum week 1	1.3	1.9	2.0
Postpartum week 2	1.1	1.6	1.3
Postpartum week 4	0.6	0.9	0.7
Enfamil Premature 67 kcal/dl (Mead-Johnson)	4.6	4.6	2.9
Similac Special Care 67 kcal/dl (Ross)	4.0	4.0	3.8
SMA Preemie 67 kcal/dl (Wyeth)	2.2	2.2	3.0

*Human milk contains d α-tocopherol (1 mg = 1.49 IU); proprietary formulas contain d,l α-tocopherol acetate (1 mg = 1 IU).
†E:PUFA ratios calculated as mg d α-tocopherol per gm linoleic acid.
**Human milk obtained from mothers delivering preterm infants: analyses performed on pooled weekly collections from 40–80 mothers.

Milk obtained from mothers of preterm infants contains a significantly greater concentration of α-tocopherol and a higher ratio of vitamin E to PUFA than does mature human milk. Therefore, vitamin E sufficiency is readily attained in preterm infants fed their own mothers milk (see Table 5). Commonly used infant formulas for preterm infants are manufactured to provide concentrations of α-tocopherol and ratios of α-tocopherol to PUFA that are in excess of estimated requirements.

± 0.18 mg/dl) than did similar infants fed mature human milk (1.38 ± 0.20 mg/dl) or premature infant formula (1.15 ± 0.20 mg/dl) (p<0.001). Ratios of serum vitamin E/total lipid at 6 weeks were also significantly higher in infants fed preterm milk than in those fed formula.

The addition of *iron* (2 mg/kg/day) to all three diets resulted in significantly lower serum vitamin E levels; however, only in the group fed formula was there evidence of vitamin E deficiency. All infants fed human milk (with or without iron supplementation) were vitamin E

sufficent by the criteria proposed above (Assessment of Status).

The Committee on Nutrition recommends that **formulas designed for preterm infants provide a minimum of 0.7 IU of vitamin E per 100 kcal and at least 1.0 IU of vitamin E per gram of linoleic acid.**[45] In addition, because of concerns about the adequacy of intestinal absorption of vitamin E, the Committee suggests that **the premature infant receive 5 to 25 IU of supplemental oral vitamin E per day** (Table 6). The vitamin E and linoleic acid composition of formulas currently used for

TABLE 5.   Comparison of Vitamin E Status in Preterm Infants Fed Human Milks or Infant Formula*

Serum values	Milks with no iron supplementation			Milks with iron supplementation		
	Preterm milk	Mature milk	Infant formula	Preterm milk	Mature milk	Infant formula
Vitamin E (mg/dl)						
Day 1	0.50 ± 0.08	0.40 ± 0.04	0.62 ± 0.04	0.37 ± 0.07	0.38 ± 0.08	0.36 ± 0.07
Week 6**	1.80 ± 0.18	1.38 ± 0.20	1.15 ± 0.20	1.52 ± 0.17	1.04 ± 0.12	0.45 ± 0.09
Vitamin E/lipid (mg/gm)						
Day 1	1.00 ± 0.15	0.83 ± 0.10	1.32 ± 0.10	0.79 ± 0.10	0.70 ± 0.12	0.71 ± 0.09
Week 6+	3.06 ± 0.26	2.38 ± 0.30	2.81 ± 0.67	3.16 ± 0.43	2.14 ± 0.44	0.79 ± 0.16

Data from Gross et al.;[24] values represent mean ± SEM.
**Preterm milk vs. formula, p<0.0001; mature milk vs. formula, p<0.02; preterm milk vs. mature milk, p<0.01. Milks without iron vs. milks with iron, p<0.05.
+Preterm milk vs. formula, p<0.001; mature milk vs. formula, p<0.05.

TABLE 6.   Enteral Vitamin E Supplements

Preparation	Form of Vitamin	Concentration
Aquasol E (Mead-Johnson)	d,l α-tocopherol acetate	50 IU/ml
Polyvisol (Mead-Johnson)	d α-tocopherol succinate	5 IU/ml
Vedaylin (Ross)	d,l α-tocopherol acetate	5 IU/ml

preterm infants are summarized in Table 4. All the formulas have been manufactured to meet requirements set forth by the Committee on Nutrition.

Parenteral Needs

Requirements for vitamin E for parenterally nourished infants are not well defined. Gutcher et al.[46] studied 10 preterm infants who received approximately 2 mg/kg/day of d, l α-tocopherol acetate as a continuous infusion with their parenteral nutrition. Mean serum α-tocopherol concentrations increased from 0.37 ± 0.09 mg/dl prior to vitamin supplementation, to 1.56 ± 0.20 mg/dl after 4 days; a further increase in mean serum concentration to 2.17 ± 0.32 mg/dl was observed 1 week later. Similar serum concentrations of α-tocopherol were reported in a small number of preterm infants who received 4.6 mg/day of d,l α-tocopherol acetate.[47] In both studies, the concomitant administration of supplemental oral vitamin E in doses from 25-150 IU per day further increased serum α-tocopherol concentrations.[46,47]

MVI Pediatric (Armour Pharmaceutical) is the currently available parenteral vitamin supplement for infants and children; this preparation contains 7 IU of d,l α-tocopherol acetate

per 5 ml vial. Based on the limited data available, 2.3 IU per kilogram of body weight per day (30% of a vial of MVI Pediatric per kilogram per day) should maintain vitamin E sufficiency in parenterally fed infants.

PHARMACOLOGIC NEEDS

There is a great deal of misinformation about vitamin E. Both lay and scientific people are exposed to extreme points of view. Some proclaim curative effects of vitamin E on a vast array of diseases; others question whether it is a vitamin. Lawrence Machlin, 1985[19]

Recently, the pharmacologic uses of tocopherol for the prevention of oxidant-induced injury to potentially susceptible tissues such as lung and retina have been investigated.

Retinopathy of Prematurity

Owens and Owens first investigated the role of vitamin E in prevention of retinopathy of prematurity (ROP) after they noted that vitamin E was the only fat-soluble vitamin not given routinely to preterm infants during an era of increasing incidence of disease. Over a 10-month period, they gave alternate infants less than 1360 gm 150 mg/day of d,l α-tocopherol acetate and found that none of 11 vitamin E treated infants developed ROP, compared to 5 of the 15 control infants.[48] Unfortunately, the "overwhelming success" of the trial prompted the investigators to discontinue their controlled study (in favor of treatment) prior to achieving results that were statistically significant. In the 1950s the role of oxygen in the pathogenesis of ROP pushed vitamin E out of the picture. Within the last few years, however, the use of vitamin E for the prevention of ROP has resurfaced for examination.

The prospective, randomized controlled clinical trials of vitamin E for the prevention of ROP reported over the past 5 years have been reviewed by Phelps.[11] All studies have concluded that prophylactic administration of pharmacologic doses of vitamin E has no effect on the incidence of retinopathy of prematurity. One of the studies[8] found that the administration of 100 mg/kg/day of d,l α-tocopherol to very low birthweight infants with respiratory distress, while not decreasing the incidence of disease, did decrease the severity of disease in affected infants; advanced fibroproliferative disease (grades III and IV) was seen in 5 of 51 control infants and none of 50 treated infants (p<0.03). The incidence of severe cicatricial disease, however, is rare. Therefore, the Committee on Fetus and Newborn of the American Academy of Pediatrics has stated:

. . . any effective prophylaxis with vitamin E in the United States would require that 22,000 surviving infants of birth weight less than 1,500 gm be treated annually to prevent approximately 2,000 infants from developing the cicatricial sequelae of retinopathy of prematurity. The treatment of 20,000 infants who would not develop retinopathy of prematurity would be acceptable if it were certain that the administration of vitamin E was completely safe or, at least, that the benefits of its use outweighed the risks by a substantial margin . . . At this time, however, the Committee regards prophylactic use of pharmacologic vitamin E as experimental and cannot recommend that high doses of vitamin E be given routinely to infants weighing less than 1,500 gm, even if such use is limited to infants who require supplemental oxygen.[49]

Bronchopulmonary Dysplasia

Based on the increased susceptibility of tocopherol-deficient animals to oxygen-induced lung injury, a pilot study was undertaken in preterm infants with respiratory distress syndrome using pharmacologic doses of parenteral tocopherol from birth.[12] The findings suggested that tocopherol shortened the time that infants required oxygen and reduced the incidence of bronchopulmonary dysplasia (BPD). The study involved small numbers of infants and had several methodological problems. When the same investigators conducted a larger, well-designed, controlled trial,[13] they could demonstrate no benefit of vitamin E in the prevention of BPD. Four other controlled clinical trials followed. All these studies have been reviewed by Bell.[50] None has shown a protective role of vitamin E in the prevention of BPD in susceptible infants.

Intraventricular Hemorrhage

In a study designed to determine the effect of parenteral vitamin E on red cell hemolysis in infants less than 32 weeks' gestational age, Chiswick et al.[51] serendipitously found that the incidence of intraventricular hemorrhage in 16 treated infants (19%) was significantly less than that of a comparable-sized control group (56%) (p<0.05). Not surprisingly, the focus of the presentation shifted from the red cell to the subependymal cell! Speer et al.[52] similarly reported that the incidence of subependymal intraventricular hemorrhage in very low birth weight infants was significantly decreased in 10 of 64 vitamin-E-treated infants (16%) compared to the 24 of 70 control infants (34%) (p<0.02).

No vitamin E story would be complete without a controversy. In this example, Phelps et al.[10] reported a higher incidence of severe intraventricular hemorrhage (hemorrhage with ventriculomegaly or parenchymal extension) in infants less than 1000 gm who received free tocopherol. In their study designed to assess the efficacy of vitamin E for the prevention of ROP, severe hemorrhages occurred in 14 of 43 (33%) treated infants and 4 of 41 (10%) controls (p<0.02). Since the incidence of subependymal/intraventricular hemorrhage is far greater than that of either retinopathy of prematurity or bronchopulmonary dysplasia, the possible benefit or risk of vitamin E with regard to cerebral hemorrhage must be further investigated.

The evaluation of the efficacy of pharmacologic administration of vitamin E for the prevention of oxygen-induced injury is further clouded by the lack of data as to desirable serum concentrations.[9,10,53] In addition, extremely variable serum tocopherol levels have been reported in low birthweight infants receiving similar pharmacologic vitamin E supplementation.[9,54] If vitamin E is given to preterm infants in excess of the recommended dose of 5-25 IU, serial serum vitamin E concentrations must be measured.

DEFICIENCY

The immature organism is particularly susceptible to vitamin-E deficiency. Nursing rats born of vitamin-E depleted mothers develop acute muscular dystrophy 17 to 29 days after birth. Young chickens, placed on a vitamin-E deficient diet at the time of hatching, suddenly develop nutritional encephalomalacia at 3 to 4 weeks of age. In each of these diseases, there is an age limit to the nutritional derangement. As they grow older the incidence of the disease steadily decreases. William and Ella Owens, 1949[48]

Human tocopherol deficiency has been recognized in two groups of patients. One group is children with prolonged and profound fat malabsorption secondary to biliary atresia, cystic fibrosis, and abetalipoproteinemia; these children may manifest a syndrome of progressive sensory and mother neuropathy that becomes apparent late in the first decade of life.[22,23] The second group of deficient patients is preterm infants who present with hemolytic anemia at 1 or 2 months of age.

In 1967, Oski and Barness[4] first described the syndrome of vitamin E deficiency in 11 premature infants. These infants presented between 6 and 11 weeks of age with anemia (mean hemoglobin 7.6 ± 1.1 gm/dl), elevated reticulocyte count (8.2 ± 2.9%), and a striking increase in sensitivity of the erythrocytes to hemolysis in hydrogen peroxide (80 ± 14%). All these infants had deficient serum vitamin E concentrations ($\leqslant 0.41$ mg/dl). These findings were confirmed by others[5-7] and the manifestations of the syndrome were expanded to include peripheral edema and thrombocytosis. All the clinical and hematologic abnormalities corrected after the initiation of oral vitamin E therapy.

It was soon recognized that **this syndrome was associated with the ingestion of formulas that were high in polyunsaturated fatty acids and low in vitamin E.** After the interrelationships of dietary PUFA, alpha tocopherol and iron were clarified,[31] infant formulas utilized for feeding preterm infants were modified appropriately. The disappearance of this syndrome soon followed.

TABLE 7.   Reported Toxicities Following Vitamin E Administration

Toxicity	Route given
Erythema, edema, and soft tissue calcification[56,57]	Intramuscular
Syndrome of pulmonary deterioration, thrombocytopenia, renal and liver failure, and death[58]	Intravenous (E-Ferol)
Sepsis[53]	Oral and intravenous
Necrotizing enterocolitis[53,61]	Oral and intravenous
Intraventricular hemorrhage[10]	Intravenous

TOXICITY

Poor vitamin E! Every time it appears to gain some respectability, it gets involved in some medical misadventure. Frank Oski, 1984[55]

A wide range of toxicities associated with vitamin E administration have been reported (Table 7). These primarily followed the pharmacologic usage of tocopherol. The mildest of these are local reactions including erythema, edema and soft tissue calcification at the site of intramuscular injection.[56,57] The most devastating toxicity was the syndrome of pulmonary deterioration, thrombocytopenia, and liver and renal failure in very low birthweight infants, which was temporally associated with the use of a parenteral d,l α-tocopherol acetate in polysorbate vehicle (E-Ferol).[58] A total of 38 reported deaths prompted the removal of E-Ferol from the market only 6 months after it was released. A retrospective analysis of this tragedy suggests a dose-related toxicity of vitamin E. Affected infants had a lower birthweight and received a higher total dose of tocopherol.[59] However, the possibility of toxicity secondary to the polysorbate vehicle also has been suggested.[60]

Other important side effects have been identified following pharmacologic vitamin E usage. Johnson et al.[53] reported that very low birthweight infants given parenteral and oral tocopherol from birth in an effort to maintain serum tocopherol concentrations at 5 mg/dl had a 2.7-fold increase in the occurrence of sepsis or necrotizing enterocolitis. The authors postulate that high serum concentrations of vitamin E may decrease the oxygen-dependent killing ability of cells.[53]

In another study, Finer et al.[61] found a twofold increase in the incidence of necrotizing enterocolitis in very low birthweight infants who received pharmacologic doses of oral vitamin E. Although not routinely measured, serum vitamin E concentrations prior to the development of disease were obtained in nine of these infants; the mean level in this group was 3.1 mg/dl and only one of these infants had a serum level greater than 3.5 mg/dl. This raises the possibility that other properties of the oral formulation, e.g., the osmolality or vehicle rather than the serum concentration per se, might be responsible for the toxicity. These data highlight the extreme caution that must be exercised before treating any infant with pharmacologic doses of a vitamin for which efficacy has not been proven.

SUMMARY OF NEEDS FOR TERM AND PRETERM INFANTS

Full-term infants demonstrate vitamin E sufficiency when fed maternal breast milk. Formula fed to term infants should contain a minimum of 0.3 IU of vitamin E/100 kcal and 0.7 IU of vitamin E/gm of linoleic acid. Term infants fed breast milk or formula manufactured to meet the above recommendations do not need supplemental vitamin E.

Preterm infants also maintain vitamin E sufficiency when fed their own mothers' milk. Formula fed to preterm infants should contain a minimum of 0.7 IU of vitamin E/100 kcal and 1.0 IU of vitamin E/gm of linoleic acid. Additionally, preterm infants should receive an oral supplement of 5–25 IU of vitamin E per day; the lower amount is adequate for those infants who are fed human milk.

Both term and preterm infants receiving total parenteral nutrition should receive approximately 2 IU/kg/day of vitamin E as a continuous infusion with other nutrients.

The use of pharmacologic doses of vitamin E should be considered experimental and, in 1988, is not recommended routinely for any group of infants.

CASE REPORT

J.E. was a 1100-gm infant born at 28 weeks' gestation to a 24-year-old primigravida. He suffered from severe respiratory distress syndrome for which he was ventilated for the first week of life. Although enteral feeds were started on day 6 of life, the baby had recurrent episodes of abdominal distention necessitating frequent periods of discontinuance of enteral feedings. He received dextrose and electrolyte fluids intravenously. J.E. is now 4 weeks old and weighs 1500 gm. His current feedings are 3/4 strength proprietary formula, which he has tolerated for 7 days at a volume of 150 ml/kg/day. He is receiving no oral iron or vitamin supplements. Routine laboratory testing reveals a hematocrit that has gradually fallen from 48% a birth to 24%.

This is a straight forward case of "anemia of prematurity" ... or is it? An astute houseofficer orders a few diagnostic tests before considering a red blood cell transfusion. Results include:

Reticulocyte count: 11.6%
Platelet count: 400,000/mm^3
Blood smear: Rare RBC fragments and moderate poikilocytosis
Serum tocopherol: 0.4 mg/dl
Serum tocopherol to total lipid ratio: 0.5

Comment: It is important in evaluating anemia in preterm infants to consider vitamin E deficiency as a cause. Although vitamin E deficiency as a result of feeding a formula with an inappropriate content of tocopherol or a low vitamin E to PUFA ratio is a historical consideration, inadequate vitamin E intake secondary to poor tolerance of enteral feeds remains a possibility.

Questions and Answers

Q.   Should this infant be treated with supplemental Vitamin E?
A.   Yes. Infants who exhibit a vitamin E dependent, hemolytic anemia should receive supplemental tocopherol. This infant was given a daily oral tocopherol dose of 25 units/kg. Repeat blood studies 4 weeks later demonstrated an increase in hematocrit to 30% in association with a decline in reticulocyte count to 3.5%, an increase in the serum concentration of vitamin E to 0.90 mg/dl and an increase in the ratio of serum vitamin E/total lipid to 0.8.

Acknowledgment. We would like to acknowledge the assistance of Pat Hammel in the preparation of this chapter.

REFERENCES

1. Evans HM, Bishop KS. On the existence of a hitherto unrecognized dietary factor essential for reproduction. Science 1922; 56:650–651.
2. Evans HM. The pioneer history of vitamin E. Vitam Horm 1962; 20:379–387.
3. Nitowsky HM, Hsu KS, Gordon HH. Vitamin E requirements of human infants. Vitam Horm 1962; 20:559–571.
4. Oski FA, Barness LA. Vitamin E deficiency: a previously unrecognized cause of hemolytic anemia in the premature infant. J Pediatr 1967; 70:211–220.
5. Hassan H, Hashim SA, Van Itallie TB, Sebrell WH. Syndrome in premature infants associated with low plasma vitamin E levels and high polyunsaturated fatty acid diet. Am J Clin Nutr 1966; 19:147–157.
6. Ritchie JH, Fish MB, McMasters V, Grossman M. Edema and hemolytic anemia in premature infants: a vitamin E deficiency syndrome. N Engl J Med 1968; 279:1185–1190.
7. Lo SS, Frank D, Hitzig WH. Vitamin E and hemolytic anemia in premature infants. Arch Dis Child 1973; 48:360–365.
8. Hittner HM, Godio LB, Rudolph AJ, et al. Retrolental fibroplasia: efficacy of vitamin E in a double-blind clinical study of preterm infants. N Engl J Med 1981; 305:1365–1371.
9. Hittner HM, Kretzer FL. Efficacy of vitamin E in retinopathy of prematurity. In McPherson AR, Hittner HM, Kretzer FL (eds): Retinopathy of Prematurity Current Concepts and Controversies. Toronto, Marcel Dekker, Inc., 1986; 89–103.

10. Phelps DL, Rosenbaum AL, Isenberg SJ, et al. Effect of IV tocopherol (vitamin E) on retinopathy of prematurity (ROP). Pediatr Res 1985; 19:375A.

11. Phelps DL. Vitamin E and retinopathy of prematurity. In Silverman W, Flynn J (eds): Contemporary Issues in Fetal and Neonatal Medicine: Retinopathy of Prematurity. Boston, Blackwell, 1985; 181-205.

12. Ehrenkranz RA, Bonta BW, Ablow RC, Warshaw JB. Amelioration of bronchopulmonary dysplasia after vitamin E administration: a preliminary report. N Engl J Med 1978; 299:564-569.

13. Ehrenkranz RA, Ablow RC, Warshaw JB. Effect of vitamin E on the development of oxygen-induced lung injury in neonates. Ann NY Acad Sci 1982; 393:452-465.

14. Scott ML. Vitamin E. In DeLuca, HL (ed): The Fat-Soluble Vitamins. New York, Plenum Press, 1978; 133-210.

15. Mandel HG, Cohn VH. Fat-soluble vitamins. In Gilman AG, Goodman LS, Gilman A (eds): The Pharmacologic Basis of Therapeutics. New York, MacMillan Publishing, Inc., 1975; 1172.

16. Farrell PM, Zachman RD, Gutcher GR. Fat soluble vitamins A, E, and K in the premature infant. In Tsang R (ed): Vitamin and Mineral Requirements in Preterm Infants. New York, Marcel Dekker, Inc., 1985; 63-98.

17. Ehrenkranz RA. Vitamin E and the neonate. Am J Dis Child 1980; 134:1157-1166.

18. Tappel AL. Vitamin E as the biologic lipid antioxidant. Vitam Horm 1962; 20:493-510.

19. Machlin L (ed): Handbook of Vitamins. Nutritional Biochemical and Clinical Aspects. New York, Marcel Dekker, 1984; 99-145.

20. Melhorn DK, Gross S. Vitamin E-dependent anemia in the premature infant. II. Relationships between gestational age and absorption of vitamin E. J Pediatr 1971; 79:581-588.

21. Filer LJ, Wright SW, Manning MP, Mason KE. Absorption of α-tocopherol and tocopherol esters by premature and full term infants and children in health and disease. Pediatrics 1951; 8:328-339.

22. Sokol RJ, Heubi JE, Iannaccone ST, et al. Vitamin E deficiency with normal serum vitamin E concentrations in children with chronic cholestasis. N Engl J Med 1984; 310:1209-1212.

23. Muller DP, Lloyd JK, Wolff OH. Vitamin E and neurologic function: abetalipoproteinemia and other disorders of fat absorption. CIBA Foundation Symposium 1983; 101:106-117.

24. Gross SJ, Gabriel E. Vitamin E status in preterm infants fed human milk or infant formula. J Pediatr 1985; 106:635-639.

25. Wright SW, Filer LJ, Mason KE. Vitamin E blood levels in premature and full term infants. Pediatrics 1951; 7:386-392.

26. Lambert GH, Papp LA, Paton JB. Megadoses of vitamin E in oxygen-dependent premature newborn infants. J Perinatol 1985; 5:44-47.

27. Gross S, Melhorn DK. Vitamin E-dependent anemia in the premature infant. III. Comparative hemoglobin, vitamin E, and erythrocyte phospholipid responses following absorption of either water-soluble or fat-soluble d-alpha tocopherol. J Pediatr 1974; 85:753-759.

28. Farquhar JW, Ahrens EH. Effects of dietary fats on human erythrocyte fatty acid patterns. J Clin Invest 1963; 5:675-685.

29. Horwitt MK, Harvey CC, Dahm CH, Searcy MT. Relationship between tocopherol and serum lipid levels for determination of nutritional adequacy. Ann NY Acad Sci 1972; 203:223-236.

30. Hashim S, Asfour RH. Tocopherol in infants fed diets rich in polyunsaturated fatty acids. Am J Clin Nutr 1968; 21:7-14.

31. Williams ML, Shott RJ, O'Neal PL, Oski FA. Role of dietary iron and fat on vitamin E deficiency anemia of infancy. N Engl J Med 1975; 292:887-890.

32. Melhorn DK, Gross S. Vitamin E-dependent anemia in the premature infant: I. Effects of large doses of medicinal iron. J Pediatr 1971; 79:569-580.

33. Dju MY, Mason KE, Filer LJ: Vitamin E (tocopherol) in human fetuses and placentae. Etudes Neonatales 1952; 1:49-62.

34. Baker H, Frank O, Thomson AD, et al. Vitamin profile of 174 mothers and newborns at parturition. Am J Clin Nutr 1975; 28:59-65.

35. Leonard PJ, Doyle E, Harrington W. Levels of vitamin E in the plasma of newborn infants and of the mothers. Am J Clin Nutr 1972; 25:480-484.

36. Straumfjord JV, Quaife ML. Vitamin E levels in maternal and fetal blood plasma. Proc Soc Exp Biol Med 1946; 61:369-371.

37. Tateno M, Ohshima A. The relationship between serum vitamin E levels in the perinatal period and the birth weight of the neonate. Acta Obstet Gynaecol Jap 1973; 20:177-181.

38. Cruz CS, Wimberley PD, Johansen K, Friis-Hansen B. The effect of vitamin E on erythrocyte hemolysis and lipid peroxidation in newborn premature infants. Acta Paediatr Scand 1983; 72:823-826.

39. Mino M, Nishimo H. Fetal and maternal relationship in serum vitamin E level. J Nutr Sci Vitaminol 1973; 19:475-482.

40. Hägä P, Lunde G. Selenium and vitamin E in cord blood from preterm and full term infants. Acta Paediatr Scand 1978; 67:735-739.

41. Horwitt MK. Interrelations between vitamin E and polyunsaturated fatty acids in adult men. Vitam Horm 1962; 20:541-559.

42. Jansson L, Akesson B, Holmberg L. Vitamin E and fatty acid composition of human milk. Am J Clin Nutr 1981; 34:8-13.

43. Quaife ML. Tocopherols (vitamin E) in milk: their chemical determination and occurrence in human milk. J Biol Chem 1947; 169:513-514.

44. Committee on Nutrition, American Academy of Pediatrics. Commentary on breast-feeding and infant formulas, including proposed standards for formulas. Pediatrics 1976; 57:278-285.

45. Committee on Nutrition, American Academy of Pediatrics. Nutritional needs for low-birth-weight infants. Pediatrics 1985; 75:976-986.

46. Gutcher GR, Farrell PM. Early intravenous correction of vitamin E deficiency in premature infants. J Pediatr Gastroenterol Nutr 1985; 4:604-609.

47. Greene HL, Moore C, Phillips B, et al. Evaluation of a pediatric multiple vitamin preparation for total parenteral nutrition II. Blood levels of vitamins A, D, and E. Pediatrics 1986; 77:539-547.

48. Owens WC, Owens EU. Retrolental fibroplasia in premature infants: II. Studies on the prophylaxis of the disease: the use of alpha tocopherol acetate. Am J Ophthalmol 1949; 32:1631-1637.

49. Committee on Fetus and Newborn, American Academy of Pediatrics. Vitamin E and the prevention of retinopathy of prematurity. Pediatrics 1985; 76:315-316.

50. Bell EF. Prevention of bronchopulmonary dysplasia: vitamin E and other antioxidants. In Farrell PM, Taussig LM (eds): Bronchopulmonary Dysplasia and Related Chronic Respiratory Disorders. Report of the Ninetieth Ross Conference on Pediatric Research, 1986; 77-82.

51. Chiswick ML, Johnson M, Woodhall C, et al. Protective effect of vitamin E (dl-alpha-tocopherol) against intraventricular hemorrhage in premature babies. Br Med J 1983; 287:81-84.

52. Speer ME, Blifeld C, Rudolph AJ, Chadda P, Holbein ME, Hittner HM. Intraventricular hemorrhage and vitamin E in the very low-birth-weight infant: Evidence for efficacy of early intramuscular vitamin E administration. Pediatrics 1984; 74:1107-1112.

53. Johnson L, Bowen F, Abbasi S, et al. Relationship of prolonged pharmacologic serum levels of vitamin E to incidence of sepsis and necrotizing enterocolitis in infants with birth weight 1,500 grams or less. Pediatrics 1985; 75:619-638.

54. Neal PR, Erickson P, Baenziger JC, et al. Serum vitamin E levels in the very low birth weight infant during oral supplementation. Pediatrics 1986; 77:636-640.

55. Oski FA, Stockman JA (eds): Yearbook of Pediatrics. Chicago, Yearbook Publishers, Inc., 1986; 72.

56. Barak M, Herschkowitz S, Montag J. Soft tissue calcification: a

complication of vitamin E injection. Pediatrics 1986; 77: 382–385.

57. Graeber JE, Williams ML, Oski FA. The use of intramuscular vitamin E in the premature infant: optimal dose and iron interaction. J Pediatr 1977; 90:282–284.

58. Lorch V, Murphy D, Hoersten L, et al. Unusual syndrome along premature infants: association with a new intravenous vitamin E product. Pediatrics 1985; 75:598–602.

59. Bove KE, Kosmetatos N, Wedig K, et al. Vasculopathic hepatotoxicity associated with E-Ferol syndrome in low-birth weight infants. JAMA 1985; 254:2422–2430.

60. Bhat R, Jiang JX, Walsh JM, et al. Effect of vitamin E and polysorbate on bile acid transport in newborn rabbit hepatocytes. Pediatr Res 1985; 19:213A.

61. Finer NN, Peters KL, Hayek Z, Merkel CL. Vitamin E and necrotizing enterocolitis. Pediatrics 1984; 73:387–393.

17

Vitamin K and the Newborn

FRANK R. GREER, M.D.
JOHN W. SUTTIE, Ph.D.

ABSTRACT

Though considerable progress has been made in the area of the physiologic function of vitamin K in the last 25 years, it remains a vitamin in which there is no true recommended dietary allowance. Its apparent deficiency worldwide remains a significant cause of infant morbidity and mortality. This chapter addresses the structure, function and metabolism of vitamin K, as well as deficiency-related hemorrhagic disease of the newborn.

INTRODUCTION

A boy on the third day of his life developed ecchymoses on his head and groin and on one foot. There was also bleeding from high up in the bowel on the 5th and 6th days, the dejections being tarry from altered blood and simulating meconium. . . . Two days later the child developed a marked paralysis of the left side of the face, and to a less degree of the left arm and leg, presumably from meningeal hemorrhage. . . . On the seventh day of the disease there was beginning improvement in the paralysis, and it was apparent that no more hemorrhages occurred. . . . The belief that the disease was self-limited, with careful artificial and wet-nurse feeding, the mother's supply proving a failure, was what saved the baby. C.W. Townsend, Arch Pediatrics, 1894.[1]

At the time that this case report was written in the late 19th century, the etiology of the hemorrhagic disease of the newborn was unknown. In fact, Townsend in his review of 50 cases thought that the most likely etiology of this bleeding disorder in the neonate was an infectious disease.[1] The truth of the matter was, it was the indeed the "artificial feeding" undoubtedly containing vitamin K which saved this infant's life.

PHYSIOLOGY

Vitamin K was first proposed as the name for a dietary antihemorrhagic factor in 1935 by Henrik Dam, a faculty member of the Biochemical Institute of the University of Copenhagen.[2] Though "K" was the first letter of the German word *Koagulation*, it was also by chance the first letter of the alphabet not in use at that time to describe an existing vitamin or vitamin-like activity.

Investigating cholesterol biosynthesis in chicks, Dam serendipitously observed a hemorrhagic disease in chicks placed on fat-free diets in 1929.[3] This hemorrhagic disease of chicks was soon described by others[4,5] and was successfully treated with ether extracts of alfalfa.[6]

At the time of Dam's discovery, the only clearly defined plasma proteins known to be involved in blood coagulation were prothrombin and fibrinogen, and he and his coworkers prepared a crude prothrombin extract from the blood of normal chicks and demonstrated that it would improve the clotting defect in vitamin K deficient chicks.[7] An understanding of the various factors involved in regulating the generation of thrombin from prothrombin did not occur until the mid 1950s, with the subsequent discovery of Factors VII, IX, and X, which were also shown to be vitamin K dependent.[8]

The vitamin was initially isolated from alfalfa as a yellow oil, and this plant form of vitamin K is now known as vitamin K_1 or phylloquinone (Fig. 1).[9] Another form of this vitamin was isolated from putrefied fish meal, which in contrast to the oil isolated from alfalfa, was a crystal.

This latter compound was originally called vitamin K_2 and is now known to be one of a series of vitamin K compounds with unsaturated side chains synthesized by bacteria, referred to as *menaquinones*.[8] The basic structure of all vitamin K compounds is *menadione*, a synthetic form that is not important in human nutrition (Fig. 1).

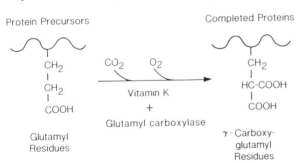

Menadione

Phylloquinone

Menaquinone-7

FIGURE 1. Biologically active forms of vitamin K. Phylloquinone is also called vitamin K_1 and is the major dietary form of vitamin K. Menaquinones are generally referred to as vitamin K_2 and are synthesized by bacteria. Menadione, a synthetic compound, is not important in human nutrition.

After its discovery, it was nearly 40 years before the metabolic function of vitamin K was determined. It is now known that plasma Factors II (prothrombin) VII, IX and X in the cascade theory of blood coagulation are dependent on the presence of vitamin K for their synthesis and that vitamin K functions postribosomally (posttranslationally) as a cofactor in the metabolic conversion of intracellular precursor proteins (produced in the absence of the vitamin) to the active forms of the plasma clotting factors.[8] This discovery was aided by the observation that the plasma of patients treated with coumarin anticoagulants contained a protein very similar to prothrombin but lacking its biological activity. The important difference between these two forms of prothrombin was subsequently shown to be the inability of the abnormal prothrombin to bind calcium ions.[10] The conversion of glutamyl residues to γ-carboxyglutamic acid residues on the prothrombin molecule creates effective calcium binding sites, and vitamin K is a necessary cofactor for the activity of this microsomal glutamyl carboxylase (Fig. 2).

Further studies of this microsomal vitamin K dependent carboxylase have not yet eluci-dated the exact molecular role of vitamin K in this reaction; however, it is apparent that during the conversion of glutamyl to γ-carboxyglutamyl residues on the vitamin K dependent peptides by carboxylase, vitamin K is converted to its 2,3-epoxide (Fig. 3).[11] Subsequently the epoxide form of vitamin K is reduced to the quinone form by an epoxide reductase and to the active coenzyme form, the hydroquinone, by various microsomal quinone reductases. It is hypothesized currently that the role of vitamin K is to abstract the hydrogen of a glutamyl (glu) residue as a proton from a vitamin K dependent protein, leaving a carbanion which is attacked by free CO_2 to form γ-carboxyglutamic acid.[11] Coumarin anticoagulants such as warfarin apparently antagonize vitamin K action by inhibiting the epoxide reductase activity as well as one of the quinone reductase activities of liver. These actions increase the concentration of vitamin K epoxide and result in an insufficient amount of reduced vitamin K for the action of carboxylase.

Other vitamin K dependent proteins include protein C, S, and Z in plasma[12] and γ-carboxyglutamic acid (gla) containing proteins in kidney, spleen, lung, uterus, placenta, pancreas, thyroid, thymus, testes and bone.[11] Carboxylase activity has also been detected in most of these tissues, including human liver.[13] Bone contains a major vitamin K dependent protein, osteocalcin, as well as lesser amounts of other gla containing proteins. The function of these skeletal gla proteins is not known but has been the subject of much speculation.[14] **All of the known vitamin K dependent proteins have in common γ-carboxyglutamic acid (gla), the unique amino acid formed by the post-ribosomal action of vitamin K dependent carboxylase.**

Vitamin K is absorbed from the intestine into the lymphatic system, requiring the presence of both bile salts and pancreatic secretions.[15] The lymphatic system is thus the major route of intestinal transport of absorbed phylloquinone in association with chylomicrons.[15]

Protein Precursors

Completed Proteins

CH_2
|
CH_2
|
COOH

CO_2 O_2

Vitamin K
+
Glutamyl carboxylase

Glutamyl Residues

CH_2
|
HC-COOH
|
COOH

γ - Carboxy-glutamyl Residues

FIGURE 2. Vitamin K functions as a cofactor with the microsomal enzyme glutamyl carboxylase to convert glutamyl residues to γ-carboxyglutamic acid residues on precursor proteins (i.e., prothrombin).

FIGURE 3.   Metabolism of vitamin K in liver. The formation of γ-carboxyglutamic acid is dependent on reduced vitamin K and is coupled to the formation of vitamin K epoxide. The regeneration of the reduced coenzyme (naphthohydroquinone) from the epoxide requires a dithiol (-SH) dependent vitamin K epoxide reductase to convert the epoxide to the quinone. Reduction of the quinone can occur by a dithiol dependent pathway or by a reduced pyridine nucleotide pathway. The two dithiol-dependent steps in vitamin K metabolism are blocked by the commonly used oral anticoagulants.

#1 Vitamin K_1 (hydroquinone)—active, coenzyme form
#2 glutamyl residue on vitamin K–dependent protein
#3 enzyme action—glutamyl carboxylase
#4 γ-carboxyglutamyl (gla) residue on vitamin K–dependent protein
#5 vitamin K_1—2–3 epoxide form
#6 enzyme action—epoxide reductase
#7 vitamin K_1—quinone form
#8 enzyme action—quinone reductase

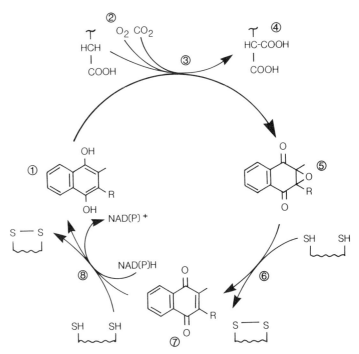

Little is known of the existence of specific carrier proteins.

In rats, phylloquinone absorption appears to be by an energy dependent process from the proximal portion of the small intestine.[16] In contrast, menaquinone absorption has been found to be a passive, non-carrier-mediated process from both the large and small intestine.[17,18] Vitamin K of bacterial origin may be absorbed from the large bowel of some mammals at a sufficent rate to prevent deficiency syndromes. There is little specific information about the intestinal absorption of vitamin K in man. In contrast to rats it has been suggested that the concentration of bile salts in the large bowel in man may not be sufficient for significant absorption of bacterial menaquinones.[19] Although it has not been possible to quantitate the contribution of menaquinone absorption from the large bowel, the rarity of dietary vitamin K deficiency in humans with normal intestinal function would suggest that the absorption of menaquinones is possible. Shearer et al. have reported that normal subjects excrete less than 20% of a 1 mg dose of phylloquinone in the feces.[19] Another report in newborn infants has recently estimated that 29% of an oral dose of phylloquinone is absorbed from the intestine.[20] The importance of the enterohepatic circulation of vitamin K in man is unknown.

Absorption of vitamin K may be inhibited by mineral oil[21] and by high dietary intakes of vitamins A[22] and E.[23-25] Vitamin K deficiency has been observed in subjects with impaired fat absorption caused by obstructive jaundice, pancreatic insufficiency (cystic fibrosis), and adult celiac disease.[19,26]

After injection of vitamin K in the rat, phylloquinone is rapidly concentrated in liver but has a short half-life (17 hours) consistent with little long-term storage by this organ.[27] Vitamin K also is concentrated by the adrenal glands, lungs, bone marrow, kidneys, and lymph nodes following injection.[28] In pigs and dogs, both phylloquinone and menaquinones (presumably of bacterial origin) are detected in the liver.[29] In adult man it has been also demonstrated with labelled phylloquinone that **the total body pool of vitamin K is replaced approximately every 2½ hours.**[30] In man, both forms of the vitamin have been found in a limited number of liver samples obtained at autopsy.[31]

There is much to be learned about the degradative products of phylloquinone and menaquinones, though some major products of phylloquinone metabolism have been identified.[8] The excretion of the various metabolites formed is radically altered by anticoagulant administration. In adult man 20% of an injected dose of either 1 mg or 45 μg of vitamin K is excreted in the urine within three days and 40-50% is excreted in the feces via the bile.[32-34]

ASSESSMENT OF NEEDS

The assessment of the vitamin K requirements of adults as well as children has been difficult because of the relative uncommonness of the deficiency state in the absence of complicating factors. **Generally, the apparent requirement of vitamin K is exceeded by almost any diet that is in other respects nutritionally adequate,** and simple dietary deficiency is of little concern. As reviewed above, vitamin K turns over rapidly and may not be stored to any significant degree. The assessment of human needs is also complicated by uncertainty regarding the extent of menaquinone utilization in man and by a lack of knowledge of the relative biopotency of the two common forms of the vitamin.

Technical difficulties have limited our knowledge of the vitamin K content of various food items. Until recently, such determinations depended on a chick biological assay that was not well suited for the small amounts of vitamin K present in most foods.[8] Almost all plant material contains phylloquinone, and animal products contain mixtures of phylloquinone and menaquinones. Recently, methods have been developed for the determination of the vitamin K content of foods by lipid extraction and HPLC analysis.[35] Satisfactory tables of the vitamin K content of various foods are not yet available and care should be taken when assessing the published data.[8]

There have been several recent reports of the vitamin K content of human milk. In a report by Haroon et al. the phylloquinone content of mature milk from 20 mothers was 2.1 ng/ml (range 1.1-6.5 ng/ml), not different from colostrum sampled from nine of the mothers (2.3 ng/ml, range 0.7-4.2 ng/ml).[36] In another study, the mean concentration of phylloquinones in the foremilk (1.4 ± 1.1 ng/ml) and hindmilk (2.5 ± 1.6 ng/ml) was reported in 10 lactating mothers.[37] Finally, the value for phylloquinones in milk from 337 lactating Japanese women was reported to be 3.8 ± 0.91 ng/ml. This latter study also reported milk levels of menaquinone-4 (0.70 ± 0.09 ng/ml) in these same mothers, which is of considerable interest, as menaquinones have not been detected in human serum.[38] There has been also a report in a single mother in whom an oral dose of 20 mg of phylloquinone increased the level in breast milk from undetectable to 140 ng/ml by 12 hours but which rapidly decreased to approximately 5 ng/ml by 48 hours.[36]

Recently, concentrations of phylloquinones have been reported as 4.9 ng/ml (range 3.6-8.9 ng/ml, n=12) in natural cow milk, 4.2 ng/ml in unsupplemented cow milk infant formulas, and 11.5 ng/ml in two vitamin K supplemented, soy-based formulas.[36] Standard 20 cal/oz formulas in the United States are routinely supplemented with 55-58 ng/ml of vitamin K_1. **Thus in the U.S. formula-fed infants have relatively high intakes of phylloquinones compared to breast-fed babies.**

The simplest assessment of the need for vitamin K in a sick neonate has been to observe whether or not a coagulopathy responds to an injection of vitamin K. Traditionally, the only way to measure the adequacy of vitamin K intake has been by the one-stage prothrombin time (PT) or by specific measurements of the plasma concentrations of the vitamin K–dependent clotting factors (Factors II, VII, IX, and X). In the newborn, these factors increase with increasing gestational age and are generally only 30-60% of normal adult values.[39] Normal adult levels are achieved by 2 to 12 months of age. Thus in the newborn, screening tests that reflect physiologic decreases in the vitamin K–dependent factors (prothrombin time, partial thromboplastin time) are prolonged compared to adult values. In all of the assays of clotting factors, the relationship between concentration of a given factor and the clotting time is non-linear, requiring the construction of careful dilution curves to standardize the activity.[8]

Human vitamin K deficiency results in the secretion into the plasma of partially carboxylated prothrombin, referred to as abnormal prothrombin or PIVKA (protein induced by vitamin K absence or antagonism).[8] As abnormal prothrombin lacks the full complement of γ-carboxyglutamic acid residues, its calcium affinity is altered, and its measurement may result in a more specific test of vitamin K deficiency. Methods for measuring this abnormal species of prothrombin based on the use of nonphysiological activators, or ratios of total prothrombin antigen to prothrombin activity have been described,[40-42] and specific antibodies for this "abnormal prothrombin" have been developed.[43,44] Recently this methodology has been adapted for measuring abnormal circulating prothrombin in infants.[43] Elevated plasma PIVKA concentrations have been reported in newborn infants and their mothers in one study,[45] but several preliminary reports have not been able to find abnormal prothrombin by less sensitive methods in cord blood.[46-48] Though abnormal PT can be utilized to detect a vitamin K deficiency, a recent report suggests that hepatic disease also may result in an impaired carboxylation of prothrombin and thus an apparent deficiency of vitamin K.[44]

Vitamin K status also may be reflected in the alterations in circulating concentrations of the vitamin. The extremely low concentration of vitamin K in serum has made measurements very difficult until recently, when high performance liquid chromatography methods for determining serum phylloquinone were developed.[35] In a preliminary study, 10 volunteer subjects on a normal diet had initial serum vitamin K concentrations of 0.85 ± 0.30 ng/ml (SD). After 3 weeks on a vitamin K–restricted diet (no green vegetables) serum vitamin K concentrations fell to 0.48 ± 0.15 ng/ml. After 7 days of the restricted diet plus 1 mg/day of vitamin K_1, the serum vitamin K concentration increased to 3.03 ± 0.96 ng/ml.[49] Thus, dietary restrictions may have some effect on circulating serum concentrations of vitamin K.

There are a number of reports measuring serum vitamin K_1 concentrations in newborn infants and their mothers.[50-53] There is a large difference in the range of values reported for reasons that are not clear. For our own data,[53] the values for maternal (1.69 ± 1.04 ng/ml [SD]) and cord blood (1.10 ± 0.58 ng/ml) concentrations are very close to values we have found for 106 blood donors from the local chapter of the Red Cross (1.29 ± 0.51 ng/ml [SD]).[54]

There are no data for serum measurements of menaquinones in adults or newborns which are not detectable by current methods of assay. On the basis of limited data showing that about 50% of the human liver vitamin K is phylloquinone and 50% menaquinones, **it has been assumed that bacterially synthesized vitamins can satisfy 50% of the daily adult requirement.**[31] There are no data to substantiate this assumption but it has been noted that the majority of vitamin K–responsive hemorrhagic episodes in adults are associated with antibiotic administration and low food intake. Presumably antibiotic administration affects gut flora and synthesis of vitamin K_2.[55]

At the present time, due to the unknown role of menaquinone in human nutrition and the apparent abundance of phylloquinone in the adult diet, the assessment of dietary requirements is very difficult. **There is no established recommended dietary allowance for vitamin K.** From limited adult studies, the vitamin K requirement can be estimated to be between 0.5 and 1.0 µg of vitamin K/kg/day.[8] The American Academy of Pediatrics recommends 0.5-1.0 mg of vitamin K_1 be given to all newborn infants because of the risk of hemorrhagic disease of the newborn.[56] They also have recommended that all milk substitute formulas containing less than 25 µg/L of vitamin K should have vitamin K added to attain a level of at least 100 µg/L.

DEFICIENCY

Though vitamin K_1 is now given to almost all newborn infants and its administration is mandated by some state governments in the United States, this was not nearly so common 15-20 years ago. Even at this earlier time, hemorrhagic disease of the newborn was recognized largely as a disease of breast-fed infants:[57]

In the 1950s there were concerns about vitamin K administration because babies who received large doses of vitamin K (water-soluble) and babies whose mothers received large doses of vitamin K developed jaundice and often kernicterus. Many practitioners and investigators stopped giving vitamin K and stated there were no apparent ill effects. It seemed that these statements emanated from centers predominantly serving middle and upper class patients. We observed that the very few infants at Cincinnati General Hospital who were not given vitamin K developed hemorrhagic disease. The General Hospital infants were from a low social economic group. Thus it seemed possible that there were low risk (mostly upper socioeconomic) populations and high risk (lower socioeconomic) populations. We, therefore, conducted a prospective study using different doses of vitamin K versus placebo in our high risk population. Vitamin K deficiency occurred only in placebo infants and only in placebo infants who were breast-fed. Artificially fed infants were protected. Since, at that time the lower social economic groups were breast feeding their infants, and the higher social economic groups were artificially feeding their infants, economic status largely determined primary risk of hemorrhagic disease if vitamin K were not administered. (As recalled by James Sutherland, M.D., Cincinnati, 1986.)

In the classic disorder, hemorrhage occurs between 2 and 10 days of life. Intracranial hemorrhage is uncommon and the disease is usually hallmarked by generalized ecchymoses or gastrointestinal hemorrhage. Bleeding from a circumcision or umbilical stump is also common. Estimates of the incidence of the classic form of this disease vary considerably, from 1 in 400 to as high as 1.7 per 100 in full-term infants.[58] Most commonly this form of the disease occurs in breast-fed infants who do not receive prophylactic vitamin K on the first day of life. As noted earlier, breast milk is very low in vitamin K.

The most common form of hemorrhagic disease of the newborn at the present time is the so-called late onset (>2 weeks of age) hemorrhagic disease. Of 89 cases of hemorrhagic disease of the newborn reported in the literature in the last three years,[38,59-74] 80 were of the late onset type (Table 1). Sixty-six of these 80 infants experienced intracranial hemorrhage, a common feature of late onset disease. The mortality rate reported in these 66 infants was high (17%) and the morbidity rate was much higher, though it was not well documented in all the reports. It is also of interest that 76 infants were exclusively breast-fed and did not receive prophylactic vitamin K at birth. Only 6 infants were reported to have been breast-fed and to have received prophylactic vitamin K at the time of birth.[63,65,71,73]

A large number of complicating factors are associated with hemorrhagic disease of the newborn (Table 3). In the 89 cases in Tables 1 and 2, low dietary intake of vitamin K (breast milk), and failure to receive vitamin K (often because of home delivery) were prominent. Disorders with fat malabsorption (cystic fibrosis, biliary atresia, α-1-antitrypsin deficiency) were not infrequently present with vitamin K deficiency in infancy.[63,66,68,73,74] The effect of antibiotic therapy and type of feeding (human milk versus formula) on bacterial flora and menaquinone production is an area for future study in newborn infants. Present information, however, indicates in Western countries that the differences in bacterial stool flora between breast-fed and formula-fed infants are not as great as previously reported.[75,76]

A peculiar form of hemorrhagic disease of the newborn occurring on the first day of life is associated with maternal anticonvulsant therapy during pregnancy.[77,78] Only two cases in Table 1 were associated with maternal drug therapy.[60] Though these cases are responsive to vitamin K administration, our understanding of the role of anticonvulsants in this hemorrhagic disorder is very limited.

TABLE 1. Hemorrhagic Disease of the Newborn 1983-1986—89 Cases

Characteristics	No. of cases
Exclusively breast-fed, no vitamin K	76
Exclusively breast-fed, with vitamin K	6
Cholestasis	8
Drugs	2
Late onset (>2 wks of age)	80
Early onset (<2 wks of age)	9
Intracranial hemorrhage	66

The rash of recent reports of hemorrhagic disease of the newborn from many parts of the world has led to speculation that this disease has experienced a resurgence. It seems more likely that there is merely renewed interest in the disease. Of great concern is the large number of cases (Table 2) of vitamin K deficiency with intracranial hemorrhage reported from the Far East,[38,65] including unofficial reports from the People's Republic of China.[79] In these countries, breastfeeding is common and vitamin K is not administered prophylactically at birth. There is little information on maternal vitamin K status in these countries, which may place this population at greater risk for late onset of hemorrhagic disease.

Despite the large number of case reports of intracranial hemorrhage in breast-fed infants without vitamin K prophylaxis, the practice of prophylactic vitamin K administration in the newborn period is not without controversy.[47,80-83] In breast-fed infants who receive vitamin K at birth, normal concentrations of vitamin K–dependent clotting factors are still found at one month of age.[84] In view of these findings and the continuing reports of hemorrhagic disease of the newborn, it seems warranted to give prophylactic vitamin K in the newborn period at the present time. When

TABLE 2. Geographic Distribution of Hemorrhagic Disease of the Newborn 1983-1986 in 89 Cases

United States	4
West Germany	5
United Kingdom	14
Canada	3
Saudi Arabia	3
Australia	6
Japan	10
Taiwan	32
Spain	1
Tunisia	2
Netherlands	9

TABLE 3.   Complicating Factors Associated
with Vitamin K Deficiency in the Newborn

Maternal Drugs—phenobarbital, diphenylhydantoin,
   primidone, warfarin
Decreased Exogenous Intake
   Home delivery—failure to receive vitamin K at birth
   Low dietary intake—breast milk
                  unfortified soy- or meat-based
                      formulas
Decreased Production (Menaquinones)?
   Antibiotic therapy—decreased gut colonization by
                  vitamin K_2–producing bacteria
Fat Malabsorption
   Diarrhea—nonspecific
   Cholestyramine therapy
   Cystic fibrosis
   Celiac disease
   Cholestasis—biliary atresia
                  α-1-antitrypsin deficiency
   Abetalipoproteinemia

---

more information becomes available regarding serum concentrations of vitamin K and abnormal circulating prothrombin, as well as the role of menaquinones in infants, then perhaps recommendations about the need for vitamin K supplementation in the newborn can be made more specifically.

TOXICITY

There is little information regarding vitamin K toxicity in humans. In the 1950s, however, menadione administration for vitamin K prophylaxis in newborn infants was associated with hyperbilirubinemia, presumably secondary to increased red cell hemolysis.[85,86] This problem was compounded by the practice of administering large doses of menadione to mothers in premature labor:[86]

Vitamin K_3 (menadione) was widely used in obstetrics in the 1950s. It was often given immediately after birth, so people decided why not give it during premature labor and prevent intraventricular hemorrhage in the infant? The drug companies could cheaply manufacture vitamin K_3 and the amount in the parenteral vial (72 mg) was chosen because it was easy to make and it "sounded like" a good substantial dose. Who wanted to package 1 mg and charge for it? It was known to cross the placenta and they wanted to be sure the fetus "got enough." It was still widely assumed at this time that the placenta was a protector of the fetus from drug toxicity. In those days vitamins were not considered dangerous and the paradoxical effects of mega-dose therapy were just becoming apparent in neonatology. I think this was the first neonatal vitamin poisoning. The vitamin D–related hypercalcemia epidemic was described soon after this in England. (Personal recollection, Jerold F. Lucey M.D., Burlington, Vermont, June 1986.)

This problem was eliminated when phylloquinone (vitamin K_1) became available for newborn prophylaxis and much smaller doses of vitamin K were utilized.

In animals, there is a report in horses of renal toxicity when large amounts of menadione are administered, though it is not clear whether or not the drug vehicle may have been the cause of the toxicity.[87]

RECOMMENDATIONS

For reasons discussed above, there is no recommended dietary allowance for vitamin K in humans. A best guess for adults is a requirement of between 0.5 and 1.0 µg/kg/day.[8] Because of the many reports of intracranial hemorrhage in newborn breast-fed infants without prophylactic vitamin K,[38,60–65,69] it seems prudent to continue prophylactic vitamin K (0.5-1 mg intramuscularly or 1.0-2.0 mg orally) in the newborn infant as recommended by the American Academy of Pediatrics.[88] More information about the vitamin K requirements of infants breast-fed exclusively for long periods of time is needed, because of occasional reports of hemorrhagic disease in these infants even when vitamin K is given in the immediate newborn period.[63,65,71] For premature infants, the minimally recommended vitamin K supplement (0.5 mg intramuscularly, 1 mg orally) would seem prudent. The practice of administering weekly injections of vitamin K (0.5-1.0 mg) to all infants (preterm and full-term) and children on total parenteral nutrition should be continued until more specific information becomes available.

CASE REPORT

A 6-week-old female infant suddenly became lethargic and unresponsive after rolling off a couch on to a carpeted floor. The infant was full-term, appropriate for gestational age, and the product of an uncomplicated pregnancy, labor, and delivery. There was no history of maternal drug ingestion. The infant received 2 mg of vitamin K_2 orally at birth. In general, the child progressed well on exclusive breast feeding without supplemental vitamins and no history of antibiotic therapy. Mild physiologic jaundice resolved by one week of age. On the day prior to presentation to the hospital emergency room the child was described as active and feeding well.

Initial physical examination revealed a comatose infant with a fixed and dilated right pupil, a bulging anterior fontanelle, abnormal posturing, slight scleral icterus, and hepatomegaly (5 cm below costal margin). Initial laboratory studies included a hemoglobin of 12.0 gm/dl, white blood cell count of 10,300/mm^3 with a normal morphologic differential. Platelet count was 300,000/mm^3. Admission coagulation studies consisted of both a prothrombin time and partial thromboplastin time of greater than 120 seconds. Fibrinogen level was normal. Liver function studies revealed total serum bilirubin of 7.8 mg/dl with a direct fraction of 3.9 mg/dl. The serum glutamic oxaloacetic transaminase was 60 IU/ml (normal <40 IU/ml) and serum glutamic pyruvic transaminase was 38 IU/ml (normal <40 IU/ml). A CT scan of the head revealed a 4×5 cm right parietal intracerebral hematoma.

The infant was treated with 15 ml/kg of fresh frozen plasma and 5 mg intramuscularly of vitamin K_1. Within 12 hours the blood clotting studies had normalized but the patient remained comatose. A subsequent workup revealed that this patient had cholestatic liver disease secondary to homozygous α-1-antitrypsin deficiency (pi-type ZZ—PiZZ). After 10 days the infant was discharged on supplemental vitamins including vitamin K. Subsequent followup at 6 months of age revealed a normal neurologic examination.

This apparently "healthy" full-term, newborn infant developed vitamin K deficiency at 6 weeks of age, clinically manifested by an acute intracranial hemorrhage following relatively minor trauma. The etiology of this deficiency is undoubtedly related to the subsequent diagnosis of cholestatic liver disease, interfering with vitamin K absorption.

Questions and Answers

Q.   What is the potential role of human milk feeding in this infant's bleeding disorder?
A.   This infant was exclusively fed human milk, which is known to be very low in vitamin K. Historically, hemorrhagic disease of the newborn has been a disease of breast-fed infants.

Q.   Was the oral administration of vitamin K at birth an additional factor?
A.   It is possible that the oral administration of vitamin K at birth contributed to the severity of the presentation, as the infant may not have retained all or part of the dose, or may not have effectively absorbed the dose. As there is no information on the half-life or hepatic storage of vitamin K in neonates, the relation of the initial dose of vitamin K to the outcome 6 weeks later is unclear.

REFERENCES

1. Townsend CW. The haemorrhagic disease of the new-born. Arch Pediatr 1894; 11:559–565.
2. Dam H. The antihaemorrhagic vitamin of the chick (letter). Nature (Lond) 1935; 135:652–653.
3. Dam H. Cholesterinstoffwechsel in Huhnereirn and Huhnchen. Biochem Zeitschs 1929; 215:475–492.
4. McFarlane WD, Graham WR, Richardson R. The fat-soluble vitamin requirements of the chick. I. The vitamin A and vitamin D content of fish meal and meat meal. Biochem J 1931; 25:358–366.
5. Holst WF, Halbrook ER. A "scurvy-like" disease in chicks (letter). Science 1933; 77:354.
6. Almquist HJ, Stokstad ELR. Dietary haemorrhagic disease in chicks (letter). Nature (Lond) 1935; 136:31.
7. Dam H, Schonheyder F, Tage-Hansen E. Studies on the mode of action of vitamin K. Biochem J 1936; 30:1075–1079.
8. Suttie JW. Vitamin K. In Diplock AT (ed): Fat Soluble Vitamins: Their Biochemistry and Applications. Lancaster, PA, Technomic Publishing Co., 1985; 225–311.

9. MacCorquodale DW, Cheney LC, Binkley SB, et al. The constitution and synthesis of vitamin K_1. J Biol Chem 1939; 131:357–370.
10. Esmon CT, Suttie JW, Jackson CM. The functional significance of vitamin K action. Difference in phospholipid binding between normal and abnormal prothrombin. J Biol Chem 1975; 250:4095–4099.
11. Suttie JW. Vitamin K-dependent carboxylase. Ann Rev Biochem 1985; 54:459–477.
12. Dahlback B. Interaction between complement component C4b-binding protein and the vitamin K-dependent protein S. Scand J Clin Lab Invest 1985; 45(Suppl 177):33–41.
13. Soute BAM, DeMetz M, Vermeer C. Characteristics of vitamin K-dependent carboxylating systems from human liver and placenta. FEBS Lett 1982; 146:365–368.
14. Price P. Vitamin K-dependent formation of bone Gla protein (osteocalcin) and its function. Vitam Horm 1985; 42:65–108.
15. Blomstrand R, Forsgren L. Vitamin K_1-^{3}H in man. Its intestinal absorption and transport in the thoracic duct lymph. Int Z Vit Forschung 1968; 38:45–64.
16. Hollander D, Rim E, Muralidhara KS. Vitamin K_1 intestinal absorption in vivo: influence of luminal contents on transport. Am J Physiol 1977; 232:E69– E74.
17. Hollander D, Rim E. Vitamin K_2 absorption by rat everted small intestinal sacs. Am J Physiol 1976; 231:415–419.
18. Hollander D, Muralidhara KS, Rim E. Colonic absorption of bacterially synthesized vitamin K_2 in the rat. Am J Physiol 1976; 230:251–255.
19. Shearer MJ, McBurney A, Barkhan P. Studies on the absorption and metabolism of phylloquinone (vitamin K_1) in man. Vitam Horm 1974; 32:513–542.
20. Sann L, Leclercq M, Guillaumond M, et al. Serum vitamin K_1 concentrations after oral administration of vitamin K_1 in low birth weight infants. J Pediatr 1985; 107:608–611.
21. Elliot MC, Isaacs B, Ivy AC. Production of "prothrombin deficiency" and response to vitamin A, D, and K. Proc Soc Exp Biol Med 1940; 43:240–245.
22. Doisy EA, Matschiner JT. In Morton RA (ed): Fat Soluble Vitamins. Pergamon Press, Oxford, 1970; 293.
23. Corrigan JJ, Marcus FI. Coagulopathy associated with vitamin E ingestion. JAMA 1974; 230:1300–1301.
24. Rao GH, Mason KE. Antisterility and antivitamin K activity of d-α-tocopherol hydroquinone in the vitamin E-deficient female rat. J Nutrit 1975; 105:495–498.
25. Corrigan JJ, Ulfers LL. Effect of vitamin E on prothrombin levels in warfarin-induced vitamin K deficiency. Am J Clin Nutr 1981; 34:1701–1705.
26. Corrigan JJ, Taussig LM, Beckerman R, Wagner JS. Factor II (prothrombin) coagulant activity and immunoreactive protein: Detection of vitamin K deficiency and liver disease in patients with cystic fibrosis. J Pediatr 1981; 99:254–257.
27. Thierry MJ, Hermodson MA, Suttie JW. Vitamin K and warfarin distribution and metabolism in the warfarin-resistant rat. Am J Physiol 1970; 219:854–859.
28. Konishi T, Baba S, Sone H. Whole-body autoradiographic study of vitamin K distribution in rat. Chem Pharm Bull 1973; 21:220–224.
29. Duello TJ, Matschiner JT. Characterization of vitamin K from pig liver and dog liver. Arch Biochem Biophys 1971; 144:330–338.
30. Bjornsson TD, Meffin PJ, Swezey SE, Blaschke TF. Disposition and turnover of vitamin K_1 in man, In Suttie JW (ed): Vitamin K Metabolism and Vitamin K-Dependent Proteins. Baltimore, University Park Press, 1980; 328–332.
31. Duello TJ, Matschiner JT. Characterization of vitamin K from human liver. J Nutr 1972; 102:331–336.
32. Shearer MJ, Barkhan P, Webster GR. Absorption and excretion of an oral dose of tritiated vitamin K_1 in man. Br J Haematol 1970; 18:297–308.
33. Shearer MJ, Mallinson CN, Webster GR, Barkhan P. Clearance from plasma and excretion in urine, faeces, and bile of an intravenous dose of tritiated vitamin K_1 in man. Br J Haematol 1972; 22:579–588.
34. Shearer MJ, Barkhan P. Studies on the metabolites of phylloquinone (vitamin K_1) in the urine of man. Biochem Biophys Acta 1973; 297:300–312.
35. Shearer MJ. High-performance liquid chromatography of K

vitamins and their antagonists. In Giddings JC, et al. (eds): Advances in Chromatography, New York, Marcel Dekker, 1983; 243–301.

36. Haroon Y, Shearer MJ, Rahim S, et al. The content of phylloquinone (vitamin K_1) in human milk, cow's milk and infant formula foods determined by high-performance liquid chromatography. J Nutr 1982; 112:1105–1117.

37. Von Kries R, Sutor A, Pollmann H, et al. Vitamin-K-Gehalt der Muttermilch bei gestillten Sauglingen mit lebensbedrohlicher Blutungsneisung infolge Vitamin-K-Mangels (abstract). Montasschr Kindesheilkd 1984; 132:725.

38. Motohara K, Matsukara M, Matsuda I, et al. Severe vitamin K deficiency in breast-fed infants. J Pediatr 1984; 105:943–945.

39. Oski FA, Naiman JL. Hematologic Problems in the Newborn, 3rd ed. Philadelphia, WB Saunders, 1982; 145.

40. Bertina RM, Van der Marel-Van Nieuwkoop W, Dubbeldam J, et al. New method for the rapid detection of vitamin K deficiency. Clin Chim Acta 1980; 105:93–98.

41. Meguro T, Yamada K. A simple and rapid test for PIVKA-II in plasma. Thromb Res 1982; 25:109–114.

42. Shah DV, Swanson JC, Suttie JW. Abnormal prothrombin in the vitamin K-deficient rat. Thromb Res 1984; 35:451–458.

43. Motohara K, Kuroki Y, Kan H, et al. Detection of vitamin K deficiency by use of an enzyme linked immunosorbent assay for circulating abnormal prothrombin. Pediatr Res 1985; 19:354–357.

44. Blanchard RA, Furie BC, Jorgensen M, et al. Acquired vitamin K-dependent carboxylation deficiency in liver disease. N Engl J Med 1981; 305:242–248.

45. Blanchard RA, Furie BC, Peck C, et al. Subclinical vitamin K deficiency in newborns and their mothers (abstract). Blood 1983; 62(Suppl):272a.

46. Van Dorm JM, Muller AD, Hemker HC. Heparin-like inhibitor, not vitamin K deficiency in the newborn (letter). Lancet 1977; 1:852–853.

47. Malia RG, Preston FE, Mitchell VE. Evidence against vitamin K deficiency in normal neonates. Thromb Haemost 1980; 44:159–160.

48. Von Kries R, Gobel A, Maase B. Vitamin K deficiency in the newborn (letter). Lancet 1985; 2:728–729.

49. Kindberg C, Mummah-Schendel L, Suttie JW. Unpublished data.

50. Shearer MJ, Barkhan P, Rahim S, Stimmler L. Plasma vitamin K_1 in mothers and their newborn babies. Lancet 1982; 2:460–463.

51. Pietersma-de Bruyn ALJM, van Haard PMM. Vitamin K_1 in the newborn, Clin Chim Acta 1985; 150:95– 101.

52. Sann L, Leclercq M, Troncy J, et al. Serum vitamin K_1 concentration and vitamin K-dependent clotting factor activity in maternal and fetal cord blood. Am J Obstet Gynecol 1985; 153:771–774.

53. Greer FR, Mummah-Schendel LL, Marshall S, Suttie JW. Vitamin K_1 (phylloquinone) and vitamin K_2 (menaquinone) status in newborn infants during the first week of life. Pediatrics 1988;137-140.

54. Mummah-Schendel L, Suttie JW. Serum phylloquinone concentrations in a normal adult population. Am J Clin Nutr 1986;44:686-689.

55. Savage O, Lindenbaum J (ed): Clinical and Experimental Human Vitamin K Deficiency. New York, Churchill Livingstone, 1983; 271–320.

56. American Academy of Pediatrics Committee Statement, Committee on Nutrition: Vitamin K supplementation for infants receiving milk substitute formulas and for those with fat malabsorption. Pediatrics 1971; 48:483–487.

57. Sutherland JM, Glueck HI, Gleser G. Hemorrhagic disease of the newborn. Am J Dis Child 1967; 113:524–533.

58. Keenan WJ, Jewett T, Glueck H. Role of feeding and vitamin K in hypoprothrombinemia of the newborn. Am J Dis Child 1971; 121:271–277.

59. Forbes D. Delayed presentation of haemorrhagic disease of the newborn. Med J Aust 1983; 2:136–138.

60. McNinch AW, Orme RLE, Tripp JH. Haemorrhagic disease of the newborn returns. Lancet 1983; 1:1089–1090.

61. O'Connor ME, Livingstone DS, Hannah J, Wilkins D. Vitamin K deficiency and breast-feeding. Am J Dis Child 1983; 137:601–602.

62. Sutor AH, Pancochar H, Niederhoff H, et al. Vitamin K deficiency haemorrhages in four entirely breast-fed infants aged 4 to 6 weeks. Deutsch Med Wochensch 1983; 108:1635–1639.

63. Verity CM, Carswell F, Scott GL. Vitamin K deficiency causing infantile intracranial hemorrhage after the neonatal period (letter). Lancet 1983; 1:1439.

64. Ware S, Mills M. Vitamin K deficiency causing infantile intracranial hemorrhage after the neonatal period (letter). Lancet 1983; 1:1439–1440.

65. Chaou W-T, Min-Lang C, Eitzman DV. Intracranial hemorrhage and vitamin K deficiency in early infancy. J Pediatr 1984; 105:880–884.

66. Payne NR, Hasegawa DK. Vitamin K deficiency in newborns: A case report in α-1-antitrypsin deficiency and a review of factors predisposing to hemorrhage. Pediatrics 1984; 73:712–716.

67. Behrmann BA, Chan W-K, Finer NW. Resurgence of hemorrhagic disease of the newborn: A report of three cases. Can Med Assoc J 1985; 133:884–885.

68. Rose SJ. Neonatal haemorrhage and vitamin K. Acta Haematol 1985; 74:121.

69. Mallouh A. Vitamin K deficiency in infants (letter). J Pediatr 1985; 107:990.

70. Von Kries R, Reifenhauser A, Gobel U, et al. Late onset haemorrhagic disease of the newborn with temporary malabsorption of vitamin K (letter). Lancet 1985; 1:1035.

71. Barnusell JB, Carnicer J, Artigas J, et al. Hemorragia intercraneal secundaria a enfermedad hemorragica tardia del recien nacido. An Esp Pediatr 1985; 23:453–455.

72. Khaldi F, Bennaceur B, Boudhina T, et al. Syndrome hemorragique tardif par hypovitaminose K. Pediatrie 1985; 40:577–580.

73. Keifer KA. Breast-feeding, α-antitrypsin deficiency, and liver disease? (letter). JAMA 1985; 254:3036–3037.

74. Widdershoven JAM, Kollee LAA, Van Oostrom CG, et al. Vitamine K deficientie by zuigelingen. Ned Tijdschr Geneeskd 1986; 130:473–476.

75. Simhon A, Douglas JR, Drasan BS, Soothill JF. Effects of feeding on infants' faecal flora. Arch Dis Child 1982; 57:54–58.

76. Lundequist B, Nord CE, Winberg J. The composition of the faecal microflora in breast-fed and bottle-fed infants from birth to eight weeks. Acta Paediatr Scand 1985; 74:45–51.

77. Mountain KR, Hirsh J, Gallus AS. Neonatal coagulation defect due to anticonvulsant drug treatment in pregnancy. Lancet 1970; 1:265–268.

78. Srinivassan G, Seele RA, Tiruvury A, Pildes RS. Maternal anticonvulsant therapy and hemorrhagic disease of the newborn. Obstet Gynecol 1982; 59:250–252.

79. Xiao-rong Chen. Personal communication. Childrens Hospital, Shanghai, First Medical College, People's Republic of China, 1986.

80. Mori PG, Bisogni C, Odino S, et al. Vitamin K deficiency in the newborn (letter). Lancet 1977; 2:188.

81. Edson JR. Vitamin K deficiency in the newborn. Lancet 1977; 2:187.

82. Gobel U, Sonnenschein-Kosenow S, Petrich C, von Voss H. Vitamin K deficiency in the newborn (letter). Lancet 1977; 2:187–188.

83. Vitamin K and the newborn (editorial). Lancet 1978; 1:755–757.

84. Jimenez R, Navarette M, Jimenez E, et al. Vitamin K dependent clotting factors in normal breast-fed infants. J Pediatr 1982; 100:424–426.

85. Meyer TC, Angus J. The effect of large doses of "Synkavit" in the newborn. Arch Dis Child 1956; 31:212–215.

86. Lucey JF, Dolan RG. Hyperbilirubinemia of newborn infants associated with the parenteral administration of a vitamin K analogue to the mothers. Pediatrics 1959; 23:553–560.

87. Rebhun WC, Tennant BC, Dill SG, King JM. Vitamin K_3-induced renal toxicosis in the horse. JAVMA 1984; 184:1237–1239.

88. American Academy of Pediatrics Committee on Nutrition. Vitamin and mineral supplement needs in normal children in the United States. Pediatrics 1980; 66:1015–1021.

18

Management of Breastfeeding

JUDY M. HOPKINSON, Ph.D.
CUTBERTO GARZA, M.D., Ph.D.

ABSTRACT

Techniques for initiating and maintaining lactation following term and preterm delivery are reviewed in this chapter. In the first section, the influence of various protocols utilized for initiation of lactation in hospital is discussed. The period of transition between hospital discharge and the first well-baby visit is a high-risk period for breastfeeding problems and is covered in detail. Differences between feeding, stool, and sleep patterns for breastfed and formula-fed infants are examined. Common problems and special situations encountered by lactating mothers are discussed in the final section of the chapter.

INTRODUCTION

The incidence of breastfeeding in the United States at 1 week postpartum has risen dramatically from its nadir of 22% in 1972. Between 1972 and 1982, the percentage of mothers who initiated breastfeeding rose to approximately 60% and has remained stable since that time.[1,2] The percentage of infants at 2 and 6 months still being breastfed also increased during that interval from levels far below 20% to approximately 45% and 28%, respectively. The distribution of breastfeeding among women in the United States is nonrandom. Breastfeeding is more prevalent among college-educated women, in upper income groups, and among whites.[1] Employed women are more likely to breastfeed (at least until their infants are 5 months of age) than are women who do not work outside the home. Geographical differences also are evident; breastfeeding is more prevalent in the western United States than in other sections of the country. The demography of breastfeeding is qualitatively similar in Australia, Western Europe, and North America.

Mothers generally decide before delivery whether or not to breastfeed their infants. Their decision is influenced by sociological and psychological factors that are poorly understood.[3] The physiological factors that influence the successful outcome of breastfeeding, however, are understood more completely. Recent research in infant feeding permits women to make an informed choice when a feeding mode is selected. When breastfeeding is chosen, the available information can be used to develop feeding skills and practices founded on physiological principles. The successful initiation and establishment of lactation are influenced by the application of these principles in perinatal hospital practices, and by the medical and paramedical support available to lactating women after discharge.

The most common reason given by women for weaning their infants prematurely is an inadequate milk supply.[3-5] An inadequate milk supply is rarely the result of primary maternal pathology. **In almost all cases lactation failure is preventable or correctable with good management.** The following discussion focuses on a single goal—the production of sufficient milk to breastfeed an infant for as long as the mother wishes. Four phases of lactation are considered: (1) breastfeeding is initiated, (2) exclusive breastfeeding is established, (3) breastfeeding is supplemented or complemented with additional foods, and (4) weaning is begun. Finally, selected problems relevant to lactation management will be discussed.

PERINATAL CONSIDERATIONS

BREAST EXAMINATION

Prepartum visits to the pediatrician should include a discussion of feeding alternatives. If breastfeeding is elected, a breast examination should be included. The nipple should be examined closely. Flat, rigid, or inverted nipples may cause problems during the initiation of lactation because the infant may not "latch-on" to the breast effectively (Fig. 1). Large-breasted women will experience greater dif-

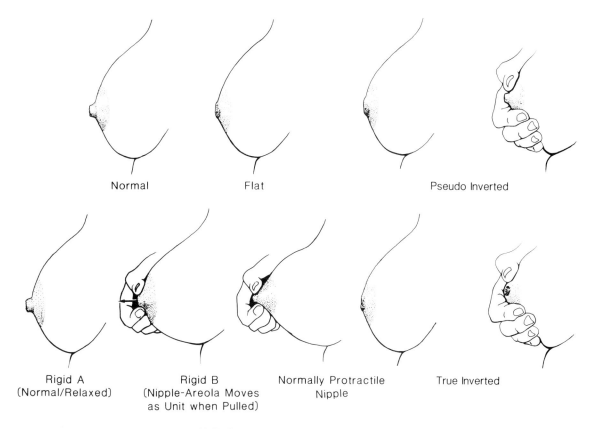

Normal   Flat   Pseudo Inverted

Rigid A
(Normal/Relaxed)

Rigid B
(Nipple-Areola Moves
as Unit when Pulled)

Normally Protractile
Nipple

True Inverted

FIGURE 1.   Nipple configurations.

ficulty nursing with flat nipples than will small-breasted women. All women with flat nipples are especially prone to experience difficulties during mammary engorgement. Rigid nipples are surrounded by an nonprotractile areola. Both move as a unit when pulled gently. Inverted nipples may be tucked into an areolar fold or may recede into the areola when the areola is compressed. Particular care is needed not to mistake pseudo- for true nipple inversion. **The pseudo-inverted nipple is dimpled in its center and does not recede inwardly when the areola is compressed.** Women with pseudo-inverted nipples may benefit from nipple exercises but will have little difficulty nursing.

Flat, rigid, or inverted nipples should be corrected before parturition. Two simple exercises ("nipple rolling" and Hoffman's exercises; see Fig. 2) or a breast shield may be used to correct these problems. The exercises may be done for a few minutes several times each day; the shield may be worn for approximately two hours at a time for one or two months before delivery. By forcing the nipple out through the breast shield's central orifice, Hoffman's ligaments are stretched or weakened and nipple

protrusion is facilitated. Nipple preparation is unnecessary for most women.[6] Some authors suggest, however, that mothers may benefit psychologically from manipulating their breasts before attempting to breastfeed their infants.[7]

Surgical interruption of nipple innervation will interfere with the hormonal response to suckling and may preclude successful breastfeeding. Mammoplasties that have interrupted nipple innervation should be noted, and patients should be monitored closely for signs of poor infant growth or poor milk production postpartum. Significant mammary disproportions and other breast anomalies have been associated with lactation failure,[8,9] but these conditions are uncommon. Discussion of these conditions is beyond the scope of this chapter, and the reader is referred to more comprehensive texts on lactation physiology and management.[7]

PLANNING THE HOSPITAL EXPERIENCE

The prenatal visit affords the opportunity to discuss infant feeding alternatives for the

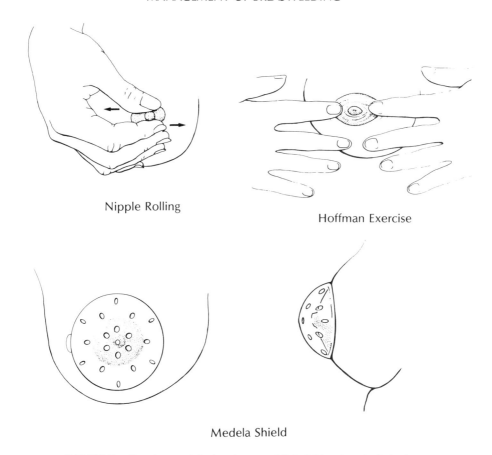

Nipple Rolling

Hoffman Exercise

Medela Shield

FIGURE 2.   Exercises and devices to correct flat, rigid, or inverted nipples.

period of hospitalization, which may directly or indirectly affect lactation. For example, will the infant be housed in the mother's room or in the nursery? Will the infant be fed on demand? Will supplementary water or formula be given? When will nursing be initiated?[3,10-15] The discussion may also include steps to be taken to minimize the use of drugs during delivery and thus increase the likelihood that the infant will be alert and able to nurse effectively.[16]

BREASTFEEDING IS INITIATED

Timing of Suckling Initiation

Although early initiation of suckling is not a prerequisite for successful breastfeeding, a **high probability of successful lactation has been documented in a number of studies if the interval between delivery and the initial nursing is short.**[13,15,17] Infants may be offered the opportunity to nurse immediately following delivery. Maternal and infant responses at the initial nursing vary. They are largely de-

pendent on the infant's alertness and general status.

Techniques for Initiation of Suckling

A variety of positions for offering the breast are used by nursing mothers. The more successful techniques like the cradle-hold characteristically allow maximum maternal comfort and close body contact between the mother and infant (Fig. 3). As the process begins, the mother places her contralateral hand against her chest wall beneath the breast and slides one or two fingers up onto the breast without actually touching the areola. She places the thumb directly above the fingers and uses it to control the placement of the nipple and areola in the infant's mouth. The infant is held facing the mother's body. The infant's head rests in the ipsilateral antecubital fossa and the mother's hand grasps the infant's upper thigh or buttocks. The nipple is brushed against the infant's lips to elicit the rooting reflex. As the infant's mouth opens wide, the mother pulls

FIGURE 3. Techniques for initiating and stopping breast-feeding. *A,* Cradle hold: Hold infant with head in cubital foci. Support breast well back of the areola, and touch the infant's lips with the nipple. *B,* When the infant opens wide, place the nipple far into the mouth to contact the upper back palate. *C,* Hold the infant close throughout the nursing and continue to support the breast as needed. *D,* Break suction prior to removing the infant from the breast by inserting a clean finger between the gums.

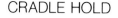

CRADLE HOLD

A
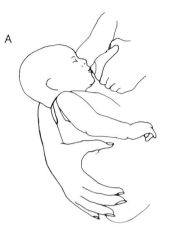

B
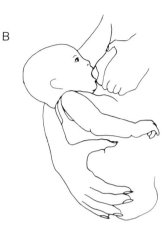

C
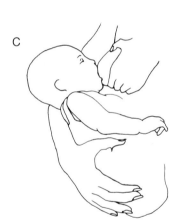

D
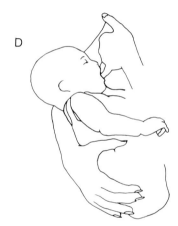

the infant close and moves the breast forward so that the nipple and areola enter the infant's mouth before he compresses his lips. If the mother has had a cesarean section or the infant cannot grasp the nipple effectively from this position, a variety of alternate positions may be tried (Fig. 4).

The sequence of events of a normal nursing episode can be divided into four steps: (1) the infant applies suction to a large area of the areola (approximately 4–6 cm in diameter), (2) the infant draws the nipple against the upper back palate (this signals the end of rooting and the initiation of suckling), (3) the infant begins a rapid, non-nutritive sucking pattern that elicits oxytocin release and milk ejection, and (4)

the infant switches to a slower, nutritive, suck-swallow pattern with a frequency of approximately 1 per second to extract milk from the lactiferous sinuses.

Suction generated by the infant holds the nipple against the upper hard palate. **This positioning allows the tongue to milk the lactiferous sinuses and drain the breast.** During effective suckling, the jaw's action is sufficiently strong to cause a brisk pulling movement of the infant's ears. The infant is removed from the breast by placing a finger between his gums to break the suction created during nursing.

If effective suckling cannot be initiated or the infant cannot be awakened for feedings at the

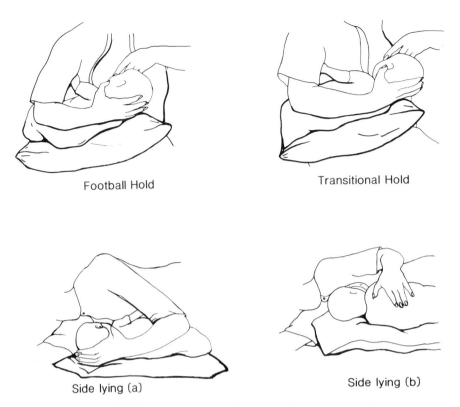

Football Hold

Transitional Hold

Side lying (a)

Side lying (b)

FIGURE 4.   Alternate positions for initiating breastfeeding.

recommended minimum mean frequency, additional counseling is required. In the interim, the mother should express milk every 3 hours to stimulate and maintain milk production.[13]

Feeding Frequencies in Hospital

Frequent suckling maximizes prolactin release and results in an earlier onset of milk production, i.e., a more rapid transition from colostrum to mature milk.[11,12] This accelerated transition is associated with greater infant weight gains and milk volumes during the first two weeks of lactation than are seen when suckling is less frequent.[12] When breast-fed infants are fed on demand, the mean frequency of feeding is approximately 10 times per day for the first 2 weeks. This results in considerably more feedings than allowed by a four-hour schedule. Infant-initiated feeding has been associated with greater weight gains than scheduled feedings when feeding frequencies were comparable in at least one study.[11] When a demand-feeding regimen is selected, the mother should be aware that at times she may have to encourage her infant to

nurse. In the early weeks of lactation, if the infant wakes for feedings less frequently than every 2 to 3 hours, the mother should initiate nursings.

Nursing frequency is inversely related to infant serum bilirubin concentrations three days postpartum: 6–8 nursings per 24 hours are associated with higher bilirubin levels than are 10–12 nursings per 24 hours.[18] If the mother and infant are separated in hospital, it may be difficult to implement high frequency, demand feedings.

Duration of Initial Nursing Episodes

Initial nursing episodes need not be timed.[14,19] The duration of initial nursings has often been limited in the past because of concern that extended nursings will result in sore or cracked nipples. Sore nipples occur with equal frequency and severity whether nursing episodes are limited or unrestricted. The onset of sore nipples is earlier, however, when nursings are unrestricted.

EXCLUSIVE BREASTFEEDING IS ESTABLISHED

Supplementary Feedings

Routine formula and water supplements are unnecessary for healthy term infants. Supplementary formula feedings in the immediate puerperium are associated with an increased incidence of feeding difficulties and/or lactation failure.[20-23] Whether such feedings cause difficulties or result from underlying feeding problems is unclear. The psychological effect of the hospital staff's implicit approval of supplementary feedings has been cited as a contributory factor in the premature cessation of breastfeeding.[24] Regardless of the rationale for the uncritical use of supplementary feedings, the extent to which they are required in hospital is an indication of existing or potential breastfeeding problems. Infants who require supplementary feedings warrant careful monitoring until exclusive breastfeeding is well established.

There are two potential physiological effects of supplementary bottle feedings that may cause problems: (1) decrease in milk supply and (2) confusion of bottle- and breast-nursing techniques (nipple confusion). Reduced milk supplies will result from decreased suckling stimulation to the breast when infant hunger is satisfied through supplementary formula feedings. **This reduction can be avoided by emptying the breasts thoroughly at least every 3 hours.** Milk may be expressed between and/or after nursings as necessary to assure thorough emptying 8 to 12 times per 24 hours.

Nipple Confusion

Anecdotal reports of nipple confusion abound as do hypothetical explanations of the phenomenon.[5,7,25] Although little scientific scrutiny has been applied to these observations, the widespread nature of these reports and the observation that even slight variations in nipple size and compressibility are known to affect the characteristics of neonatal suckling[26,27] suggest that **caution is necessary in switching between breast- and bottle-feeding.**

The same oral musculature is used to nurse from either a breast or a bottle. However, the spatial arrangement of the tongue and nipple differs between the two feeding modes. Skills required for nursing from a breast are not interchangeable with those required for bottle-feeding. When a newborn infant nurses from an artificial nipple, the first and second steps of the four-step sequence previously outlined for breastfeeding are accomplished by a caretaker. The infant does not have to open his mouth widely to grasp the artificial nipple effectively. Suction is applied and milk flows rapidly from the artificial nipple.

An infant who attempts to use bottle-feeding skills to nurse from his mother's breast may drain the lactiferous sinuses inadequately and consequently will be unlikely to empty the breast effectively.[27] The magnitude of resulting difficulties depends on several factors, e.g., maternal breastfeeding skills and the precise location of the mother's ampullae. When milk is not removed effectively, the result is milk stasis, decreased milk production, and poor infant weight gain. If the infant's tongue and dental ridges push against the mother's nipple rather than the areola, sore or fissured nipples may result.

Bottle-feeding may be introduced after lactation has been established (two weeks postpartum is a reasonable estimate). If the infant has difficulty nursing the breast after receiving a bottle, the mother should insure that the infant has his mouth positioned well over the lactiferous sinuses and his lower lip turned outward.[27]

Nipple confusion may also operate in reverse. Older infants who have never received bottle-feedings often refuse to nurse from a bottle. Women who anticipate the occasional need to bottle-feed their infants should be advised to initiate feeding from a bottle approximately within the first month and to maintain such feedings on a relatively frequent basis. Approximately once per week is usually enough.

Stool Characteristics

The characteristics of the stools of breastfed infants often alarm mothers. The normal breastfed infant often will have an evacuation at each nursing. Therefore, **10 or more stools per day are common in this population.** The frequency of evacuations may decrease suddenly to one stool per week or even fewer in later lactation. **A low stool frequency in early lactation, however, suggests an inadequate intake of milk.** Stools of breastfed infants are most often unformed, may be yellow, brown, or green, are seedy in appearance, and do not have an offensive smell until after the introduction of supplementary foods.

Jaundice

Elevated concentrations of serum bilirubin in the newborn period occur more often in breast- than in formula-fed infants. **Feeding frequency during the first three days of life of breastfed infants is related inversely to the serum concentration of bilirubin at hospital discharge.**[18] Although cause and effect have not been established, frequent feedings are a reasonable and prudent precaution for reducing the incidence of neonatal jaundice. In contrast, the routine use of water supplements in breastfed infants has no impact on serum bilirubin concentrations.[28]

If the concentration of serum bilirubin rises sufficiently to be of clinical concern, formula supplements may be used and will serve several purposes. Supplementing the infant's diet with formula prevents increments in bilirubin levels associated with hypocaloric intake and reduces the enterohepatic circulation of bilirubin.[29,30]

Discontinuation of breastfeeding for 24-72 hours also is of diagnostic value in differentiating breast-milk jaundice from other causes of elevated serum bilirubin concentrations. A rapid drop of serum bilirubin levels following the transient discontinuation of breastfeeding is pathognomonic of this condition. It is not clear if the discontinuation of breast milk has a direct effect on the liver or if the substitution of formula increases bilirubin excretion. Formula-feeding appears to increase stool volume and net bilirubin elimination. Slight elevations in serum bilirubin are observed commonly when breastfeeding is resumed, and jaundice may persist for several weeks. **No detrimental effects of breast-milk jaundice have been reported.** Discontinuation of breastfeeding is of no known therapeutic value during this condition.

If formula-feeding is introduced to supplement or replace breastfeeding, the mother's milk production can be maintained by frequent milk expression. Both breasts should be emptied approximately 8 times per 24 hours.

Maternal Anxiety

Increased activity of the sympathetic nervous system appears to reduce the pituitary release of prolactin and oxytocin and the effects of these hormones on the mammary gland. Laboratory experiments have used pain and cold to demonstrate the negative effects of physical stress on lactation. In one study, the influence of the hospital setting alone was sufficiently stressful to reduce milk output.[31] Both physical and psychological stress can influence lactation. Positive reinforcement of breastfeeding by hospital personnel may assist the mother in coping with stress, and brief relaxation routines before nursing or milk expression may be helpful. Support personnel can instill confidence by making positive observations about the patient's mothering skills, the infant's responsiveness to the mother, or the value of breast milk. A particular challenge arises when the temporary termination of breastfeeding is suggested as a diagnostic tool to evaluate jaundice in the newborn period.

Breastfeeding Consultation Services

The health professional is in a unique position to provide the information and teach the skills needed for successful lactation. This support is particularly important in the first few days postpartum. Both the incidence and the long-term success of breastfeeding are increased when breastfeeding consultation services are available during hospitalization and after discharge.[3,32-34]

Discharge Planning

If the mother is aware of the nursing problems that usually arise shortly after release from the hospital and is prepared to manage them, many cases of lactation failure may be averted. The decision to terminate breastfeeding early, or to introduce formula prematurely, frequently is made within the first two weeks postpartum.[15] Among the factors that precipitate these decisions are **two predictable events: (1) the onset of breast engorgement on approximately the third day postpartum and (2) the infant's first "appetite spurt" on the 8th to 10th day of postnatal life.** The inappropriate use of formula in the management of these problems significantly lessens the probability of long-term breastfeeding.[20] Women who receive free formula at discharge are more likely to introduce supplementary feedings prematurely when nursing difficulties are encountered.[15,20]

Breast Engorgement

The primiparous woman generally experiences breast engorgement on day 3 postpartum, although engorgement may not occur for several days after delivery. The breasts become hard and often are painful, the areola is nonprotractile, and the mother's temperature may increase slightly. The traditional symptomatic treatments for breast engorgement include breast binding or the application of ice or heat packs. Either ice or heat reduces local discomfort, but **the best management is to enhance milk flow during suckling.** Swelling and discomfort can be reduced but not eliminated during initial engorgement, since they result from increased blood flow and lymphatic congestion, as well as increased milk production.

If severe engorgement occurs, the mother should not rely solely on the infant to empty engorged breasts because areolar rigidity often prevents the infant from drawing the nipple and areola into the proper position. As a consequence, the child receives little milk and the mother experiences inadequate symptomatic relief. **The application of moist heat packs and the expression of milk before nursing decreases intralobular pressure, increases the areolar pliability, and facilitates appropriate "latch-on" and milk flow.** When the infant nurses, special attention to proper "latch-on" and hand massage of the breast are necessary adjuncts to assist complete drainage and to minimize nipple trauma, which may result in cracked or bleeding nipples.

Appetite Spurts

So-called "spurts" in the infant's appetite are reported at various ages. The first is usually noted at 8 to 10 days of life. Mothers report an increase in the frequency with which the infant demands to be fed.[7] Studies of infants fed on demand from birth, however, do not indicate an increase in nursing frequency at this time. In the authors' clinical experience, the behavior is reported frequently and constitutes one of the more common complaints during that stage of lactation. Adherence to a demand-feeding routine is appropriate management during an appetite spurt. Although the impact of increasing nursing frequencies above a baseline of 8–12 times per 24 hours has not been clinically assessed, increases in milk expression frequencies above baselines of 3–5 pumpings per day

result in augmented milk volumes over a few days.[35,36] The appetite spurt may serve a similar function. Such episodes are characteristically brief; if a demand for increased nursing frequency persists for more than a few days, and this behavior is accompanied by inadequate weight gain, other measures to increase the milk production should be considered. **Importantly, infants with faltering growth should receive supplemental feedings while milk production is augmented.** Nursing devices are available to provide both supplemental milk for the infant and simultaneous stimulation to the mother's breasts.[5,9] One simple guideline for assessing the adequacy of an infant's intake is to evaluate his or her hydration status.

A well-hydrated infant voids at least 6–8 times per day. Each voiding should be sufficient to soak, not merely moisten, a diaper. Mothers should be advised to contact the infant's pediatrician if the infant voids a dark yellow urine less than 6 times per day. The advisability of using formula supplements should be discussed if this occurs. Preparing the mother for the infant's first appetite spurt reduces maternal anxiety, provides skills for managing the problem, and prevents the unnecessary additon of supplements.

Transition to Office-Based Pediatric Care

After discharge from the hospital, mothers tend to become more dependent on the pediatrician, obstetrician, their respective office staffs, and others for help with lactation management. Timely interventions can establish excellent rapport between physician and the family, and enhance a mother's confidence in the health care persons with whom she has contact. Telephone follow-up during the two-week interim between discharge and the first pediatric visit to monitor the progress of lactation is helpful and often productive.[7,9] **For example, a call on the third day postpartum to help in the management of breast engorgement is appropriate.** If problems cannot be managed by telephone, a home visit by a lactation consultant may be arranged. A second call at approximately 8 or 10 days postpartum will detect problems associated with the infant's first "appetite spurt."

For the breastfed infant, it is recommended that the first pediatric visit occur at two weeks of age to allow the physician to evaluate the mother's lactation status and to implement appropriate interventions when necessary. Although initial weight loss in the neonatal period is greater in the breastfed than in the bottle-fed infant, birthweight generally is regained by approximately two weeks of age with good lactation management.

Nursing Frequency and Infant Sleep Patterns

The mean nursing frequency of exclusively breastfed infants is approximately 8–12 times per day during the first two weeks postpartum and 8–9 times per day at 4 weeks postpartum.[37,38] Feeding frequencies may decline with age to approximately 6–7 times per day by 4 months. Frequencies, however, of over 10 nursings per day are reported in nursing infants 12 months or over.[39] **Mothers should be cautioned not to reduce feeding frequency to 6 nursings per day or less during the first 3 months.** Basal serum prolactin concentrations fall and the duration of breastfeeding appears shortened when this low frequency is adopted early in lactation.[40]

At 4 weeks, nursings usually are distributed evenly through a 24-hour period; the mean inter-nursing interval is approximately 3 hours.[38] Night feedings are less common after 3 months of age; however, many breastfed infants do not "sleep through the night" until they are weaned. For the older breastfed infant, the usual period of continuous sleep each night is approximately 6–7 hours. When breastfeeding is discontinued, the sleep period increases to approximately 8 hours.[40]

Normal Nursing Durations

The usual duration of nursing is 4 to 20 minutes per breast. Nursings of 25–30 minutes or more per breast may be an adaptation to inadequate milk production or ineffective "latch-on." Eighty percent of milk usually is consumed in approximately the first 4 minutes of nursing at each breast.[41] However, because the caloric density of milk increases nonlinearly throughout a feeding, **the infant consumes disproportionately fewer calories in the early phases of each nursing.** Therefore, if a nursing is terminated before the breast is emptied, the infant has received a disproportionately decreased amount of energy. If the infant's weight gain is inadequate or the mother objects to prolonged nursings, the mother may be referred to a trained lactation counselor.

Milk Volume

Milk volume increases rapidly during the first two weeks after parturition. The physiological factors that regulate milk production have been reviewed in Chapter 2. Mean milk production in exclusively breastfeeding women is approximately 750 ± 130 ml/day. This level of production is maintained during exclusive breastfeeding through 4 6 months.[37,38] Milk volume usually declines after solid foods have been added to the infant's diet, even when the frequency of nursing remains unchanged.[42] Although the published nutritional requirements of infants are higher than the amounts provided by the volumes of milk consumed normally by breast-fed infants, growth remains within normal limits.

Maternal and infant behaviors are strong determinants of milk volume. Specific determinants likely operate through their effects on maternal prolactin and oxytocin release and intramammary milk pressure. Tactile stimulation of the nipple and areola and maternal sleep and exercise appear to stimulate prolactin release. Although tactile stimulation to the nipple and areola and maternal sleep patterns are mentioned frequently as adjuncts to increasing milk volume, the effect of maternal exercise has received little attention. Tactile stimulation of the nipple and areola, maternal grooming or stroking the infant prior to suckling, or any behavior associated with nursing may elicit the release of oxytocin. **The effect of conditioning is so powerful that in early lactation infant cries are sufficient to initiate milk ejection in many women.**

Increased intramammary gland pressure is associated with glandular involution and subsequently decreased milk volumes.[43] The frequency of nursing, milk expression, and binding of the breasts all influence this variable. Effective emptying of the breast reduces intramammary pressure. Breast emptying is enhanced by raising the temperature of the breast or by breast massage. The former may dilate blood vessels and mammary ducts; breast massage may aid in propelling milk toward the lactiferous sinuses and may initiate the contraction of myoepithelial cells surrounding the acini of the mammary gland. Frequent and complete emptying of the breast is associated with increased milk production.

Various drugs also may influence milk volume.[44-47] Bromocriptine will prevent milk production because of its inhibitory effects on prolactin; metoclopramide and chlorpromazine will stimulate prolactin release; oxytocin delivered as a nasal spray promotes breast emptying; decongestants and antihistamines may reduce milk production through mechanisms understood incompletely; and progesterone and estrogen have varying effects on milk production, depending on their dose and the time of administration.

SUPPLEMENTARY FOODS ARE INTRODUCED

The introduction of supplementary feedings from a bottle of expressed breast milk after the second week postpartum and at weekly intervals thereafter aids the infant in retaining the skill and disposition to nurse from a bottle. Mothers may minimize the possibility of "nipple confusion" by monitoring carefully nursings that follow a supplementary feeding (see section on nipple confusion). If the infant is under 4 months of age when supplementary feedings are introduced on a regular basis, infant formula should be given. Breast- and bottle-feeding can be integrated successfully if milk volumes are maintained. Periodic increases in nursing frequency (e.g., on weekends, particularly for the woman working outside the home) may be sufficient to maintain milk volume. The range of nursing frequencies when both modes of feeding are integrated is broad; some women maintain desired milk volumes with only a few nursings per day.

If the infant is over 4 months of age, solid foods may be added to the diet. From present data it appears that **the limiting nutrients in the diet of the exclusively breastfed infant 4 to 6 months of age are likely to be energy, protein, iron, and zinc.** Meats may be the most appropriate food to add first to the diet of exclusively breastfed infants; meats could be followed by cereals and vegetables or fruits. The introduction of supplementary foods does not appear to increase the infant's caloric intake per kg body weight for at least 3 months after their addition to the diet.[42] Human milk intake declines after solid foods have been added, regardless of the feeding pattern the mother adopts; she may elect to nurse first and offer other foods only after nursing, or offer solid foods and breast milk at alternate meals. Single ingredient foods should be introduced initially (to identify adverse reactions to specific foods). Each new food should be fed for 2 or 3 days before the next new food is added, thus permitting the identification of foods that may not be tolerated by the infant.

WEANING IS BEGUN

Weaning may be initiated either by the infant or the mother. The process should be gradual to minimize the occurrence of breast engorgement or mastitis. Several days should be allowed to lapse before successively decreasing the frequency of nursing. If abrupt weaning is not avoidable, milk may be expressed to reduce discomfort and the possibility of mastitis. The introduction of supplementary foods ideally should precede weaning by several months. The American Academy of Pediatrics recommends **breastfeeding for 12 months with the introduction of supplementary foods at 4 to 6 months.** With this schedule, the infant is allowed ample time to develop necessary feeding skills.

SELECTED TOPICS RELEVANT TO LACTATION MANAGEMENT

BREAST PUMPS AND SAFETY PRECAUTIONS FOR MILK COLLECTION, STORAGE AND TRANSPORT

A variety of breast pumps are available. They range in complexity from inexpensive hand pumps to electric pumps that provide oscillating positive and negative pressure.[48] Bulb-type pumps are the least expensive. However, cleaning them is a problem and significant contamination of milk may result.[48,49] Whether the mother uses a breast pump or chooses to express her milk manually, contamination of expressed milk can be reduced by:

(1) scrubbing hands and fingernails before collection,[43]

(2) using sterile equipment,

(3) discarding the first 10 ml of milk from each breast,[50,51] and

(4) storing milk in a refrigerator's or freezer's far end to minimize temperature fluctuations.

Milk may be refrigerated for 24 hours before use or frozen immediately after collection and stored for approximately 3 months. All milk, whether fresh or frozen, should be transported on ice. Milk may be thawed or warmed by gentle shaking under warm running water immediately before feeding. Thawing in this manner reduces the probability that milk will be left at inappropriate temperatures for extended periods during preparation for feeding. **Heating milk in a microwave oven is inadvisable because such heating produces uneven temperatures that can cause severe burns.**[52] Temperature differentials of up to 30°C have been reported within 4-ounce bottles of milk heated in a microwave oven.[53] Human milk is damaged easily by excessive heating. The secretory IgA of human milk, for example, is rapidly destroyed by incubating milk for 15 minutes at temperatures above 60°C.[54]

PREMATURE DELIVERY

Maintenance of Milk Production Following Premature Delivery

Premature delivery presents special problems to the breastfeeding woman. In the interim preceding the infant's suckling, lactation must be initiated and adequate volumes of milk maintained. Prolonged delays in the initiation of milk expression (> 4 days) result in temporary reductions in milk production or possibly involution of the mammary gland. It is not necessary to initiate milk expression during the first 24 hours after delivery. The Lactation Support Program at Texas Children's Hospital in Houston, Texas uses the following protocol with considerable success:

(1) Begin milk expression within 2 or 3 days after delivery.
(2) Express milk 6 or more times per day, approximately every 3 hours.
(3) Empty both breasts thoroughly at each expression (10–15 minutes per side).
(4) Skip one pumping at night to allow a 6-hour interval for sleep.

If milk volumes are low or begin to decline, mothers are advised to increase their expression frequencies to 8 times per 24 hours. Metoclopramide has been used with some success to increase milk production in mothers of premature infants.[55]

Initiation of Suckling Following Premature Delivery

Although premature infants have been reported to suckle successfully at body weights as low as 1300 gm,[56,57] most are unable to coordinate suckling and swallowing until they are at least 1500–1800 gm. The capacity to nurse adequately is dependent on a variety of factors: coordination by the infant of the suck/swallow reflex, no ventilatory support requirements, strength, wakefulness of the infant, maternal milk volumes and nipple anatomy, and the mother's nursing skills. The decision to initiate suckling should be made after careful evaluation of both infant and maternal readiness.[58-60] (See Chapter 19).

Discharge Planning for the Nursing Preterm Infant

If the mother is either not producing sufficient milk or expresses significant doubt that the infant is receiving enough milk, a supplemental nursing device presents a viable alternative to supplemental bottle-feeding. Such a device delivers milk through a small tube leading from a milk reservoir to the side of the mother's nipple as the infant nurses. It provides a mechanism for the infant to stimulate increased milk production through suckling, while receiving supplementary feeds at the breast. Moreover, the visual confirmation of milk intake reduces maternal anxiety. Supplementary feedings, whether fed via bottles or nursing devices, may be discontinued gradually as the mother's milk supply and the infant's nursing skills improve.

Elements of Lactation Support for Mothers of Preterm Infants

Practical support for the lactating mother of a preterm infant includes clear instructions for collecting, labeling, storing, transporting, and delivering expressed milk and the provision of (or identification of sources for) breast pumps and collection and storage containers. It also includes dedicated space for use by mothers to express milk during hospital visits. **Appropriate use and cleaning of milk collection equipment are best reviewed with each mother,** since equipment rental agencies frequently provide little or inadequate information in these important areas. Finally, records of milk delivered by mothers for their infants should be maintained by the support service helping the mother initiate and maintain lactation.

Psychological support for the preterm mother is more difficult to define. Certainly the provision of a logistical framework for milk expression as described above will afford both validation and encouragement of the mother's efforts. Lactation consultants at Texas Children's Hospital additonally assist the mother at the initiation of suckling. Prior to breastfeeding, the infant is allowed non-nutritive suckling at the mother's breast. During this time, a consultant helps the mother to distinguish an appropriate from an inappropriate "latch-on" and to identify infant behaviors that indicate the need to interrupt suckling to eructate or pass gas. Later, the consultant helps the mother to recognize infant hunger and to distinguish nutritive from non-nutritive suckling. Specific feedings are frequently reserved by nursery personnel for the mother to nurse her infant as soon as the child's maturity and clinical condition permit. Finally, the mother of the preterm infant is allowed to test her perceptual skills and care for her infant in the hospital for one or two days prior to discharge. These practices are intended to enhance mothering skills and to reinforce the mother's sense of competence. In addition, the period of rooming-in before discharge allows the physician to evaluate the need for supplementary feedings post discharge and home visits by the lactation support staff.

MANAGEMENT OF OTHER COMMON PROBLEMS

The problems most commonly encountered by breastfeeding women are sore nipples, localized milk stasis, mastitis, other illnesses in the mother or infant, maternal medications, and the coordination of maternal employment outside the home with breastfeeding. Sound patient education can either prevent problems of this type or provide the skills for their successful resolution.

Sore Nipples

Sore nipples occur frequently during the first two weeks postpartum. The prenatal preparation of the breast reduces neither the incidence nor severity of this problem.[6] Appropriate "latch-on" and positioning of the infant help to prevent sore nipples and are essential in its treatment.[20] **Successful management of sore, fissured, or bleeding nipples includes:**

(1) repositioning the infant at the breast,
(2) frequent short nursings,
(3) rinsing nipples after nursing with water only,
(4) air-drying the nipples after each nursing, and
(5) daily exposure of nipples to direct sunlight.

The use of plastic-lined brassiere pads or heavy ointments can maintain an inappropriately moist environment that promotes bacterial growth between nursings. If a fissured nipple becomes infected it may form a superficial ulcer; topical antibiotics are valuable in treating persistently inflamed, fissured nipples. Cracked nipples can bleed sufficiently to cause the infant to pass a dark stool; infants also may regurgitate blood when nipples bleed significantly. In severe cases, it may be advisable to interrupt nursings from a few hours to a few days to allow healing of damaged tissues. If this is necessary, regular milk expression should continue to maintain the mother's milk supply and prevent mastitis. During this interim, steps should be taken to minimize and/or correct the occurrence of nipple confusion.

Nipple soreness may not respond to usual treatments if the etiologic agent is *Candida albicans*. In these cases, nipples may appear unremarkable on visual inspection, but cultures of the nipples' surfaces will be positive for *C. albicans.*[7] **Women often describe shooting pains at the end of a nursing when C. albicans is the etiologic agent.** Onset of nipple soreness late in lactation, maternal history of monilial vulvovaginitis, recent antibiotic therapy, or signs of thrush in the infant are associated with *C. albicans* infection of the nipple. Treatment includes topical antifungal agents. Both the infant and other sites of maternal infection should be treated when appropriate.

Milk Stasis and Localized Tenderness

In most women initial breast engorgement, typically observed on the third or fourth day postpartum, is followed by the cyclic filling and emptying of the breast with no discomfort. In a few women, however, milk production is sufficiently rapid that uncomfortably full breasts are reported soon after each nursing for longer periods. Tight-fitting brassieres are often successful in modulating milk production and analgesics may provide pain relief. If milk expression is necessary to relieve discomfort, frequency of breast stimulation can be minimized by expressing just before or just after nursing. Breast engorgement also may be associated with prolonged interfeeding intervals and blocked mammary ducts. Localized distention of the breast may result from external localized pressure, trauma, or incomplete or uneven drainage of the breast. Tenderness and inflammation are common sequelae when drainage is uneven or incomplete. If the conditon remains untreated, mastitis may follow. Symptoms of mastitis include fever, chills, and generalized aching.

Distention may be relieved by applying hot, moist compresses to the breast, massaging the painful breast, and expressing milk effectively by either positioning the infant appropriately or by using a breast pump. When pain is localized, nursing with the infant's chin next to the painful area facilitates drainage of that part of the breast by focusing the pressure exerted by the tongue on the ampullae contiguous with the blocked duct. Nursing or pumping should be frequent and the mother should maintain a schedule of adequate rest. Her temperature and general condition should be monitored for a few days to identify any early signs of mastitis.

Mastitis

If mastitis develops, subjective reports by the mother focus on fever and generalized aching. Mammary symptoms are often not the basis of her primary complaint. **Whenever a lactating woman reports flu-like symptoms, mastitis should be considered a possible cause.** Treatment of mastitis includes frequent and complete emptying of the breast. Breastfeeding should not be stopped. Effective emptying of the breast is the primary objective in the management of this condition and is best accomplished by increased nursings. Nursing from a mastitic breast has no adverse effects on the healthy infant,[61] although at times the infant may refuse to take milk from a mastitic breast.

Appropriate antibiotic therapy is indicated. Less virulent strains of *Staphylococcus aureus* are the predominant etiologic agents in spontaneous mastitis. In the rare event of epidemic puerperal mastitis, a highly virulent *Staphylococcus aureus* strain or other pathogen may be involved. Either dicloxacillin or one of the cephalosporins is effective in most cases.[7] Women should be cautioned to complete the course of antibiotics even though symptoms may disappear within a few days of initiating treatment. Recurrent mastitis is more common when treatment is incomplete.

Abscess

Untreated mastitis may progress to a breast abscess. If an abscess is diagnosed, breastfeeding should be discontinued from the affected breast until the condition is treated successfully. Milk expression from the affected breast should continue, but expressed milk should be discarded. Bacterial proliferation and potential accumulation of toxins in the milk may present significant risks to the infant.

Maternal or Infant Illness

As a general rule, nursing should be continued throughout most illnesses. The "homing" of immunologic cells from gut- and bronchially-associated lymphatic tissue to the breast provides specific protection in milk against offending pathogens. Nonspecific protective components in the milk also are available. The dynamics of maternal protective responses are understood incompletely; clinical signs of illness in either the mother or infant are preceded by mutual exposure to the offending pathogen. Maternal AIDS (acquired immune deficiency syndrome); active untreated tuberculosis; herpes lesions on the nipple, areola, or other regions of the breast; and primary disseminated herpes are exceptions to the general rule that nursing should be continued through illness. While it has been suggested that nursing should also be discontinued for maternal hepatitis, from a practical standpoint, infant exposure preceding clinical illness in the mother is very likely. When maternal tuberculosis is diagnosed, breastfeeding may be reinstated following the initiation of treatment.

Drugs

This topic is too broad to be reviewed adequately within the constraints of this discussion. The reader is referred to review articles on this topic.[45,46] These or other pertinent references should be consulted if there is any question regarding safety to the infant. Special concern is appropriate when the recipient infant was born prematurely. Preterm infants may be particularly sensitive to a number of drugs because of a reduced ability to clear durgs systemically or convert them to inactive metabolites. The possibility of drug interactions in the preterm infant also should be considered carefully if the infant is undergoing any medical therapy.[7]

The mother should be advised against the use of unprescribed drugs including alcohol, nicotine, caffeine, marijuana or other "street drugs." Although alcohol commonly has been promoted to enhance the "let down" reflex, it has been shown to inhibit oxytocin release.[62] Its positive effects are probably limited to its enhancement of relaxation. Alternative, non-drug-dependent approaches for stress reduction may be utilized more effectively. Cigarette smoking appears to inhibit milk production in mothers[63] and to alter suckling patterns of neonates.[64]

WORKING MOTHERS

Breastfeeding and work outside the home are not mutually exclusive. Most working women in the United States are required to return to work within 4 to 8 weeks after delivery. If a mother plans to breastfeed after she returns to work and does not intent to introduce other foods to the infant diet, she can begin to express and store milk approximately 2 weeks before her return to the workplace.

Initiating milk collection at the early morning nursing usually is best. Mothers may begin by nursing the infant on one breast and pumping the other breast either simultaneously or as soon as possible after the infant has finished nursing. The infant's stimulation of the milk-ejection reflex increases the effectiveness of milk expression and assists in conditioning the reflex to pump use. **After expressing milk, the infant should be allowed to nurse at the breast from which milk has been expressed to stimulate additonal production.** Expressed milk should be frozen and the date of collection recorded on the container.

Meanwhile the mother can identify when and where she will express milk at work. The return to work may be followed by mastitis when milk expression routines differ markedly from previous nursing patterns. Intervals between milk expressions should be short (3 to 5 hours) and regular, especially in the first few days. The mother may nurse her baby before she leaves home or at the child care facility. She may then (ideally) express milk two or three times during the day and nurse as soon after work as possible. Nursing at lunch or during a break will assist in maintaining the breast-feeding relationship.

CASE REPORTS

A term female infant was born January 5, 1986 after an uncomplicated pregnancy to a 29-year-old gravida 2, para 1 mother. Apgar scores were 8 and 9 at 1 and 5 minutes, respectively. The birthweight was 3180 gm. The infant was put to breast immediately after delivery but did not suckle. The first successful nursing occurred 38 hours after delivery. The infant was discharged 79 hours after birth. Discharge weight was 2930 gm. Formula supplements were offered in hospital after unsuccessful breastfeeding attempts, and water supplements were given between feedings. The infant was a slow feeder consuming an average of 45 cc over 35 minutes when formula was offered. In the final 24 hours, the infant nursed six times, had six stools, eight wet diapers, and three supplemental water bottles. The mother was experiencing the onset of breast engorgement at discharge.

The parents discontinued supplements after discharge with the onset of milk production. Increased irritability was noted by the parents on the seventh postpartum day. They called the pediatrician's office on the ninth day and reported that the infant was nursing about every 3 hours. The decision was made to bring the baby to the office for an examination on the 14th day postpartum, as scheduled, and to give water supplements between feedings if the child was fussy. Examination on the 14th postpartum day showed a well-hydrated infant weighing 2790 gm. The parents' 24-hour-recall of feeding times indicated an actual feeding frequency of 5 times per 24 hours. The last feeding occurred 3 hours before the examination. Feeding durations were 50 to 75 minutes per feed. Stool frequency was 3 per 24 hours. The mother's nipples were sore with a slight fissure on the tip of the left nipple. A nursing was observed. The infant took the nipple and base of the areola into the mouth. Suckling was sporadic. The mother reported nipple pain throughout the 20 minutes of nursing on the right breast. The infant consumed 15 cc of milk in that period. Before nursing the infant on the left breast, correct latch-on was demonstrated. The mother was instructed to use hand massage on the breast during nursing to maintain milk flow. The infant consumed 30 cc of milk in 15 minutes. Nipple pain decreased within 1 minute of latch-on, and the mother reported greater comfort during the remainder of the nursing. Following nursing, an additional 35 cc of milk was expressed from the right breast and 10 cc from the left breast using an electric pump. The mother reported that the infant's suck was slightly weaker than the suction exerted by the pump. Expressed milk was fed to the infant using a supplemental nursing device.

The mother was advised to nurse 10 to 12 times per day using good latch-on and hand massage throughout. She was further advised to give 3 or more ounces of formula at each of two p.m. nursings using a supplemental nursing device. Supplementation was continued for two weeks, and the infant was weighed at four-day intervals (see accompanying chart). The infant's growth rate decreased inappropriately following the elimination of supplements. Subsequently, the mother was advised to express residual milk following each nursing and to feed collected milk to the infant with formula ad libitum. The use of a supplemental nursing device was continued. The volume of residual milk increased over the following week, and supplemental formula was discontinued. Pumping was discontinued at 2 months postpartum. Subsequent weight gain was rapid, and the infant's growth and development were normal at one year of age.

Comment. The parent's perception underestimated the infant's feeding frequency by approximately 40%. The low feeding frequency may have inhibited milk production in early lactation. Corrected latch-on and use of hand massage reduced maternal discomfort and improved breast emptying. The infant's feeding difficulties persisted beyond the hospital confinement and may have been responsible for the low breast milk intake. The additional stimulation and/or the effective reduction of intramammary pressure afforded by the pump apparently helped to increase the mother's milk production to levels adequate for infant growth and development. Subsequent to these interventions the child was able to suckle effectively, and milk production was maintained with no added stimulus.

DATE	WEIGHT	DATE	WEIGHT
1/5	3180 (birth)	2/7	3690 (discontinue formula)
1/9	2930	2/10	3660
1/20	2790 (supplement)	2/14	3700 (pump & formula)
1/24	2990	2/17	3790
1/27	3170	2/22	3980 (discontinue formula)
1/31	3330	3/1	4160
2/3	3510	3/12	4560 (discontinue pump)

REFERENCES

1. Martinez GA, Krieger FW. 1984 milk-feeding patterns in the United States. Pediatrics 1985; 76:1004–1008.
2. Hendershot GE. Trends in breastfeeding. Pediatrics 1984; 74(Suppl):591–602.
3. Simopoulos AP, Grave GD. Factors associated with the choice and duration of infant-feeding practice. Pediatrics 1984; 74(Suppl):603–614.
4. Martin J. Infant Feeding 1975: Attitudes and Practice in England and Wales. London, Office of Population Censuses and Surveys, Social Survey Division, Her Majesty's Stationery Office, 1978.
5. Newman J. Breast-feeding: The problem of "not enough milk." Can Fam Phys 1986; 32:571–574.
6. Brown MS, Hurlock JT. Preparation of the breast for breast-feeding. Nurs Res 1975; 24:448–451.
7. Neville NC, Neifert MR, (ed). Lactation: Physiology, Nutrition and Breastfeeding. New York, Plenum Press, 1983.
8. Neifert MR, Seacat JM, Jobe WE. Lactation failure due to insufficient glandular developement of the breast. Pediatrics 1985; 76:823–301.
9. Neifert MR, Seacat JM. A guide to successful breastfeeding. Contemp Pediatr 1986; 3:26–45.
10. Verronen P, Visakorpi JK, Lammi A, et al. Promotion of breast feeding: effects of a campaign.In Freier S, Eidleman AI (eds): Human Milk; Its Biological and Social Value. International Symposium on Breast Feeding. Amsterdam, Excerpta Medica, 1980; 305–308.
11. Illingsworth RS, Stone DG. Demand feeding in a maternity unit. Lancet 1952; 1:683–687.
12. De Carvalho M, Robertson S, Friedman A, Klaus M. Effect of frequent breast-feeding on early milk production and infant weight gain. Pediatrics 1983; 72:307–311.
13. Salariya EM, Easton PM, Cater JI. Duration of breast-feeding after early initiation and frequent feeding. Lancet 1978; 2(8100):1141–1143.
14. Slaven S, Harvey D. Unlimited suckling time improves breast feeding. Lancet 1981; 1(8216):392–393.
15. Samuels SE, Margen S, Schoen EJ. Incidence and duration of breast-feeding in a health maintenance organization population. Am J Clin Nutr 1985; 42:504–510.
16. Dubignon J, Campbell D, Curtis M, Partington MW. The relation between laboratory measures of sucking, food intake, and perinatal factors during the newborn period. Child Dev 1969; 40:1107–1120.
17. Taylor PM, Maloni JA, Brown DR. Early suckling and prolonged breast-feeding. Am J Dis Child 1986; 140:151–154.
18. De Carvalho M, Klaus MH, Merkatz RB. Frequency of breast-feeding and serum bilirubin concentration. Am J Dis Child 1982; 136:737–738.
19. De Carvalho M, Robertson S, Klaus MH. Does the duration and frequency of early breastfeeding affect pain? Birth 1984; 11:82–84.
20. Bergevin Y, Dougherty C, Kramer MS. Do infant formula samples shorten the duration of breast-feeding? Lancet 1983; 2(8334):1148–1151.
21. Feinstein JM, Berkehamer JE, Gruszka ME, et al. Factors related to early termination of breast-feeding in an urban population. Pediatrics 1986; 78:210–2151.
22. Loughlin HH, Clapp-Channing NE, Gehlback SH, et al. Early termination of breast-feeding: identifying those at risk. Pediatrics 1985; 75:508–513.
23. Gray-Donald K, Kramer MS, Munday S, Leduc DG. Effect of formula supplementation in the hospital on the duration of breast-feeding: a controlled clinical trial. Pediatrics 1985; 75:514–518.
24. Reiff MI, Essock-Vitale SM. Hospital influences on early infant-feeding practices. Pediatrics 1985; 76:872–879.
25. Frantz KB. An easy solution to an early problem. In Freier S, Eidelman AI (eds): Human Milk, Its Biological and Social Value. Amsterdam, Excerpta Medica, 1980.
26. Christensen S, Dubignon J, Campbell D. Variations in intra-oral stimulation and nutritive sucking. Child Dev 1976; 47:539–542.
27. Dubignon J, Campbell D. Intraoral stimulation and sucking in the new born. J Exp Child Psychol 1968; 6:154–166.
28. De Carvalho M, Hall M, Harvey D. Effects of water supplementation on physiological jaundice in breast-fed babies. Arch Dis Child 1981; 56:568–569.
29. Gartner LM, Lee K, Moscioni AD. Effect of milk feeding on intestinal bilirubin absorption in the rat. J Pediatr 1983; 103:464–471.
30. Lascari AD. "Early" breast-feeding jaundice: clinical significance. J Pediatr 1986; 108:156–158.
31. Lindblad BS, Ljungquist A, Gebre-Medhin M, Rahimtoola RJ. The composition and yield of human milk in developing countries In Hambraeus L, Hanson LA, McFarlane H (eds): Food and Immunology: Symposium of the Swedish Nutrition Foundation XIII. Uppsala, Sweden, Almquist & Wiksell, 1977;125.
32. Jones DA, West RR. Lactation nurse increases duration of breast feeding. Arch Dis Child 1985; 60:772–774.
33. Auerbach KG. The influence of lactation consultant contact on breastfeeding duration in a low-income population. Nebraska Med J 1985; 55:341–346.
34. Naylor AJ, Johnson DD, Wester RA. Teaching health professionals how to promote lactation: Example of a successful program. International Symposium on Human Milk Banking. Czechoslovakia, Hradec Kralove, May 18–21, 1982.
35. De Carvalho M, Anderson DM, Giangreco A, Pittard WB. Frequency of milk expression and milk production by mothers of nonnursing premature neonates. Am J Dis Child 1985; 139:483–485.
36. Egli GE, Egli NS, Newton M. The influence of the number of breast feedings on milk production. Pediatrics 1961; 27: 314–317.
37. Butte NF, Garza C, Smith EO, Nichols BL. Human milk intake and growth in exclusively breast-fed infants. J Pediatr 1984; 104:187–195.
38. Butte NF, Wills C, Jean CA, et al. Feeding patterns of exclusively breast-fed infants during the first four months of life. Early Hum Dev 1985; 12:291–300.
39. Elias MF, Nicolson NA, Bora C, Johnston J. Sleep/wake patterns of breast-fed infants in the first 2 years of life. Pediatrics 1986; 77:322–329.
40. Delvoye P, Demaegd M, Delogne-Desnoeck J, Robyn C. The influence of the frequency of nursing and of previous lactation experience on serum prolactin in lactating mothers. J Biosoc Sci 1977; 9:447–451.
41. Lucas A, Lucas PJ, Baum JD. Pattern of milk flow in breast-fed infants. Lancet 1979; 2(8133):57–58.

42. Stuff JE, Garza C, Boutte C, et al. Sources of variance in milk and caloric intakes in breast-fed infants: implications for lactation study design and interpretation. Am J Clin Nutr 1986; 43:361-366.

43. Peaker M. The effect of raised intramammary pressure on mammary function in the goat in relation to the cessation of lactation. J Physiol 1980; 301:415-428.

44. Lawrence RA. Breastfeeding: a guide for the medical profession, St. Louis, C.V. Mosby Co., 1980; 315-331.

45. Peterson RG, Bowes WA, Jr. Drugs, toxins and environmental agents in breast milk. In Neville NC, Neifert MR (eds): Lactation: Physiology, Nutrition and Breast-feeding. New York, Plenum Press, 1983; 367-403.

46. Roberts RJ (ed): Drug Therapy in Infants. Philadelphia, W.B. Saunders, 1984; 346-353.

47. Kochenour NK. Lactation suppression. Clin Obstet Gynecol 1980; 23:1045-1059.

48. Liebhaber M, Lewiston NJ, Asquith MT, Sunshine P. Comparison of bacterial contaminatiion with two methods of human milk collection. J Pediatr 1978; 92:236.

49. West PA, Hewitt JH, Murphy OM. The influence of methods of collection and storage on the bacteriology of human milk. J Appl Bacteriol 1979; 46:269-277.

50. Carroll L, Osman M, Davies DP. Does discarding the first few ml of breast milk improve the bacteriological quality of bank breast milk. Arch Dis Child 1980; 55:898-899.

51. Tibbetts E, Cadwell K. Selecting the right breast pump. Maternal Child Nurs 1980; 5:262-264.

52. Pujczynski M, Rademaker D, Gatson RL. Burn injury related to improper use of microwave oven. Pediatrics 1983; 72:714-715.

53. Sigman MJ, Burke KI, Register UD, et al. Effects of microwaving on the bacterial and IgA content of human milk. J Am Diet Assoc 1987; in press.

54. Ford JE, Law BA, Marshall VME, Reiter B. Influence of the heat treatment of human milk on some of its protective constituents. J Pediatr 1977; 90:29-35.

55. Ehrenkranz RA, Ackerman BA. Metoclopramide effect on faltering milk production by mothers of premature infants. Pediatrics 1986; 78:614-620.

56. Bowen-Jones A, Thomas C, Drewett RF. Milk flow and sucking rates during breastfeeding. Dev Med Child Neurol 1982; 24:626-633.

57. Pearce JL, Buchanan LF. Breast milk and breast feeding in very low birthweight infants. Arch Dis Child 1979; 54:897-899.

58. Boggs KR, Rau PK. Breastfeeding the premature infant. Am J Nurs 1983; 83:1437-1439.

59. Meier P. A program to support breast-feeding in the high risk nursery. Perinatol/Neonatol 1980; 4(2):43-49.

60. Yu VYH, Jamieson J, Bajuk B. Breast milk feeding in very low birthweight infants. Aus Paediatr J 1981; 17:186-190.

61. Marshall BR, Heppler JK, Zirbel CC. Sporadic puerperal mastitis, an infection that need not interrupt lactation. JAMA 1975; 233:1377-1379.

62. Cobo E. Effect of different doses of ethanol on the milk ejecting reflex in lactating women. Am J Obstet Gynecol 1973; 115:817-819.

63. Counsilman JJ, Mackay EV. Cigarette smoking by pregnant women with particular reference to their past and subsequent breast feeding behavior. Aust NZ J Obstet Gynaecol 1985; 25:101-107.

64. Martin DC, Martin JC, Streissgath AP, Lund CA. Sucking frequency and amplitude in newborns as a function of maternal drinking and smoking. Curr Alcohol 1978; 5:359-366.

19

Special Methods in Feeding the Preterm Infant

RICHARD J. SCHANLER, M.D.

ABSTRACT

Enteral nutrition is available for the preterm infant. Gavage feeding is necessary before the infant develops coordinated sucking and swallowing mechanisms. The advantages and disadvantages of the various forms of gavage feeding (continuous vs. intermittent, nasogastric or orogastric vs. transpyloric) are described in this chapter. In addition to immature neurological, developmental, and gastrointestinal systems, preterm infants particularly are prone to superimposed conditions that either arise from the type and method of feeding or affect their ability to feed enterally. Methods to evaluate the tolerance to feedings are described. As the infant matures, breast- and bottle-feedings are introduced. A suggested feeding protocol for preterm infants begins with a period of parenteral nutrition until postnatal adjustment is completed. Following this period, infants weighing less than 1500 gm are given continuous enteral infusions of milk, infants weighing between 1501 and 1800 gm are fed by intermittent bolus, and infants weighing more than 1800 gm are breast- or bottle-fed. A schedule for graded increments in milk intake is included.

INTRODUCTION

"Next to the maintenance of body temperature the premature infant needs adequate feeding...two of the most valuable items in their care are incubators and gavage feeding." Thomas E. Cone, Jr.[1]

"When infants are feeble, (however), they sometimes refuse to suck. Milk is then made to trickle into their mouths directly from the nipple, by exerting pressure upon it, or they are fed from a small spoon, till they become strong enough to take the breast; but, if they allow the milk to dribble out of their mouths, if they do not want to swallow, or if they reject what is given to them gavage feeding, by stomach tube, must be considered." B. Corner[2]

Although Marchant described gavage feeding of preterm infants in 1850, it was not until 1885 that Tarnier reintroduced the technique to feed the "weaklings" (preterm infants) at the Maternite Hospital in Paris. Later, at the turn of the century, another technique, the nasal spoon, was developed for feeding preterm infants (Fig. 1). This dangerous method, advocated as late as 1939, utilized a curved spoon that allowed milk to drip into the infant's nostril.[1]

Both Tarnier and his pupil Budin recommended that "weaklings" be fed human milk supplied by the mother or by wet nurses. If human milk was not used, they advocated milk from the goat or ass, because they believed that cow milk was too difficult for the preterm infant to digest. If cow milk was selected, however, a formula that consisted of boiled milk and sugar water was fed to the infant. Human milk was recommended for feeding preterm infants until the 1940s, when Gordon's studies that compared human milk with cow milk were reported.[3] When evaluating growth and nutrient absorption, he found that a significant proportion of the fat from human and cow milk was unabsorbed and that the preterm infants fed human milk failed to gain weight. Although not his intention, these studies resulted eventually in a transition to cow milk formula feeding.[4] The proponents of human-milk feeding argued for its role in the nutrition of the preterm infant, but reports of improved weight gain and fat absorption with the feeding of half-skimmed cow milk were hard to ignore. Investigations that compare human and cow milk have been ongoing for the last 40 years and continue to be an important controversial topic in the nutrition of the preterm infant.

The 1940s also initiated another controversy, the timing of the initial feeding for a preterm infant. Before this period, the consensus was that milk feedings should be given within the first hours of life.[5]

"These feeble infants must not be allowed to wait 2 or 3 days for regular feeding with mothers' milk: the loss of weight and . . . rise in temperture . . . may be the last straw for some . . . who are fighting a feeble struggle for existence, wrote Goodhart in 1913."

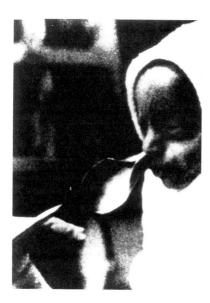

FIGURE 1.   The nasal spoon for feeding preterm infants, circa 1900.

The practice to delay the introduction of feedings for preterm infants, however, became a routine in the 1940s. Feedings for stressed infants begun on the second or third day or even later were thought to avoid potential gastroesophageal reflux and its complication of aspiration pneumonia.[5,6] A second reason cited for the delay in feedings was the excessive retention of extracellular fluids in the preterm infant, which was thought to be alleviated by starvation. The consensus at that time was to initiate feedings on the third day of life so that the metabolic derangements brought on by starvation would be overcome without adverse effects![5] The period of obligatory starvation generally depended upon birthweight. Crosse's schedule delayed nutritional intervention for three days if birthweight was 1360–1800 gm and four days if <1360 gm.[7]

Not until the early 1960s did investigators become convinced that early starvation impaired growth and neurologic development.[5,8,9] Drillien concluded that the incidence of handicap was related to this early period of undernutrition.[5,8] The highest incidence of cerebral palsy and mental retardation was observed in infants born in 1953–1954, a period when delayed feeding was practiced. Drillien further concluded that the 21% weight loss and the 33 days to regain birthweight were significant predictors of abnormal outcome in that population.[5,8] These clinical data prompt-

ed the groups led by Widdowson and Winick to investigate the effects of undernutrition on brain and body growth.[5] In the 1960s Smith suggested that the delay in nutrition be abandoned and that early feedings be reinstituted.[6]

The early initiation of human-milk feeding in preterm infants resulted in lower serum bilirubin values, greater blood glucose values, reduction in the incidence of hypernatremia, and shortened time to regain birthweight.[5,9,10] A lower rate of handicap also was observed in preterm infants following the reinstitution of early feedings.[5]

Enteral nutrition for the preterm infant is unique. In addition to their immature neurological and gastrointestinal systems, preterm infants particularly are prone to superimposed conditions such as necrotizing enterocolitis, nonspecific feeding intolerance, malabsorption, patent ductus arteriosus, and episodes of apnea and bradycardia, all of which affect their ability to deal with enteral nutrition (Table 1). Furthermore, attempts to compensate for the immature development may result in complications (Table 2). Repeated passage and use of indwelling tubes for gavage feeding may perforate the gastrointestinal tract.[11] Complications such as lactobezoars may arise from the type of milk and method of its administration.[12]

TABLE 1.   Conditions in Preterm Infants That May Affect Tolerance to Enteral Nutrition

Birth asphyxia
Circulatory instability
hypotension, patent ductus arteriosus
Apnea and bradycardia
Necrotizing enterocolitis

TABLE 2.   Complications of Enteral Nutrition

Milk aspiration
Laryngospasm
Perforation of gastrointestinal tract
Perforation of renal pelvis
Lactobezoar
Necrotizing enterocolitis
Hematochezia
Malabsorption
Poor growth

DEVELOPMENTAL CONSIDERATIONS

Several considerations regarding developmental immaturity that limit the feeding of preterm infants should be mentioned. Mechanical methods for feeding often are required because of the fatigability of the sucking and swallowing reflexes and the lack of coordination of these actions with breathing. The coordination of sucking and swallowing is present in the healthy infant at a gestational or postconceptional age of 32–34 weeks.

The components of sucking develop early in fetal life. Non-nutritive sucking (rapid rate) develops before nutritive sucking (slower rate).[13] Mouth opening is first observed at 7 to 8 weeks' gestation, oral reflexes in response to trigeminal nerve stimulation at 12-13 weeks, protrusion of the lips and tongue motion at 13-16 weeks, lip puckering at 22 weeks, and actual nonnutritive sucking at 24 weeks.[13,14]

The development of swallowing actually may precede sucking.[13] This may be related to the large amount of amniotic fluid that the fetus swallows during gestation.[13] Historically, the clinical correlate of this early development of swallowing is reflected in the use of eyedroppers for feeding the preterm infant. The current practice of using "preemie" nipples that allow easy flow of milk also reflects this developmental pattern.

Postnatal studies in preterm infants report rhythmic non-nutritive sucking bursts as early as 28 weeks postconception and a more consistent pattern at 31 to 32 weeks.[14] **The onset of "true" or nutritive sucking is reported between postnatal days 10 and 26 (3 to 10 days after initiation of feedings) in infants born at 32-34 weeks' gestation.**[15]

Gastric capacity may limit the ability of the preterm infant to tolerate enteral feedings. Estimates of gastric capacity in fullterm infants date back to 1920 when Scammon and Doyle reported the relative physiologic capacity of the stomach to be less than the anatomic capacity until after the fourth day of life.[16] Silverman calculated that the average physiologic gastric capacity of the 2-2.5 kg preterm infant was 2-27 ml/kg birthweight, from day 1 to 10, respectively.[16]

Delayed gastric emptying, often observed in preterm infants, may be associated with conditions of gastroesophageal reflux, respiratory distress syndrome, and congenital heart disease.[17] The type of feeding can influence gastric emptying, e.g., human milk promotes faster emptying than cow milk.[18] Individual nutrients affect gastric emptying; long-chain triglycerides and glucose delay emptying, medium-chain triglycerides and fructose enhance emptying.[17] Milk osmolality and energy density may affect gastric emptying, e.g., hyperosmolar formulas delay emptying.[19,20] Continuous nasogastric milk infusion and frequent small feedings enhance emptying. Opiates and β-adrenergic drugs delay and metoclopramide promotes gastric emptying.[17]

Diminished gastrointestinal motility may limit feeding of the preterm infant. Milk, paradoxically, may decrease motility, a response that may be related to diminished maturation of peristalsis.[21] The maturation of duodenal motility has been evaluated by indwelling manometry in preterm infants from 26 to 42 weeks postconception.[22] Morriss et al. showed that the duodenal contraction rate and force of contraction were low before 29 weeks, increased abruptly between 29 and 32 weeks, and increased gradually thereafter until the adult pattern was achieved at 40 weeks. This pattern matured more quickly when antenatal steroids were given to mothers in preterm labor.[22]

EARLY VERSUS LATE INITIATION OF ENTERAL FEEDING: CURRENT STATUS

"In 1949 Smith et al. wrote that 'premature infants at the Boston Lying-in and Children's Hospitals are given no food or water for two or three days after birth'. This regimen, according to Dr. Smith, 'was introduced by Dr. Stewart Clifford, not only to avoid the danger of aspiration but also because clinical observation of these patients had revealed the frequency of generalized edema, often associated with other disturbances and usually disappearing with the first few days.'"[1]

With the advent of safe methods for short courses of parenteral nutrition, the decision to introduce enteral nutrition in the first weeks of life is, once again, a focus of considerable debate. Delayed introduction of enteral nutrition has been proposed to enable the very low birthweight preterm infant to adjust to extrauterine life and to reduce the incidence of necrotizing enterocolitis. In a recent survey of neonatal intensive care unit practices, 20% of the responders provided enteral nutrition during the first week of life, but only in combination with parenteral nutrition, to infants with birthweights below 1000 gm.[23] Approximately

67% of the responders provided this combination to infants with birthweights greater than 1000 gm. Only 30% of the responders provided enteral nutrition alone to infants if the birthweights were greater than 1500 gm. The units that based their decision for starting enteral nutrition at specific postnatal ages began feeds of sterile water at seven days for infants with birthweights less than 1000 gm, at five days for infants 1001–1500 gm, and at three days for infants 1501–2499 gm.[23]

Enteral nutrition, however, does play a role in stimulating metabolic and gastrointestinal adaptations.[24] Hormonal responses have been evaluated. When compared to unfed infants, human milk–fed preterm infants at 6 days of age demonstrated significantly greater serum concentrations of selected gastrointestinal hormones (enteroglucagon, glucagon, gastrin, motilin, neurotensin, and gastric inhibitory polypeptide).[24] The unfed preterm infants had greater concentrations of secretin and lower levels of β-hydroxybutyrate, glycerol, and alanine.[24] The speculation was made that lower serum concentrations of certain hormones may retard the development of the gastrointestinal tract. The presence of milk in the lumen also affects gastrointestinal tract development.[25]

As mentioned, a delay in enteral nutrition has been suggested as a measure to reduce the incidence of necrotizing enterocolitis. A recent study, however, reported that the delay in enteral nutrition did not prevent necrotizing enterocolitis.[26] In a prospective study of high-risk very low birthweight infants, the institution of feedings on postnatal day 1 or day 7 did not affect the rate of this devastating condition.[27]

Because the best time to initiate enteral nutrition is unknown, the decision frequently is based on clinical criteria that suggest satisfactory achievement of extrauterine adaptation. These criteria generally include the normalization of vital signs, the absence of stress from severe illness and instrumentation, and the presence, on physical examination, of a nondistended, soft abdomen with normal bowel sounds.

VOLUME, ENERGY DENSITY, AND CHOICE OF MILK

Few data exist concerning the enteral fluid requirements of the preterm infant. Most evaluations consider either parenteral needs or a combination of parenteral and enteral

fluid needs. In an early statement concerning the fluid needs for these infants, Silverman suggested that 130-150 ml/kg/day of milk would be appropriate for preterm infants and that this volume could supply 120 kcal/kg/day.[16] Bell evaluated the combined parenteral and enteral fluid intakes of preterm infants during the first 30 days of life.[28] While receiving a high fluid intake (above approximately 150-160 ml/kg/day), the preterm infants in his study experienced a greater rate of patent ductus arteriosus and necrotizing enterocolitis.[28] Two European groups, however, concluded that enteral intakes of 200-250 ml/kg/day were tolerated by preterm infants without ill effects.[29,30] Those infants demonstrated appropriate growth that mimicked intrauterine standards.

Most authorities consider an energy intake of 120 kcal/kg/day appropriate for preterm infants.[16,31,32] This energy intake can be achieved with 180 ml/kg/day of a 20 kcal/oz (67 kcal/dl) formula, or 150 ml/kg/day of a 24 kcal/oz (81 kcal/dl) formula. Formulas designed for preterm infants generally supply 24 kcal/oz (81 kcal/dl), and 150 ml/kg/day of the formula will provide 120 kcal/kg/day. The volume of human milk that will provide this energy intake generally is 180 ml/kg/day.[33]

"Homemade" preparations of formulas with nutrient supplements may have a high renal solute load and osmolality and may not be indicated. Formulas of high osmolality may be associated with necrotizing enterocolitis.[34] **The current 24 kcal/oz formulations are iso-osmolar and have a relatively low renal solute load.** The renal solute load, however, is greater than that of human milk. For these reasons, the formula usually is diluted to one-half strength for the initial feedings of the very low birthweight infants.

A combination of parenteral and enteral nutrition often is used during the first postnatal weeks. If enteral feedings are introduced gradually and cautiously, the infant does not suffer from malnutrition because nutritional needs will be met by the parenteral route.[32,34,35] The infant then may be maintained on a protocol of enteral nutrition by gavage methods that provides 120 kcal and 150 ml/kg/day (see Tables 3 and 4).

Feeding human milk to the very low birthweight preterm infant is controversial.[33] Despite high intakes of human milk, these infants may fail to mineralize their bones and also manifest protein inadequacy.[33,36] For infants

TABLE 3.   Suggested Feeding Guidelines

	Birthweight Groups			
	<1250 gm	1250–1500 gm	1501–1800 gm	>1800 gm
NPO (days)*	5–7	3–5	0–3	0–1
Method	gavage continuous infusion	gavage continuous infusion	gavage or oral† intermittent bolus	oral or gavage intermittent bolus
Human milk	Until "full" feeds only	yes, unless fluid restricted	yes	yes
Specialized formulas for VLBW‡ infants	yes	yes	yes	no
Routine infant formulas	no	no	no	yes
Breastfeeding	no	no	yes	yes
Pacifier	yes	yes	yes	yes

*NPO: No enteral feeding until postnatal adjustment is completed.
†Oral: Refers to breastfeeding or bottle-feeding.
‡VLBW: Very low-birth-weight infants.

<1250 gm birthweight, once enteral feeding with human milk is "well tolerated," a switch to a specialized formula designed for the very-low-birthweight infant seems prudent. For infants >1250 gm, the decision to change to a specialized formula should be based on clinical criteria, e.g., the need to restrict enteral fluids and the development of early signs compatible with poor bone mineralization. Any switch to formula must be made as a temporary maneuver, lactation should continue, and human-milk feeding should resume when the infant's clinical course improves and a satisfactory weight gain is achieved for 3-5 weeks. Although lacking the protective, inductive, and digestive functions of human milk, these specialized commercial formulas provide sufficient minerals and protein to meet the estimated needs of these infants.[31,36-38] Recent experience shows that the fortification of

TABLE 4.   Suggested Schedule of Feedings for Infants <1800 gm*

Day of Feeding	Birthweight Groups:					
	<1250 gm		1250–1500 gm		1501–1800 gm	
	Continuous infusion		Continuous infusion		Intermittent bolus†	
	Human Milk	Special‡ Formula	Human Milk	Special‡ Formula	Human Milk	Special‡ Formula
	(ml/hr)		(ml/hr)		(ml/kg/day)	
1§	1.0//	1.0//	1.0	1.0	25	25
2	1.0	1.0**	1.0	1.0**	25	25**
3	1.0	1.0	2.0	1.0	50	25
4	2.0	1.0	3.0	2.0	75	50
5	2.0	1.0	4.0	3.0	100	75
6	3.0	2.0	5.0	4.0	125	100
7	3.0	2.0	6.0	5.0	150	125
8	4.0	3.0	7.0	6.0	175	150
9	4.0	3.0	7.0	6.0	180	150
10	5.0	4.0				
11	5.0	4.0				
12	6.0	5.0				
13	6.0	5.0				
14	7.0	6.0				
15	7.0	6.0				

*If any intolerance to feeding occurs, go back to earlier day on schedule. Supplemental parenteral nutrition is used until "full" enteral feedings are achieved.
†Oral or gavage feedings every 3 hours.
‡Specialized formula designed for preterm infants, 24 kcal/oz.
§Sterile water is fed on the first day if <1500 gm and first feeds if >1500 gm.
//May use smaller increments (e.g., 0.5 ml/hr) for infants with birthweights below 800 gm.
**Half-strength formula.

human milk is a promising means of providing an infant with his mother's milk.[36]

Once the infant demonstrates an effective gag reflex and an ability to coordinate sucking, swallowing, and breathing, usually at a body weight of approximately 1800 gm or postconceptional age of 34-35 weeks, breast-feeding or a "routine" infant formula (20 kcal/oz, 67 kcal/dl) can be introduced. At this time, the infant may feed "on demand." The infant should be allowed to consume ad libitum volumes of milk every 2-3 hours if breastfeeding, and every 3-5 hours if bottle-feeding (see Tables 3 and 4).

METHODS OF GAVAGE FEEDING

"Small infants too weak to nurse at the breast have been fed by medicine dropper or pipette for more than two hundred years and since 1884 by gavage feeding. The latter method was first described by Marchant in 1850, but was not commonly used until introduced by Tarnier at the Maternite in Paris . . . .Nasal spoon feeding, a bizarre technique, was practiced successfully by the French and was used as late as the 1940s by Madame Recht who was Couney's nurse."[1]

INTERMITTENT BOLUS

The nasogastric or orogastric method may be used for infants who are unable to suck, either because they are immature or have had neurologic insults. First introduced in 1951, this technique has proven successful for the feeding of "weak" preterm infants.[32] The intermittent bolus method is used most often in neonatal units today, possibly because it mimics "normal" bolus feeding patterns and because most nurseries have the largest experience with this modality.[23]

The *nasogastric tube* may interfere with respiration because neonates are obligatory nose breathers. It also may contribute to excessive nasal secretions and produce ulceration or erosion of the nasal septum and mucosa.[32] With repeated insertion of a nasogastric tube, excessive vagal stimulation and bradycardia may result.[32] The *orogastric tube,* on the other hand, is difficult to secure and prone to dislodgment. Because of the problems with intolerance to the feeding tubes, gastrostomy has been suggested for the bolus feeding of very low birthweight infants.[39] This technique, however, is associated with greater mortality in this population.[39]

The size of the feeding tube is selected according to the body weight: 3.5 or 5 F for infants < 1000 gm, 5 or 8 F for 1000-1500 gm, and 8 F for larger infants. For nasogastric feeding, the catheter is measured from the tip of the nose, around the ear, to the xiphoid.[40] For orogastric feeding, the catheter is measured from the nasal bridge to the xiphoid process.[32] When the tube is inserted, the infant is observed for choking or gasping, indications that the catheter is in the trachea. Once in the stomach, the volume and pH (< 5) of gastric residuals are assessed. If bilious material is aspirated (pH >6.5), the tube is withdrawn 2 cm and the gastric residual is rechecked.

The feeding is allowed to flow, by gravity, into the stomach. At the end of the feeding, the catheter is pinched and withdrawn and the infant is placed in the prone position or on his right side. If the catheter is indwelling, the tube is clamped and the infant positioned. Feedings generally are administered every 3 hours. Occasionally, a schedule of every 2-4 hours is necessary. An indwelling gavage tube may remain in place for 2-4 days before removal. Most nurseries use indwelling nasogastric tubes to avoid repeated passage of the catheter. The orogastric tube is used for repeated passage, but in our experience it may be left in place for 2-4 days to prevent the unnecessary stress that accompanies frequent catheter changes.

CONTINUOUS INFUSION

Continuous Nasogastric Infusion

The continuous nasogastric infusion, first reported in 1972 by Valman, has several advantages over intermittent feeding.[32,41] The infant is disturbed less often and has fewer problems from gastric distention.[32] The infant that does not tolerate handling (for example, the very low birthweight infant who has apneic episodes) may do better with this method of feeding. The continuous milk drip potentially may give the infant a greater volume of milk each day than that obtained from intermittent feedings. A disadvantage, however, is that the tube may be dislodged, resulting in aspiration of milk into the trachea. Milk aspiration, however, was not reported in the 56 low birthweight infants in Valman's original series.[41] If the tube is taped to the cheek and an additional piece of tape is placed on the tube at the nose, the position can be verified frequently.

Continuous Transpyloric Infusion

The continuous transpyloric infusion, which gained popularity in the mid-1970s,[42] attempts to circumvent the slow gastric emptying of the preterm infant by passing the tube directly into the duodenum or jejunum. An additional advantage of this method is the reduced danger of reflux and potential milk aspiration into the trachea. Complications from this method, including perforations of the intestine and renal pelvis and impaired fat absorption, may be signficant.[11,32,43,44] Abdominal distention, diarrhea, necrotizing enterocolitis, pyloric incompetence with gastric reflux, and a change in gastrointestinal flora also are reported following transpyloric feeding.[11,45,46]

The time required to intubate the jejunum successfully is lengthy and may be a disadvantage.[44,47] In one method of tube insertion, two catheters are used.[32] A 5 F nasogastric catheter is passed and **the stomach is inflated with air.** A second catheter, whose length is measured from the forehead to the heel, is inserted slowly through the nostril into the stomach. Once the entire length is inserted, proper placement is verified by aspiration of intestinal contents with pH > 6.5. The first tube is removed. An abdominal radiograph may be needed if placement is not assured; however, this results in radiation exposure unnecessary with other modalities.[47] The tube should be replaced every three days. Another method of tube insertion uses a 24-karat gold weight to guide a soft silicone feeding tube into position![46]

Rhea and colleagues, in Saudi Arabia, used a highly polished, 24-karat gold plug to guide a soft, limp, silicone feeding tube into the duodenum or jejunum . . . A competent dental laboratory technician readily cast these gold plugs whose weights varied from 246-842 mg for a 1 and 3 kg infant, respectively![46] The other current methods for transpyloric feeding are available at a fraction of the cost!

TECHNICAL PROBLEMS WITH CONTINUOUS INFUSION

Technical problems may be encountered when milk is administered by continuous infusion. The prolonged exposure of milk to synthetic tubing, infusion pumps, ambient light and phototherapy, and room temperature possibly may alter nutrient composition. **Significant losses of calcium, iron, and zinc are reported following continuous infusion of formulas designed for preterm infants.[48,49]** These losses, which are not observed following intermittent bolus feeding of the same formulas, suggest that the stability of various infant formulas should be evaluated for their use in continuous milk infusions.[49]

Technical problems arise from the use of continuous infusions of human milk. Because human milk is not homogenized, the cream separates from the body of the milk upon standing. **This cream tends to adhere to the extensive array of tubing and cassettes frequently used for infusions.** We have found that 50% of the fat (and therefore the energy) may be lost in a system employing continuous infusions of human milk (unpublished data). The rate of infusion correlates inversely with the degree of fat loss.[50] The problem may be corrected with improved mixing techniques and with the design of a delivery system that eliminates most of the "dead space" tubing. The use of a design employing a simple infusion pump, an attached syringe, and a feeding tube reduces fat losses dramatically (Fig. 2). We used a small syringe pump (AutoSyringe, Hookset, NH) that was positioned vertically, with the nozzle up, within the infant's incubator.[36] Implementation of this design change for continuous infusion of human milk reduced the losses of fat following infusion from 50% to <4% (unpublished data).

Feeding tubes made of polyvinylchloride may stiffen after long-term placement.[45] This change in texture may lead to gastric and intestinal tract perforations. Silicone tubes are softer and may reduce this hazard; however, they are more difficult to insert.[45]

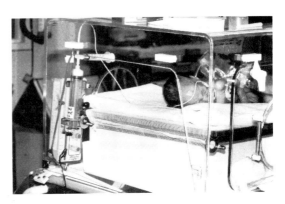

FIGURE 2. System for continuous infusion of milk.

COMPARISON OF METHODS

Intermittent vs Continuous Delivery of Milk

Krishnan[51] and Parker[52] have compared the intermittent and continuous nasogastric methods. An energy intake of 90 kcal/kg and a steady pattern of weight gain are achieved more rapidly in very low birthweight infants fed by the continuous nasogastric method.[51] A crossover study of infants less than 7 months of age with intestinal diseases fed via continuous nasogastric infusion and oral, intermittent boluses of milk reported that the former method resulted in **greater absorption of fat, nitrogen, copper, zinc, and calcium, and greater increments in weight gain during the period of evaluation.**[52] Differences also are reported in the pattern of hormonal responses following intermittent and continuous nasogastric feedings.[24] Preterm infants fed by continuous infusion do not experience cyclical changes in insulin secretion that are observed in bolus-fed infants.[24]

Published studies that compare intermittent nasogastric and continuous transpyloric methods reveal conflicting results. During the first 15 days of life, the implementation of the nasojejunal method reportedly improves weight gain and enables greater intake of energy and fluid in preterm infants.[45] The use of this method, however, is related to greater fat and potassium malabsorption, greater stool frequency, and diminished increments in skinfold thickness compared to that of the intermittent nasogastric method.[43] Other investigators report that the use of this method resulted in lower caloric intakes during the first week of life and slower gains in weight and head measurements than those observed with the intermittent methods.[53,54]

Continuous Nasogastric vs Transpyloric Infusions

Van Caillie reported that transpyloric (nasoduodenal) feedings in preterm infants provided a greater caloric intake and resulted in a greater weight gain in the first week of life compared with continuous nasogastric infusion.[55] This study described three cases of diarrhea and no aspiration pneumonia in the six infants fed by transpyloric tube, and one case of diarrhea and two of aspiration pneumonia in the five infants fed by nasogastric tube. In a brief report, the use of the continuous nasogastric method appeared to provide a greater caloric intake at 7 and 14 days compared with that of the nasojejunal method.[56]

In summary, the disagreement as to the appropriate method for feeding the preterm infant is the reason for the disparity in the feeding methods chosen for these preterm infants.[23] The practical matters of the time required for insertion and of radiation exposure with the transpyloric method make it a less than optimal choice. Because several methods for gavage feeding are available, the protocol chosen should be consistent at each institution to generate sufficient experience.

INTRODUCTION OF BREASTFEEDING

"Home care of babies weighing less than 1500 gm in Bogota, Colombia has become famous. Instead of being placed in an incubator, low birthweight babies are packed close to their mothers right next to the breast . . . the kangaroo position . . . breastfeeding on demand . . . dropping the death rate from 70% to 10%."[57]

A somewhat different approach to breastfeeding preterm infants is taken in the United States. Healthy infants born at a gestational age of 35 weeks generally have the ability to feed directly from the breast. If "rooming-in" is not possible, every effort should be made to bring the mother and infant together to allow breastfeeding. Infants with gestational ages less than 35 weeks, infants with birthweights less than 1800 gm, or infants who are more mature at birth, but are ill and unable to suck, generally are in a transition between gavage and breastfeeding.

Gavage-fed infants can begin to feed at the breast if they have established (1) a good pattern of weight gain, (2) tolerance of complete enteral nutrition, (3) a proximity to 34 weeks postconception, (4) appropriate control of body temperature, and (5) coordination of suck-swallow-breathing mechanisms.[58] This approach may be conservative because there are accounts of very low birthweight infants feeding at the breast at 11 days of life (body weights of 1300 ± 100 gm).[59]

Appropriate lactation counseling in the early days after delivery should be provided to mothers whose infants are unable initially to breastfeed. Mothers are taught the techniques for milk expression. Lactation management personnel evaluate milk production from records maintained by the mother. The initiation of breastfeeding begins with several days of nonnutritive sucking by the infant at mother's breast. During this period of bonding, the infant's "latch-on" and sucking reflexes are evaluated and the mother's anxieties are acknowledged and alleviated.[58,60] The initiation of breastfeeding before bottle-feeding results in an easier transition to exclusive breastfeeding at home.[60] Efforts should be made to provide nursery areas for breastfeeding, and "rooming-in" should be encouraged when the infant's clinical condition is stable. This "early" introduction of breastfeeding also stimulates milk production in situations where milk output is low.

After the initial stages, the infant may breastfeed in lieu of one gavage feeding. Each day for several consecutive days, one breastfeeding should be encouraged in place of a gavage feeding. The indicators of successful breastfeeding are the maintenance of the infant's pattern of weight gain, evidence of satiety, and the mother's subjective impression of breast emptying. When these are achieved, additional breastfeedings are substituted for gavage feedings. Weighing the infant before and after nursing to determine the amount of milk consumed is unnecessary, because this method is inaccurate and will serve only to increase maternal anxiety.[61]

With successful intervention programs, preterm infants are able to begin breastfeeding early and to continue breastfeeding after hospital discharge. One center that uses a standardized lactation program reports that a very low birthweight infant population (less than 1500 gm at birth) maintained a 75% rate of breastfeeding in the hospital and a 44% rate on follow-up examination at 3 months.[62]

EVALUATING THE TOLERANCE OF FEEDINGS

The infant's tolerance to feedings is evaluated frequently to identify the potential hazards of a particular feeding method and also to decide on increments in milk intake. Vomiting, abdominal distention, significant gastric residual volumes, and abnormal stool patterns are used to assess this tolerance.[32] Systemic illness and necrotizing enterocolitis may present with a combination of any or all of these signs of feeding intolerance.

Vomiting may indicate too rapid an increase in the infant's feeding volumes, or too great a volume for the infant's size and maturity. Systemic illness also may manifest with vomiting.

If bile-stained material is vomited, a more ominous problem may be present.

Abdominal distention is a nonspecific sign that may occur if feedings are given too rapidly or volumes are too large, if the infant has swallowed an excessive amount of air, or if the infant has been resuscitated using face-mask ventilation. Occasionally, a dislodged endotracheal tube with gas leakage to the stomach may be discovered because of the infant's distended abdomen.

Gastric residual volumes should be measured before each intermittent gavage feeding and frequently (every 2-4 hours) during continuous infusions of milk. When using transpyloric infusions, the presence of a significant amount of gastric residual (determined from the tube in the stomach) indicates pyloric incompetence. In general, during intermittent gavage feedings, no residual volume is present 3 hours after the feeding. If a significant volume is present at that time, the next feeding should be reduced accordingly. If residual volumes are still present with subsequent evaluations, the feedings should be stopped for 6-12 hours and then resumed at a lower rate. Gastric residual volumes during continuous milk infusions should not exceed the sum of the hourly infusion rate and the volume of milk in the feeding tube. The infant generally serves as his own "control." A deviation from a consistent pattern of gastric residual volumes when the same milk intake has been maintained should be a cause for concern.

The character of the stools also may be a clue to the tolerance of the feedings. Normal stools are described as seedy, soft, and yellow. Watery stools suggest too rapid an increase in feeding volume, increased gastrointestinal motility, intolerance to lactose, and infection. The presence of reducing substances generally suggests incomplete absorption of sugar, either due to feeding an excessively large volume, decreased gastrointestinal transit time, lactose intolerance, or impending necrotizing enterocolitis. The presence of gross or occult blood in the stool always is a concern. The most common cause, however, is blood swallowed at delivery. An Apt test on the stool may differentiate maternal from fetal blood.[32] A simple rectal fissure is the second most common cause. The frequency of stools also may be of concern.

Infrequent stooling may lead to abdominal distention and vomiting. When clinical signs are present, a small glycerine suppository may help stool evacuation.

TABLE 5.   Routine Nutritional Assessment of the Preterm Infant

Measurement	Frequency of Determination
Milk intake (ml/kg/d)	daily
Caloric intake (kcal/kg/d)	daily
Body weight (gm)	same time each day
Length (cm)*	weekly
Head circumference (cm)†	weekly
Skinfold thickness (mm)‡	weekly

*Measurements of recumbent crown-heel length should be performed using a rigid board with immobile head support and movable foot support; however, paper tape is used frequently because it is clean, easily available and reproducible.

†Measurements of head circumference should be made with a flexible stainless steel tape; however, paper tape is used frequently.

‡Calipers should be read at a constant time interval after applying pressure to sites selected (triceps, subscapular, periumbilical, thigh) for skinfold measurements. This measurement generally is not performed routinely.

TABLE 6.   Suggested Biochemical Monitoring of Nutritional Status in Enterally-Fed Preterm Infants

Laboratory Test	Frequency of Determination
Hemoglobin, hematocrit	weekly
Reticulocyte count	weekly
Serum electrolytes	weekly ×2, then as indicated
Calcium, phosphorus	weekly ×2, then every 2 wk*
Alkaline phosphatase	weekly ×2, then every 2 wk*
Albumin, blood urea nitrogen	weekly ×2, then every 2 wk*

*Assumes feeding appropriate volumes of specialized formulas designed for preterm infants: Enfamil Premature Formula, Similac Special Care, or "Preemie" SMA. If fed human milk, may need more frequent evaluations.

A complete nutritional assessment to determine the impact of feeding upon the infant and the infant's tolerance to the feedings is made by measurements of growth parameters and selected biochemical indices of nutritional status (Tables 5 and 6). A discussion of these measurements is beyond the scope of this chapter.

NON-NUTRITIVE "FEEDING"

The use of gavage feedings raises the concerns that bypassing the mouth prevents stimulation of lingual lipase and perhaps other factors that may aid digestion, and also that this technique may impair mandibular development and sucking. Bernbaum reported that the use of a simple nipple pacifier during gavage feedings facilitated the maturation of the sucking reflex and the transition to oral feedings.[63] This non-nutritive sucking method results in greater weight gain, decreased intestinal transit time, and shorter hospital stays.[63,64]

SUGGESTED FEEDING PROTOCOL

The protocols in Tables 3 and 4 were derived from those currently in use in the neonatal nurseries at Texas Children's Hospital and Jefferson Davis Hospital in Houston, Texas. Table 3 provides the feeding guidelines for four groups of preterm infants, classified by birthweights <1250 gm, 1250-1500 gm, 1501-1800 gm, and >1800 gm. The most conservative protocol is depicted for infants with birthweights <1250 gm. In a majority of cases, after the first few days of feeding, the schedule is advanced more rapidly. In these cases, a change in volume may be made each day. A protocol for nutritional assessment and monitoring also is included (Tables 5-6).

Table 4 provides a daily schedule for feeding. If continuous infusions of human milk are selected, the use of the feeding system described in the text is suggested (Fig. 2). For all infants <1800 gm, "formula" refers to a specially designed formula for preterm infants, 24 kcal/oz.

Beyond 1800 gm body weight and/or birthweight, the use of either expressed human milk, breast-feeding, or routine infant formula (20 kcal/oz) is advised. These infants generally are >34 weeks postconception and will take feedings by mouth. It is suggested, generally, to begin with 25 ml/kg/day and advance, as tolerated, by this amount each day. The concept of "full feeds" usually is an ad libitum volume of milk, ≥180 ml/kg/day.

Acknowledgments. I thank Dr. Arnold J. Rudolph for his critique of this chapter, Y. Garza for editorial advice, and N. Hayley for secretarial assistance. This work is a publication of the USDA/ARS Children's Nutrition Research Center, Department of Pediatrics, Baylor College of Medicine and Texas Children's Hospital. This project has been funded in part with federal funds from the U.S. Department of Agriculture, Agricultural Research Service, under Cooperative Agreement #58-7MNI-6-100. The contents of this publication do not necessarily reflect the views or policies of the U.S. Department of Agriculture, nor does mention of trade names, commercial products, or organizations imply endorsement by the U.S. Government.

REFERENCES

1. Cone TE Jr. History of the Care and Feeding of the Premature Infant. Boston, Little, Brown and Co., 1985;32–34.
2. Corner B (ed): Prematurity. Springfield, IL, Charles C Thomas, 1960;260.
3. Gordon HH, Levine SZ, McNamara H. Feeding of premature infants. Am J Dis Child 1947;73:442–452.
4. Davidson M. The feeding of prematurely born infants—a critique of current status. J Pediatr 1960;57:604–610.
5. Davies DP. The first feed of low brithweight infants. Arch Dis Child 1978;53:187–192.
6. Smith CA. Prenatal and neonatal nutrition. Pediatrics 1962; 30:145–156.
7. Crosse VM, Hickmans EM, Howarth BE, Aubrey J. The value of human milk compared with other feeds for premature infants. Arch Dis Child 1954;29:178–195.
8. Drillien CM (ed): The Growth and Development of the Prematurely Born Infant. Baltimore, Williams & Wilkins, 1964; 302–308.
9. Wharton BA, Bower BD. Immediate or later feeding for premature babies? Lancet 1965;2:969–972.
10. Smallpiece V, Davies PA. Immediate feeding of premature infants with undiluted breast-milk. Lancet 1964;2: 1349–1352.
11. Heird WC. Nasojejunal feeding: a commentary. J Pediatr 1974;85:111–112.
12. Erenberg A. Lactobezoar. In Sunshine P (ed): Feeding the Neonate Weighing Less Than 1500 Grams—Nutrition and Beyond. Columbus, Ross Laboratories, 1980;99–102.
13. Herbst JJ. Development of suck and swallow. J Pediatr Gastroenterol Nutr 1983;2(Suppl):S131–S135.
14. Hack M, Estabrook MM, Robertson SS. Development of sucking rhythm in preterm infants. Early Hum Devel 1985;11: 133–140.
15. Gryboski JD. Suck and swallow in the premature infant. Pediatrics 1969;43:96–102.
16. Silverman WA (ed): Dunham's Premature Infants, 3rd ed. New York, Paul B. Hoeber, Inc., 1961;151–159.
17. Lebenthal E, Siegel M. Understanding gastric emptying: implications for feeding the healthy and compromised infant. J Pediatr Gastroenterol Nutr 1985;4:1–3.
18. Cavell B. Gastric emptying in infants fed human milk or infant formula. Acta Paediatr Scand 1981;70:639–641.
19. Pascale JA, Mims LC, Greenberg MG, Alexander JB. Gastric response in low birth weight infants fed various formulas. Biol Neonate 1978;34:150–154.
20. Siegel M, Lebenthal E, Krantz B. Effect of caloric density on gastric emptying in premature infants. J Pediatr 1984; 104:118–122.
21. Walker WA. Development of gastrointestinal function and selected dysfunctions. In Mead Johnson Symposium on Perinatal and Developmental Medicine. No. 11, Selected Aspects of Perinatal Gastroenterology. Evansville, IN, Mead Johnson Co. 1977;3–10.
22. Moriss FH, Moore M, Weisbrodt NW. Duodenal motility in preterm infants: ontogeny and effects of antenatal corticosteroids. Pediatr Res 1986;20:356A.
23. Churella HR, Bachhuber WL, MacLean WC. Survey: methods of feeding low-birth-weight infants. Pediatrics 1985;76: 243–249.
24. Aynsley-Green A. Metabolic and endocrine interrelations in the human fetus and neonate. Am J Clin Nutr 1985;41: 399–417.
25. Hughes CA. Intestinal adaptation. In Tanner MS, Stocks RJ (eds): Neonatal Gastroenterology, Contemporary Issues. Newcastle-upon-Tyne, Intercept Ltd, 1984;69–91.
26. LaGamma EF, Ostertag SG, Birenbaum H. Failure of delayed oral feedings to prevent necrotizing enterocolitis. Am J Dis Child 1985;139:385–389.
27. Ostertag SG, LaGamma EF, Reisen CE, Ferrentino FL. Early enteral feeding does not affect the incidence of necrotizing enterocolitis. Pediatrics 1986;77:275–280.
28. Bell EF, Warburton D, Stonestreet BS, Oh W. Effect of fluid administration on the development of symptomatic patent ductus arteriosus and congestive failure in premature infants. N Engl J Med 1980;302:598–604.
29. Järvenpää AL, Raiha NCR, Rassin DK, Gaull G. Preterm infants fed human milk attain intrauterine weight gain. Acta Paediatr Scand 1983;72:239–243.
30. Lewis MA, Smith BAM. High volume milk feeds for preterm infants. Arch Dis Child 1984;59:779–781.
31. Committee on Nutrition, American Academy of Pediatrics. Nutritional needs of low-birth-weight infants. Pediatrics 1985;75:976–986.
32. Benda GIM. Modes of feeding low-birth-weight infants. Semin Perinatol 1979;3:407–415.
33. Schanler RJ. Human milk for the very low birthweight infant. Perinatol Neonatol 1983;7:17–26.
34. Book LS, Herbst JJ, Atherton SO, Junq AL. Necrotizing enterocolitis in low-birth-weight infants fed an elemental formula. J Pediatr 1975;87:602–605.
35. Benda GI, Babson SG. Peripheral intravenous alimentation of the small premature infant. J Pediatr 1971;79:494–498.
36. Schanler RJ, Garza C, Nichols BL. Fortified mothers' milk for very low birth weight infants: results of growth and nutrient balance studies. J Pediatr 1985;107:437–445.
37. Shenai JP, Reynolds JW, Babson SG. Nutritional balance studies in very-low-birth-weight infants: enhanced nutrient retention by an experimental formula. Pediatrics 1980;66: 233–238.
38. Ehrenkranz RA, Chamberlin MA, Gettner PA, Nelli CM. Nutritional adequacy of fortified preterm human milk (PTHM) in VLBW infants. Pediatr Res 1984;18:195A.
39. Vengusamy S, Pildes R, Raffensperger JF, et al. A controlled study of feeding gastrostomy in low birth weight infants. Pediatrics 1969;43:815–820.
40. Fanaroff AA, Klaus MH. Feeding and selected disorders of the gastrointestinal tract. In Klaus MH, Fanaroff AA (eds): Care of the High Risk Neonate, 3rd ed. Philadelphia, W.B. Saunders, 1986;113–146.
41. Valman HB, Heath CD, Brown RJK. Continuous intragastric milk feeds in infants of low birth weight. Br Med J 1972; 3:547–550.
42. Cheek JA, Staub GF. Nasojejunal alimentation for premature and fullterm newborn infants. J Pediatr 1973;82: 955–962.
43. Roy RN, Pollnitz RP, Hamilton JR, Chance GW. Impaired assimilation of nasojejunal feeds in healthy low-birth-weight newborn infants. J Pediatr 1977;90:431–434.
44. Loo SWH, Gross I, Warshaw JB. Improved method of nasojejunal feeding in low-birth-weight infants. J Pediatr 1974; 85:104–106.
45. Wells DH, Zachman RD. Nasojejunal feedings in low-birth-weight infants. J Pediatr 1975;87:276–279.
46. Rhea JW, Ghazzawi O, Weidman W. Nasojejunal feeding: an improved device and intubation technique. J Pediatr 1973;82:951–954.
47. Laing IA, Lang MA, Callaghan O, Hume R. Nasogastric compared with nasoduodenal feeding in low birthweight infants. Arch Dis Child 1986;61:138–141.
48. Antonson DL, Smith JL, Nelson RD, et al. The stability of vitamin and mineral concentrations of a low-birth-weight infant formula during continuous enteral feeding. J Pediatr Gastroenterol Nutr 1983;2:617–621.
49. Bhatia J, Fomon SJ. Formula for premature infants: fate of the calcium and phosphorus. Pediatrics 1983;72:37–40.
50. Greer FR, McCormick A, Loker J. Changes in fat concentration of human milk during delivery by intermittent bolus and continuous mechanical pump infusion. J Pediatr 1984; 105:745–749.
51. Krishnan V, Satish M. Continuous vs. intermittent nasogastric feeding in very low birth weight infants. Pediatr Res 1981; 15:537, abstract.
52. Parker P, Stroop S, Greene H. A controlled comparison of continuous versus intermittent feeding in the treatment of infants with intestinal disease. J Pediatr 1981;99: 360–364.
53. Pereira GR, Lemons JA. Controlled study of transpyloric and intermittent gavage feeding in the small preterm infant. Pediatrics 1981;67:68–72.
54. Whitfield MF. Poor weight gain of the low birthweight infant fed nasojejunally. Arch Dis Child 1982;57:597–601.
55. Van Caillie M, Powell GK. Nasoduodenal versus nasogastric

feeding in the very low birthweight infant. Pediatrics 1975;
56:1065-1072.

56. Pyati S, Ramamurthy R, Pildes RS. Continuous drip nasogastric feedings: a controlled study. Pediatr Res 1976;
10:359.

57. Whitelaw A, Sleath K. Myth of the marsupial mother: home care of very low birthweight babies in Bogota, Colombia. Lancet 1985;2:1206-1209.

58. Meier P, Pugh EJ. Breast-feeding behavior of small preterm infants. Matern Child Nurs 1985;10:396-401.

59. Pearce JL, Buchanan LF. Breast milk and breast feeding in very low birthweight infants. Arch Dis Child 1979;54:897-899.

60. Boggs KR, Rau PK. Breastfeeding the premature infant. Am J Nurs 1983;83:1437-1439.

61. Stuff J, Garza C, Boutte C, et al. Sources of variation in milk and calorie intakes in breast-fed infants: implications for lactation study design and interpretation. Am J Clin Nutr 1986;43:361-366.

62. Yu VYH, Jamieson J, Bajuk B. Breast milk feeding in very low birthweight infants. Aust Paediatr J 1981;17:186-190.

63. Bernbaum JC, Pereira GR, Watkins JB, Peckham GJ. Nonnutritive sucking during gavage feeding enhances growth and maturation in premature infants. Pediatrics 1983;71:41-45.

64. Field T, Ignatoff E, Stringer S, et al. Nonnutritive sucking during tube feedings: effects on preterm neonates in an intensive care unit. Pediatrics 1982;70:381-384.

20

Parenteral Nutrition
for the Neonate

WILLIAM B. PITTARD, III, M.D.
ABNER H. LEVKOFF, M.D.

ABSTRACT

As is true of many facets of neonatal care, the modern use of parenteral nutrition has evolved through several years of experience and numerous observations, leading to a vastly broadened physiologic understanding of infant growth needs. Although originally designed to support the growth and development of full-term infants who could not be fed enterally as a result of gastrointestinal abnormalities, parenteral nutrition has become a fundamental support for the extremely premature neonate. In this chapter, the principles of infant parenteral nutrition are covered in a developmental sequence. These principles have been divided into those unique to the first week of life in both the full-term and premature infant, and those more generally applicable to growth among all infants following the initial transition from intrauterine to extrauterine life. Specifically, a detailed discussion of water and electrolytes, calories, urinary solute, and minerals during the first week of life, divided into three physiologic phases of development, is given. The "period of growth" is developed first by defining the goals of parenteral nutrition and secondly by discussing basic nutrient components, including amino acids, carbohydrates, and lipids. Two major medical complications of parenteral nutrition, cholestasis and osteopenia, and their proposed etiology are reviewed. Finally, three case studies have been added to provide clinical insight.

INTRODUCTION

The challenge of providing optimal nutrition for low birthweight infants is to satisfy their growth needs in the face of physiologic and biochemical immaturity. In the smallest of preterm infants with marked gastrointestinal immaturity, it is often necessary to provide parenteral nutrition for 2-4 weeks, either as the sole source of nutrition or as a supplement to enteral feeding. It is the purpose of this chapter to describe some of the physiologic principles involved in supplying parenteral nutrition for infants during these first weeks of life, with emphasis placed on infants under 1500 gm, or the very low birthweight (VLBW) infant.

HISTORICAL PERSPECTIVE

The first documented success of total parenteral nutrition (TPN) in an infant was reported by Helfrick and Abelson in 1945. A 5-month-old infant with extreme marasmus showed dramatic improvement in nutritional status after 5 days of infusions of 50% dextrose, 10% casein hydrolysate, and olive oil lecithin emulsion.[1]

Twenty years passed before Dudrick and coworkers[2] in 1968 provided the breakthrough that made TPN a practical reality. These investigators showed first in Beagle puppies and subsequently in a newborn infant that satisfactory growth could be achieved with central venous nutrition. An infant girl with short bowel syndrome maintained adequate growth for over a year when infused with parenteral nutrition. The method of delivery devised by Dudrick was a catheter placed in the superior vena cava for continuous infusion of hypertonic glucose, protein hydrolysate, electrolytes, minerals and vitamins.

In 1972, in a series of publications, the team of Heird, Driscoll, and Winters[3-5] described their success with intravenous alimentation in pediatric patients. The types of patients they thought would benefit from parenteral nutrition included neonates with congenital malformations or extensive resections of their intestinal tracts, infants with chronic diarrhea and malabsorption, and small preterm infants whose immaturity made feeding difficult and predisposed them to pulmonary aspiration.

FIRST WEEK OF LIFE

The early period from birth to full enteral feedings may be divided into the first week of extrauterine adjustment and the ensuing weeks of postnatal growth. The first week may be further subdivided into three successive phases: the first is characterized by minimal urinary salt and water excretion; the second is characterized by negative salt, water and caloric balance; and the third is defined by the equilibration of body fluids and attainment of nutrient balance. These phases of postnatal water and sodium homeostasis are summarized in Table 1.

THE PRETERM INFANT

Water and Electrolytes

Important in the early adjustment to extrauterine life is the redistribution of body fluids associated with contraction of extracellular fluid volume.[6] In the very-low-birth-weight infant, this change is accompanied by weight loss, diuresis and enhanced urinary excretion of sodium (natriuresis). Sodium deficits of up to 16 mEq/kg[7] may be incurred during this time, and a weight loss of 10–15% of birth weight may be observed. **On the first day of life, in the smallest of preterm infants, the fractional sodium excretion may be as high as 10%** (of the filtered load) and may not recede to rates under 1% until the second week of life.[8]

In the presence of this obligatory natriuresis, it is not obvious when the parenteral administration of sodium should be started. Usually, none is provided during the first 24 hours of life when urinary sodium excretion is minimal. After that time, sodium usually is given in amounts that will not overcome the early negative sodium balance but will prevent hyponatremia and eventually will allow optimal

growth when the fractional sodium excretion "bottoms out." A quantity of 2–3 mEq/kg/day given as sodium chloride normally permits appropriate growth and the maintenance of a serum sodium concentration between 130 and 150 mEq/L. Some small preterm infants whose fractional sodium excretion remains high into the second week may require 2–3 times this amount of sodium.

During intrauterine life, the "large" extracellular fluid volume, the "high" fractional sodium excretion, and the "elevated" urine flow (10 ml/kg/hour)[9] serve the fetus well, perhaps providing him with an amniotic fluid volume that permits optimal growth and development. Like old soldiers, however, these features must fade away after birth. It may be inadvisable to provide fluid and electrolytes in quantities to match these losses in view of the reported associations with an increased incidence of necrotizing enterocolitis and patent ductus arteriosus.[10]

Unlike sodium, there is no obligatory potassium diuresis (kaluresis) in the first few days after delivery.[7] Intracellular fluid volume remains fairly constant during the adjustment to extrauterine life.[7] The potassium requirement, however, must be considered in the light of the low glomerular filtration rate in VLBW infants, the frequent presence of acidosis, and the release of nitrogen and potassium secondary to negative caloric balance. These factors predispose the infants to hyperkalemia in the first two days of life, and potassium administration usually can be omitted. Once serum potassium concentrations are documented to be normal and a normal urine flow rate has been established, potassium can be started at a rate of 2 mEq/kg/day.

TABLE 1.   Postnatal Phases of Water and Sodium Homeostasis

Age*	Birth–36 hrs	12–96 hrs	After 2–4 days
Renal function	GFR is low	GFR increases abruptly	GFR decreases slightly, then continues to slowly increase with maturation
	FENa† is low	FENa increases	FENa slowly decreases
Urinary output	Minimal regardless of intake—ability to excrete water and Na is most limited	Diuresis/natriuresis occurs independent of intake	Excretion of water and Na varies appropriately with intake
Balance	Water and Na balance remain unchanged on restricted intake	Water and Na balance become negative regardless of intake	Water and Na balance stabilize and then become positive with growth

*Time course is variable among infants and may be altered by disease. A detailed explanation of these phases is given in Chapter 4.
†FENa—fractional excretion of sodium.

The fact that the major source of evaporative water loss in the human is the skin surface rather than the respiratory tract places the small premature neonate at a disadvantage. The stratum corneum, the skin's vapor barrier, is underdeveloped in the immature newborn and permits increased rates of water loss in the first weeks before cornification takes place. Fluid losses are even more excessive if these infants are placed under radiant heat or phototherapy. **The effects of these two interventions are additive and can approximately triple the evaporative water loss in the VLBW infant.**[11] Thus, the environment, the gestational age, and the postpartum age are significant determinants of insensible water loss.

This large solute free-water loss seen in the first days of life, especially in infants under 27 weeks gestational age, threatens them with hypertonic dehydration when diuresis occurs. Fluid replacement during this time, while allowing for an average of 1-3% weight loss per day to a maximum of 8-15%, as the extracellular fluid volume contracts, must at least compensate for evaporative water loss.

Infants 25-27 weeks' gestational age, weighing between 700 and 900 gm and nursed in incubators with an ambient humidity of 50%, have transepithelial water losses (TEWL) as great as 125 ml/kg/day in the first 24 hours of life.[12] While the TEWL can be reduced with an increase in the environmental humidity beyond 50%, such levels of humidity are impractical because of "rainout" on incubator walls. Surprisingly, by the fifth day of life the TEWL decreases dramatically to a low of 50 ml/kg/day even at 50% humidity. In contrast, the small for gestational age (SGA) infant of the same weight but at 28–30 weeks of gestational age has a TEWL of less than 40 ml/kg/day even during the first 24 hours of life. Corneal layer thickness presumably accounts for these observations.

For fluid replacement in VLBW infants during the first days of life, when incubator humidity is approximately 50%, it is reasonable to follow the recommendations of Bell et al.[13] as modified by Nash,[14] utilizing 105 ml/kg/day (Table 2). The recommendation by Lorenz et al.[15] starting with 80 ml/kg/day in infants less than 1000 gm were derived from studies of infants cared for in "maximally" humidified incubators.

The appropriateness of neonatal fluid therapy is, in the clinical setting, most commonly monitored with daily weight assessments. In

TABLE 2. Fluids (ml/kg/day) During the First Weeks of Life*

Birthweight (g)	Day 1–2	Day 3	Day 15–30
750–1000	105	140	150
1001–1250	100	130	140
1251–1500	90	120	130
1501–1700	80	110	130
1701–2000	80	110	130
Term infant	70	80	100

*(Nash MA. Fluid and Electrolyte Disorders in the Neonate. Clin Perinatol 1981;8:2, 251.)

the most premature infant this weight assessment may need to be more than once a day. Weight losses from birth amounting to more than 10-15% are considered excessive and suggest an uncompensated TEWL. Similarly, there may be an associated increase in hematocrit, serum sodium, BUN and osmolality, or a decrease in urine output and increase in its concentration associated with negative water balance. There may also be an increased frequency of apneic episodes with negative water balance. On the other hand, if weight loss is less than 2% per day for the first 4-5 days, this may suggest excessive fluid administration.

Although it is not clear whether excess free-water administration in the absence of additional sodium chloride, particularly in the presence of high free water (insensible) losses, will predispose VLBW infants to necrotizing enterocolitis and patent ductus arteriosus,[10] it seems wise to practice restraint. To reduce the need for free-water administration, many nurseries use plastic heat shields and/or double walled isolettes. The use of plastic heat shields will significantly reduce (by almost half) the insensible water loss in infants of less than 1000 gm nursed in incubators.[16]

Calories

Energy reserves in the small premature infant as might be expected, are scant. Fat deposits are less than 5% of total body weight compared to over 15% in term infants.[17] What is perhaps even more critical is the diminished glycogen content of the liver. This glucose precursor can be depleted within hours after birth, leaving the brain deprived of its major source of metabolic fuel. An ameliorating factor is the infant's low, near-fetal, metabolic rate during the first week of life of 35-40 kcal/kg/day in a neutral thermal environment. This rate increases to approximately 50-55 kcal/kg/day in the second week of life. The cause of this increase is thought to be the increase in energy devoted to tissue synthesis.[18]

The organ of the body requiring the largest portion of metabolic expenditure is the brain. Further, the brain is able to utilize only glucose and ketone bodies as substrates. Reduced fat stores limit ketone body production in the VLBW infant. Thus, provision of exogenous glucose is as imperative as replacement of insensible water loss. Fortunately, the two are combined as the strategic fluid of parenteral nutrition during the first days of life. Optimal amounts of glucose during this time support normoglycemic blood concentrations between 40 and 125 mg/dl, provide calories to approximate resting metabolic rate (35-40 kcal/kg/day), and reduce negative nitrogen balance. In spite of the urgent need for glucose, there is a relative intolerance to intravenously administered glucose in the preterm infant.[19] This poor glucose tolerance is associated with a state of insulin resistance, especially in infants who are under 1000 gm. In these tiny neonates, rates of glucose administration exceeding 6 mg/kg/min are often not tolerated. Serum hyperosmolarity associated with hyperglycemia can produce an osmotic diuresis. A rise in blood sugar of 18 mg/dl will increase the serum osmolarity by 1 mOsm. Tolerance to glucose improves in the days following delivery. Thus, depending upon birth weight and postpartum age, **the usual rate of glucose administration is 5-9 mg/kg/min.** Interestingly, when amino acids are added to glucose, glucose tolerance improves.[20]

With diminishing rates of insensible water loss and the termination of the obligatory contraction of extracellular fluid, the period of negative water balance comes to an end on the third or fourth day of life. During this third phase, provision of adequate water for urinary solute excretion becomes a major consideration.

Urinary Solutes

The quantity of solutes to be excreted by the kidney varies from 7.5–15 mOsm/kg/day[21]: the lesser amount for infants actively growing, the greater amount for starving infants with endogenous catabolism. The solute sparing effect of growth reduces the renal solute load by

approximately 1 mOsm for each gram of weight gain.

The potential daily renal solute load of the parenteral infusate for a 1-kg infant is: sodium, 3 mOsm; potassium, 2 mOsm; chloride, 5 mOsm (assuming 1 mOsm = 1 mEq); and protein (2.5 gm), 13.2 mOsm (5.7 mOsm urea/g protein). If there is growth, the actual solute load presented to the kidney for excretion will be reduced proportionally from the potential renal solute in the intake. This results from some of the solute being retained in the new tissue (growth).

Minerals

Although calcium, magnesium, phosphorous, trace minerals and vitamins are often routinely added to parenteral alimentation fluid by the third day, the need for these nutrients in the first week of extrauterine adaptation is not well defined. During the first days of life, in the absence of growth, calcium requirements for normal neuromuscular stability and myocardial contractility are of concern. Classical signs of tetany, however, are difficult to diagnose in the small preterm infant. Normal serum calcium concentrations are needed for adequate calcium homeostasis.

The use of serum calcium concentrations for assessment of calcium homeostasis requires that one be aware of the normal decrease and spontaneous increase in serum calcium present in the first week of life.[22] In the preterm infant a level of less than 7.0 mg/dl has been defined as hypocalcemia, a value lower than that considered hypocalcemic in the term infant. The relationship during the first hours between ionized calcium, the physiologically active component, and total calcium may not be constant. Without the ability to determine ionized calcium, excessive treatment with this mineral is possible. Because of the number of adverse reactions associated with calcium infusion, especially local tissue injury, it may be the best decision to monitor serum concentration closely and administer this mineral when the concentration is below 6 or 7 mg/dl. Using recent highly specific electrodes, the lower limit of normal ionized calcium among infants born at term at the nadir of 24 hours of age has been proposed as 4.6 mg/dl.[23] Even lower ionized calcium concentrations (less than 3 mg/dl) have been observed in totally asymptomatic VLBW infants.[24]

Summary

In summary, for infants of birth weight 750-1500 gm nursed in incubators with an ambient humidity of 50%, it is reasonable to begin parenteral alimentation with 100 ml/kg/day of 7.5% dextrose. A larger quantitiy of fluid and a lower concentration of glucose are to be used in preterm infants weighing under 1000 gm, with careful observation of weight, serum glucose, serum electrolyte concentration and urine specific gravity.

By the third day, a 120-140 ml/kg infusion of 10% dextrose can be administered, with sodium and potassium having been added on the second or third day (Table 1). At this point, when caloric intake is 50 to 60 kcal/kg/day, amino acids are generally added in 0.5 gm/kg/day increments until the rate of 2.5 gm/kg/day is reached. At this level of nonprotein and protein nutrient intake, positive nitrogen balance can be achieved. It is important that one realize that the delivery of nonprotein calories should be about 60 kcal/kg/day prior to the initiation of protein. If fewer nonprotein calories are given and protein is added to the infusate, the protein will be utilized for energy and will not facilitate growth. A nutritional intake of 60 nonprotein kcal/kg/day plus 2.5 gm/kg/day of protein is a reasonable goal for the end of the first week. The amounts of nutrients are reduced proportionately if enteral feeding has been started during this time.

If total parenteral nutrition is to be maintained, additional calories are needed for growth; these calories are generally supplied in the form of lipids. Intrauterine accretion rates of 15 gm/kg/day can be observed when nonprotein calories reach approximately 80 kcal/kg/day in conjunction with 2.5-3.0 gm protein/kg/day.[25] It is important to keep in mind that small preterm infants cared for in incubators receiving more than 150 ml/kg/day are at risk for necrotizing enterocolitis and patent ductus arteriosus.[10]

TERM INFANT

In contrast to the VLBW infant, the appropriately grown newborn at term is blessed with nature's best intentions. His well-developed stratum corneum limits insensible water loss via the skin. Goodly stores of fat and liver glycogen provide reserves for metabolic fuel. The extracellular fluid content at birth is closer to the volume intended for extrauterine life. Renal tubular function, with a lower fractional sodium excretion, is in tune with the smaller postpartum change in extracellular fluid volume.[7] Gestational maturation has also led to an improved glomerular filtration rate that will facilitate the excretion of catabolic solutes and undue water loads. Thus, like a sailboat whose beam is broad, the well-endowed term infant (unlike the precarious preterm infant) is forgiving in matters of salt and water.

During the initial days of the first week, 70 ml/kg/day of water are adequate (Table 1). In term infants on the first day of life, the insensible water loss is only 0.5 ml/kg/day if the infant is in a neutral thermal environment at 50% relative humidity.[12] This amount of infusate will permit the usual postpartum contraction of body fluids, which is about one half that seen in the VLBW infants. Given as 10% dextrose, this amount of glucose plus the presence of endogenous fuel stores will usually maintain normoglycemia. The addition of electrolytes is timed as it is for the preterm infant as noted above. However, with a fractional sodium excretion of less than 1%, only 2 mEq/kg/day of sodium is necessary. At this point, toward the end of the first week when the infant is receiving 100 ml/kg/day of 10% dextrose with electrolytes, the decision to add amino acids must be made. If feedings are more than a few days away and the continuation of negative nitrogen balance appears inadvisable, amino acids should be started.

As previously stated 60 kcal/kg/day of nonprotein fuel are necessary to prevent the catabolism of nitrogenous nutrients. If the route of administration is to remain via peripheral vein, then 10% dextrose in the amounts of 150 ml/kg/day must be provided as the amount of amino acids infused reaches 2 gm/kg/day. This amount of water, though more than the term infant requires, can easily be handled by the normal kidney in the second week of life.

Though essential fatty acid deficiency does not threaten the term well-nourished infant as early as the VLBW infant, intravenous fats are necessary to supply additional calories for growth. Zlotkin has determined that intravenously fed term infants receiving 2 gm/kg/day of amino acids will accrete nitrogen at the same rate as the breastfed infant as long as a total of approximately 87 kcal/kg/day are being infused.[25]

Perhaps the decision to advance to total

parenteral nutrition at the end of the first week in the term infant should be based on the infant's nutritional status, as reflected by his ponderal index at birth. It is reasonable to assume that the growth-retarded infant is unable to tolerate continuing negative nitrogen balance. One must remember that perinatal asphyxia is one of the common nonsurgical conditions that necessitates short term parenteral alimentation in the term infant. Two common complications of this catastrophy are acute tubular necrosis and inappropriate secretion of antidiuretic hormone. In both instances it may be necessary to restrict fluid intake to amounts that do not exceed insensible water loss.

PERIOD OF GROWTH AND PARENTERAL NUTRITION

REFERENCE STANDARDS FOR GROWTH

The amount and composition of weight gain seen in the term newborn who is breastfed can be reasonably used as a reference standard for growth in gestationally mature infants.[26] No such yardstick exists for VLBW infants. In its place fetal accretion rates of nutrients factored for specific gestational age have been used as the measure for optimal postpartum growth.[27,28]

Whether this standard is appropriate is open to argument. It is reasonable to think that once "aquatic" life with its direct line to maternal energy deposits is over, a less turgid individual with increased fat reserves could better face the vicissitudes of extrauterine life.

The VLBW preterm infant, appropriately grown for gestational age (AGA), when fed standard cow-milk formula in amounts that provide 130 kcal/kg/day of metabolizable energy (ingested calories minus those lost in stool and urine), gains 17 gm/kg/day, a rate that is comparable to the fetus of similar gestational age.[18] **In the preterm neonate, the amount of daily fat accreted is approximately three times that of the fetus;** protein accretion is approximately the same and water accretion is less. Of interest is the fact that **the small for gestational age (SGA) infant of similar size accretes significantly less fat and less protein, but more water, on the same diet, while gaining the same amount of weight.**[29] The 130 kcal/kg/day of metabolizable energy provides the AGA neonate with approximately 60 kcal/kg/day for energy of oxidation, which satisfies his resting metabolic needs. The remainder of the nutrient energy is stored as tissue increment, 4 kcal/gm. Energy for the actual synthesis of tissue, which is a part of the energy of oxidation, amounts to appoximately 0.7 kcal/gm.[18]

TOTAL AND SUPPLEMENTAL PARENTERAL NUTRITION

Growth

Growth comparable to that seen in formula-fed infants can be achieved when all nutrients are provided by intravenous infusion. However as noted above, the composition of this growth remains a concern. Bone mineralization is frequently deficient. Of greater concern but difficult to evaluate is the effect of TPN on the growth and development of the central nervous system. In a controlled trial, Yu et al. demonstrated in immature infants whose birth weight was approximately 950 gm that TPN during the first 2 weeks of life was as safe and effective as formula feedings.[30] Mortality rates were the same in both groups. The premature neonates given TPN grew faster in the second week post-delivery and had a lower incidence of necrotizing enterocolitis than those who were formula-fed. Neurodevelopmental outcome was not assessed. The present trend toward the management of smaller and less mature infants will no doubt be associated with longer periods of TPN. Finding reliable ways to assess the effect of TPN on neurodevelopmental outcome in very small neonates is one of today's major unresolved questions.

Supplemental parenteral nutrition is commonly used in small preterm infants as they progress to full enteral feeding in the first weeks of life. In 1966, Cornblath et al.[31] reported that in infants under 1250 gm, intravenous infusion of 10% dextrose and 0.22% saline in the first 72 hours of life significantly reduced the mortality rate compared to two control groups who were given either formula, as tolerated, or only 10% glucose and .22% saline by nasogastric tube. Pildes et al.[32] in 1973 showed that infants under 1500 gm, supplemented with glucose, electrolytes and amino acids until full feedings were tolerated, gained weight faster and were discharged earlier than infants supplemented with only 5% glucose and 0.2% saline. There was no difference in mortality rates. Finally, Bryan et al.[33] in a similar study involving infants of 1300 gm birthweight, demonstrated not only more rapid growth but fewer apneic spells when nitrogen was supplemented.

Cashore et al.[34] utilized glucose, casein hydrolysate, and lipid to supplement formula feeding in infants under 1500 gm. They emphasized the importance of supplemental alimentation, since it required an average of 14 days for infants over 1000 gm and 25 days for those under 1000 gm to achieve full enteral feeding. Most infants gained weight at the fetal growth rate. Plasma amino acids were not measured in this study.

In all likelihood, the majority of neonatal intensive care units currently supplement preterm neonates with parenteral nutrition until full enteral feeding is achieved. The desire to reach fetal growth rates perhaps, in part, stems from Winick's work showing that malnutrition adversely effects the developing central nervous system.[35]

Amino Acid Solutions

The source of nitrogen today is a solution of crystalline amino acids, whereas 20 years ago it was the hydrolysate of either fibrin or casein.[3,36] Protein hydrolysates have several disadvantages compared to crystalline amino acids that have lead to the almost exclusive use of the latter. These disadvantages include (1) fixed amino acid composition, (2) large amounts of free ammonia, and (3) insoluble forms of cystine and tyrosine. When compared to newborns receiving protein hydrolysates, newborns receiving crystalline amino acids demonstrated improved growth and nitrogen retention.[37] Furthermore, there were fewer biochemical aberrations (abnormal blood pH, elevated serum ammonia concentrations, and abnormal plasma amino acid concentrations) seen in newborns receiving crystalline amino acids.

Present day amino acid solutions, which Stegink[36] classifies as third generation mixtures, differ from earlier solutions in that the metabolically inactive D-stereoisomer of alpha amino acids has largely been eliminated, leaving the L-form, which is the only form utilized by humans (Table 3). Compared to human milk and fetal growth models, present mixtures are still heavily weighted with glycine but low in tyrosine and cystine. On the other hand, the inappropriate balance of hydrogen-ion-absorbing amino acids and hydrogen-ion-producing amino acids that previously led to metabolic acidosis in small preterm infants has been corrected by increasing the content of acetate salts. Indeed, a tendency to develop mild alkalosis has been reported with the use

TABLE 3. Development of Amino Acid Solutions for Parenteral Use

Generation	Composition
I	Protein hydrolysates
II	Early solutions of crystalline amino acids
III	Current solutions of crystalline amino acids
IV	Amino acid solutions currently under development and testing

of newer amino acid solutions containing increased amounts of acetate salts.[38] Future amino acid mixtures may be tailored for LBW infants controlling for gestational age.

Glucose

The establishment of positive nitrogen balance is dependent on nonprotein calories as well as nitrogenous nutrients. Early attempts at total parenteral nutrition depended almost exclusively on glucose for nonprotein energy. Supplemental transfusions were used as a source of essential fatty acids and trace minerals. More recently, intravenous infusion of lipid has been used as a supplemental energy source that also provides essential fatty acids.

Although hepatic injury has been associated with the use of glucose as the sole source of energy,[39] the most obvious limitation to the use of glucose in parenteral nutrition is its osmolality. Most nurseries limit the concentration of glucose infusion in peripheral parenteral nutrition to 10-12 gm/dl, because greater concentrations result in necrosis of tissue and even full-thickness slough if subcutaneous tissue infiltration occurs. Further, as noted above, glucose tolerance is limited in the most preterm infants. Hyperglycemia and its attendant osmotic diuresis occur regularly in VLBW infants with initial infusion rates in excess of 8 mg/kg/min.

Lipids

Currently available lipid products are marketed as a 10% lipid emulsion of soybean or safflower oil containing 1.1 kcal/ml (1.0 kcal/ml from the lipid and 0.1 kcal/ml from the lipid glycerol carrier). These lipid solutions provide essential fatty acids primarily as linoleic acid. This form of nonprotein calories has minimal osmolality and, although complications with its use have been reported,[40-42] it is in general tolerated metabolically by the neonate and has been shown to facilitate positive nitrogen balance as well as glucose.[43]

Metabolism of infused fat emulsions is similar to that of enterally derived chylomicrons and is dependent on lipoprotein lipase activity. This lipase activity is the rate-limiting enzymatic step in the hydrolysis of circulating protein-bound triglycerides. The infusion of lipid is generally started at 0.5 gm/kg/day and is slowly increased to 2-3 gm/kg/day. Essential fatty acid deficiency can be prevented when linoleic acid is given in amounts that constitute 1-2% of total caloric input. This amount can be provided by 0.5 gm/kg/day of lipid.[44]

Fattyacidemia can be avoided by intermittent intravenous fat administration at the rate of 0.15 gm/kg/hr for 18 hours each day.[45] The 6 hours of interrupted infusion ensures cyclic regeneration of necessary enzymes. Although no absolute numbers have been reported, serum triglyceride concentrations probably should be monitored at least biweekly and lipid infusion reduced if the triglyceride concentration is greater than 200 mg/dl after the 6 hours of interrupted infusion. Hyperlipidemia has been more commonly reported in preterm (less than 32 weeks' gestation) than in full term infants.[46] Similarly, hyperlipidemia has been noted to be more common in intrauterine growth-retarded neonates than in appropriately grown infants. Although hyperlipidemia has in the recent past been monitored by visual inspection of serum in a spun hematocrit tube, this practice has been shown to be unreliable.[47] Hyperlipidemia may adversely affect pulmonary gas exchange, which is a particularly significant concern for the preterm neonate who already may have major difficulty in this area related to his immature lung status.[42] Finally, one interesting report describes lipid deposits in the wall of the pulmonary artery in three preterm infants treated with intravenous lipid infusion.[48]

COMPLICATIONS OF PARENTERAL ALIMENTATION

Perhaps the two major clinical concerns today regarding parenteral nutrition in the VLBW infant are cholestasis and osteopenia. Discussion of these two nutritional dilemmas occupies much of the time currently expended during nursery rounds.

Cholestasis

Parenteral-nutrition cholestasis, like necrotizing enterocolitis, appears to be the end result of a disease process stemming from a multifactorial etiology. It is clearly more common in smaller, more immature, and more asphyxiated infants,[49-50] and it is more frequently observed with prolonged periods of parenteral nutrition than with shorter periods of support. Hepatic injury may well result from one or more components in the nutrient infusate. This injury appears to be superimposed on a "transient cholestasis" present normally in neonates and manifested by reduced hepatocyte uptake and conjugation of bile acids.[51,52] The primary physiologic derangement of cholestasis with parenteral nutrition is thus an exacerbation of a normally transient hepatocyte dysfunction of neonates. This results in both an increase in serum bile acid concentration and a decrease in intestinal bile salt concentration, with an overall impairment in biliary secretion. Perhaps the earliest clinical manifestation of this hepatic injury is direct hyperbilirubinemia (greater than 2 mg/dl).

Although the dextrose content of parenteral alimentation fluid has been implicated as a cause of this exacerbated hepatic dysfunction and cholestasis, the protein or more specifically the amino acids in the infusate clearly have been shown to be detrimental to hepatocyte function.[53] In one clinical study, the onset of cholestasis was earlier and more severe in neonates parenterally receiving greater amounts of amino acids.[54] Further, a significant correlation has been reported between the total amount of amino acids infused in neonates and their serum bile acid concentration.[55] Finally, in laboratory animals, a reduction in bile flow has been reported with the continuous infusion of amino acid solutions.[56] An interesting but probably infrequent mechanism for parenteral nutrition associated cholestasis is "bile sludge" in the gall bladder and secondary obstruction in the common bile duct.[57] Although bile sludge may be one mechanism for cholestasis, the current speculation is that a continuous infusion of amino acids in neonates results in competition between the amino acids and bile acids for hepatocellular uptake and secondarily results in reduced bile secretion. This scenario perhaps is worsened by the frequent lack of enteral feeding for these neonates, since fasting decreases gut hormones such as secretin and motilin that normally stimulate biliary secretion.[58]

Osteopenia

Osteopenia and even pathologic bone fractures in VLBW infants are associated with inadequate bone mineralization. This observation is commonly made in immature infants receiving prolonged parenteral alimentation. The etiology of the change in bone density is probably multifactorial. Inadequate concentrations of infused calcium, phosphorus or vitamin D can be potentially at fault.

Currently, the optimal calcium and phosphorus composition of parenteral fluid for VLBW infants is not known. If placental transfer of calcium from mother to fetus is evaluated, one finds that fetuses of 800-1200 gm birthweight receive calcium and phosphorus at 100-150 mg/kg/day and 60-80 mg/kg/day, respectively.[59] The delivery of this amount of calcium and phosphorus without infusing large (unsafe) volumes of fluid is difficult secondary to the tendency of these minerals to precipitate in solution at greater concentrations. This precipitation is largely related to the physical and chemical properties of the alimentation fluid, such as pH and temperature, and dextrose, amino acid, and most emphatically mineral concentration. Recently, it has been shown that a 2% amino acid solution (Aminosyn) containing 10% dextrose at a pH range of 5.5-5.8 can maintain in solution adequate amounts of calcium and phosphorus to provide fetal amounts of mineral in a volume of 150 ml/kg/day.[60]

Finally, a 2 to 1 ratio between calcium and phosphorus content has long been a goal for enteral feeding, and this goal has been rightly or wrongly extended to parenteral nutrition fluid. Perhaps because this ratio is observed in human milk and bone deposition, it has been teleologically accepted as optimal. The validity of this reasoning has been questioned.[61-63] The true optimal calcium/phosphorus ratio for neonatal parenteral fluid is not known, but for VLBW infants the placental delivery rates of 100-150 mg/kg/day for calcium and 40-60 mg/kg/day for phosphorus appear reasonable.

An even more interesting question regarding calcium homeostasis is the need for vitamin D and the form of vitamin D needed. Although vitamin D_2 and D_3 are both efficiently absorbed by VLBW infants, the hepatic conversion of either one to the 25 hydroxy metabolite may be limited in these small infants.[64] These data are derived from studies involving enteral alimentation and their relevance for parenteral alimentation is speculative.

Interestingly, the data that are available regarding parenteral administration of vitamin D are contradictory and are derived from older children and adults rather than neonates. These data raise questions concerning the need or safety of adding vitamin D to parenteral nutrition fluids. In a few adult patients with severe bone demineralization, when vitamin D was removed from the parenteral fluid, urinary calcium excretion decreased, serum calcium normalized, and patients returned to a positive calcium balance.[65] Since data indicating differing results have also been published,[66] and no neonatal data are readily available, the vitamin D issue for neonatal parenteral nutrition is currently unclear. Nevertheless, the current practice in many nurseries is to include 400-800 IU vitamin D/liter of fluid.

SUMMARY

Providing optimal nutrition by parenteral alimentation for VLBW infants remains a major challenge. However, there is now a clear understanding of salt and water needs in the first week of life, when large insensible water losses and obligatory changes in body fluid spaces are occurring. The needs and apportionment of nitrogen and nonprotein calories have been well analyzed in growing preterm infants. With the evolution of lipid emulsions and crystalline amino acid preparations, satisfactory methods of providing these basic needs by safe peripheral infusion are in place. On the other hand, parenteral provision of minerals and vitamins that will support normal bone growth requires further elucidation.

Perhaps the remaining enigma is the effect of TPN on the developing central nervous system. It will be necessary to find ways to evaluate brain function as affected by nutrition versus other environmental stresses. Perhaps newer techniques of brain imaging, evoked responses, or spectral analysis of the electroencephalogram will be useful tools.

It must be remembered that optimal nutrition may be more critical to the recovery of the injured brain than any treatment modality in use today.

Challenges remain.

1mg Ca = ¼ mmol Ca   25 mmol - 37.5 mmol.

CASE REPORTS

Case 1. A 1020-gm male infant was born by spontaneous vaginal delivery at 29 weeks' gestation to a 20-year-old mother whose pregnancy was complicated by mild hypertension and premature rupture of membranes of 2 hours' duration. The one-minute Apgar was 2. The infant was resuscitated with endotracheal intubation and was assigned a 5-minute Apgar of 7. Ventilator support was continued, an umbilical artery catheter was positioned, and a blood culture was obtained. Parenteral administration of 7.5% dextrose in water was begun at a rate of 100 ml/kg/day. Laboratory values revealed a serum sodium of 135 mEq/L, potassium 6.1 mEq/L, and calcium 7.5 mg/dl. Blood glucose was 88 mg/dl. A complete blood count (CBC) and differential were unremarkable and a chest x-ray revealed no intrathoracic pathology. Intravenous ampicillin and gentamicin were begun.

The infant's weight was 980 gm at 24 hours of age. Urine output was 2.2 ml/kg/hour. He was extubated at 14 hours of age and required no oxygen therapy thereafter. Serum electrolytes and BUN as well as calcium and glucose were within normal limits. The umbilical artery catheter was removed during the first day and a solution of 10% dextrose containing 2 mEq NaCl per 100 ml was administered at a rate of 110 ml/kg/day via peripheral vein after 24 hours.

At the beginning of the third day, the infant weighed 955 gm. Urine output was normal and admission blood culture was negative. Serum sodium was 133 mEq/L, potassium 4.8 mEq/L, calcium 8.2 mg/dl and glucose 105 mg/dl. Parenteral fluids were increased to 130 ml/kg/day and 1.5 mEq of potassium chloride per 100 ml was added. Antibiotics were discontinued.

On day 4, the infant's weight was 930 gm. Several short episodes of apnea without bradycardia occurred. There was no cyanosis or color change and perfusion was good. There was also a report of a heme positive stool, but no abdominal distention. X-ray of the abdomen revealed a normal gas pattern; platelet count, CBC and differential were within normal limits. Serum indirect bilirubin was 8.0 mg/dl. Serum electrolytes, calcium and blood urea nitrogen (BUN) were unremarkable. Blood glucose was 105 mg/dl. A polyionic solution* containing 10% dextrose, 0.5% crystalline amino acids, calcium, phosphorus, magnesium, trace minerals and multiple vitamins was administered at a rate of 150 ml/kg/day.

On day 5, the infant's weight was 920 gm. His condition was stable. Serum indirect bilirubin was 9 mg/dl. One out of three stools was reported heme positive. Blood chemistries were within normal limits. BUN was 12 mg/dl and creatinine was 1.1 mg/dl. The polyionic solution was continued with 1% crystalline amino acid at a rate of 160 ml/kg/day.

On day 6, the infant's weight was 930 gm. All stools were negative for occult blood. Serum bilirubin was 6.2 mg/dl. BUN was 14 mg/dl. The polyionic solution with 10% dextrose was continued at a rate of 150 ml/kg/day with 1.5% crystalline amino acids.

On day 7, the infant's weight was 935 gm. Laboratory values included hematocrit 42%, BUN 15 mg/dl and blood glucose 110 mg/dl. The polyionic solution was increased to 2% crystalline amino acids and was given at a rate of 150 ml/kg/day. A 10% lipid emulsion was started at a rate of 1 gm lipid/kg/day infused over a period of 18 hours.

On day 8, the infant's weight was 945 gm. Serum bilirubin was 7.2 mg/dl, BUN 15 mg/dl, blood glucose 115 mg/dl. Serum electrolytes and calcium were within normal limits. The polyionic solution was continued at 150 ml/kg/day containing 10% dextrose and 2% crystalline amino acid. The 10% lipid emulsion was increased to provide 2 gm lipid/kg/day. On the ensuing days, enteral feedings were gradually increased with a comparable decrease in parenteral nutrition.

Questions and Answers

Q.   When would positive nitrogen balance have been anticipated in this neonate?
A.   The data in current literature indicate that a positive nitrogen balance can be achieved in a neonate with parenteral nutrition when the infant is receiving 2.5 gm/kg/day of protein and a total nonprotein calorie intake of 60 kcal/kg/day. This should have been achieved in this infant between day 6 and day 7, when he received a polyionic solution containing 10% dextrose and 1.5-2% crystalline amino acid at a rate of 150 ml/kg/day. This intravenous therapy delivered to this 1-kg neonate was 16 gm of glucose or about 64 kcal/kg/day and simultaneously 2-2.5 gm/kg/day of protein.

Q.   What factors regulated initiation of protein infusion?
A.   In this case, other than the obvious lack of enteral feeding, the major regulatory factors for initiation of protein infusion were nonprotein calorie intake to meet the basal energy needs of the infant and the routine practice of allowing fluid changes associated with intrauterine to extrauterine transition (contraction of extracellular fluid space, obligate sodium diuresis, increase in glomerular filtration rate and decrease in transepidermal water loss) to occur.

Q.   Is lipid infusion necessary?
A.   Essential fatty acids are required for normal body metabolism; however, as an energy source per se, lipids were not required in this infant to achieve a positive nitrogen balance.

---

*Polyionic solution composition per 100 ml:
Sodium   2.2 mEq
Potassium   1.3 mEq
Chloride   2.2 mEq
Acetate   0.6 mEq
Phosphate   0.5 mmol (equivalent to 15.5 mg P)
Calcium Gluc.   1.0 mEq (equivalent to 20 mg Ca)
Magnesium SO4   0.3 mEq (equivalent to 37 mg Mg)
Heparin   0.5 unit/cc
Neonatal trace minerals   0.2 cc
Multivitamin pediatric

Case 2. A 2750-gm, 43-week gestation female infant was delivered through heavily meconium-stained amniotic fluid. She had her oropharynx suctioned via a DeLee catheter on the mother's perineum but was depressed with minimal tone and no respiratory effort. The infant was briefly dried and placed in a heat-gaining environment. There was rapid improvement in color and respiration with blow-by oxygen (100%), although the tone continued to be somewhat depressed. The Apgar scores were assigned as 4 at 1 minute and 6 at 5 minutes. The initial chest x-ray revealed bilateral pulmonary infiltrates and cardiomegaly.

An umbilical arterial catheter was positioned in the delivery room and an arterial blood gas was obtained that revealed a mixed respiratory/metabolic acidosis with pH 7.24, PCO_2 56 mmHg, and a bicarbonate of 13 mEq/L. Blood glucose and hematocrit were normal. Intravenous fluid of 10% dextrose in water was begun at 70 ml/kg/day and the child was transferred to the intermediate care nursery. In the nursery a complete blood count and white blood cell differential were drawn and cultures were obtained. The infant was started on antibiotics, and parenteral fluids were continued at 70 ml/kg/day of 10% dextrose. Clear urine was observed 4 hours after birth and output continued at a rate of approximately 2 ml/kg/hr. Urinalysis revealed no red blood cells. Normal abdominal peristaltic sounds were heard.

After 30 hours the child was started on 20-ml feeds of half-strength standard infant formula every 3 hours. Progressively, the enteral feeds were increased to full strength and full volume (60–90 ml every 3 hours), and the parenteral fluids were reduced and then discontinued commensurate with increasing the enteral feeds. Urine output was consistently greater than 1 ml/kg/hour and no proteinuria or hematuria were ever detected. By 3 days of age the infant was on full feeds, all cultures were negative, and she was deemed ready for discharge.

Questions and Answers

Q.   Why was no enteral feeding begun in the first 30 hours of the neonates life?
A.   Asphyxiated term infants are assumed to have experienced limited oxygen and blood flow to organs such as the kidneys and gut, as oxygen is preferentially supplied to other organs, such as the heart, adrenal glands, and brain in such circumstances. Thus, until a period of stabilization has occurred, all enteral feeding is withheld and fluid and energy (glucose) are supplied intravenously as 10% dextrose in water at approximately 70 ml/kg/day.

Q.   Why was 70 ml/kg/day of 10% dextrose in water given to this infant in the first 24 hours of life?
A.   The normal physiologic hepatic output of glucose is about 5–7 mg/kg/min. Intravenous 10% dextrose in water delivered at 70 ml/kg/day will supply 4–5 mg/kg/min to the infant. This infusion should prevent hypoglycemia in the neonate and simultaneously allow mild fluid restriction.

Q.   Why was half-strength, rather than full-strength, formula started when enteral feeding was begun?
A.   Half-strength formula is commonly used clinically to feed neonates when there is concern about the presence of gut injury (as in this case) and secondary feeding intolerance. The assumption is that the half-strength feeding will be better tolerated than full-strength formula by the injured intestine, perhaps due to its lower osmolality.

Case 3. A 2400-gm, 37-week gestation male infant was delivered by emergency cesarean section following acute onset of painful vaginal bleeding in the mother. The infant was severely depressed with Apgar scores assigned as 0 at 1 minute and 2 at 5 minutes. The infant was placed in a heat-gaining environment, was quickly dried, and had an umbilical aterial catheter (UAC) positioned at T-10. Initial

blood hematocrit was 58% and blood glucose was 40 mg/dl. Arterial blood gas on 40% FiO_2 revealed pH 7.14, PCO_2 48, PO_2 56 mmHg, and a bicarbonate level of 17 mEq/L. Intravenous delivery of 10% dextrose via UAC was started at 70 ml/kg/day and the infant was transferred to the intensive care nursery.

Initially, he did well; however, he subsequently had oliguria with 0.6 ml/kg/hr urine output in which there were significant amounts of blood and protein. Fluids were continued at 80 ml/kg/day after 24 hours, providing approximately 5 mg/kg/min of glucose. The blood glucose remained at 45 mg/dl.

After 48 hours the urine output increased to approximately 1.5 ml/kg/hour and the parenteral infusion was increased from 80-120 ml/kg/day. Enteral feeds were initiated on day 3 of life with half-strength 20 calorie/ounce feeds at 20 ml every 3 hours. Parenteral fluids were reduced proportionally. By day 6, the infant was on oral feeds of full-strength 20 calorie/ounce formula receiving 45-60 ml every 3 hours, or 170 ml/kg/day. His urine output was well above 1 ml/kg/hr and he had only trace proteinuria with no hematuria. He was ready for discharge.

Questions and Answers

Q.   Why was the urine production reduced initially, and why was there blood and protein in the urine?
A.   When blood flow is limited to the kidney, as in neonatal asphyxia, the associated hypoxia and ischemia are often also associated with renal tubular injury. This renal injury is clinically manifest by oliguria, proteinuria, and/or hematuria.

Q.   Why was parenteral nutrition, including protein and fat, not begun initially?
A.   Initially nutrition was supplied with 10% dextrose in water delivered at 70 ml/kg/day. This is a bit beyond the estimated newborn maintenance requirement for fluid of 40 ml/kg/day and was elected secondary to the asphyxia with renal injury, which was confirmed by his initial 24-hour urine output of 0.6 ml/kg/hour. Since enteral feeding was well tolerated on day 3, parenteral fat and protein were not required.

REFERENCES

1. Helfrick FW, Abelson NM. Intravenous feeding of a complete diet in a child: Report of a case. J Pediatr 1944;25:400–403.
2. Dudrick SJ, Wilmore DW, Vars HM, Rhoads JE. Long-term total parenteral nutrition with growth, development, and positive nitrogen balance. Surgery 1968;64:134–142.
3. Heird WC, Winters RW. Total parenteral nutrition: The state of the art. J Pediatr 1975;86:2–16.
4. Heird WC, Driscoll JM Jr, Shullinger JN, et al. Intravenous alimentation in pediatric patients. J Pediatr 1972;80:351–372.
5. Driscoll JM Jr, Heird WC, Schullinger JN, et al. Total intravenous alimentation in low-birth-weight infants: A preliminary report. J Pediatr 1972;81:145–153.
6. Shaffer G, Bradt S, Hall R. Postnatal changes in total body water and extracellular volume in the preterm infant with respiratory distress syndrome. J Pediatr 1986;109:509–514.
7. Butterfield J, Lubchenco LO, Bergstedt J, O'Brien D. Patterns in electrolyte and nitrogen balance in the newborn premature infant. Pediatrics 1960;26:777–791.

8. Engelke SC, Shah BL, Vasan U, Raye JR. Sodium balance in very low-birth-weight infants. J Pediatr 1978;93: 837–841.
9. Campbell S, Wladimiroff JW, Dewhurst CJ. The antenatal measurement of fetal urine production. J Obstet Gynaec Br Common 1973;80:680–686.
10. Bell EF, Warburton D, Stonestreet BS, Oh W. Effect of fluid administration on the development of symptomatic patent ductus arteriosus and congestive heart failure in premature infants. N Engl J Med 1980;302:598–604.
11. Wu PYK, Hodgman JE. Insensible water loss in preterm infants: Changes with postnatal development and non-ionizing radiant energy. Pediatrics 1974;54:704–712.
12. Hammarlund K, Sedin G, Stromberg B. Transepidermal water loss in newborn infants: Relation to gestational age and postnatal age in appropriate and small for gestational age infants. Acta Paediatr Scand 1983;72:721–728.
13. Bell FB, Warburton D, Stonestreet BS, Oh W. High-volume fluid intake predisposes premature infants to necrotizing enterocolitis. Lancet 1979;2:90.
14. Nash MA. The management of fluid and electrolyte disorders in the neonate. Clin Perinatol 1981;8:251–262.
15. Lorenz JM, Kleinman LI, Kotagal UR, Reller MD. Water balance in very low-birth-weight infants: Relationship to water and sodium intake and effect on outcome. J Pediatr 1982;101(3):423–432.
16. Fanaroff AA, Wald M, Gruber HS, Klaus MH. Insensible water loss in low birth weight infants. Pediatrics 1972;50:236–245.
17. **Widdowson E. Changes in body proportion and composition during growth. In Davis JH, Dobbing J (eds): Scientific Foundations of Paediatrics. London, William Heinemann Medical Books Ltd., 1974; 123.**
18. Chessex P, Reichman BL, Verellen GJE, et al. Influence of postnatal age, energy intake, and weight gain or energy metabolism in the very low-birth-weight infant. J Pediatr 1981;99:761–766.
19. Goldman SL, Hirata T. Attenuated response to insulin in very low birthweight infants. Pediatr Res 1980;14:50–53.
20. Chance GW. Results in very low birth weight infants (1300 gm birth weight). In Winters RW, Hasselmeger EG (eds): Intravenous Nutrition in the High Risk Infant. New York, John Wiley and Sons. 1975;79.
21. Roy RN, Sinclair JC. Hydration of the low birth-weight infant. Clin Perinatol 1975;2:393–417.
22. Salle BL, David L, Chopard JP, et al. Prevention of early neonatal hypocalcemia in low birth weight infants with continuous calcium infusion: Effect on serum calcium, phosphorus, magnesium, and circulating immunoreactive parathyroid hormone and calcitonin. Pediatr Res 1977;11:1180–1185.
23. Longhead J, Mimouni F, Tsang RA. Redefinition of neonatal hypocalcemia (in press).
24. Koo WWK, Tsang RC, Steichen JJ, et al. Parenteral nutrition for infants: Effects of high versus low calcium and phosphorus content. J Pediatr Gastroent Nutri (in press).
25. Zlotkin SH, Bryan MH, Anderson GH. Intravenous nitrogen and energy intakes required to duplicate in utero nitrogen accretion in prematurely born human infants. J Pediatr 1981;99:115–120.
26. AAP, CON: Commentary on breast-feeding and infant formulas, including proposed standards for formula. Pediatrics 1976;57:278–285.
27. Ziegler EE, O'Donnell AM, Nelson SE, Fomon SJ. Body composition of the reference fetus. Growth 1976;40:329–341.
28. Ziegler EE, Biga RL, Fomon SJ. Nutritional requirements of the premature infant. In Suskind RM (ed): Textbook of Pediatric Nutrition. New York: Raven Press, 1981.
29. Chessex P, Reichman B, Verellen G, et al. Metabolic consequences of intrauterine growth retardation in low birthweight infants. Pediatr Res 1984;18:709–713.
30. Yu VYH, James B, Hendry P, MacMahon RA. Total parenteral nutrition in very low birth weight infants: A controlled trial. Arch Dis Child 1979;54:653–661.
31. Cornblath M, Forbes AE, Pildes RS, et al. A controlled study of

early fluid administration on survival of low birth weight infants. Pediatrics 1966;38:547–554.
32. Pildes RS, Ramamurthy RS, Cordero GV, Wong PWK. Intravenous supplementation of L-amino acids and dextrose in low-birth-weight infants. J Pediatr 1973;82:945–950.
33. Bryan MH, Wei P, Hamilton JR, et al. Supplemental intravenous alimentation in low-birth-weight infants. J Pediatr 1973;82:940–944.
34. Cashore WJ, Sedaghatian MR, Usher RH. Nutritional supplements with intravenously administered lipid, protein hydrolysate, and glucose in small premature infants. Pediatrics 1975;56:8–16.
35. Winick M. Malnutrition and brain development. J Pediatr 1969;74:667–679.
36. Stegink LD. Amino acids in pediatric parenteral nutrition: Solutions infused—lessons learned. Am J Dis Child 1983; 137:1008–1016.
37. Duffy B, Gunn T, Collinge J, Pencharz P. The effect of varying protein quality and energy intake on the nitrogen metabolism of parenterally fed very low birthweight (1600 g) infants. Pediatr Res 1981;15:1040–1044.
38. Heird WC. Studies of pediatric patients receiving Aminosyn as the nitrogen source of total parenteral nutrition. In Barlow AL (ed). Current Approaches to Nutrition of the Hospitalized Patient. North Chicago, Illinois, Abbott Press, 1975;45–49.
39. Thaler MM. Liver dysfunction and disease associated with total parenteral alimentation. ASPEN Sixth Clinical Conference, San Francisco, 1982;67.
40. Greene HL, Hazlett D, Demaree R. Relationship between Intralipid-induced hyperlipemia and pulmonary function. Am J Clin Nutr 1976;29:127–135.
41. Levene MI, Wigglesworth JS, Desai R. Pulmonary fat accumulation after intralipid infusion in the preterm infant. Lancet 1980;2:815–818.
42. Friedman Z, et al. Effect of parenteral fat emulsion on the pulmonary and reticuloendothelial systems in the newborn infant. Pediatrics 1978;61:694–698.
43. Rubecz I, Mestyan J, Varga P, Klujber L. Energy metabolism, substrate utilization, and nitrogen balance in parenterally fed postoperative neonates and infants: The effect of glucose, glucose + amino acids, lipid + amino acids infused in isocaloric amounts. J Pediatr 1981;98:42–46.
44. Kerner JA. Fat requirements. In Kerner JA (ed): Manual of Pediatric Parenteral Nutrition. New York, John Wiley and Sons, 1983;103.
45. Das JB, Joshi ID, Philippart AI. Depression of glucose utilization by Intralipid in the post-traumatic period: An experimental study. J Pediatr Surg 1980;15:739–745.
46. Shennan AT, Bryan MH, Angel A. The effect of gestational age on Intralipid tolerance in newborn infants. J Pediatr 1977;91:134–137.
47. Schreiner RL, Glick MR, Nordschow CD, Gresham EL. An evaluation of methods to monitor infants receiving intravenous lipids. J Pediatr 1979;94:197–200.
48. Dahms BB, Halpin TC Jr. Pulmonary arterial lipid deposit in newborn infants receiving intravenous lipid infusion. J Pediatr 1980;97:800–805.
49. Pereira GR, et al. Hyperalimentation-induced cholestasis: Increased incidence and severity in premature infants. Am J Dis Child 1981;135:842–845.
50. Dosi PC, Raut AJ, Bhaktharai P, et al. Perinatal factors underlying neonatal cholestasis. J Pediatr 1985;106:471–474.
51. Balistreri WF, Heubi JE, Suchy FJ. Immaturity of the enterohepatic circulation early life: Factors predisposing to "physiologic" maldigestion and cholestasis. J Pediatr Gastroenterol Nutr 1983;2:346–354.
52. Suchy FJ, Balistreri WF, Heubi JE, et al. Physiologic cholestasis: Elevation of the primary serum bile acid concentrations in normal infants. Gastroenterology 1981; 80:1037.
53. Vileisis RA, Inwood RJ, Hunt CE. Prospective controlled study of parenteral nutrition-associated cholestatic jaundice: Effect of protein intake. J Pediatr 1980;96:893–897.
54. Preisig R, Rennert O. Biliary transport and cholestatic effects

of amino acids (abstract). Gastroenterology 1977; 73:1240.

55. Touloukian RJ, Downing SE. Cholestasis associated with long-term parenteral hyperalimentation. Arch Surg 1973; 106:58–62.

56. Zahavi I, Shaffer EA, Gall DG. Total parenteral nutrition (TPN) associated cholestasis in infant and adult rabbits (abstract). Gastroenterology 1982;82:1217.

57. Enzenauer RW, Montrey JS, Bareia PJ, Woods J. Total parenteral nutrition cholestasis: A cause of mechanical biliary obstruction. Pediatrics 1985;76:905–908.

58. Rager R, Finegold MJ. Cholestasis in immature newborn infants: Is parenteral alimentation responsible? J Pediatr 1975;86:264–269.

59. Delivoria-Papadopoulos M, et al. Total, protein-bound, and ultrafilterable calcium in maternal and fetal plasmas. Am J Physiol 1967;213:363–366.

60. Poole RL. Problems with preparation of parenteral nutrition solutions. In Kerner JA (ed): Manual of Pediatric Parenteral Nutrition. New York, John Wiley and Sons, 1983;177.

61. Moya M, Domenech E. Role of calcium phosphate ratio of milk formulae on calcium balance in low birth weight infants during the first three days of life. Pediatr Res 1982;16:675–681.

62. Senterre J, Putet G, Salle B, Rigo J. Effects of vitamin D and phosphorous supplementation on calcium retention in preterm infants fed banked human milk. J Pediatr 1983; 103:305–307.

63. Widdowson E, McCance R, Harrison G, Sutton A. Effect of giving phosphate supplements to breastfed babies on absorption and excretion of calcium, strontium, magnesium, and phosphorous. Lancet 1963;2:1250–1251.

64. Hollis BW, Pittard WB III. Evidence for a maturational change in the ability to convert vitamin D to 25-hydroxy vitamin D in neonates (abstract). Pediatr Res 1986;20:412A.

65. Shike M, et al. Metabolic bone disease in patients receiving long term total parenteral nutrition. Ann Intern Med 1980;92:343–350.

66. Klein GL, et al. Infantile vitamin D-resistant rickets associated with total parenteral nutrition. Am J Dis Child 1982;136: 74–76.

21

Special and Therapeutic Formulas for Inborn Errors of Metabolism

HELEN K. BERRY

ABSTRACT

The successful prevention of mental retardation, death, or serious disease as a consequence of early detection and treatment of inborn errors of metabolism will surely stand as a milestone in medicine equal to the prevention of diseases caused by nutritional deficiencies and infections.

"The course of metabolism along any particular path should be pictured as in continuous movement rather than a series of distinct steps. If any one step in the process fail, the intermediate production being at the point of arrest will escape further change just as when the film of a biograph is brought to a standstill the moving figures are left foot in air." Sir Archibald Garrod[1]

The concept of inborn errors of metabolism was introduced by Sir Archibald Garrod in 1908 based on studies of alkaptonuria, albinism, cystinuria and pentosuria.[1] He reasoned that these defects were present at birth and persisted throughout life. They resulted from failure of some step in the series of chemical changes that constitute metabolism, and he viewed them as biochemical counterparts of structural malformations. He also noted that the disorders often occurred in several members of the same family, frequently in collateral relatives of the same generation, and that parents of affected individuals were often related. We now recognize Garrod's description as that of autosomal recessive inheritance.

Garrod's concept of inborn errors of metabolism is still relevant, though it has been greatly expanded from the original four disorders to several hundred entities. Experimental evidence of the blocking of specific metabolic reactions due to defective or missing enzymes came later. Thirty years passed before the first instance of a particular gene being related to a specific and known biochemical reaction was discovered.

A substance in serum from normal individuals can break down homogentisic acid (the metabolite found in alkaptonuria); the substance was not present in serum from alkaptonurics. From these observations Beadle proposed the hypothesis that gene action can be interpreted in terms of one gene-one reaction, or one gene-one enzyme.[2] In alkaptonuria, for the first time, a specific enzyme was found that intervened between gene and trait.

This was the beginning of the science of biochemical genetics. Much of our present knowledge of metabolic pathways has come from study of these chemical mutations known as inborn errors of metabolism.

The human body is a vast chemical factory. Each of the several thousand molecules in a cell is capable of reacting with other cellular molecules. Unaided, the reactions are slow, but they can be speeded up by enzymes, which are proteins with a unique catalytic function. Enzymes are so specific that they catalyze a single type of reaction. Synthesis of each enzyme is controlled by a single gene made up of deoxyribonucleic acid (DNA).

DNA is a large molecule put together from smaller molecules, adenine, guanine, cytosine, and thymine. Specific arrangements of these four bases within the molecule, the genetic code, correspond to specific amino acids. The genetic code specifies the order in which amino acids go together to make up a protein when it is synthesized in the body. A change in the sequence of bases within the gene can lead to production of an altered protein or enzyme that cannot carry out its catalytic function. The result is an alteration of the ability of the cell to carry out a particular reaction, hence a metabolic block.

The consequence of a metabolic block is usually that the substrate of the inactivated enzyme accumulates and may be "shunted" into alternate pathways. There may be increased amounts of metabolites, which are normally present as minor components. Substances normally produced after the block may be deficient. Inborn errors of metabolism can be identified by finding increased amounts of normal substrates in blood, urine, or tissues or by finding decreased amounts of normal products.

"No study which helps to throw light on the complex processes which are carried out in the human organism can fail in the long run to strengthen our hand in the combat with the pathogenic influences which make for its destruction."[1]

Phenylketonuria (PKU)

INTRODUCTION

The PKU story began quite by accident in 1934 when Dr. Asbjorn Folling tested urine from two mentally retarded children with ferric chloride and obtained an unusual blue-green color. The source of the color was identified as phenylpyruvic acid, and within 5 months Dr. Folling published a report in which he postulated an inherited disorder of phenylalanine metabolism.[3]

Dr. Folling identified eight additional patients by testing a group of 430 children in an institution for mentally retarded individuals.[4] Later Folling found that blood from these individuals contained increased amounts of phenylalanine.[5] Penrose[6] gave the disorder its name, derived from the "phenylketonic" acid found in the urine.

Folling noted the familial incidence of phenylketonuria in the first patients he described.[3] Studies of Penrose,[6] Jervis,[7] and Monroe[8] showed beyond doubt that phenylketonuria is inherited as a simple autosomal mendelian recessive trait. Not until 1953 was it shown that the enzymatic system for conversion of phenylalanine to tyrosine is absent in phenylketonuria.[9] This was the first member of the group of many inherited diseases that are described collectively as "inborn errors of metabolism." Discovery of the biochemical basis for phenylketonuria provided the first complete demonstration of the relationships postulated by Garrod.

PHYSIOLOGY AND PATHOLOGY

The biochemical defect in phenylketonuria is a deficiency of the liver enzyme phenylalanine hydroxylase, which catalyzes the parahydroxylation of phenylalanine to yield tyrosine (Fig. 1). The hydroxylase system is complex, consisting of a cofactor, tetrahydrobiopterin, and another enzyme, dihydropteridine reductase, which keeps the cofactor in its active (tetrahydro) form.[10-12] Metabolic blocks may occur in any component of the system, although

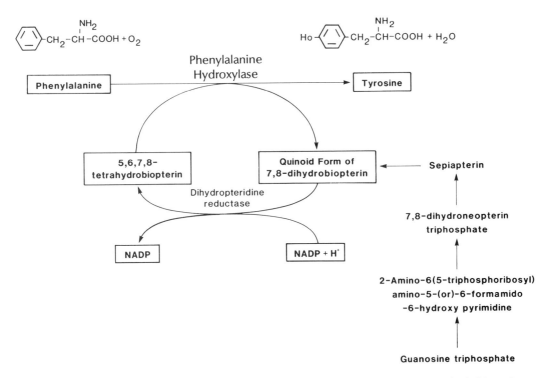

FIGURE 1.   Conversion of phenylalanine to tyrosine is dependent on a pterin cofactor. Tetrahydrobiopterin, synthesized from guanosine triphosphate, donates an electron to convert molecular oxygen to water and hydroxylate the ring of phenylalanine to produce tyrosine. The resulting dihydrobiopterin is recycled by dihydropteridine reductase via NADPH.

dihydropteridine reductase deficiency and defects in tetrahydrobiopterin synthesis are rare.[13]

In normal individuals most of the phenylalanine in the diet is converted to tyrosine, with minor routes for decarboxylation to phenylethylamine, some being used for protein synthesis and some excreted unchanged in the urine. When the pathway to tyrosine is blocked, phenylalanine accumulates in body fluids and tissues. More phenylalanine is channeled through other pathways. Increased decarboxylation leads to increased production of phenylethylamine, which is further oxidized to phenylacetic acid. Normally minor pathways such as transamination to form phenylpyruvic acid, acetylation to N-acetylphenylalanine, and others become significant. Production of phenylpyruvic acid and its metabolites, phenyllactic and orthohydroxyphenyl acetic acids, progressively increases as blood phenylalanine rises (Fig. 2).

Phenylalanine acts as a competitive inhibitor of tyrosinase, the enzyme responsible for melanin production; this accounts for the reduced pigmentation of skin, hair, and eyes seen in phenylketonuria. Excess phenylalanine interferes with hydroxylation of tyrosine to dihydroxyphenylalanine (DOPA) and tryptophan to 5-hydroxytryptophan (5-HT), as well as with their subsequent decarboxylation, so that the production of catecholamines from tyrosine and serotonin from tryptophan is diminished. In addition, active transport systems that carry phenylalanine across membranes also carry other large neutral amino acids, such as the branched chain amino acids, tyrosine, and tryptophan. **When the transport system is overloaded by excess phenylalanine, other amino acids are excluded from transport, particularly across the blood-brain barrier.**

Accumulation of phenylalanine leads to a series of direct and indirect biochemical changes that occur during early stages of development of the central nervous system and contribute to a pathogenic pattern that usually results in severe mental retardation by a still unknown mechanism. Other symptoms include diminished pigmentation, eczema, hypertonicity, seizures, and an abnormal electroencephalogram. Untreated patients may be irritable, subject to temper tantrums, and have erratic, aggressive behavior. Many never learn to walk nor talk.

DIETARY MANAGEMENT

Phenylketonuria remained a somewhat obscure biochemical curiosity for nearly 20 years. In 1951 Woolf and Vulliamy pointed out that there might be a relation between excess

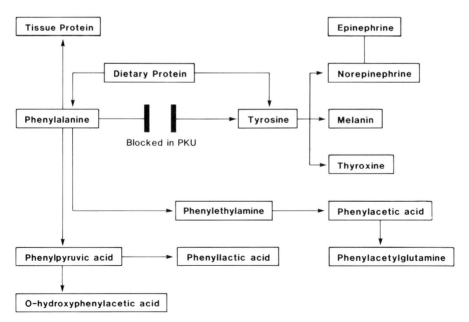

FIGURE 2. Normally 80% of phenylalanine from dietary protein is converted to tyrosine, also derived from dietary protein. When this reaction is blocked in phenylketonuria the excess phenylalanine enters other, normally minor, pathways.

phenylalanine and brain damage. If the amount of phenylalanine in the diet could somehow be decreased, phenylalanine might not accumulate and normalization of serum phenylalanine concentrations should improve the condition of patients with phenylketonuria.[14] A method for treating protein hydrolysates with charcoal to remove aromatic amino acids (phenylalanine, tyrosine, and tryptophan) had been described in 1943.[15]

Dent was the first to use a phenylalanine-restricted diet in 1951.[16] About the same time Woolf in Oxford, England and Armstrong in Utah began studies on the effects of phenylalanine-restricted diets. Woolf described the diet preparation to Bickel, who was caring for a 2-year-old patient recently found to have phenyketonuria. Bickel prepared the diet, fed the patient on it and in 1953 published the first report describing marked clinical improvement in a patient fed a phenylalanine-restricted diet.[17] Other reports followed quickly,[18-20] describing darkening of hair, clearing of eczema, improved behavior, and normalization of electroencephalogram associated with decreased serum and urinary phenylalanine and decreased excretion of phenylpyruvic acid. Return to phenylalanine-containing diet resulted in regression of behavior and return of biochemical abnormalities.

Unfortunately, it soon became clear that there was little improvement in intellectual functioning.[21-23] Brain damage that occurred before the start of the diet therapy was irreversible. It seemed reasonable to presume that the pathologic effects might be prevented or at least minimized if treatment were begun in in-

fancy.[24] Clinical interest quickened and attention centered on the younger patient.[25]

With few exceptions, prior to 1962, the only instance in which phenylketonuria was recognized early in infancy occurred when a child was born into a family in which an older sibling had been identified as having PKU. Urine screening programs, so effective in detecting PKU in the mentally retarded population, were ineffective when applied to infants, since phenylpyruvic acid was not present in urine of some phenylketonuric infants until as late as 6 weeks of age.[26]

In 1963 Guthrie and Susi[27] described a bacterial inhibition assay for phenylalanine in blood which made possible screening of large populations and led to comprehensive screening programs in most states (48 in 1984) of the U.S. and many developed countries of the world.

The first diets for treatment of PKU were prepared from acid hydrolyzed casein treated with charcoal[17,19] or from crystalline amino acids.[18] Tyrosine and tryptophan were restored to the charcoal-treated amino acid hydrolysate and starch, glucose, fat, minerals and vitamins were added to prepare a complete diet. By 1958, several commercial low-phenylalanine products were available that appeared to be nutritionally adequate, excepting, of course, for their low content of phenylalanine (Table 1).

NEEDS OF TERM INFANTS

The dietary treatment of phenylketonuria consists of providing a nutritionally balanced

TABLE 1.   Nutrient Composition of Human Milk and Formulas for Treatment of PKU*

Nutrient	Human Milk†	Lofenalac‡	Phenylfree‡	PKU-1‡	PKU AID§
Weight (gm)	1033	67	49	29	16.7
Energy (kcal)	700	307	202	54	40
Protein (gm)	10	10	10	10	10
Fat (gm)	46.6	12	3.35	0	0
Carbohydrate (gm)	69.9	40	32.5	3.52	0

*Values for human milk shown in Tables 1–4 were taken from references 28–30. Compositions of low-phenylalanine products were from literature furnished by manufacturers.
†Lofenalac and Phenylfree are products of Mead Johnson and Co. Evansville, IN.
‡PKU-1 is a product of Milupa International Scientific Dept, distributed in the United States by Milupa Corp, Darien, CT.
§PKU AID is a product of Milner Scientific and Medical Research Co., Roscrea, Ireland, distributed in the United States by Anglo Dietetics, Wilton, CT.

Formulas may be selected for low fat, low calorie, or low volume, while still providing low phenylalanine protein source.

diet containing enough phenylalanine to meet the needs of a growing child without exceeding his limited capacity to utilize it. The diet includes low-phenylalanine or phenylalanine-free protein substitutes, phenylalanine-containing foods to provide the requirement for phenylalanine, and low-protein products. The objective of treatment is to reduce serum phenylalanine from concentrations above 20 to a range between 3 and 8 mg/dl.

Protein Requirement

The protein requirement is provided by a semi-synthetic diet derived either from a modified protein hydrolysate or from a mixture of L-amino acids. Needs for carbohydrate, fat (including essential fatty acids), minerals and vitamins are met by the special dietary products and by supplements of natural foods. Composition of formulas for treatment of PKU, and of human milk, are shown in Tables 1-4. The recommendation for protein (Table 5) should be met from the low-phenylalanine formula. The amounts shown are somewhat higher than the current recommended daily allowance[31] to allow for individual differences in protein requirements and to offset any differences in protein utilization due to amino acid composition of the hydrolysates. For example, Lofenalac is low in sulfur amino acids

compared to human milk. This may lower its biological quality for some individuals.

It must be emphasized that none of these formulas is nutritionally complete and should never be used for nutrition of normal infants. They should never be administered without first having confirmed a diagnosis of phenylketonuria and then only with close biochemical monitoring of phenylalanine and other plasma amino acids, frequent measurements of weight and height, and periodic assessment of other nutritional parameters.

The dietary products can be used separately or in combinations. The variety of products is particularly valuable in prescribing appropriate protein and calorie intakes at different ages. This is significant, because treatment of PKU is a *lifelong* commitment. Recent reports suggest that termination of the low-phenylalanine diet in most patients is accompanied by deterioration in intellectual and neuropsychological functioning.[32-37]

Phenylalanine Requirement

In the late 1940s pure amino acids became available in quantities to permit study of amino acid requirements in man, and phenylalanine was shown to be essential in the diet.[38] Since tyrosine could be formed from phenylalanine, its presence in the diet reduced by 70-75% the

TABLE 2.   Amino Acid Composition of Human Milk and Formulas for Treatment of PKU

Amino Acids (mg/10 gm of protein)	Human Milk	Lofenalac	Phenylfree	PKU-1	PKU AID
Isoleucine	570	580	540	680	430
Leucine	975	1110	850	1140	1020
Lysine	700	1100	930	800	1020
Methionine	210	360	310	280	250
Phenylalanine	470	75	0	0	0
Threonine	478	520	460	540	800
Tryptophan	170	130	138	200	150
Tyrosine	540	530	460	680	1000
Valine	645	920	620	800	770
Histidine	235	320	232	290	300
Arginine	440	373	340	400	520
Alanine	390	450	0	480	630
Aspartate	853	930	2610	1140	1350
Cystine	205	40	172	280	250
Glutamate	1950	2670	940	2400	1550
Glycine	277	253	1630	280	520
Proline	846	950	0	1080	600
Serine	459	630	0	600	600
Taurine	33	0	0	0	0
Glutamine	85	0	2360	0	0

Low-phenylalanine formulas and human milk provide comparable amounts of essential amino acids except for phenylalanine.

TABLE 3.   Vitamin Composition of Human Milk and Formulas for Treatment of PKU

Vitamins (per 10 gm of protein)	Human Milk	Lofenalac	Phenylfree	PKU-1	PKU AID
Vitamin A (IU)	1898	770	600	1660	0
Vitamin D (IU)	22	193	75	200	0
Vitamin E (IU)	2	4.8	5	6.8	0
Vitamin K (µg)	15	48	50	33	0
Vitamin C (mg)	43	25	26	47	0
Thiamin (µg)	150	240	300	540	333
Riboflavin (µg)	365	287	500	800	420
Pyridoxine (µg)	140	193	450	440	330
Niacin (mg)	1.65	3.87	4	10.8	4.1
Biotin (µg)	2	24	15	20	98
Pantothenic acid (mg)	2	1.5	1.5	5	3.3
Choline (mg)	—	41	42	87	0
Inositol (mg)	—	15	15	100	0
Folic acid (µg)	52	48	63	67	65
Vitamin B12 (µg)	.3	.93	1.23	1.34	4.2

When comparable amounts of protein are fed, low-phenylalanine formulas provide adequate amounts of vitamins, except for PKU AID, which contains no fat-soluble vitamins.

TABLE 4.   Mineral Composition of Human Milk and Formulas for Treatment of PKU

Minerals (per 10 gm of protein)	Human Milk	Lofenalac	Phenylfree	PKU-1	PKU AID
Sodium (mEq)	7.3	6.4	8.8	9.3	10.2
Potassium (mEq)	13.6	8	17.2	12	11.2
Chlorine (mEq)	11	6	12.8	9.3	13.2
Calcium (mg)	333	287	251	480	420
Phosphorus (mg)	140	213	251	372	250
Magnesium (mg)	35	33	75	104	50
Sulfur (mg)	140	—	—	—	—
Iron (mg)	.50	5.7	6	6.8	4.2
Zinc (mg)	2	1.9	3.5	5.2	2.5
Copper (µg)	450	287	300	1340	420
Selenium (µg)	25	—	3	—	—
Manganese (µg)	10	480	500	460	580
Iodine (µg)	45	21	23	47	25
Fluorine (µ)	110	—	—	—	—

Adequate amounts of minerals and trace elements are present in low-phenylalanine formulas, though they vary widely in their content.

amount of phenylalanine otherwise required. The phenylalanine requirement by normal adults in the presence of tyrosine was 0.3 gm/day.[38]

Amino acid requirements of a growing infant are determined by the amino acid composition of tissue protein formed, superimposed upon the requirements for replacement of endogenous losses of nitrogenous material through skin, urine and stool, and for obliga-tory catabolism; that is, upon growth and maintenance. Snyderman and others estimated normal infant requirements for phenylalanine, in the presence of tyrosine, to be 47-90 mg/kg/day.[39] As the child grows older the relative requirement of an essential amino acid for growth decreases while other uses account for an increasingly larger proportion of the total requirement. This means that the total requirement for a given child may remain relatively

TABLE 5.   Recommended Daily Intakes of Nutrients for Children with Phenylketonuria and Normal Children

Age	Phenylalanine (mg/kg)	Protein (gm/kg)	Calories/kg
NORMAL			
12 d-9 mo[39]	47–90		
8-112 d[40]	63–91		
PKU			
0–3 mo	50–60	2.2–2.5	110–120
4–6 mo	40–50	2.0–2.5	110–120
7–12 mo	30–40	2.0–2.5	110
2 yr	25–30	1.8–2.0	100
3 yr	20–25	1.8–2.0	100
4–6 yr	15–25	1.5–2.0	85
7–10 yr	15–25	1.0–1.5	75
11–15 yr	10–25	1.0–1.5	50–60
15–18 yr	5–15	1.0–1.3	40–45
Adult	5–10	1.0–1.3	40

d = days; mo = months; yr = years

The recommendations for protein and phenylalanine are based on our own experiences as well as those of others;[41-44] that for calories is based on the RDA.[31] The amounts may have to be varied depending on responses of individual patients.

> In well children fed the appropriate phenylalanine intake, the serum phenylalanine concentration will usually fall in a range from 3–10 mg/dL, provided protein and calorie intakes are maintained.

constant. Study of patients with phenylketonuria have provided approximate requirements for age ranges between infancy and adulthood (see Table 5).[41-44]

Use of amino acid–restricted diets provides examples of the necessary balance among nutrients that make up normal diets. If intake of formula by a baby with phenylketonuria drops such that there is insufficient nitrogen in the diet, or if an amino acid other than phenylalanine is present in insufficient amounts to meet requirements for that amino acid, tissue catabolism occurs. This releases phenylalanine along with the deficient nutrient. Hence, there may be a *paradoxical rise* in serum phenylalanine concentration as a consequence. Similarly, if insufficient calories are provided, protein sources may be utilized for energy, again resulting in increase of serum phenylalanine.

PRETERM INFANTS

The tyrosine oxidizing system is functionally deficient in preterm infants due to slow maturation of the enzymes involved (Fig. 3). The first enzyme in the pathway, tyrosine aminotransferase, is reduced in fetal liver, and tyrosine may accumulate. The second enzyme, p-hydroxyphenylpyruvic acid oxidase, is inactivated by its substrate, but the activity of the enzyme may be restored by ascorbic acid.

Preterm infants with phenylketonuria present special problems. Serum phenylalanine concentrations only slightly above normal may have inhibitory effects on myelin protein synthesis in the developing brain. Since the production of tyrosine from phenylalanine is blocked in patients with phenylketonuria, it becomes an essential amino acid and must be provided in the diet if normal growth is to ensue. Additional protein and energy may be needed for "catch-up" growth, and **the phenylalanine requirement may be greater than 90 mg/kg/day, depending on growth rate.** Shortland et al.[45] reported that phenylalanine intake of 100 mg/kg/day and tyrosine of 270-290 mg/kg/day was required for a 1560 gm infant with PKU to achieve catch-up growth of 20 gm/kg/day.

PHENYLALANINE DEFICIENCY

In the first reported use of restricted phenylalanine intake for treatment of a phenylketonuric child, Bickel and coworkers[17] described rapid weight loss, vomiting, and generalized aminoaciduria. Supplementation of the diet with tyrosine slowed the decline in weight, but other symptoms persisted. Follow-up studies on the same child were reported by Blainey and Gulliford in 1956.[46] Weight remained stationary from age 2-4 years in spite

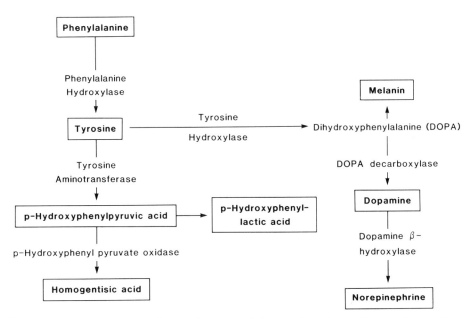

FIGURE 3.   Metabolism of tyrosine is disturbed in preterm infants and in patients with phenylketonuria. In preterm infants transamination of tyrosine with glutamic acid is reduced because of immaturity of liver enzymes. p-Hydroxyphenylpyruvate oxidase is inhibited by its substrate. In phenylketonuria excess phenylalanine inhibits tyrosine hydroxylase and DOPA decarboxylase (aromatic acid decarboxylase).

of what was regarded as adequate calorie and carbohydrate intake.

In 1958 Woolf and others described the treatment of a phenylketonuric infant beginning at age 5 weeks.[24] They noted poor weight gain, refusal to eat, anemia requiring blood transfusions, repeated infections, decrease in serum protein concentrations and elevated blood urea nitrogen. Weight gain occurred only after milk was added to the diet. It was not clear whether phenylalanine deficiency or lack of other essential nutrients was responsible for the syndrome. The first signs of an amino acid deficiency are failure to gain weight and refusal to eat.[39,42] Other reports appeared of these clinical symptoms, along with anemia and hypoproteinemia, in patients on phenylalanine-restricted diets. Sherman and others described a patient with phenylketonuria in whom striking bone marrow vacuolizations of the erythroid series occurred with blood hemoglobin content of 8.2 gm/dl.[47] Addition of phenylalanine to the diet was followed by weight gain and increase in hemoglobin content.

Feinberg and Fisch reported calcified spicules projecting into the epiphyseal area of long bones, associated with early cupping of the metaphysial plate, in young children treated with phenylalanine-restricted diets.[48] The changes were seen as early as 3 months of age. With growth the cupping disappeared and the spicules shortened, broadened, and were incorporated into the metaphysial spongiosa. Ultimately they were seen in the diaphysis. In spite of the resemblance to rickets, there was no reversal upon adding 25,000 units daily of vitamin D to the diet.

Murdoch and Holman described similar changes in long bones suggestive of rickets with osteoporosis and epiphyseal spiculation in patients maintained on a diet severely restricted in phenylalanine.[49] They found a striking correlation between phenylalanine intake and the bone lesions. When sufficient phenylalanine was fed, there was dissolution of roentgenologic bone changes, with spicules being absorbed into the diaphysis.

Deaths of 8 children, which occurred while the patients were on treatment with low-phenylalanine diets, were described in a symposium on deficiency syndromes held in 1969.[50]

These early experiences led to much criticism of the low-phenylalanine diet for treatment of phenylketonuria as ineffective and hazardous.[51,52]

Finally, it was recognized that normal brain development as well as normal physical growth was dependent on providing appropriate phenylalanine intake for infants and children with phenylketonuria. **Overtreatment (too rigid biochemical control) was responsible for mild to moderate retardation in some PKU patients in spite of early diagnosis and early treatment.**[53,54]

The need to treat children with phenylketonuria is no longer questioned.[55,56] Normal intellectual attainment is found in phenylketonuric children maintained since infancy on low-phenylalanine diets.[57-60] However, as noted earlier, behavior and performance may be adversely affected by termination of the diet,[32-37] and it is recommended that children with PKU should continue to follow the phenylalanine-restricted diet.[37]

TOXICITY

It is difficult to assess the toxic effects of phenylalanine or its metabolites because the evidence is so varied. **It is generally agreed that excess phenylalanine exerts a permanent deleterious effect on the brain during development and a reversible toxic effect subsequently.** There are several hypotheses for the pathogenic mechanism that produces the brain damage in phenylketonuria.[61-64]

Postmortem material from patients with untreated phenylketonuria has shown reduced myelination, reduction of lipid content of brain white matter, and deficient cerebrosides in white matter lipid.

The monoamine neurotransmitters, epinephrine, norepinephrine, dopamine and serotonin are involved in transmission of nerve impulses in both the peripheral and the central nervous systems. Patients with PKU have low plasma concentrations of the catecholamines and serotonin, and low concentrations of homovanillic acid and 5-hydroxyindoleacetic acid in cerebrospinal fluid, secondary to inhibition by phenylalanine of tyrosine hydroxylase, dihydroxyphenylalanine decarboxylase and tryptophan-5-hydroxylase.

Decreased concentrations of essential amino acids in brains of patients with PKU have been attributed to overloading of a common amino acid transport mechanism, from blood to brain, by phenylalanine. This overload may lead to a relative deficiency of substrates for brain protein synthesis.

The specific link between a deficient liver enzyme and the mental defect in PKU is still unknown. There may be no single cause but rather a combination of the known abnormalities. Monoamine depletion is reversed by lowering plasma phenylalanine levels. Neurotransmitter deficiency may account for the deterioration in performance which follows termination of the diet.

A "justification" theory proposed by Bessman[65] conjectured that tyrosine deficiency rather than phenylalanine excess was responsible for the mental defect in PKU. He further suggested that the heterozygous mother could harm her non-PKU offspring through tyrosine deficiency *in utero*.[66] The theory has not gained wide support, and there is evidence against it. Berry et al.[67] found similar cord blood tyrosine concentrations in 5 infants of heterozygous mothers and normal full-term infants. Scriver et al.[68] likewise found no significant difference in cord blood tyrosine concentrations measured in 14 infants with hyperphenylalaninemia and 56 control infants born in the same hospital on the same day as the affected infants. Cabalska et al.[69] studied the development of 82 unaffected siblings of PKU patients. Intellectual development was normal (mean intelligence quotient 104) and there were no deficits that might reflect intrauterine damage. Treatment of an affected child with tyrosine (1 mmol/kg/day) for four years in lieu of a low-phenylalanine diet diet not prevent development of the neurological sequelae characteristic of untreated PKU.[70]

MATERNAL PKU

The harmful effects of PKU are not limited to those who inherit the disease directly. Retrospective surveys indicated that maternal phenylalanine concentrations >20 mg/dl during pregnancy were associated with increased frequency of fetal complications, including intrauterine growth retardation, microcephaly, mental retardation, and a high incidence of heart defects.[71] Lipson et al. described a peculiar facial appearance in children of mothers with untreated PKU, characterized by facial bone hypoplasia, especially maxillary hypoplasia, underdeveloped philtrum, small upturned nose, thin upper lip and epicanthic folds.[72] The appearance was not unlike that of infants of alcoholic mothers.[73]

In the past women with PKU were severely retarded and a few had children. The success of nationwide neonatal PKU screening programs created an unexpected problem as women with PKU reached childbearing age. Although data are limited, control of maternal blood phenylalanine concentrations during the entire pregnancy seems to offer some protection to the fetus.[74] Dietary treatment begun after conception may not be sufficient to protect the fetus.[75] The National Institute of Child Health and Human Development is sponsoring a Maternal PKU Collaborative Study to evaluate the efficacy of a phenylalanine-restricted diet in reducing the morbidity associated with maternal PKU/hyperphenylalaninemia. The project began in November, 1984 and is designed to last 7 years. Clinics from 50 states and Canada are involved.

There was some concern that phenylalanine concentrations in the blood of pregnant heterozygous mothers of phenylketonuric children might increase to the degree that fetal damage could occur.[76] Phenylalanine concentrations in the female carrier do not rise sufficiently during pregnancy to harm the infant *in utero*.[67]

SUMMARY

Treatment of inborn errors of metabolism using dietary modification represented an experiment in nutrition that required courage—to feed to young infants a diet of known composition, lacking an essential nutrient, with the hope of preventing mental retardation. For the first time in history nutritional modification altered the outcome of a genetic disease. The experiment has been successful in that infants with PKU are now detected and treated early in life, and the majority achieve intellectual ability consistent with other family members. Outcome of treatment of metabolic disorders other than PKU has been less optimistic; treatment begun early in life for galactosemia or maple syrup urine disease is not always successful in achieving normal development. New information gained through molecular genetics may provide other opportunities for treatment in the future.

CASE REPORTS

Case 1. A male infant, the first child, was born 12/22/1960 to a 31-year-old mother. Pregnancy and birth were unremarkable. Birthweight was 3.6 kg. Although there were minor feeding problems during the first month, he weighed 4.1 kg at 6 weeks. When the baby was 6 weeks old, a urine specimen, dried on filter paper and mailed to our laboratory in a newborn screening program, was tested with ferric chloride and found to be positive for phenylpyruvic acid.

Serum phenlalanine was 45 mg/dl, confirming a diagnosis of phenylketonuria. Phenylalanine intake from evaporated milk formula was 280-300 mg/kg/day. Treatment with a low-phenylalanine diet was begun on 2/4/61.

The diet consisted of 100 gm of Lofenalac to provide 112 calories, 3.6 gm of protein and 18 mg of phenylalanine per kg per day. Within 5 days serum phenylalanine concentration dropped to 10 mg/dl and milk was added to the diet. Serum phenylalanine concentrations ranged from 1-3 mg/dl during the first few months. Phenylalanine intake was 25-35 mg/kg/day between 6 weeks and 4 months, and growth was at the 10th percentile. When phenylalanine intake was increased to 40 mg/kg/day, there was rapid weight gain and growth continued at the 90th percentile.

The patient has remained on the low-phenylalanine diet throughout his life. At age 25 years he weighs approximately 90 kg and is over 180 cm tall. Intellectual, emotional and social development is normal; he works as a firefighter and paramedic.

Questions and Answers

Q.   Is this course typical for treatment of an infant with PKU?
A.   This was the first infant in our program to be diagnosed by newborn screening and treated early in life. From the beginning normal growth was a major factor in assessing adequacy of the diet. In our experience, growth rate decreased with inadequate phenylalanine intake and increased when phenylalanine intake was raised. Each new patient must be watched carefully to balance dietary phenylalanine intake with desired serum phenylalanine concentrations and growth rates.

Q.   What are the problems that may occur at age 25 years?
A.   Maintaining the diet is the chief problem. By this age the amount of phenylalanine which can be permitted in the diet is 500-1000 mg/day, principally derived from fruits and vegetables. The low-phenylalanine formula must be taken in amounts to furnish 90% of the protein needs. If Lofenalac or Phenylfree are used, calorie intake is likely to be excessive and weight control becomes a problem. When this occurs the formulas such as PKU AID and PKU 1 are useful. The diet becomes monotonous, but return to an unrestricted diet may bring about changes in performance and behavior which interfere with a job or other aspects of daily living.

Q.   Does PKU in a man affect his offspring?
A.   The only abnormalities seen in children of men with PKU have been PKU or hyperphenylalaninemia. In fact, 10% of the children of both men and women with PKU also have PKU or hyperphenylalaninemia.

Case 2. A female infant was born 2/10/86 at 35 weeks' gestation, weighing 2440 gm. She was breast-fed for 3 days while in the hospital and was fed Similac formula (Ross Laboratories) thereafter. Blood collected on 2/13/86 and mailed to the Ohio Department of Health Newborn Screening Laboratory was positive for phenylalanine at 10 mg/dl (normal <4 mg/dl). Serum phenylalanine at 10 days of age was 40 mg/dl. The baby was referred to the Cincinnati Metabolic Disease Center on 2/21/86 at 11 days of age. Repeat serum phenylalanine was 42.3 mg/dl; tyrosine was 0.68 mg/dl (normal <1.5 mg/dL); and weight was 2.6 kg. Urine was negative for phenylpyruvic acid and other metabolites of phenylalanine, although urinary phenylalanine was increased above normal limits. Measurements of dihydropteridine reductase (DHPR) in blood and urinary biopterin/neopterin ratio were within normal limits, ruling out a defect other than phenylalanine hydroxylase deficiency.

Treatment with a low-phenylalanine formula was begun at 12 days of age. Diet consisted of 80 gm of Lofenalac made up to 480 ml with water. This formula provided 132 calories, 4.2 gm of protein and 22 mg of phenylalanine per kg per day. Serum phenylalanine concentration declined to 10 mg/dl within 72 hours and to <0.5 mg/dl within 5 days. Phenylalanine was added to the diet in the form of cow milk to furnish increasing amounts of phenylalanine up to a maximum of 110 mg/kg/day until serum phenylalanine concentrations were above 1.0 mg/dl. The baby gained rapidly and weighed 3.8 kg at 4 weeks. By 5 weeks of age serum phenylalanine concentrations were >10 mg/dl; phenylalanine intake was reduced stepwise to 55 mg/kg/day. At age 9 weeks an episode of fever with vomiting and refusal to take formula was associated with increased serum phenylalanine concentrations. Subsequently serum phenylalanine concentrations were between 3 and 8 mg/dl. Growth was at the 50th percentile for height and 75th percentile for weight by age 4 months.

Questions and Answers

Q.   Is the course described for this child typical?
A.   This illustrates treatment of a low birthweight infant and demonstrates the relatively high intake of phenylalanine needed for a few weeks to achieve "catch-up" growth. A more typical pattern at initial stages of treatment would be a phenylalanine intake of 50-60 mg/kg/day.

Q.   What is the significance of dihydropteridine reductase and urinary biopterin/neopterin ratio? Were you considering a diagnosis other than PKU?
A.   Defects in the synthesis and regeneration of the cofactor, tetrahydrobiopterin (BH_4) have been recognized as a cause of high blood phenylalanine concentrations. Diseases caused by deficient concentrations of BH_4 require treatment different from that for PKU; screening for cofactor defects is recommended. DHPR activity, necessary for regeneration of the cofactor, can be measured directly in blood. Neopterin is a precursor of BH_4; defects in synthesis of the cofactor can be recognized by finding accumulation of neopterin in urine and deficiency of BH_4.

Q.   Do illnesses in infancy complicate dietary management, and if so, why?
A.   Febrile illnesses may complicate treatment because of associated protein catabolism. Formula intake usually decreases at the same time, either because of lack of appetite or vomiting; protein synthesis is diminished. Increased release of phenylalanine from tissue protein together with decreased utilization for protein synthesis leads to its accumulation.

Q.   Can a PKU infant be breast-fed?
A.   Phenylketonuria cannot be treated effectively with a low protein diet. Even though the phenylalanine content of human milk is low (454 mg/L), phenylalanine accumulates in breast fed infants. The proportion of phenylalanine compared to other amino acids in the diet must be restricted. After control of serum phenylalanine concentration is achieved with Lofenalac, human milk can be used to meet phenylalanine requirements. An infant

may be able to consume 300-600 ml day of human milk (135-225 mg phenylalanine) in addition to 60-80 gm/day of Lofenalac. The amount of milk consumed can be determined by weighing the baby before and after nursing. The milk supply may have to be maintained by pumping.

More information on breastfeeding can be found in Ernst AE, McCabe ERB, Neifert MR, O'Flynn ME: Guide to Breast Feeding the Infant with PKU, which can be obtained from the Superintendent of Documents, U.S. Government Printing Office, Washington DC.

Case 3. A 26-year-old woman with PKU was referred to our clinic for dietary treatment when she was 8 weeks' pregnant. Serum phenylalanine concentration decreased from 27 to 7 mg/dl within a week after beginning a diet consisting of 320 g/day of Phenylfree (Mead Johnson) and 450 mg/day phenylalanine from all other foods. Serum phenylalanine concentration was monitored twice weekly and remained between 7 and 10 mg/dl for two weeks, after which the patient was unable to tolerate the low-phenylalanine formula without vomiting; serum phenylalanine concentrations increased to 16-21 mg/dl by 12 weeks' gestation. Because of the risk to the fetus the patient elected to terminate the pregnancy.

Questions and Answers

Q.   What effects does hyperphenylalaninemia have on the fetus?
A.   Most babies born to untreated phenylketonuric mothers have a pattern of malformations consisting of prenatal and postnatal growth retardation, microcephaly and central nervous system dysfunction, and increased incidence of malformations, particularly of the heart.

Q.   How high does phenylalanine have to affect the fetus?
A.   The teratogenic effects of phenylalanine are variable; there is a direct relation between the severity of the defects and maternal blood phenylalanine concentration. The highest frequency of defects occurs in women with blood phenylalanine concentrations above 20 mg/dl (1.21 mmol/L; the lowest, with phenylalanine concentrations below 10 mg/dl (.606 mmol/L). A "safe" range cannot be specified.

REFERENCES

1. Garrod A. Croonian lectures: Inborn errors of metabolism. Lancet 1908;2:1-7, 73-79, 142-148, 214-220.
2. Beadle GW. Biochemical genetics. Chem Rev 1945;37:15-96.
3. Folling A. Uber Ausscheidung von Phenylbrenztraubsaure in den Harn als Stoffwechselanomalie in Verbindung mit Imbezillitat. Hoppe-Seylers Z Physiol Chem 1934;227:169-176.
4. Folling A. Phenylpyruvic acid as a metabolic anomaly in connection with imbecility. Nord Med Tidskr 1934;8:1054-1059.
5. Folling A, Closs K. Uber das vorkommen von L-Phenylalaninin in Harn und Blut bei Imbecillitas phenylpyruvica. Hoppe-Seylers Z Physiol Chem 1938;254:115-116.
6. Penrose LS. Inheritance of phenypyruvic amentia (phenylketonuria). Lancet 1935;2:192-194.
7. Jervis GA. The genetics of phenylpyruvic oligophrenia. (A contribution to the study of the influence of heredity on mental defect.) J Ment Sci 1939;85:719-762.

8. Monroe TA. Phenylketonuria. Data on forty-seven British families. Ann Eugenics 1947;14:60–88.
9. Jervis GA. Phenylpyruvic oligophrenia: deficiency of phenylalanine oxidizing system. Proc Soc Exp Biol Med 1953;82:514–515.
10. Kaufman S. Studies on the structure of the primary oxidation product formed from tetrahydropteridines during phenylalanine hydroxylation. J Biol Chem 1964;239:332–338.
11. Kaufman S. The phenylalanine hydroxylating system in PKU and its variants. Biochem Med 1976;15:42–54.
12. Kaufman S. Differential diagnosis of variant forms of hyperphenylalaninemia. Pediatrics 1980;65:840–844.
13. Dhondt J-L. Tetrahydrobiopterin deficiencies: preliminary analysis from an international survey. J Pediatr 1984; 104:501–508.
14. Woolf LI, Vulliamy DG. Phenylketonuria with a study of the effect upon it of glutamic acid. Arch Dis Child 1951;26:487–494.
15. Knox WE. Phenylketonuria. In Stanbury JB, Fredrickson DS, Wyngaarden JB (eds): The Metabolic Basis of Inherited Disease. New York, McGraw Hill, 1960;321–382.
16. Schramm G, Primosigh J. Uber die quantitative Trennung der nuetralen Aminosauren durch Chromatographie. Ber Dtsch Chem Ges 1943;76:373–375.
17. Bickel H, Gerrard J, Hickmans EM. Influence of phenylalanine intake on phenylketonuria. Lancet 1953;2:812–813.
18. Armstrong MD, Tyler FH. Studies on phenylketonuria. I. Restricted phenylalanine intake in phenylketonuria. J Clin Invest 1955;34:565–580.
19. Woolf LI, Griffiths R, Moncrieff A. Treatment of phenylketonuria with a diet low in phenylalanine. Br Med J 1955;1:57–64.
20. Bickel H, Gerrard J, Hickmans EM. The influence of phenylalanine intake on the chemistry and behavior of a phenylketonuric child. Acta Pediatr 1954;43:64–77.
21. Horner FA, Streamer CW, Clader DE, et al. Effect of phenylalanine restricted diet in phenylketonuria. Am J Dis Child 1957;93:615–618.
22. Berry HK, Sutherland BS, Guest GM and Umbarger B. Chemical and clinical observations during treatment of children with phenylketonuria. Pediatrics 1958;21:929–940.
23. Hsia DY-Y, Knox WE, Quinn KV, Paine RS. A one-year controlled study of the effect of low phenylalanine diet on phenylketonuria. Pediatrics 1958;21:178–202.
24. Woolf LI, Griffiths R, Moncrieff A, et al. The dietary treatment of phenylketonuria. Arch Dis Child 1958;33:31–45.
25. Brimblecombe FSW, Stoneman M, Maliphant R. Dietary treatment of an infant with phenylketonuria. Lancet 1959; 1:609–611.
26. Armstrong MD, Centerwall WR, Horner FA, et al. The development of biochemical abnormalities in phenylketonuric infants. In Folch-Pi J (ed): Chemical Pathology of the Nervous System. Pergamon Press, New York, 1961;38–50.
27. Guthrie R, Susi A. A simple phenylalanine method for detecting phenylketonuria in large populations of newborn infants. Pediatrics 1963;32:338–343.
28. McLaren DS, Burman D. Textbook of Paediatric Nutrition. Edinburgh, Churchill Livingstone, 1976;23.
29. Suskind RM. Textbook of Pediatric Nutrition. New York, Raven Press, 1981;58–59.
30. Packard VS. Human Milk and Infant Formula. New York, Academic Press, 1982;231–233.
31. Recommended Dietary Allowances, 9th ed. Committee on Dietary Allowances, Food and Nutrition Board, National Research Council, Washington, DC, National Academy of Sciences, 1980.
32. Brunner RL, Jordan MK, Berry HK. Early-treated phenylketonuria: neuropsychologic consequences. J Pediatr 1983;102:831–839.
33. Krause W, Halminski M, McDonald L, et al. Biochemical and neuropsychological effects of elevated plasma phenylalanine in patients with treated phenylketonuria. J Clin Invest 1985;75:40–48.
34. Seashore MR, Friedman E, Novelly RA, Bapat V. Loss of intellectual function in children with phenylketonuria after relaxation of dietary phenylalanine restriction. Pediatrics 1985;75:226–232.
35. Lou H, Guttler F, Lykkelund C, et al. Decreased vigilance and neurotransmitter synthesis after discontinuation of dietary treatment for phenylketonuria (PKU) in adolescents. Eur J Pediatr 1985;144:17–20.
36. Pennington BF, van Doorninck WJ, et al. Neuropsychological deficits in early treated phenylketonuric children. Am J Ment Def 1985;89:467–474.
37. Holtzman NA, Kronmal RA, van Doorninck W, et al. Effect of age at loss of dietary control on intellectual performance and behavior of children with phenylketonuria. N Engl J Med 1986;314:593–598.
38. Rose WC, Wixom RL. The amino acid requirements of man. XIV. The sparing effect of tyrosine on the phenylalanine requirement. J Biol Chem 1955;217:95–101.
39. Snyderman SE, Pratt EL, Cheung MW, et al. The phenylalanine requirement of the normal infant. J Nutr 1955; 56:253–263.
40. Fomon SJ, Filer LJ. Amino acid requirements for normal growth. In Nyhan WL (ed): Amino Acid Metabolism and Genetic Variation. New York, McGraw-Hill, 1967; 391–401.
41. Paine RS, Hsia DY-Y. The dietary phenylalanine requirements and tolerances of phenylketonuric patients. Am J Dis Child 1957;94:224–230.
42. Holt LE Jr, Snyderman SE. The amino acid requirements of children. In Nyhan WL (ed): Amino Acid Metabolism and Genetic Variation. New York, McGraw-Hill, 1967; 381–390.
43. Berry HK. Hyperphenylalaninemias and tyrosinemias. Clin Perinatol 1976;3:15–40.
44. Ruch T, Kerr D. Decreased essential amino acid requirements without catabolism in phenylketonuria and maple syrup urine disease. Am J Clin Nutr 1982;35:217–228.
45. Shortland D, Smith I, Frances DEM, et al. Amino acid and protein requirements in a preterm infant with classic phenylketonuria. Arch Dis Child 1985;60:262–265.
46. Blainey JD, Gulliford R. Phenylalanine restricted diets in the treatment of phenylketonuria. Arch Dis Child 1956;31: 452–466.
47. Sherman JD, Greenfield JB, Ingall D. Reversible bone marrow vacuolizations in phenylketonuria. N Engl J Med 1964; 270:810–814.
48. Feinberg SB, Fisch RO. Roentgenologic findings in growing long bones in phenylketonuria: a preliminary study. Radiology 1962;78:394–398.
49. Murdock MM, Holman GN. Roentgenologic bone changes in phenylketonuria. Am J Dis Child 1964;107:523–532.
50. Rubin MI. Deficiency syndromes or hypophenylalaninemias. In Cohen BE, Rubin MI and Szeinberg A (eds): International Symposium on Phenylketonuria and Allied Disorders. Tel Aviv, Translators' Pool, 1971;166–199.
51. Bessman SP. Legislation and advances in medical knowledge-acceleration or inhibition. J Pediatr 1966;69:334–338.
52. Birch HG, Tizard J. The dietary treatment of phenylketonuria: not proven? Dev Med Child Neurol 1967;9:9–12.
53. Hackney IM, Hanley WB, Davidson W, Lindsao L. Phenylketonuria: mental development, behavior and termination of low phenylalanine diet. J Pediatr 1968;72:646–655.
54. Hudson FP, Mordaunt VL, Leahy I. Evaluation of treatment begun in first three months of life in 184 cases of phenylketonuria. Arch Dis Child 1970;45:5–12.
55. Scriver CR, Clow CL. Phenylketonuria: epitome of human biochemical genetics. N Engl J Med 1980;303: 1394–1400.
56. Genetic screening programs: Principles and research. National Research Council Committee for the Study of Inborn Errors of Metabolism, Washington DC, National Academy of Sciences, 1975.
57. Smith I, Wolff OH. Natural history of phenylketonuria and influence of early treatment. Lancet 1974;2:540–544.
58. Berry HK, O'Grady DO, Perlmutter LJ, Bofinger MK. Intellectual development and academic achievement of children treated early for phenylketonuria. Dev Med Child Neurol 1979;21:311–320.
59. Bickel H. Phenylketonuria: past, present, future. J Inherited Metab Dis 1980;3:123–132.
60. Williamson ML, Koch R, Azen C, Chang C. Correlates of in-

telligence test results in treated phenylketonuric children. Pediatrics 1981;68:161–167.

61. Blau K. Phenylalanine hydroxylase deficiency: biochemical, physiological and clinical aspects of phenylketonuria and related hyperphenylalaninemias. In Youdin MBH (ed): Aromatic Amino Acid Hydroxylases and Mental Disease. New York, John Wiley and Sons 1979;77–139.

62. Vorhees CV, Butcher RE, Berry HK. Progress in experimental phenylketonuria: a critical review. Neurosci Behav Rev 1981;5:177–190.

63. Sandler M. Inborn errors and disturbances of central neurotransmission (with special reference to phenylketonuria). J Inherited Metab Dis 1982;5(Suppl 2):65–70.

64. Pratt OE. Transport inhibition in the pathology of phenylketonuria and other inherited metabolic diseases. J Inherited Metab Dis 1982;5(Suppl 2):75–81.

65. Bessman SP. Genetic failure of amino acid "justification". A common basis for many forms of metabolic, nutritional and "nonspecific" mental retardation. J Pediatr 1972;81:834–842.

66. Bessman SP, Williamson ML, Koch R. Diet, genetics and mental retardation interaction between phenylketonuric heterozygous mother and fetus to produce nonspecific diminution of IQ: evidence in support of the justification hypothesis. Proc Natl Acad Sci USA 1978;75:1562–1566.

67. Berry HK, Poncet IB, Sutherland BS, Burkett R. Serum amino acid concentrations during pregnancy of women heterozygous for phenylketonuria. Biol Neonate 1975;26:102–108.

68. Scriver CR, Cole DEC, Houghton SA, et al. Cord-blood tyrosine levels in the full-term phenylketonuric fetus and the "justification" hypothesis. Proc Natl Acad Sci USA 1980;77:6175–6178.

69. Cabalska B, Miesowicz I, Zorska K, et al. Influence of phenylketonuric heterozygote on the developing fetus. J Inherited Metab Dis 1982;5:129–131.

70. Batshaw ML, Valle D, Bessman SP. Unsuccessful treatment of phenylketonuria with tyrosine. J Pediatr 1981;99:159–160.

71. Lenke RR, Levy HL. Maternal phenylketonuria and hyperphenylalaninemia. An international survey of the outcome of untreated and treated pregnancies. N Engl J Med 1980;303:1202–1208.

72. Lipson A, Beuhler B, Bartley J, et al. Maternal hyperphenylalaninemia fetal effects. J Pediatr 1984;104:216–220.

73. Lipson AH, Yu JS, O'Halloran MT, Williams R. Alcohol and phenylketonuria. Lancet 1981;1:717–718.

74. Lenke RR, Levy HL. Maternal phenylketonuria: results of dietary therapy. Am J Obstet Gynecol 1982;142:548–553.

75. Levy HL, Kaplan GN, Erickson AM. Comparison of treated and untreated pregnancies in a mother with phenylketonuria. J Pediatr 1982;100:876–880.

76. Kang E, Paine RS. Elevation of plasma phenylalanine levels during pregnancies of women heterozygous for phenylketonuria. J Pediatr 1963;63:283–289.

Maple Syrup Urine Disease

INTRODUCTION

Maple syrup urine disease (MSUD) is the prototype of disorders of organic acid metabolism which have the common feature of presenting as a metabolic emergency in the newborn. The symptoms and signs are not unlike those of neonatal sepsis in that metabolic acidosis is present and there is central nervous system dysfunction.

PHYSIOLOGY AND PATHOLOGY

Maple syrup urine disease results from a defect in branched-chain amino acid metabolism.[1,2] The initial transamination of leucine, isoleucine, and valine to alpha-keto acids occurs normally, but the second step, **oxidative decarboxylation of the keto acids, is defective** (Fig. 4). The consequence of the defect is accumulation of amino acids and their corresponding keto acids in blood, cerebrospinal fluid and urine.[3,4]

The unusual name comes from the odor, reminiscent of maple syrup or burnt sugar, which appears in the urine, breath and skin of affected infants. The odor is believed to come from the ketoacids or hydroxy acids derived from isoleucine.

Affected infants are normal at birth, but during the first days of life they become listless, refuse to eat, and vomit. This progresses to loss of reflexes, alternating hypertonicity and hypotonicity, convulsions and irregular respiration. Untreated infants are first lethargic, then comatose.[1,4–6] **Unless the diagnosis is made promptly, infants may die of respiratory disturbances.** If diagnosis is delayed beyond one to two weeks of age, those who survive the acute neonatal period show severe mental retardation and cerebral palsy.

Emergency treatment may be required for infants with acute symptoms: peritoneal dialysis, hemodialysis, or "exchange" blood transfusion can produce dramatic, temporary improvement.[5,7,8] Chronic management entails restriction of the intake of branched-chain amino acids.

Patients with the severe clinical course usually have no demonstrable alpha-ketoacid decarboxylase activity in leukocytes and cultured fibroblasts[9–12] and are designated as having classical MSUD. Variant forms of MSUD have been described with reduced levels of decarboxylase activity compared to normal, though higher than in the classical form.[13–15] Enzymatic activity is sufficient to maintain plasma branched-chain amino acids in the

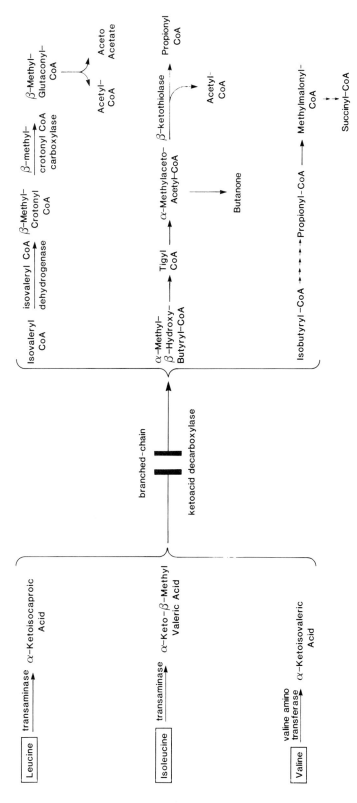

FIGURE 4.   Conversion of leucine, isoleucine, and valine to their corresponding keto acids, via transamination, occurs normally. In patients with MSUD the branched-chain keto acid decarboxylase is deficient, and the ketoacids and amino acids accumulate.

normal range except during stress. **Acute episodes may be triggered by infections, vaccinations, surgery, or a sudden increase in protein intake, and death can occur.**[13] Emergency measures and a restricted diet may be necessary during acute episodes in patients with variant MSUD, similar to patients with the classical form.

The first diets for treatment of MSUD consisted of mixtures of crystalline L-amino acids, omitting leucine, isoleucine, and valine.[6,16] Vitamins, minerals, fat, and carbohydrate were added, and the requirements for branched-chain amino acids were provided by small amounts of natural foods in the form of milk, gelatin, and low-protein fruits and vegetables.[17] *Gelatin* is one of the few proteins which has a relatively low content of branched chain amino acids.

Clow et al.[18] described in detail their experience in using MSUD-Aid® to treat four patients in whom the diagnosis of MSUD was made at 10 and 11 days of age. They combined MSUD-Aid® with a protein-free diet powder (Mead Johnson Product 80056^R) as a source of calories and other nutrients. Natural foods were used to meet other total and specific nutrient requirements. Home management was aided by daily monitoring of urinary ketoacids using the 2,4-dinitrophenylhydrazine reaction. Ketoacid excretion was estimated by the time interval at which yellow turbidity appeared after adding the reagent to urine. Intake of leucine from foods ranged from 250-600 mg/day; most children averaged about 400 mg of leucine per day. The amounts of isoleucine and valine in the diet were 60% and 70% of the leucine intake. Patients had normal intellectual development, with intelligence quotients ranging from 89 to 117 at ages 15 months to 9 years.

These data are in contrast to those of Naughten et al.[19] and Leonard et al.[20] who reported results of 14 patients with classical MSUD diagnosed at 1 day to 9 months of age (median age 7 days). Five patients with classical and one with variant MSUD died between the ages of 2 and 13 years, two after short severe illnesses and the other four during the recovery phase of apparently minor infections; three of the survivors had cerebral palsy and spastic quadriplegia; four others had abnormal neurological signs. Only one child was clearly normal. Long-term results reported by Rousson and Guibaud[21] were similar: only 3 of 20 patients with MSUD had normal psychomotor development.

NEEDS OF TERM AND PRETERM INFANTS

The dietary management of MSUD is complicated because the intake of three essential amino acids (leucine, isoleucine, and valine) must be carefully regulated. Enough of each of these amino acids must be included in the diet to meet needs for growth (net body protein accretion). Excess of any one of the three will permit the reappearance of symptoms and signs of MSUD. Similarly, deficiency of any one of the three can bring about tissue catabolism with consequent accumulation of the other two.

The nutritive composition of dietary products free of branched-chain amino acids which are commercially available for treatment of children with MSUD are shown in Tables 6 to 9.[22] During early stages of treatment many investigators prefer to use mixtures of synthetic L-amino acids. The mixtures, free of branched-chain amino acids, are fed in amounts and proportions found in human breast milk. Energy needs, essential fatty acids, vitamins and minerals can be provided through parenteral nutrition while the small amount of amino acids can be fed enterally, through a nasogastric tube if the infant is unable to suck.

Table 6 also shows the composition of a protein-free diet powder (Product 80056, Mead Johnson Co) that can be used with crystalline amino acid mixtures to produce a suitable infant formula. Vitamin and mineral contents of the protein-free diet powder are similar to those shown for MSUD Diet Powder (Mead Johnson Co.) Table 10 shows the recommended intake of nutrients for patients with MSUD. From our experience it is preferred that the RDA for protein come from the amino acid–modified formula. Protein-containing foods to provide the requirements for isoleucine, valine, and leucine are considered supplemental to the formula intake.

DEFICIENCY

The first infant to be treated for MSUD was born to a family in which a previous child had died with the disease.[26] Plasma amino acids showed high concentrations of leucine, isoleucine, valine, and methionine. The latter was identified only through its position on plasma aminograms. Although treatment to reduce plasma concentrations of the elevated amino acids was begun at two weeks of age, the neonatal course was stormy with many episodes of vomiting, metabolic acidosis and failure to grow.[27]

Methionine as well as leucine, isoleucine and valine was eliminated from the diet, which was made up from synthetic L-amino acids, corn oil, dextrimaltose, minerals and vitamins. Plasma concentrations of the branched chain amino acids fell to normal, but restriction of methionine intake had no effect on that amino acid. After 7 months of therapy, weight gain ceased. A trial with ordinary milk formula, undertaken in an effort to supply some unidentified deficiency resulted in rapid biochemical and clinical relapse. The infant became ataxic and could no longer sit. This was followed by alternate periods of ataxia and hypertonicity, somnolence, and finally by a generalized clonic convulsion. She was returned to the original, amino acid modified, diet. At 23 months of age a decision was made to ignore the high plasma "methionine." Weight gain improved and the frequency of acidotic episodes declined. Subsequently brewer's yeast was added to the diet, and the weight curve finally crossed the third percentile curve. The child was discharged to her parents after spending her first four years in the hospital.[28]

Data obtained with an early version of an automatic amino acid analyzer suggested that methionine was elevated as well as the branched-chain amino acids. Dietary methionine was therefore restricted. More sophisticated instrumentation for amino acid analysis led to separation of an unknown substance that was identified as alloisoleucine, a substance produced by transamination of keto-isoleucine and which previously had coeluted with methionine.[29]

The preceding illustrates the consequences of a amino acid deficiency. If an infant is fed a diet deficient in a specific amino acid, within one to two days growth ceases and the plasma concentration of the specific amino acid decreases. Holt and Snyderman showed an interesting relationship between the metabolism of branched-chain amino acids and their plasma concentrations; normal infants fed diets deficient in leucine showed decreased plasma concentrations of leucine, while concentrations of isoleucine and valine increased to 3-4 times normal.[30] Conventional foods contain a fixed ratio of branched-chain amino acids and the balance may not be adequate to meet requirements of patients with MSUD. In a number of children with MSUD, supplements of valine or isoleucine are required. If one of the three becomes limiting in the diet, the plasma concentration of that amino acid decreases and concentrations of the others rise markedly along with their corresponding keto-acids. Eventually body protein is catabolized to release the limiting amino acid, and even the limiting amino acid increases in plasma. The metabolic response to any episode that causes tissue catabolism and breakdown of body protein releases a normal complement of branched-chain amino acids and the consequence is the same as though that amount of protein were fed.

TOXICITY

The basis for the cerebral dysfunction in patients with MSUD has not been determined. **Among the theories proposed for pathogenesis are decreased energy sources for brain, decreased neurotransmitters, and interruption of myelin production.**

Severe to moderate fasting hypoglycemia results from relatively short periods of fasting. Haymond et al. investigated the etiology of hypoglycemia in patients with classic MSUD.[31] There was no difference between MSUD and control subjects in insulin, glucose, or ketone bodies following a fast of 24-30 hours. Alanine flux was lower in MSUD patients. They concluded the hypoglycemia was the conse-

TABLE 6.   Nutrient Composition of Formulas for Treatment of Maple Syrup Urine Disease*

Nutrient	Protein-Free Diet Powder†	MSUD Powder†	MSUD-Aid‡	MSUD-1§
Powder (gm)	100	122	16.1	24.4
Energy (kcal)	490	473	40	68.2
Protein (gm)	0	10	10	10
Fat (gm)	22.5	24.4	0	0
Carbohydrate (gm)	71.8	77.2	0	7

*Compositions of products free of branched-chain amino acids are from literature furnished by manufacturers.
†MSUD Powder and Product 80056, Protein-Free Diet Powder, are products of Mead Johnson Co., Evansville, IN.
‡MSUD-Aid is a product of Milner Scientific, Roscrea, Ireland, distributed in the United States by Anglo Dietetics, Wilton, CT.
§MSUD-1 is a product of Milupa International Scientific Dept., distributed in the United States by Milupa Corp, Darien, CT.

Formulas for treatment of MSUD vary greatly in their energy content for the same amount of protein. MSUD Powder may cause excessive weight gain if used for older children and adolescents to meet protein needs.

TABLE 7.   Amino Acid Composition of Formulas for Treatment of Maple Syrup Urine Disease

Amino Acids (mg/10 gm of protein)	MSUD Powder	MSUD-Aid	MSUD-1
Isoleucine	0	0	0
Leucine	0	0	0
Lysine	622	1150	978
Methionine	305	306	342
Phenylalanine	671	613	587
Threonine	671	532	660
Tryptophan	244	194	244
Valine	0	0	0
Arginine	598	823	489
Alanine	537	1150	587
Aspartate	1390	1950	1390
Cystine	305	339	342
Glutamate	2560	2150	2930
Glycine	732	629	342
Proline	1090	371	1320
Serine	732	387	733
Tyrosine	793	613	709

Formulas for treatment of MSUD provide comparable amounts of essential and non-essential amino acids, other than isoleucine, valine, and leucine, which are missing in all.

TABLE 8.   Vitamin Composition of Formulas for Treatment of Maple Syrup Urine Disease

Vitamins (per 10 gm of protein)	MSUD Powder	MSUD-Aid	MSUD-1
Vitamin A (IU)	1440	0	2280
Vitamin D (IU)	336	0	244
Vitamin E (IU)	9.02	0	8.31
Vitamin K (μg)	90.2	0	40.8
Vitamin C (mg)	46	0	57
Thiamin (μg)	451	323	660
Riboflavin (μg)	537	403	978
Pyridoxine (μg)	366	323	538
Niacin (mg)	7.2	4.03	13.2
Biotin (μg)	48.8	36.8	24.4
Pantothenic acid (mg)	2.66	3.23	6.11
Choline (mg)	76.8	0	105
Inositol (mg)	26.8	0	122
Folic acid (μg)	90.2	64.5	81.7
Vitamin B12 (μg)	1.93	3.23	1.64

Adequate amounts of vitamins are present in the formulas except that MSUD-Aid does not contain fat-soluble vitamins or vitamin C.

quence of defective gluconeogenesis from amino acids.

Keto-isocaproic acid (KIC), derived from leucine, has been shown to inhibit transport of pyruvate and 3-hydroxybutyrate into mitochondria.[32] Bowden et al. using rat brain and Patel et al. using human and rat brain mitochondria found that KIC inhibited pyruvate dehydrogenase and alpha-ketoglutarate dehydrogenase.[33,34] These effects would lead to reduced production of substrates for the tricarboxylic acid cycle. Decreased energy metabolism and decreased biosynthesis of lipids from glucose and ketone bodies in the developing brain may contribute to the poor prognosis in patients with MSUD.

Tashian showed that KIC, keto-isovalerate, and the hydroxy acids derived from the corresponding ketoacids, compete with L-glutamate for decarboxylation by rat brain homo-

TABLE 9.   Mineral Composition of Formulas for Treatment of Maple Syrup Urine Disease

Minerals (per 10 gm of protein)	MSUD Powder	MSUD-Aid	MSUD-1
Sodium (mEq)	9.76	9.84	11.3
Potassium (mEq)	15.2	10.6	14.7
Chloride (mEq)	12.7	11.8	11.3
Calcium (mg)	596	403	587
Phosphorus (mg)	329	242	455
Magnesium (mg)	63.4	46.4	127
Iron (mg)	10.9	6.06	8.31
Zinc (mg)	3.66	2.42	6.36
Copper (μg)	524	403	1640
Manganese (μg)	3.66	2.42	6.36
Iodine (μg)	40.2	24.2	57.2

Adequate amounts of minerals are present in the formulas, though the content varies.

TABLE 10.   Recommended Daily Intakes of Nutrients for Children with Maple Syrup Urine Disease

Age	Calories*	Protein*	Leucine†	Isoleucine‡	Valine‡
0–2 mo	120/kg	2.2 gm/kg	90–110 mg/kg	60–70 mg/kg	70–85 mg/kg
2–5 mo	110/kg	2.2 gm/kg	65–90 mg/kg	40–60 mg/kg	50–70 mg/kg
6–12 mo	105/kg	2.0 gm/kg	50–65 mg/kg	33–40 mg/kg	40–50 mg/kg
1–2 yr	1100	25 gm	35–55 mg/kg	23–35 mg/kg	27–45 mg/kg
2–3 yr	1300	25 gm	400–500 mg	240–300 mg	280–350 mg
3–4 yr	1400	30 gm	400–500 mg	240–300 mg	280–350 mg
4–6 yr	1700	30 gm	400–550 mg	240–330 mg	280–385 mg
6–8 yr	2200	35 gm	400–600 mg	240–360 mg	280–420 mg
8–10 yr	2400	40 gm	400–700 mg	240–420 mg	280–490 mg

*Recommended Dietary Allowances, revised 1980.[23]
†Calculated from data in Snyderman,[5] Clow et al.,[18] Dickinson et al.,[24] and Ruch and Kerr.[25]

Metabolic control can usually be achieved by feeding the age-appropriate amounts of the branched-chain amino acids. Metabolic control is considered good when plasma concentrations are in these ranges (μmol/L):

Leucine	180 to 700
Isoleucine	70 to 280
Valine	200 to 800

genates.[35] He suggested reduced GABA production would be the consequence. Yuwiler found that excess dietary leucine reduces brain serotonin in rats.[36]

In cultures of myelinating newborn rat cerebellum, KIC caused delay in myelin formation.[37] Failure of myelinization, but not demyelinization, was found at autopsy of MSUD patients, along with general reduction in proteolipids and cerebrosides.[2,38]

SUMMARY

Patients with MSUD present complications in diagnosis, treatment and long-term management. Childhood illness, minor in a normal child, can become major crises. Dietary treatment has been life-saving for affected children.

Nevertheless, many children with MSUD have severe handicaps, both physically and neurologically. Preventive approaches should continue to focus on early diagnosis and treatment, genetic counseling, and prenatal monitoring.

CASE REPORT

A female infant, born 8/17/76 following an uncomplicated pregnancy and delivery, weighed 3.7 kg. No neurologic or breathing difficulties were noted. She did well the first 3 days on Similac formula (Ross Laboratories). By the end of the first week she was lethargic and refused formula. She was hospitalized at age 2 weeks. "Metabolic screen" done while on intravenous fluids with **no protein intake** was normal. Neurologic damage of unknown etiology was diagnosed. The child had many formula changes. She continued to vomit even with gavage feeding. Following the onset of projectile vomiting at age 4 months she was again hospitalized. An unusual odor was noted;

blood and urine specimens showed increased concentrations of branched chain amino acids; urinary keto acids were abnormal. Enzyme studies of leukocytes and fibroblasts showed absence of ketoacid decarboxylase activity.

She was started on a diet of crystalline L-amino acids lacking valine, isoleucine, and leucine, and Mead Johnson Product 80056 was used to furnish calories, fat, carbohydrate, vitamins and minerals. Concentrations of branched-chain amino acids decreased in blood and urine. Within 48 hours plasma concentrations of isoleucine and valine were near normal, and both were added to the formula as solutions of crystalline amino acids. By 72 hours concentration of plasma leucine decreased from 2500 µmol/L to less than 1000 µmol/L. Leucine solution was then added to the diet, and the formula was adjusted to provide per kg per day: 2.0 gm of protein from the amino acid mixture, 100 calories from MJ80056, 28 mg of valine and, 14 of mg isoleucine from solutions of the amino acids. Milk was not used at this stage because it has a fixed ratio of the amino acids, and the amount of milk needed to provide the recommended amounts of isoleucine and leucine did not provide a sufficient amount of valine. Fruits (apple sauce and pears) were fed in small amounts. (Details on diagnosis and early treatment of this patient are courtesy of Dr. Paul Wong, Rush-Presbyterian Hospital, Chicago.)

The patient moved from Chicago to the Cincinnati area at age 18 months. The formula was changed from one based on crystalline amino acids to MSUD-Aid. The requirement for branched-chain amino acids was provided by milk and other foods, together with supplement of valine solution to provide an additional 5 mg/kg/day.

At age 10 years the patient is mentally retarded with cerebral palsy. She has had many episodes of acidosis requiring hospitalizations. On these occasions branched-chain amino acids are omitted from the dietary formula. Plasma concentrations of isoleucine and valine decline before leucine. Usually plasma leucine decreases to less than 1 mol/L within 48-72 hours after omission of branched-chain amino acids from the diet. Isoleucine and valine are added first and then leucine, as described above.

Questions and Answers

Q.   How could the diagnosis of MSUD be made earlier in this and other patients?

A.   A high degree of suspicion on the part of the physician helps. **Routine metabolic screening of blood and urine from sick infants at the time of admission to the hospital would reveal the elevation of branched-chain amino acids and keto acids.** In this instance the test was not performed until after some period on intravenous fluids without protein. An unexplained anion gap might have alerted the physicians to the possibility of an organic acidemia.

Q.   Would newborn screening be of value in MSUD?

A.   It is feasible to test for increased concentrations of leucine in the same blood specimen collected for PKU screening. However, clinical signs will probably be present before the test is completed and death may occur in the first week of life, prior to diagnosis. In the patient described here, newborn screening would most likely have permitted an early diagnosis.

Q.   What is the key to dietary management in these subjects?

A.   The key to successful management of MSUD as well as other organic acidemias is in maintaining the necessary balance of amino acids in the diet; both excesses and deficiencies of branched-chain amino acids must be avoided, since both lead to accumulation of amino acids and ketoacids.

REFERENCES

1. Menkes JH, Hurst PL, Craig JM. New syndrome: progressive familial infantile cerebral dysfunction associated with unusual urinary substance. Pediatrics 1954;14:462–470.
2. Westall RG, Dancis J, Miller S. Maple syrup urine disease—a new molecular disease. Am J Dis Child 1957;94:571–572.
3. Dancis J, Levitz M, Westall RG. Maple syrup urine disease: Branched-chain ketoaciduria. Pediatrics 1960;25:72–79.
4. Tanaka K, Rosenberg LE. Disorders of branched chain amino acids and organic acids. In Stanbury JB, Wyngaarden JB, Fredrickson DS, Goldstein JL, Brown MS (eds): The Metabolic Basis of Inherited Disease, 5th ed. New York, McGraw Hill Book Co, 1983;440–473.
5. Snyderman SE. Medical and nutritional aspects of maple syrup urine disease. In Koch R, Shaw KNF, Durkin F (eds): Maple Syrup Urine Disease Symposium: Issues and Perspectives. Rockville, MD, DHEW Publication No. (HSA) 79-5294, 1979;18–33.
6. Westall RG. Dietary treatment of a child with maple syrup urine disease (branched-chain ketoaciduria). Arch Dis Child 1963;38:485–491.
7. Gaull GE. Pathogenesis of maple syrup urine disease: observations during dietary management and treatment of coma by peritoneal dialysis. Biochem Med 1969;3:130–149.
8. Saudubray JM, Ogier H, Charpentier C, et al. Neonatal management of organic acidurias. Clinical update. J Inherited Metab Dis 1984;7(Suppl 1):2–9.
9. Dancis J, Hutzler J, Levitz M. The diagnosis of maple syrup urine disease (branched chain ketoaciduria) by the in vitro study of the periphral leukocyte. Pediatrics 1963;32:234–238.
10. Dancis J, Jansen V, Hutzler J, Levitz M. The metabolism of leucine in tissue culture of skin fibroblasts of maple syrup urine disease. Biochim Biophys Acta 1963;77:523–524.
11. Wendel U, Wohler W, Goedde HW, et al. Rapid diagnosis of maple syrup urine disease (branched chain ketoaciduria) by micro-enzyme assay in leukocytes and fibroblasts. Clin Chim Acta 1973;45:433–440.
12. Chuang DT, Niu WL, Cox RP. Activities of branched-chain 2-oxo acid dehydrogenase and its components in skin fibroblasts from normal and classical maple syrup urine disease subjects. Biochem J 1981;200:59–67.
13. Kiil R, Rokkones T. Late manifesting variant of branched-chain ketoaciduria (maple syrup urine disease). Acta Pediatr 1964;53:356–364.
14. Schulman JD, Lustberg TJ, Kennedy JL, et al. A new variant of maple syrup urine disease (branched chain ketoaciduria). Am J Med 1970;49:118–124.
15. Dancis J, Hutzler J, Snyderman SE, Cox RP. Enzyme activity in classical and variant forms of maple syrup urine disease. J Pediatr 1972;81:312–320.
16. Snyderman SE, Norton PM, et al. Maple syrup urine disease with particular reference to dietotherapy. Pediatrics 196; 434:454–472.
17. Snyderman SE. Maple syrup urine disease. In Raine DN (ed): The Treatment of Inherited Metabolic Disease. Baltimore, University Park Press, 1975;71–90.
18. Clow CL, Reade TM, Scriver CR. Outcome of early and long term management of classical maple syrup urine disease. Pediatrics 1981;68:856–862.
19. Naughten ER, Jenkins J, Francis DEM, Leonard JV. Outcome of maple syrup urine disease. Arch Dis Child 1982;57:918–921.
20. Leonard JV, Daish P, Naughten ER, Barltett K. The management and long term outcome of organic acidemias. J Inherited Metab Dis 1984;7(Suppl 1):13–17.

21. Rousson R, Guibaud P. Long term outcome of organic acid-urias: survey of 105 French cases (1967–1983). J Inherited Metab Dis 1984;7(Suppl 1):10–12.
22. Committee on Nutrition, American Academy of Pediatrics. Report of the task force on the dietary management of metabolic disorders, June, 1985.
23. Food and Nutrition Board. Recommended Dietary Allowances, 9th ed. Washington DC, National Academy of Sciences, 1980.
24. Dickinson JP, Helton JB, Lewis GM, et al. Maple syrup urine disease: four years experience with dietary treatment of a case. Acta Pediatr Scand 1969;58:341–350.
25. Ruch T, Kerr D. Decreased essential amino acid requirements without catabolism in phenylketonuria and maple syrup urine disease. Am J Clin Nutr 1982;35:217–228.
26. Holt LE Jr, Snyderman SE, Dancis J. The treatment of a case of maple syrup urine disease. Fed Proc 1960;19:10.
27. Snyderman SE. Maple syrup urine disease. In Nyhan WL (ed): Amino Acid Metabolism and Genetic Variation. New York, McGraw Hill, 1967;171–183.
28. Snyderman SE. Personal communication.
29. Norton PM, Roitman E, Snyderman SE, Holt LE Jr. A new finding in maple syrup urine disease. Lancet 1962;1:26–27.
30. Holt LE Jr, Snyderman SE. The amino acid requirements of children. In Nyhan WL (ed): Amino Acid Metabolism and Genetic Variation. New York, McGraw Hill, 1967; 381–390.
31. Haymond MW, Karl IE, Feigen RD, et al. Hypoglycemia and maple syrup urine disease-defective gluconeogenesis. Pediatr Res 1973;7:500–508.
32. Land JM, Mowbray J, Clark JB. Control of pyruvate and beta-hydroxybutyrate utilization in rat brain mitochondria and its relevance to phenylketonuria and maple syrup urine disease. J Neurochem 1976;26:823–830.
33. Bowden JA, McArthur CL. The inhibition of pyruvate decarboxylation in rat brain by alpha-ketoisocaproic acid. Biochem Med 1971;5:101–108.
34. Patel MS. Inhibition by the branched-chain 2-oxo acids of the 2-oxoglutarate dehydrogenase complex in developing rat and human brain. Biochem J 1974;144:91–97.
35. Tashian RE. Inhibition of brain glutamic decarboxylase by phenylalanine, leucine and valine derivatives. A suggestion concerning the neurological defect in phenylketonuria and branched-chain ketoaciduria. Metabolism 1961;10: 393–402.
36. Yuwiler A, Geller E. Serotonin depletion by dietary leucine. Nature (London) 1965;208:83–84.
37. Silberberg DH. Maple syrup urine disease metabolites studied in cerebellum cultures. J Neurochem 1969;16: 1141–1146.
38. Prensky AL, Moser HW. Brain lipids, proteolipids and free amino acids in maple syrup urine disease. J Neurochem 1966;13:863–874.

Galactosemia

INTRODUCTION

Galactosemia is an inborn error in metabolism of galactose. It is a serious disease frequently leading to death in infancy. Untreated survivors suffer from mental and physical retardation, cataracts, and varying degrees of damage to liver and kidney. The disease was first described by von Reuss in 1908.[1] Mason and Turner provided the first detailed description of the syndrome.[2]

Their patient, a 6 month old black infant, failed to gain weight, had hepatosplenomegaly, jaundice, anemia, a generalized osteoporosis, albuminuria, and mellituria. The sugar in the urine was shown to be galactose and the infant improved markedly on a soy formula, free of lactose. Liver damage and cataracts appeared to be reversible, but mental retardation was persistent. This patient, when reassessed at age 16 years, had an intelligence quotient of 64 and galactose tolerance test showed a flat blood glucose curve.[3]

New interest was generated by the finding of aminoaciduria and proteinuria, which fluctuated in relation to presence or absence of galactose in the diet.[4,5] The aminoaciduria appeared to result from failure of renal reabsorption rather than from overflow.[6]

PHYSIOLOGY AND PATHOLOGY

Infants with galactosemia are unable to convert galactose, a component of milk sugar, into glucose, the form in which the body can utilize it. The inability to metabolize dietary galactose leads to a variety of clinical signs within the first few days of life, including some at birth. Jaundice persisting beyond the usual period is an early sign along with neonatal bleeding, hepatomegaly, splenomegaly, leading to ascites and cirrhosis. There may be cataracts, hypoglycemia, feeding difficulties, coagulation problems and decreased immunity. Without treatment, infants often die of *Escherichia coli* sepsis. Those who survive the liver disease and hemorrhagic episodes have cataracts and are physically and mentally retarded.

The pathway for conversion of galactose to glucose is shown in Figure 5. The liver is the primary site of galactose metabolism, although other also tissues have the capacity for metabolism.

Schwarz and associates found that there was an abnormal accumulation of galactose-1-phosphate in red blood cells when milk was fed to a child with galactosemia.[6] Isselbacher et al. showed that blood and liver of patients with

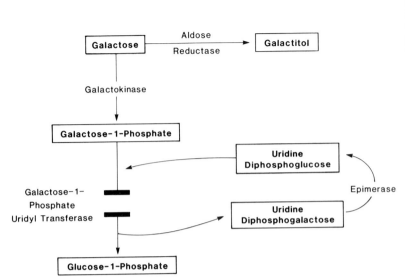

FIGURE 5.   Normally galactose is converted to glucose via galactose-1-phosphate and glucose-1-phosphate. In galactosemia this conversion is blocked, and galactose, galactitol and galactose-1-phosphate accumulate.

the disorder lacked galactose-1-phosphate uridyl transferase, the enzyme catalyzing the second step in the pathway.[7] This enzyme lack accounts for the accumulation of galactose-1-phosphate in red cells and galactose in blood. Galactose is converted by a pyridine nucleotide–dependent, nonspecific, aldose reductase to galactitol, which accumulates in tissues and is excreted in urine.[8]

Galactosemia is inherited as an autosomal trait. Heterozygous parents have no clinical symptoms but have approximately half the normal transferase activity. There are clinically nonsignificant variants with reduced enzyme activity (50% to 75% of normal).[9] Rare patients with clinical symptoms of galactosemia have variant forms of the enzyme with measurable activity in the range of 10% to 20% of normal.[9]

Galactose ingestion by affected infants can be fatal; removal of the offending carbohydrate from the diet can bring about dramatic recovery. Exchange transfusion may be an appropriate emergency measure in the jaundiced and toxic galactosemic baby, since it not only removes ammonia and other waste products associated with liver failure, but the small amount of transferase supplied by donor blood, together with removal of red blood cells containing galactose-1-phosphate, may hasten improvement of the baby.[10]

NEEDS OF TERM AND PRETERM INFANTS

The prescribed treatment for galactosemia is immediate removal from the diet of foods that contain lactose and other oligosaccharides incorporating galactose. The principal source of lactose is milk and products made from milk. **It is not easy to formulate a diet entirely free of galactose.** Hydrolyzed casein and soy protein are standard protein sources for infant formulas. It is not always certain that all galactose is removed from casein prepared from milk. Galactose-containing oligosaccharides (raffinose, a trisaccharide; stachyose, a tetrasaccharide; and verbascose, a pentasaccharide) are found in soybean products and in dry leguminous seeds. The alpha-D-galactopyrariosyl group present in these substances is not readily digested since human small intestinal mucosa contains no alpha-galactosidase activity. Soy protein isolates are free of galactose-containing oligosaccharides.

Table 11 shows the composition of commercially available products that are suitable for infants with galactosemia. Foods to which lactose or milk solids are added should be strictly avoided. **Careful attention to labels showing additives can prevent inadvertent feeding of lactose and galactose. Antibiotics and other medications that have lactose as filler or sweetener must be avoided.**

TABLE 11.   Composition of Lactose-Galactose Free Products

Nutrient (per 100 calories 5 fl oz)	Nutramigen*	Prosobee*	Isomil†
Protein (gm)	2.8	3	3
Fat (gm)	3.9	5.3	5.3
Carbohydrate (gm)	13.4	10	10
Protein source:	Casein, enzymatically hydrolyzed and charcoal treated	Soy protein isolate	Soy protein isolate
Carbohydrate source	Corn syrup solids	Corn syrup solids	Corn syrup sucrose

*Nutramigen and Prosobee are products of Mead Johnson Co., Evansville, IN; data are from manufacturer's literature.
†Isomil is a product of Ross Laboratories, Columbus, OH; data are from manufacturer's literature.

> Formulas for treatment of galactosemia, while varying in source of protein and carbohydrate, are equally effective as the basis for a lactose-, galactose-restricted diet.

The effectiveness of dietary galactose restriction can be monitored by measurement of accumulation of galactose-1-phosphate by erythrocytes and urinary galactitol excretion.

Galactose restriction is advised during pregnancy in heterozygous women. Their reduced enzyme activity together with the usual high intake of milk advised during pregnancy leads to accumulation of high concentration of galactose-1-phosphate by fetal cells. Intrauterine effects of galactosemia may account for the low birthweight and cataracts found in infants with galactosemia.[11] Galactose-1-phosphate is present in liver of aborted fetuses with galactosemia as early as 21 weeks' gestation.[12,13] Galactitol may be responsible for lenticular damage in the developing fetal eye.[13] Morever, galactose-1-phosphate may accumulate in an affected fetus even with strict control of the mother's diet.[14-15]

DEFICIENCY

No ill effects have ever been described of feeding infants a diet free of galactose. The great bulk of galactose residues, which are an essential part of cerebrosides, gangliosides, mucopolysaccharides, and many glycoproteins, are derived from glucose. Galactose is incorporated into these structures via uridine-5'-diphosphogalactose (UDP galactose). The epimerase that converts uridine-5'-diphos-phoglucose (UDPG) to UDP-galactose is normal in galactosemic infants.

TOXICITY

Early diagnosis and prompt treatment by feeding a lactose-galactose-free diet prevent or reverse the clinical complications. However, the long-term response to dietary intervention in galactosemia has not been uniformly satisfactory in preventing intellectual and language deficits. Komrower[14] found below average intelligence in early diagnosed and well-treated patients. Fishler et al.[16] found intellectual function within normal range in children identified and treated prior to 1 month of age (mean intellectual quotient 95) or between 1 and 3 months (mean intellectual quotient 91). Visual-perceptual difficulties and problems with social adjustment were described by both investigators. Waisbren et al.[17] found significantly lower verbal than performance score in a group of seven early-treated patients with galactosemia, identified initially through newborn screening. All the children had delays or early speech difficulties and subsequent language disorders. Gitzelmann and Steinmann[18] confirmed that early-treated patients made reasonable though suboptimal progress, were prone to speech defects and had visual-perceptual deficits, in spite of strict early treatment. Lo et al.[19] described a unique and progressive neurologic syndrome of mental retardation, tremor, and ataxia in two siblings treated with lactose restriction since the neonatal period.

The biochemical basis for the toxicity of galactose may differ in different organs. **Galactose-1-phosphate is thought to be responsible for many of the toxic effects of galactosemia.** Blood glucose concentrations are subnormal. Although galactose tolerance tests were used earlier to aid in diagnosis of galactosemia, they are not recommended, because irreversible hypoglycemia may follow these tests. Among the reactions reported to be disturbed by galactose-1-phosphate are: the phosphoglucomutase which converts glucose-6-phosphate to glucose-1-phosphate, the dehydrogenase which oxidizes glucose-6-phosphate to glucuronic acid and pyrophosphorylase which functions in formation of uridine-5'-diphosphoglucose from glucose-1-phosphate. The accumulation of galactitol in the lens leads to osmotic swelling, drop in glutathione content of lens and changes in lens permeability.

Female patients with galactosemia have a high incidence of acquired ovarian failure in spite of dietary galactose restriction.[20] The age at which treatment began appeared to be a factor in the initial study by Kaufman et al.,[20] although in another series of patients, the symptom was independent of age of diagnosis.[21] Hypergonadotropinism has been found as early as 2 years of age.[22] Ovarian failure is acquired after ovarian differentiation and initiation of follicularogenesis,[23] although Chen[24] found a striking reduction in oocyte number of offspring of pregnant rats fed a 50% galactose diet from the third day after conception until birth.

SUMMARY

Patients with galactosemia have been treated with galactose-restricted diets for over 30 years, yet information about outcome is sparse. The assumption was made that the diet was easy to follow and essentially curative, so there was no need for detailed follow-up. A collaborative effort is clearly needed to measure outcome of early treatment of galactosemia which takes into account effects of family background, socioeconomic status, and genetic factors other than the metabolic defect.

CASE REPORT

A female infant was born at term on 9-1-62 after an uncomplicated pregnancy and delivery. Birthweight was 3.24 kg. She was admitted to Cincinnati Children's Hospital at age 3 weeks because of weight loss to 2.9 kg. She was fed an evaporated milk formula, but vomiting, present since birth, had increased. On admission hepatomegaly was noted, and she bled from venipuncture sites. Bilateral, central cataracts were noted. Urine showed a reducing substance which was not glucose. Assay for galactose-1-phosphate uridyltransferase in erythrocytes showed no activity, suggesting galactosemia. Both parents had approximately 50% of normal activity, characteristic of heterozygotes for galactosemia. The baby was placed on a meat-base formula (no longer commercially available), free of lactose and galactose. Vomiting ceased. Within a week hepatomegaly was reduced and weight was 3.60 kg. Erythrocyte galactose-1-phosphate, monitored monthly remained < 25 µg/ml packed cells. Ophthalmologic exam at 3 months of age showed no cataracts.

The patient has remained on a lactose, galactose-free diet. Menses began at age 14; periods are regular, lasting about 5 days. Intellectual and social development were normal (intelligence quotient 100) at 18 years of age. She graduated from high school in 1980 and works as a clerical assistant in a hospital laboratory.

Questions and Answers

Q.   Isn't it unusual to have such a good prognosis for this condition?
A.   This patient seems to be an exception to the usual outcome reported in the literature. We have no ready explanation. Other patients in the clinic have not fared so well: intelligence quotients range from 75 to 100 with mean of 88, similar to other studies.

REFERENCES

1. von Reuss A. Zuckerausscheidung im Sauglingsalter. Wien Med Wchnschr 1908;58:799–803.
2. Mason HH, Turner ME. Chronic galactosemia: report of a case with studies on carbohydrates. Am J Dis Child 1935;50:359–374.
3. Townsend EH Jr, Mason HH, Strong PS. Galactosemia and Laennec's cirrhosis and presentation of 6 additional cases. Pediatrics 1951;7:760–763.
4. Holzel A, Komrower GM, Wilson VK. Aminoaciduria in galactosemia. Br Med J 1952;1:194–195.
5. Cusworth DC, Dent CE, Flynn FU. The aminoaciduria in galactosemia. Arch Dis Child 1955;30:150–154.
6. Schwarz V, Goldberg L, Komrower GM, Holzel A. Some disturbances of erythrocyte metabolism in galactosemia. Biochem J 1956;62:34–40.
7. Isselbacher KJ, Anderson EP, Kurahashi K, Kalkar HM. Congenital galactosemia, a single enzymatic block in galactose metabolism. Science 1956;123:635–636.
8. Wells WW, Pittman TA, Egan TJ. The isolation and identification of galactitol from the urine of patients with galactosemia. J Biol Chem 1964;239:3191.
9. Segal S. Galactosemia. In Stanbury JB, Wyngaarden JB, Fredrickson DS, Goldstein JL, Brown MS (eds): The Metabolic Basis of Inherited Disease. 5th ed. New York, McGraw Hill, 1983;174–194.
10. Haworth JC, Coodin FJ. Liver failure in galactosemia successfully treated by exchange blood transfusion. Can J Med Assoc 1971;105:301–312.
11. Hsia DY-Y, Walker FA. Variability in the clinical manifestations of galactosemia. J Pediatr 1961;59:872–883.
12. Ng WK, Donnell GN, Bergren WR, et al. Prenatal diagnosis of galactosemia. Clin Chim Acta 1977;74:227–235.
13. Allen JT, Gillett MG, Holton JB, et al. Evidence of galactosemia in utero. Lancet 1980;1:603.
14. Komrower GM. Galactosemia—thirty years on. The experience of a generation. J Inherit Metab Dis 1982;5(Suppl 2):96–104.

15. Irons M, Levy HL, Pueschel S, Castrece K. Accumulation of galactose-1-phosphate in the galactosemic fetus despite maternal milk avoidance. J Pediatr 1985;107:261–263.
16. Fishler K, Koch R, Donnell GN, Wenz E. Developmental aspects of galactosemia from infancy to child hood. Clin Pediatr 1980;19:38–44.
17. Waisbren SE, Norman TR, Schnell RR, Levy HL. Speech and language deficits in early treated children with galactosemia. J Pediatr 1983;102:75–77.
18. Gitzelmann R, Steinmann B. Galactosemia: how does long-term treatment change the outcome? Enzyme 1984;32:37–46.
19. Lo W, Packman S, Nash S, et al. Curious neurologic sequelae in galactosemia. Pediatrics 1984;73:309–312.
20. Kaufman FR, Kogut MD, Donnell GN, et al. Hypergonadotropic hypogondadism in female patients with galactosemia. N Engl J Med 1981;304:994–998.
21. Steinmann B, Gitzelmann R, Zachmann M. Hypogonadism and galactosemia (letter). N Engl J Med 1981;305: 464–465.
22. Kaufman FR, Donnell GN, Roe TF, Kogut MD. Gonadal function in patients with galactosemia. J Inherit Metab Dis 1986;9:140–146.
23. Levy HL, Driscoll SG, Porensky RS, Wender DF. Ovarian failure to galactosemia. N Engl J Med 1984;310:50.
24. Chen Y-T, Mattison DR, Feigenbaum L, et al. Reduction in oocyte number following prenatal exposure to a diet high in galactose. Science 1981;214:1145–1147.

APPENDIX

Special and Therapeutic Formulas for Inborn Errors of Metabolism

Since many pediatricians complete their training without ever seing a case of PKU, maply syrup urine disease or galactosemia, it is recommended where possible that physicians take advantage of centers combining multidisciplinary skills of pediatrics, social work, psychology, nutrition, and nursing for assistance in diagnosis, treatment, follow-up care ad study of patients with inborn errors of metabolism. (From Committee on the Handicapped Child, American Academy of Pediatrics, March, 1965.)

State Treatment Centers for Metabolic Disorders

City, STATE	Clinic Director	Telephone
Birmingham, AL	Dr. Gary Myers	205-934-5471
Mobile, AL	Dr. Paul R. Dyken	205-471-2159
Juneau, AK	Dr. David Spence	907-465-3100
Scottsdale, AZ	Dr. Frederick Hecht	602-945-4363
Tucson, AZ	Dr. Burris Duncan	802-626-6303
Little Rock, AR	Dr. Sam Shultz	501-661-2251
Little Rock, AR	Dr. Jocelyn Elders	501-661-6412
Davis, CA	Dr. Matthew Connors	916-453-3112
Fresno, CA	Dr. Susan Winters	209-225-3000 X 234
Loma Linda, CA	Dr. Constance Sandlin	714-796-7311 X 2838
Los Angeles, CA	Dr. John Barranger	213-669-2178
Los Angeles, CA	Dr. Richard Fefferman	213-667-5316
Los Angeles, CA	Dr. Miriam Wilson	213-226-3816
Los Angeles, CA	Dr. Stephen Cederbaum	213-825-0402
Oakland, CA	Dr. Richard Umansky	415-428-3351
Oakland, CA	Dr. Edgar Schoen	415-428-5783
Orange, CA	Dr. Kenneth Dumars	714-634-5791
San Diego, CA	Dr. Raymond Peterson	619-576-2932
San Francisco, CA	Dr. Seymour Packman	415-476-2871
Stanford, CA	Dr. Raymond Hintz	415-723-5791
Torrance, CA	Dr. Larry Shapiro	213-533-3751
Denver, CO	Dr. Michael Hambidge	303-394-7037
Farmington, CT	Dr. Suzanne Cassidy	203-674-2676
New Haven, CT	Dr. Margretta Seashore	203-785-2660
Wilmington, DE	Dr. Douglas Spencer	302-651-4500
Washington, DC	Dr. Wellington Hung	202-745-2121
Washington, DC	Dr. Nina Scribanu	202-625-2348
Washington, DC	Dr. John Downing, Jr.	202-745-1592
Gainesville, FL	Dr. Harry Ostrer	904-392-4104

Miami, FL	Dr. Paul Benke	305-547-6091
Tampa, FL	Dr. John Malone	813-974-4214
Atlanta, GA	Dr. Louis Elsas II	404-727-5840
Augusta, GA	Dr. David Flannery	404-828-4159
Honolulu, HI	Dr. Y.E. Hsia	808-948-6834
Boise, ID	Dr. Zsolt Koppanyi	208-334-5968
Chicago, IL	Dr. Reuben Matalon	312-996-5305
Chicago, IL	Dr. Margaret O'Flynn	312-880-4012
Chicago, IL	Dr. Paul Wong	312-942-6299
Indianapolis, IN	Dr. Ira Brandt	317-274-3966
Iowa City, IA	Dr. James Hanson	319-356-2674
Kansas City, KS	Dr. Leona Therou	913-588-5908
Wichita, KS	Dr. Sechin Cho	316-261-2622
Lexington, KY	Dr. C. Charlton Mabry	606-233-5404
Louisville, KY	Dr. Billy Andrews	502-562-8825
New Orleans, LA	Dr. Flora Cherry	504-568-5075
New Orleans, LA	Dr. Emmanuel Shapira	504-588-5229
Bangor, ME	Dr. Laurent Beauregard	207-945-7354
Scarborough, ME	Dr. Thomas Brewster	207-883-4362
Baltimore, MD	Dr. Miriam Blitzer	301-528-3480
Baltimore, MD	Dr. David Valle	301-955-3071
Boston, MA	Dr. Mary Ampola	617-956-5531
Boston, MA	Dr. Harvey Levy	617-735-7945
Ann Arbor, MI	Dr. Richard Allen	313-763-4697
Detroit, MI	Dr. Henry Nadler	313-745-6035
Minneapolis, MN	Dr. Robert Fisch	612-626-6777
Rochester, MN	Dr. Virginia Michels	507-284-8397
Jackson, MS	Dr. Hans-Georg Otto Bock	601-984-1900
Columbia, MO	Dr. Calvin Woodruff	314-882-3996
Kansas City, MO	Dr. David Harris	816-234-3290
St. Louis, MO	Dr. Roger Sharp	314-391-6300
St. Louis, MO	Dr. Richard Hillman	314-454-6093
Helena, MT	Dr. Sidney Pratt	406-444-4740
Omaha, NE	Dr. Hobart Wiltse	402-559-7350
Carson City, NV	Richard C. Bentnick	702-885-4885
Concord, NH	Charles Alabano	603-271-4517
Camden, NJ	Dr. Chester Minarcik	609-342-2226
Camden, NJ	Dr. Ernest Post	609-343-2260
Newark, NJ	Dr. Anna Haroutunian	201-268-8763
Newark, NJ	Dr. Ling-Yu Shih	201-456-5278
New Brunswick, NJ	Dr. Max Salas	201-745-8600 X 8574
Albuquerque, NM	Dr. John Johnson	505-277-4842
Albany, NY	Dr. Marilyn Cowger	518-445-5723
Buffalo, NY	Dr. Robert Cooke	716-878-7595
New York, NY	Dr. Selma Snyderman	212-340-6266
Rochester, NY	Dr. Kenneth McCormick	716-275-7744
Stony Brook, NY	Dr. David Hyman	516-444-2700
Chapel Hill, NC	Dr. Henry Kirkman	919-966-4202
Charlotte, NC	Dr. James Parke, Jr.	704-338-3156
Durham, NC	Dr. Charles Roe	919-684-2036
Winston-Salem, NC	Dr. Barbara Burton	919-748-4321
Fargo, ND	Dr. Alan Kenien	701-237-2431
Grand Forks, ND	Dr. Douglas Knowlton	701-780-2477
Akron, OH	Dr. Daryl Steiner	216-753-0345
Cincinnati, OH	Dr. John Hutton	513-559-4451
Cleveland, OH	Dr. Geoffrey Redmond	216-444-6238

Columbus, OH	Dr. Carolyn Romshe	614-461-2115
Dayton, OH	Dr. Harold Chen	513-226-8408
Toledo, OH	Dr. Paul Delamater	419-259-1369
Oklahoma City, OK	Dr. Owen Rennert	405-271-4401
Tulsa, OK	Dr. James Coldwell	918-664-6600 X 264
Portland, OR	Dr. Neil Buist	503-225-8344
Hershey, PA	Dr. Cheston Berlin	717-531-8412
Philadelphia, PA	Dr. Warren Grover	215-427-5464
Pittsburg, PA	Dr. Jane Breck	412-647-5097
San Juan, PR	Dr. L. Torres de Jiminez	809-763-1093
Providence, RI	Dr. Siegfried Pueschel	401-277-5071
Columbia, SC	Dr. William Kemick	803-734-8959
Greenwood, SC	Dr. Roger Stephenson	803-223-9311
Pierre, SD	Allen Krom	605-773-3737
Memphis, TN	Dr. Jewel Ward	901-528-6514
Dallas, TX	Dr. Charles Mize	214-920-2085
Galveston, TX	Dr. Bobbye Rouse	409-761-2355
Houston, TX	Dr. Arthur Beaudet	713-791-3261
Houston, TX	Dr. Rodney Howell	713-797-4555
Salt Lake City, UT	Dr. Claire Leonard	801-581-3461
Burlington, VT	Dr. Christopher Kus	802-863-7315
Charlottesville, VA	Dr. William Wilson	804-924-2665
Richmond, VA	Dr. Karl Roth	804-786-9617
Seattle, WA	Dr. Ronald Scott	206-543-3370
Dunbar, WV	Dr. Mary Skinner	304-768-6295
Morgantown, WV	Dr. William Klingberg	304-293-4451
Madison, WI	Dr. Stanley Berlow	608-263-5787
Marshfield, WI	Dr. Sharon Mabry	715-387-5185
Milwaukee, WI	Dr. June Dobbs	414-931-4069
Cheyenne, WY	Dr. Larry Meuli	307-777-6297

The information listed above was taken from: *State Treatment Centers for Metabolic Disorders,* National Center for Education in Maternal and Child Health, 38th and R Streets, N.W., Washington, DC 20057, September, 1986. The Directory, which contains the complete listing of names and addresses, can be obtained by writing to the address.

THE MATERNAL PKU COLLABORATIVE STUDY

Coordinating Center:

Dr. Richard, Koch, Principal Investigator
Children's Hospital of Los Angeles
Los Angeles, California 90027
213-669-2152

Contributing Centers

Northeast Region

Dr. Harvey Levy
Children's Hospital Medical Center
Gardner 6, Room 650
283 Longwood Avenue
Boston, Massachusetts 02115
617-735-7945

Southeast

Dr. Bobbye Rouse
Department of Pediatrics
University of Texas Medical Branch
Galveston, Texas 77550
409-761-2355

Midwest	Dr. Reuben Matalon Department of Pediatrics Room 1220 CSB 840 South Wood Street Chicago, Illinois 312-996-6714
Western	Dr. Richard Koch (See Coordinating Center)
Canada	Dr. William Hanley The Hospital for Sick Children 555 University Avenue Toronto, Ontario Canada M5G 1X8 416-597-1500

For additional information contact the Coordinating Center in Los Angeles or the Contributing Center for your region.

22

Infant Feeding Practice

BUFORD L. NICHOLS, M.D.

ABSTRACT

Significant changes in infant feeding practice over the last 30 years are highlighted, with emphasis on the development of special-purpose formulas for infants with various milk intolerances or to meet specific therapeutic needs.

"Of all the fatal affections that occur in the first year of life, forty per cent are diseases of the digestive, and twenty per cent diseases of the respiratory organs. Mortality diminishes with every day of advancing life: every additional hour improves the baby's chances for preservation. Almost one-half of the infants who die before the end of the first year, do so before they are one month old. The causes of disease are the more active, the earlier they are brought to bear upon the young with their defective vitality. Two grave conclusions are to be drawn from this fact. First. That diminution of early mortality depends upon avoiding diseases of the digestive organs by insisting on normal alimentation. This is particularly important in the first few months. While it has been shown that breast milk lowers the rate of infant mortality through the entire first year, it does so much more in the first few months; thus, although infants may not be fed on breast milk through the whole of the normal period for nursing, very great gain is accomplished by insisting that they shall be nursed for at least a limited time, if only a few months. There are few mothers but are capable of nursing during that brief period, and all contribute to the illness or death of their babes by refusing to nurse them through at least the first dangerous weeks. Second. The hygienic rules for infants concern the digestive organs mainly—so much so, that infant hygiene, and the hygiene of the digestive organs in infants, appear to be nearly identical." A. Jacoby, 1890.[1]

During the past century the mortality rate of infants in Europe and North America has decreased from approximately 150/1000 live births to less than 15/1000. This is a measure of the contribution of science to human welfare.[2,3] While it is impossible to isolate individual factors responsible for this progress, one notable accomplishment during the past century has been the development of safe artificial infant feeding practices (Fig. 1). To illustrate the progress in infant feeding in the U.S., in 1922 the *mortality rate* in artificially fed infants was five times higher than that in completely breast-fed infants.[4] Since then, the fall in total mortality rate has made such a comparison impossible to design. A recent study of *morbidity* in the United States suggests that the incidence of illness among artificially fed infants is no greater than in breast-fed infants.[5]

FORMULA FEEDING OF INFANTS

Infant mortality rates in the United States declined to 50/1000 live births by 1950. This change resulted from a major decline in postneonatal death in infants up to 28 days of age. Two-thirds of all residual infant deaths occurred during the neonatal period. The proportion of infants who weighed 2500 gm or less at birth was 7.5%, but these infants accounted for two-thirds of the neonatal deaths. Since 1950, the proportion of infants with low birthweight has declined only slightly. Today, 7.0% of all infants born in the United States weigh 2500 gm or less at birth. The infant mortality rate during the years 1977-1979 fell to 13.6%/1000. At the present, infants who weigh 1500 gm or less at birth account for only 1.15% of births but represent one-half of all neonatal deaths.[6]

A substantial change in feeding practices occurred in the United States since 1955. This is illustrated in Figure 2, which demonstrates types of infant feeding at one week of age.[8] Evaporated milk formulas were common in 1955. By 1970, nearly all hospitals in the U.S. were utilizing ready-to-use formulas. Exclusive or partial breastfeeding accounted for 90% of infant feeding at one month of age in 1922.[4] This had fallen to 25% by 1955. Since 1970, the rate of breastfeeding of young infants has increased two-fold. The decline in postneonatal mortality occurred before the current increase in breastfeeding. The early improvement reflects the superiority of prepared milk formulas over evaporated milk formulas.

In Figure 3, the distribution of intake in 1983 is divided according to the percentage of infants receiving different dietary sources of calories: human milk, prepared formula, whole cow milk, baby foods, and table foods. Only

367

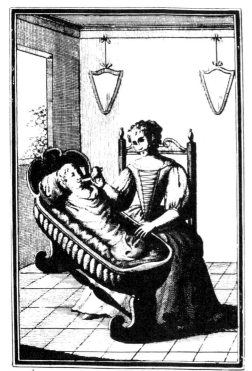

Ficta teneris immulget ubera labris.

FIGURE 1.   Artificial feeding practice in 1787. The infant feeding apparatus is made of leather with a silver nipple. (Rossi, G. Metado di Allattare a Mano I Bambini Del Dottor Filippo Baldini, 1787. Napoli, Vicenza.)

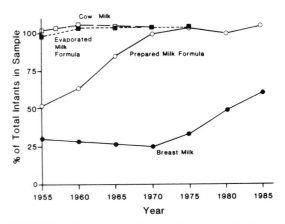

FIGURE 2.   Distribution of types of infant milk feedings during the past 30 years. Prepared milk formulas were commercially available. Cow milk and evaporated milk formulas were prepared in the home.[7]

on modified cow milk.[4] A few displayed signs and symptoms suggestive of milk intolerance. As a result, continuing research resulted in improved quality and acceptability of infant formulas. In addition to formulas for term infants (Table 1, part A and B), special-purpose formulas were developed for low birthweight infants (Table 1, part C) and infants with gastrointestinal or metabolic disturbances (Table 1, part D and E). In the U.S. cow milk based infant formulas comprise 80% of total present

20% of infants were exclusively breast-fed at three months of age. Fifteen percent of calories came from baby foods after four months of age. Table foods and whole cow milk were introduced after six months of age. Milks were the major source of dietary calories for infants. Human milk contributed 22% of all caloric intake during the first year of life. Prepared milk formulas accounted for 35% of all caloric intake for the same period.[9] The generally accepted recommendation for energy intake during infancy is 115 kcal/kg/day at birth and 105 kcal at the end of infancy. The total energy intake of infants revealed in Figure 3 does not meet this recommendation. From current evidence it appears that the average child is ingesting about 80 cal/kg during the period of four to eight months of life.[10]

COMPLETE COW MILK FORMULAS

The nutrient composition and quality of ingredients of infant formulas have improved over many years. With the home-prepared formulas available in 1922, most infants thrived

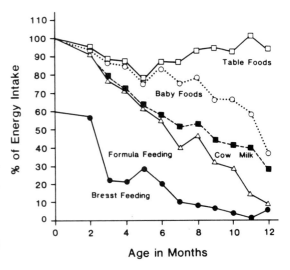

FIGURE 3.   Infant feeding as a function of age in 1983. The data are expressed as percent of total calories from various sources. Formulas are prepared commercially from cow milk or soy. Cow milk includes full fat and partially defatted commercial dairy products. The baby foods are prepared from pureed and strained foods. Table foods are those foods normally eaten by the family at mealtime.[8]

day prepared formulas used by infants.[11] These formulas are composed of reconstituted skimmed cow milk or mixtures of skimmed cow milk and electrolyte-depleted cow milk whey and casein. The dietary fat is a mixture consisting of soy, palm, coconut, corn, oleo, safflower, or butter designed to resemble human milk fat. All contain lactose. The current cow milk based formulas have been tested intensively under experimental and field conditions and are equal to human milk in promoting rapid growth during the first six months of life.

COMPLETE SOY FORMULAS

Based on the concept that cow milk formula intolerance is a manifestation of either protein hypersensitivity or lactose intolerance, soy-protein-based formulas were introduced in 1909.[12,13] These formulas evolved through a series of production refinements and today represent a nutritionally sound and safe alternative to cow milk based formulas (Table 1, part B). Soy-protein-based formulas now make up 20% of the total infants formulas sold in the United States.[11] The soy protein is isolated and treated to improve its nutritional qualities. **L-Methionine is added to improve the quality of protein in comparison to casein in cow milk.** The carbohydrate in these formulas is sucrose, glucose oligomers (smaller molecular weight starches), or a mixture of the two. The fat mixture is similar to that used in cow milk formulas. The frequency of use of soy formulas in the United States increases from 3% in newborns to 10% of formula-fed infants between 2 and 12 months of age.[11]

Early studies suggested that the use of soy protein formulas could prevent the development of allergic disorders in later life.[12,13] Seventy-five years of clinical experience with soy formulas have not confirmed this hypothesis. The frequency of clinical intolerance to soy or cow milk formulas is not different.[14,15] The perceived benefits of soy protein formula might be due to the substitution of sucrose or glucose oligomers for lactose. Clinical studies of infants fed these formulas have seldom differentiated between intolerance of carbohydrate or of protein. Soy protein formulas can be recommended for use in vegetarian families where animal protein formulas are not desired, and for the management of galactosemia, primary lactase deficiency, secondary lactose intolerance and cow milk protein hypersensi-

tivity. All of these indications require close supervision by the pediatrician.

COMPLETE FORMULAS FOR PRETERM INFANT

Infant mortality in the United States currently is higher than in 10 other countries. This difference in infant mortality is due to a higher incidence of low birthweight infants in the U.S. However, the U.S. mortality rate associated with birthweights of 1500-2500 gm is equal to that of term infants. In addition, survival among infants between 800 and 1500 gm is 60-70% in most nurseries in the United States. Improved nutrition for the preterm infant has played a substantial role in improved survival. Immaturity of the digestive and excretory systems and the high growth rates of preterm infants led to specific modifications in these formulas (Table 1, part C). A major modification was the addition of medium chain triglycerides (MCT) to the fat mixture because of superior digestibility. Glucose oligomers were added to reduce the relative dietary lactose and osmolar loads.

THERAPEUTIC FORMULAS

The composition of specific components in infant formulas have been modified or refined to meet specific therapeutic requirements (Table 1, part D and E). Complete therapeutic formulas designed to bypass digestive insufficiency or protein hypersensitivity are based upon hydrolyzed casein, whole casein, and soy protein as a source of amino acid nitrogen. All of these formulas are lactose-free, some contain glucose oligomers and soluble starches, and some contain MCT. The modular formulas allow stepwise introduction of specific carbohydrates and fats into the diet in a logical sequence for the purpose of therapeutic feeding trials. All of these therapeutic formulas have been used in the management of children with formula intolerances. **The modular formulas are incomplete and should only be used under close professional supervision.** This is especially true of the locally made modular formulas.[15,16]

"The pernicious folly of making phyfic precede food at an infant's birth is, I hope, fufficiently expofed in the former fection; and notice is there taken of the admirable manner, in which the thin, diluted, and gently opening properties of the mother's milk, are adapted to every medicinal as well as alimentary purpofe. Nature does not afford, nor

TABLE 1. Classification and Composition Per 100 Kcal of Available Infant Formulas

A. Complete Cow Milk Based Infant Formulas

	Mother	Mead Johnson	Ross	Ross	Wyeth	Nestlé	Nestlé
Manufacturer: Product:	Human milk	Enfamil	PM 60/40	Similac	S.M.A.	NAN	Lactogen
Protein, gm whey:casein source	1.46 70:30 human milk	2.20 60:40 cow milk+ whey	2.22 60:40 cow whey+ casein	2.22 18:82 cow milk	2.20 60:40 cow milk+ whey	2.25 60:40 cow whey+ casein	2.55 18:82 cow milk+ whey
Fat, gm source	5.42 human milk	5.60 coconut+ soy	5.59 coconut+ corn	5.30 coconut+ soy	5.37 oleo+coconut safflower+soy	6.9 butter+corn	6.9 butter+corn +oleo
Carbohydrate, gm source	10.00 lactose	10.30 lactose	10.20 lactose	10.60 lactose	10.70 lactose	11.4 lactose	11.1 lactose

B. Complete Soy Based Infant Formulas (soy formulas are enriched with L-methionine)

	Mead Johnson	Ross	Ross	Wyeth	Loma Linda	Loma Linda	Nestlé
Manufacturer: Product:	Prosobee	Isomil	Isomil SF	Nursoy	Soyalac	I-Soyalac	Alsoy
Protein, gm source	3.00 soy isolate	2.66 soy isolate	2.96 soy isolate	3.10 soy isolate	3.10 soy isolate	3.10 soy isolate	1.90 soy isolate
Fat, gm source	5.30 coconut+ soy	5.46 coconut+ soy	5.33 coconut+ soy	5.30 coconut+ safflower+ soy+oleo	5.50 coconut+ soy	5.50 soy	3.30 coconut+ soy+palm
Carbohydrate, gm source	10.00 gluc oligomers	10.00 gluc oligomers +sucrose	10.00 gluc oligomers	10.20 sucrose	10.00 gluc oligomers +sucrose	10.00 gluc oligomers +sucrose	7.40 gluc oligomers

C. Complete Preterm Infant Formulas (MCT = medium chain triglyceride)

	Mead Johnson	Ross	Ross	Wyeth	Nestlé
Manufacturer: Product:	Enfamil Premature Formula	Similac Special Care	Similac LBW	S.M.A. Preemie	Pre NAN
Protein, gm whey:casein source	3.00 60:40 cow milk+ whey	2.71 60:40 cow whey+ casein	2.71 18:82 cow milk	2.40 60:40 cow milk+ whey	2.00 60:40 cow milk+ whey

Fat, gm source	5.10 coconut+soy +MCT	5.43 corn+soy +MCT	5.53 coconut+ corn+MCT	5.40 coconut+soy+ oleo+MCT	3.40 corn+butter +MCT
Carbohydrate, gm source	11.00 lactose+gluc oligomers	10.60 lactose+gluc oligomers	10.50 lactose+gluc oligomers	10.50 lactose+gluc oligomers	8.00 lactose+gluc oligomers

D. Complete Therapeutic Formulas

Manufacturer: Product:	Mead Johnson Portagen	Mead Johnson Nutramigen	Mead Johnson Pregestimil	Nestlé AL 110	Nestlé Alfare
Protein, gm source	3.50 sodium caseinate	2.80 casein hyrolysate	2.80 casein hydrolysate	1.90 casein	2.50 whey hydrolysate
Fat, gm source	4.80 corn+MCT	3.90 corn	4.10 corn+MCT	3.30 butter+corn	3.60 butter+corn +MCT
Carbohydrate, gm source	11.50 gluc oligomers +sucrose	13.40 gluc oligomers +starch	13.50 gluc oligomers +starch	7.40 gluc oligomers	7.80 gluc oligomers +starch

E. Modular Therapeutic Formulas

Manufacturer: Product:	Mead Johnson Mono-Disaccharide	Mead Johnson Protein Free Diet	Ross RCF	Ross RMF	Local[16] Eiweissmilch	Local[17] Chicks
Protein, gm source	2.80 casein hydrolysate +amino acids	0.00	2.95 soy isolate	2.2 casein	3.00 casein	3.75 chicken
Fat, gm source	4.20 corn+MCT	3.90 corn	5.31 coconut+ soy	0.00	2.50 butter	1.50 chicken
Carbohydrate, gm source	4.20 starch	12.50 gluc oligomers +starch	0.00	0.00	1.50 lactose	5.00 gluc oligomers

can art contrive, any effectual fubftitute for that delicious fluid. By degrees the milk acquires confiftence, and affords greater nourifhment to the child, as he becomes more capable of degefting it. At length, his bodily ftrength increafing, and his teeth burfting through his gums, he can take more folid and fubftantial food, which requires ftill greater powers of digestion. These changes are fo obvious, that they cannot be mistaken. Ignorance is pleaded in vain, and the leaft deviation from fo plain a road to health, is punifhed with lafting injury. The infant, after having derived its whole fluftenance and growth, while in the womb, from the mother's juices, cannot without the greateft danger have its fupplies totally altered at its birth. It muft ftill be fed from the fame congenial fource, or the fhock of a fudden and unnatural change will prove very trying to its tender conftitution." W. Buchan, 1811.[18]

INDICATIONS FOR FORMULA USE

There are three basic applications of complete cow milk based infant formulas: (1) substitution for infants whose mothers do not choose to or cannot breastfeed; (2) supplementation for infants whose mothers choose to omit occasional breastfeeding; and (3) complementation of formula if the mother's milk productiion is inadequate. The substitution of formula feeding is indicated in the presence of infectious diseases such as cavitary tuberculosis or herpetic or syphilitic lesions of the breast. In some women with metabolic disorders, breastfeeding may not be indicated. If the mother has thyrotoxicosis and is on antithyroid medication, care should be exercised in surveillance of the breast-fed infant's thyroid status. Lists of maternal medications that contraindicate breastfeeding should be consulted for details.[19,20] Complementation of the breastfeeding with cow milk formula is common from the third or fourth month of life. Clinical assessment is required during the first six months to determine if growth has faltered and to detect other signs of malnutrition. When growth faltering occurs, if the mother wishes to continue breastfeeding, formula must be offered as a temporary supplement, but unless effective steps are taken to increase her milk production, the mother's milk supply will fail. Complete cow milk based infant formula is an appropriate complement to the diet of a growth-faltering breast-fed infant.

As previously indicated, complete soy formulas are most often described by physicians suspicious that cow milk protein intolerance is present in young infants. This is frequently in response to family concerns about formula adequacies. Marketing data indicate that the majority of parents with concerns believe the infant to have been benefited by a change

from cow milk to soy milk formula.[11] However, similar responses are frequently seen when the infants are switched from one brand of cow milk formula to another.

The lactose-free characteristics of these soy formulas provide an important rationale for their use in congenital or acquired lactose intolerance. It has become common practice to refeed infants recovering from acute diarrhea with complete soy formulas and to keep them on this diet from 30-60 days after recovery.

Failure to tolerate sucrose or glucose oligosaccharide formulas during refeeding leads to the use of hydrolyzed casein formulas in suspected cow milk protein hypersensitivity and modular formulas in suspected carbohydrate intolerances. See the subsequent case report for an example of the approach to complex formula intolerances.

WHOLE COW MILK

Whole cow milk is introduced into the diet of some infants after six months of age. The appropriate time for introduction of whole cow milk and other adult dietary items to the infant's diet is unclear. It is evident that by 12 months of age, infants tolerate whole cow milk as part of a mixed diet. Three lines of concern are reflected in the recommendation that infants not receive whole cow's milk before one year of age: (1) the occurrence of whole milk protein; (2) the occurrence of iron deficiency anemia in infants fed whole cow milk; (3) and the high level of solute requiring renal excretion present in whole cow milk.[22]

The introduction of skimmed cow milk to infant feeding should never be proposed to control excessive weight gain during infancy. Although studies suggest that the use of 2% fat cow milk as part of a mixed diet during the last half of infancy can be satisfactory, the concerns associated with its use are similar to those for whole cow milk, but with the additional potential for exaggerated impact on renal water requirements.[24]

"The indication for Eiweissmilch is diarrhea, due to indigestion or fermentation. The action of Eiweissmilch is based upon inhibition of fermentation and the promotion of protein decomposition in the intestine. It is accomplished by lessening of the milk-sugar, and of the whey salts, as well as by the relative increase in the amount of protein and calcium. As a consequence of the changes thus produced in the intestine it becomes possible to add a carbohydrate which less readily undergoes fermentation (a dextrin-maltose preparation), a very important consideration in avoding a carbohydrate starvation. The technique of feeding with Eiweissmilch can be varied as one gathers experience, depending upon the exact nature and degree of the disturbance. The beginner will do well to accept the dogmatic directions laid down by Finkelstein and Meyer, until that experience is gained. The Charybdis of starvation lies on one side, the Scylla of overfeeding and return of diarrhea, on the other, and the mariner who sails without a pilot to guide him is very likely to come to grief on one or the other. In the cases where Eiweissmilch is most indicated, in severe marasmus with rapid loss in weight and diarrhea ('Decomposition,' Finkelstein); and in severe alimentary intoxications, these dangers are so real that life is seriously threatened by either one. Langstein and Meyer give the following direction for the treatment of the former of the two conditions: 'After 12 hours of a tea diet (a longer time is not necessary, and may be even harmful; a shorter time does not always accomplish the purpose) one begins to give small amounts of Eiweissmilch, to which has been added 3 per cent of a dextrin-maltose preparation. The initial dose is 300 gm. given in 6 to 10 feedings a day, and continued for three or four days. During this time the primary aggravation of symptoms takes place and generally this is followed by convalescence with cessation of diarrhea. After convalescence is established one proceeds briskly to an increase of food of 50 to 60 gm every second day until a total quantity of 200 gm. Eiweissmilch per kg of body-weight daily is reached, but never more than one liter a day. Depending upon the severity of the disturbance and the nature of the stool, one hastens or retards the beginning of an increase in carbohydrate. Gain in weight is attained by the addition of carbohydrates up to 5 per cent of the dextrin-maltose preparation, and in the case of infants over three months old, by the further addition of 1 to 2 per cent of flour (wheat, or oat). An increase beyond 5 per cent is permitted in those cases in which the gain in weight does not begin with 5 per cent . . . It is, therefore, permissible in certain cases in which a gain in weight does not occur with less to increase the carbohydrate to 8 or even 10 per cent. The duration of Eiweissmilch feeding should be six weeks in the younger infant and four weeks in the older, but in the older infant one can often get along with less time.' The child is then put on the usual milk mixtures. In cases of less severity and in simple dyspepsia with diarrhea, one can proceed much more rapidly. In severe intoxications the initial dosage and progress must be much slower, unless the child has at the same time a severe marasmus (Decomposition) which calls for food at the earliest possible time." J. Brennemann, 1923.[23]

CASE REPORT

Jose F. was admitted to Ben Taub General Hospital at 36 days of age. He had been delivered of the first pregnancy of a 20-year-old woman. His birthweight was 3060 gm. He was started on breastfeeding but was discharged at two days of age on Similac. After three weeks, he was changed to whole cow milk and was also fed bananas and peaches. Three days before admission, he developed vomiting followed by diarrhea. He weighed 200 gm less than at birth at the time he was admitted. Physical examination demonstrated

severe malnutrition and dehydration. His arm/head circumference ratio was 0.24; triceps skinfold thicknesses were 3 mm. His stool at the time of admission was positive for shigella and rotavirus. Following intravenous hydration, he was given Pedialyte, a 5% glucose electrolyte solution, which he tolerated well (Fig. 4). He then was advanced to half-strength and then full-strength Prosobee, a soy formula that contains glucose polymers. He tolerated this and after three days on the pediatric ward was transferred to the convalescent ward where he was managed for the following eight days.

During hospitalization on the convalescent ward, glucose began to appear in his stool. He received an adequate caloric intake but failed to gain weight; his weight fell gradually for several days. He was determined to be dehydrated and was transferred back to the pediatric ward. When he was fasted during intravenous rehydration, the stool volume dropped and no glucose was present in the stool. The following day he was given Pedialyte, which he tolerated well. There was no increase in the number of stools and he then was started on Ross carbohydrate free formula, a soy formula without carbohydrate (RCF). The formula was offered with 3, then 4, then 5% glucose. He tolerated the 3% and 4%, but at 5% diarrhea recurred with an increase in the number of stools and reappearance of glucose in the stools. This prompted a change to Ross Modular Formula (RMF). RMF is a casein base to which carbohydrate and fat are added. At this time the infant was placed on 1% glucose RMF and continued to have glucose in the stools. He was again placed on Pedialyte and this time demonstrated an intolerance to dietary intake of 5% glucose. There was a simultaneous increase in the number of stools. Figure 4 shows the number of stools per day, the intake of formula (cc/hr) and body weight. Notice that he continud to lose weight with the exception of the early period when he was on the RCF formula. Subsequently, he lost weight acutely. He was subsequently given peripheral TPN and began to show some weight gain. He then received "central line" TPN for 36 days.

When he was readmitted from the convalescent ward, the characteristic distended abdomen with depletion of muscle mass and subcutaneous fat was evident (Fig. 5A). Small bowel mucosal biopsy taken before the central line TPN was started revealed almost complete villus atrophy (Fig. 6). Normally the ratio of villus length to crypt depth is approximately 4 to 1. No villous structures were visible. Notice

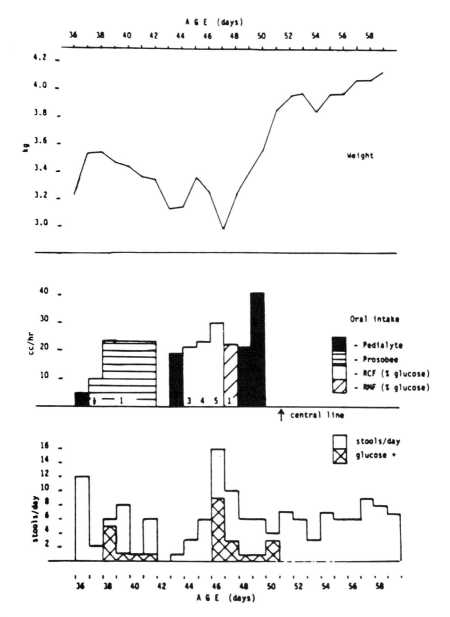

FIGURE 4.   Clinical course of a patient who developed a complex formula intolerance during hospitalization for acute diarrhea. For the periods when he was fed a modular formula, the percent concentration of glucose in the formula is shown at the bottom of the middle panel. The number of stools per day and the presence of glucose are indicated in the bottom panel. Central line total parenteral nutrition was begun at 51 days of age. See text for the clinical course.

the increased cellularity, a lack of goblet cells and a reduced number of mitotic figures. Subcutaneous fat and muscle mass filled out after 36 days of TPN (Fig. 5B). He was subsequently discharged home tolerating a normal diet, and on follow-up was thriving.

The general strategy utilized in refeeding this patient is summarized in Figure 7. This approach is limited to those infants whose diarrhea on admission responded to rehydration and fasting with a remission.

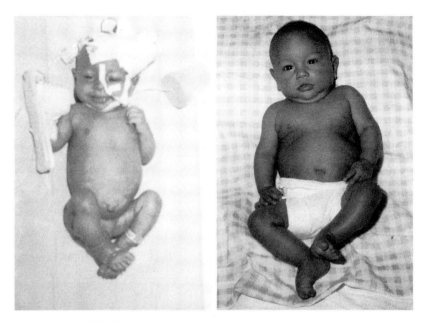

FIGURE 5.   The same patient at 46 days of age (left) and
at 82 days of age (right) after 36 days of total parenteral
nutrition.

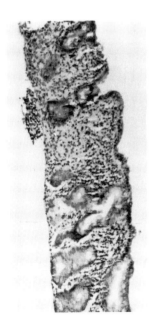

FIGURE 6.   Mucosal biopsy taken at 50 days of age.
Note the lack of villous structure. The normal villus to
crypt ratio of 4:1 has been lost.

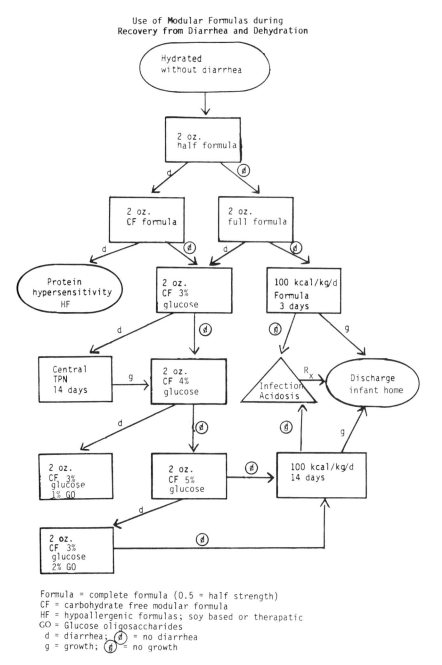

Use of Modular Formulas during
Recovery from Diarrhea and Dehydration

Formula = complete formula (0.5 = half strength)
CF = carbohydrate free modular formula
HF = hypoallergenic formulas; soy based or therapatic
GO = Glucose oligosaccharides
d = diarrhea; Ø = no diarrhea
g = growth; Ø = no growth

FIGURE 7.   Approach to the use of modular formulas
during recovery from diarrhea and dehydration. This is the
technique used in the case report.[25]

REFERENCES

1. Jacobi A. Intestinal Diseases of Infancy and Childhood, 2nd ed. Detroit, G.S. Davis; Detroit, New York Academy of Medicine, 1890;vii–viii.
2. Bloom BS. Changing infant mortality: The need to spend more while getting less. Pediatrics 1984;73:862–866.
3. Russell B. The Scientific Outlook. London, George Allen & Unwin Ltd., 1931;202.
4. Woodbury RM. The relation between breast and artificial feeding and infant mortality. Am J Hyg 1922;2:668–687.
5. Bauchner H, Leventhal JM, Shapiro ED. Studies of breast feeding and infections: How good is the evidence? JAMA 1986;256:887–892.
6. McCormick MC. The contribution of low birth weight to infant mortality and childhood morbidity. N Engl J Med 1985; 312:82–89.
7. Wegman ME. Annual summary of vital statistics—1984. Pediatrics 1985;76:861–871.
8. Martinez GA, Krieger FW. 1984 Milk-feeding patterns in the United States. Pediatrics 1985;76:1004–1008.
9. Johnson GH. Unpublished information collected by Gerber Products Company, 1983 (270 infants aged 2-12 months).
10. Whitehead RG, Hall AA, Black AE, Wiles SJ. Recommended diet for the first 6 months of life. Food Nutr Bull 1981;Suppl 5:242–246.
11. Stahle DA. Hypoallergenic formula usage by infant age (unpublished). Available from Ross Laboratories, Columbus, Ohio 43216, 1982.
12. Ruhrah J. The soy bean as an article of diet for infants. JAMA 1910;54:1664–1665.
13. Ruhrah J. The soy bean in infant feeding. Arch Pediatr 1909;26:496–501.
14. Taitz LS. Soy feeding in infancy. Arch Dis Child 1982; 57:814–815.
15. Gruskay FL. Comparison of breast, cow and soy feedings in the prevention of onset of allergic disease. Clin Pediatr 1982;21:486–491.
16. Finkelstein H. Lehrbuch der Sauglingskrankheiten. In Dritte Vollstandig Umgearbeitete Auglage. Berlin, 1924;323.
17. Larcher VF, Shepherd R, Francis DEM, Harries JT. Protracted diarrhoea in infancy. Arch Dis Child 1977;52:597–605.
18. Buchan W. Advice to Mothers . . . The second edition. London, T. Cadell and W. Davies, 1811;208–210.
19. Lawrence RA. Breast-feeding: A Guide for the Medical Profession. St. Louis, C.V. Mosby Co., 1980.
20. Goldfarb J, Tibbetts E. Breast-feeding Handbook: A Practical Reference for Physicians, Nurses, and Other Health Professionals. Hillside, N.J., Enslow Publishers, 1980; 119–120.
21. Crumpacker CS. Hepatitis. In Remington JS, Klein JO (eds): Infectious Diseases of the Fetus and Newborn Infant. Philadelphia, W.B. Saunders Co., 1983.
22. American Academy of Pediatrics Committee on Nutrition. The use of cow's milk in infancy. In press, 1983.
23. Brennemann J. Artificial feeding of infants. In Abt IA (ed): Pediatrics, Vol. II, chapter XXII. London, W.B. Saunders Co., 1923;749–750.
24. Yeung DL, Pennell MD, Leung M, Hall J. The effects of 2% milk intake on infant nutrition. Nutr Res 1982;2:651–660.
25. Klish WJ, Potts E, Ferry GD, Nichols BL. Modular formula: An approach to management of infants with specific or complex food intolerances. J Pediatr 1976;88:948–952.

23

Human Milk Substitutes

JAMES W. HANSEN, M.D., Ph.D.
DAVID A. COOK, Ph.D.
ANGEL CORDANO, M.D., M.P.H.
STANLEY G. MIGUEL, Ph.D.

ABSTRACT

The interesting history of the development and use of human milk substitutes proclaims the need for such products and the critical nature of their composition. The necessary nutrient characteristics of these substitutes require a complex mixture of the highest quality food grade ingredients to meet infant needs without exceeding metabolic capacities. Meticulous quality control systems must be in place to assure the reliable manufacture of products which will be the sole item of diet for several months in fragile newborns. Prior to distribution for general use, however, thorough preclinical and clinical testing of new formulations is essential to establish their safety and nutritional adequacy for supporting normal health and physiologic growth. Modern infant formulas are a nutritionally complete substitute for human milk and, for many infants with specific medical conditions, can safely provide life-giving nutrition that may not otherwise be available.

NEED FOR MILK SUBSTITUTES

Human milk is believed to be the most nearly complete and perfect food for the human infant, and breastfeeding the preferred mode of delivery.[1] It is the most natural nutrition available and is generally suited to the individual needs of the infant.

Importance of Breast Milk

The importance of breastfeeding before modern sanitary methods was emphasized by Buchanan who declared in 1812:

"Nothing can shew the disposition which mankind have to depart from nature more that their endeavoring to bring up children without the breast. The mother's milk or that of a healthy nurse is unquestionably the best food for an infant. Neither art nor nature can afford a proper substitute for it. Children may seem to thrive for a few months without the breast; but when teething, the small-pox, and other diseases incident to childhood come on they generally perish."[2]

As early as the first century, discussions were written concerning the "goodness" of human milk. Soranus of Ephesus (A.D. 98-138) described a "fingernail" test by which one could ascertain whether or not milk was good. Phaire repeated it in his "Boke of Children" in 1545:

"That mylke is goode that is whyte and sweete; and when you droppe it on your nayle and do move your finger, neyther fletheth abrod at every stiring nor will hange faste upon your naile, when ye turn it downeward, but that whyche is betwene bothe is beste."[2]

Myths flourished about breast milk including the thought that the characteristics of the source of the milk would be passed on to the suckling. This attitude stems at least in part from the early Roman writer, Phayorinus, whom Phaire quoted as affirming that

" . . . if the lambes be nourished with the milk of goates, they shall have course wool lyke the heare of goates; and if kiddes in lyke manner suck upon shepe, the heare of them shall be soft lyke wolle."[2]

This prevailing thought led to the careful selection of a wet nurse when an alternative to the mother's milk was sought. Phaire recommended that much attention be given to the qualities of the wet nurse chosen to suckle an infant.

" . . . such shall be sobre, honeste, and chaste, well-formed, amyable, and cheerefull, so that she may accustome the infant into mirth, no dronkarde, vicious, sluttyshe, for such corrupteth the nature of the chylde."[3]

Alternatives to Breast Milk

Alternatives to breastfeeding infants have been sought and used at least since the stone age. The earliest known infant feeding vessel

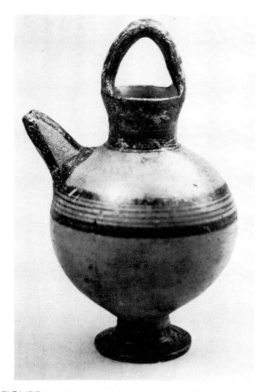

FIGURE 1.   Early infant feeding vessel. Throughout history, pottery, metal, wood, porcelain, glass, plastic and even hollowed-out gourds and cow horns have been used as infant feeding vessels. The nipples were made out of the same material as the bottle until the last half of the 1800s when softer substances were used. The feeding vessel pictured here is of Greek origin (circa 500 B.C.) and was found on Cyprus. It is now a part of the Mead Johnson collection of infant feeding devices.

was found in Phoenikas, Cyprus and is dated circa 2000 B.C.[3] It is of similar shape to the Greek vessel circa 500 B.C. shown in Figure 1.

There are several reasons why an alternative to breast milk is chosen. In some cases the mother is unwilling or unable to nurse due to factors such as employment or illness, and in other cases the mother's milk supply is insufficient. Thomson and Hytten cite two studies, one conducted in 1957 and one conducted in 1977, that examined the reason for stopping breastfeeding before the infant reached 3 months of age. In both studies, conducted 20 years apart, the most common reason given by the mothers was "my milk was insufficient."[4] In other situations, psychosocial ideas prevent the mother from breastfeeding. She may feel that breastfeeding would be too demanding or it may not be totally acceptable to peers. Cultural trends dictate the number of infants breast-fed or formula-fed. Underwood et al.[1] cite a study of Asian women who immigrated

to England. While their native culture supported breastfeeding, their adopted culture did not and they abandoned the practice. Figure 2 charts the trends in feeding breast milk, prepared formula and evaporated milk over the last 30 years.

That cultural ideas have long played a role in determining whether a mother would breastfeed her infant is obvious from the following quote from the novel, *Dr. Thorne,* by the Victorian novelist Trollope. "Of course Lady Arabella could not suckle the young heir herself. Ladies Arabella never can. They're gifted with the powers of being mothers but not nursing mothers. Nature gives them bosoms for show but not for use."[2]

As early weaning occurred or the milk supply was found inadequate, the historical practice was to begin administering "pap," usually a mixture of bread, toast, or baked flour and water. When milk, butter, and or broth was added, the mixture was referred to as "panada" and was obviously more nourishing. Other ingredients frequently included sugar, raw meat juices, beer, wine, Castile soap and occasionally drugs "to soothe the baby."[3] In 1784, Underwood criticized this practice:

TRENDS IN INFANT FEEDING

1955-1984

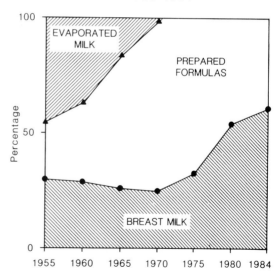

FIGURE 2.   Infant feeding patterns 1955-1984. The pattern of feeding choices for a one-week-old infant has changed considerably since 1955. Then, the ratio of feeding breast milk to milk substitutes was 30:70; by 1984, this ratio was 60:40. The use of evaporated milk, once a popular substitute, has been supplanted by prepared formulas. (All data are for infants 1 week of age.)

It was indeed been a wonder to me how the custom of stuffing newborn babies with and such like could become so universal, or the idea first enter the mind of a parent that such heavy food could be fit for the babies' nourishment at the age of six or seven months. This food may be justly considered a poison, which, if not puked up, or very soon voided by stool, may occasion sickness, gripes (inward fits), and all the train of bowel complaints, which may terminate in Worms, Convulsions, Rickets, Scrofula, Slow Fevers, Purging and a fatal Marasmus.[2]

He recommended cow milk for the healthy infant with barley water as a diluent; this is perhaps the beginning of milk dilution for infant feedings. He was also one of the first to mention the importance of cleansing the vessel used to feed the baby.[2]

In the mid-nineteenth century, the German chemist Justus Von Liebig, who also studied infant nutrition, tried to more closely emulate human milk by proposing an infant formulation consisting of one part malt flour, one part wheat flour, two parts water, and 10 parts cow milk with the addition of some potassium

	ALLERGY RISK	LACTOSE INTOLERANCE	SUCROSE INTOLERANCE	GALACTOSEMIA
PROSOBEE	⊘	⊘	⊘	⊘
ISOMIL	⊘	⊘		⊘
ISOMIL-SF	⊘	⊘	⊘	⊘
NURSOY	⊘	⊘		⊘
SOYALAC	⊘	⊘		⊘
i-SOYALAC	⊘	⊘		⊘

FIGURE 4. Soy formula uses. Because they do not contain the lactose of cow milk formulas, soy formulas are useful human milk substitutes for infants with lactose intolerance, galactosemia, or an allergy risk to cow milk. Sucrose-free soy formulas are also useful for infants with sucrose intolerance.

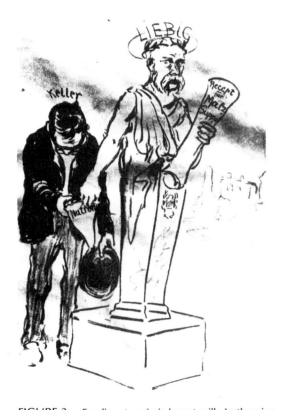

FIGURE 3. Feedings to mimic breast milk. In the nineteenth century, Justus von Liebig, a German chemist, analyzed human milk and proposed a recipe for "Malz Suppe" made from malt flour, wheat flour, water, and cow milk in an early scientific attempt to nutritionally mimic human milk.

chloride.[5] This need to dilute the protein content of cow milk and to increase the proportion of carbohydrate in order to prepare a human milk substitute that would more closely emulate human milk continued to be recognized in the German medical community throughout the latter half of the century. In 1903, Dr. Ernst Moro of Vienna published his observations on the response of infants to various formulations and asserted his preference for a carbohydrate supplement of higher dextrin to maltose ratio than was present in the widely used "Liebig-Suppe" and other preparations of the day.[6]

There are modern situations that indicate use of a breast milk substitute. An infant may have a specific condition such as lactose intolerance, inborn errors of metabolism, prematurity or protein hypersensitivity that may require the use of a specialized formula. Figures 4 and 5 depict formulas available today to meet these specific needs.

EVOLUTION OF HUMAN MILK SUBSTITUTES

While the search for human milk substitutes has been conducted since the dawn of mankind, it was not until sanitation practices developed in the late 19th century that feeding milk or milk substitutes to infants could be safely accomplished. Much credit is due Pasteur, Koch and others for providing the methods to eliminate bacteria from the milk. The period from 1890 to 1915 saw popular

	PROTEIN INTOLERANCE	FAT MALABSORPTION	LACTOSE INTOLERANCE	SUCROSE INTOLERANCE	GLUCOSE INTOLERANCE
PORTAGEN		⊘	⊘		
NUTRAMIGEN	⊘		⊘	⊘	
PREGESTIMIL	⊘	⊘	⊘	⊘	
MONO- AND DI-SACCHARIDE FREE DIET POWDER[1]	⊘	⊘	⊘	⊘	⊘
RCF[1] ROSS CHO-FREE			⊘	⊘	⊘
PROTEIN FREE DIET POWDER[2]	⊘				

1. Supplemental carbohydrate required

2. Supplemental protein/amino acids required

FIGURE 5. Specialized formulas. Formulas to meet the special dietary needs of infants with protein intolerance, fat malabsorption or intolerance to lactose, sucrose or glucose are available either as complete diets or as diets requiring supplementation.

Sidebar 1

NECESSITY—THE MOTHER OF INVENTION

A sick son and the desire to reduce the intolerably high infant mortality rate prevailing at the turn of the century led to the development of the first effective carbohydrate milk modifier and the emergence of one of the leaders in the infant formula world. Edward Mead Johnson incorporated his own business, Mead Johnson & Company, in 1905.

Little was known about infant feeding in those days but Edward remembered how the life of his eldest son, Ted, had been saved by the use of dextrinized gruel when he developed a food intolerance. Determined to pursue this lead, Edward consulted with Dr. Jerome Leopold who explained how starch is dextrinized in cereal grains to produce "dextrins" and "maltose." Early experiments with these ingredients produced only a messy gruel, but Lambert, the second eldest son, fortuitously discovered how to produce a product that could be powdered. Serendipity played a role in this development. One day Lambert left on the steam cooker containing the gruel mixture while he was called away for an extended time. To his amazement, upon his return, he found the material had floated to the top, producing a dry porous layer that could be made into a powder.

Dextri-maltose, introduced in 1911, was hailed as the first effective carbohydrate milk modifier. It enjoyed a market history spanning six decades, attesting to its long-term continued usefulness.

use of the feeding method of Thomas Morgan Rotch. This method was based on the supposition that **each infant required a feeding tailored to its digestive capacity and that the percentage composition, not the amount, was the critical factor. Rotch's approach led to use of the term "formula."**[3] The extreme precision demanded by the method eventually led to its demise. However, a fundamental tenet of the procedure which has persisted is that cow milk protein must be diluted and supplemented with additional energy.[2]

These early formulations had a relatively high curd tension in comparison to breast milk. When fresh, unprocessed cow milk enters the stomach, it forms a hard curd of casein and minerals, which is difficult for some infants to digest. A striking clinical manifestation of this is the problem of lactobezoars, which some preterm infants develop when given a high protein, high calorie formula; the incidence of lactobezoars has been markedly reduced since the introduction of whey-predominant formulas for these infants. Breast milk has a relatively small casein component, hence, a low curd tension; the curds it forms are soft and easily digested. Cow milk can be processed by acidification or heating to reduce curd tension; thus, curd formation from infant formulas is similar to that of human milk.

A series of formulations were developed and used over the next several years based on buttermilk, high protein milk, soybean flour, and acidified milk. In 1927, Marriott pointed out that evaporated milk was already sterilized and heated sufficiently to ensure very fine curds and thus provided a convenient, inexpensive base from which to make an acceptable infant formula. He recommended equal parts of evaporated milk and an acid-sugar mixture (90 ml Karo syrup + 5 ml lactic acid + water to 250 ml).[2] Sobee, using the soybean as a source of protein and the forerunner of current ProSobee, was originally introduced in 1929 to meet the needs of cow milk hypersensitive infants. It was also about this time that Mead Johnson introduced Oleum Percomorphum (fish liver oil) as a source of vitamins A and D as increasing attention was given to infant vitamin needs.

In this same period, the first nutritionally *complete* infant formulas were made. These were designed to imitate mother's milk as closely and practicably as possible at that time. Gerstenberger blended various animal and vegetable oils together in an effort to mimic the fat in mother's milk and combined them with protein and sugar to make Synthetic Milk Adapted, the forerunner of today's S.M.A. Another formulation was introduced by the Franklin Infant Food company which even-

tually became today's Similac. Mead Johnson & Company marketed several formulas leading to the current Enfamil infant formula. These three brands of infant formulas for healthy term infants are currently available in the United States.

NUTRIENT CHARACTERISTICS OF INFANT FORMULAS

The major goal in preparing human milk substitutes is to formulate an acceptable product that is nutritionally as close to human milk as possible. Figure 6 depicts the percentage of the four major macronutrients—protein, fat, carbohydrate, and ash—in cow milk, carbohydrate modified cow milk, milk-based infant formula and human milk. Modern milk-based infant formulas closely approximate the macronutrient composition of human milk.

A much more detailed look at the composition of the major human milk substitutes, including the specialized formulas, is provided in the Appendix to this book. Formulas specifically designed to meet unique nutritional needs may differ substantially from the composition of human milk. Due to a smaller market volume and higher manufacturing costs, these specialized formulas cost more than those for routine use. Table 1 depicts a few of the types of formulas available and provides a cost index relative to milk-based infant formula.

MACRONUTRIENT COMPOSITION

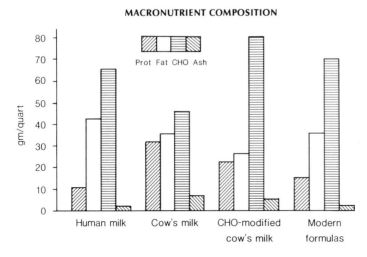

FIGURE 6. Macronutrient composition comparison. Ideally, a human milk substitute would have the same macronutrient composition as breast milk. As is evident, cow milk differs considerably; modifying it with carbohydrate improves the comparison, but still does not attain the comparability of modern formulas. Efforts continue to provide a formula closer to human milk.

TABLE 1.   Types of Formulas Available
and Relative Cost Index*

Type of Formula	Relative Cost Index†
Milk based infant formula	1.0
Soy protein formula	1.1
Protein hydrolysate formula	1.7
Banked human milk	17.6

*Adapted from Lifshitz F: Nutrition for Special Needs
in Infancy. New York, Marcel Dekker, 1985.
†Approximate.

The protein, vitamin and mineral contents of infant formulas are usually somewhat higher than the average levels of these nutrients in human milk. This helps to assure adequate nutrient intake by essentially all infants consuming these products. An example of this aspect of infant formula design is illustrated in Figure 7.

The example used here is protein; the principle applies to other nutrients. If a formula contained only the *average* nutrient level in human milk, then by definitioin half of all infants fed this formula would get less than what they would from breastfeeding. Increasing the amount of nutrient to greater than the average amount in human milk means that *most* infants will get at least as much as they would from human milk. **Thus, many nutrient levels in formula are higher than the average level in human milk.**

Some nutrient contents vary in formula ingredients and others may decrease during processing or storage through shelf life. **Extra amounts (overages) of such nutrients above those specified on the label are included to ensure that the appropriate nutrient contents are present at the end of shelf life.** Addition of nutrients is carefully controlled during manufacture to assure that none is present at or near toxic levels.

PROTEIN

The period of most rapid growth occurs during the last fetal trimester and in the newborn stages of development. This rapid growth occurs at a time when the organ systems are still immature and of limited functional capacity. Sufficient protein must be provided to support optimal growth without overloading the metabolic capacity of the liver, kidneys, and other organs to utilize it and dispose of excess nitrogen. The quality of the protein (proportiion of each amino acid) must be high enough that an overabundance of one or several amino acids does not stress the solute handling capabilities of the liver and kidneys or allow the blood concentrations of potentially toxic amino acids to become excessive. These considerations are even more important in the case of preterm infants, who are even more sensitive and vulnerable to nutrient deficiencies or excesses.

Milk proteins have been divided into two classes based on their relative solubilities in acid: whey (soluble) and casein (insoluble). Human milk protein is approximately 60-70%

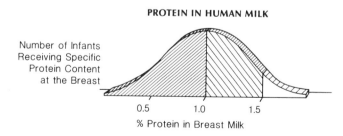

PROTEIN IN HUMAN MILK

Number of Infants
Receiving Specific
Protein Content
at the Breast

0.5   1.0   1.5
% Protein in Breast Milk

- Feeding average human milk content means 1/2 would get less than they would at the breast.

- Feeding higher than average human milk content means most would get at least as much as they would at the breast.

- Same principle applies to other nutrients.

FIGURE 7.   Choice of nutrient levels in formulas. The "average" content of nutrient (protein in this example) in human milk means half of the population would receive less than they would if breastfeeding and half would get more. To ensure that all infants, including those who would have received more than the average, receive an adequate nutrient intake, modern infant formulas generally contain larger amounts of nutrients than the average provided by human milk.

whey and 30-40% casein and, accordingly, forms a very small, soft curd in acid. It is relatively rich in cysteine. Cow milk protein is approximately 20% whey and 80% casein and forms a larger, firmer curd in acid. Casein has somewhat less cysteine than whey protein. **Commercial formulas made with cow milk proteins are heat-treated and as a consequence form smaller, softer curds than raw or pasteurized cow milk.** This is an important factor in acceptability of infant formula. Formulas in which the whey fraction constitutes the major portion of the formula protein are even more similar to human milk in this regard.

Figure 8 is a schematic diagram of how cow milk formulas using a 50:50 mixture of whey and milk can actually approximate the whey:casein ratio of human milk.

Prior to the use of whey-predominant protein in the high-protein formulas for preterm infants, those fed by slow intragastric infusion would occasionally form "lactobezoars." These were large hard curds that could not be easily digested and sometimes required surgical removal. With the utilization of whey-predominant formulas, the incidence of lactobezoars has been essentially eliminated. It is reasonable to believe that it was the relatively large casein protein component that was responsible for the formation of lactobezoars.

> **A point of controversy**
>
> "... all formulas and human milk have been associated [with lactobezoars], although casein predominant formulas have been more of a problem in the premature infant.... The curd tension of whey-predominant and casein dominant formulas is no different."
>
> William C. MacLean, Jr., M.D.
> Medical Director, Pediatric Nutrition
> Ross Laboratories

Today the protein in commercially produced formulas in the U.S. designed for preterm infants is whey-predominant to optimize tolerance and provide increased cysteine; the risk of lactobezoars is thus reduced as is dependence upon the preterm infant's immature cysteine biosynthetic pathway.

Plasma and serum amino acid concentrations in infants fed formulas with whey predominant or casein predominant protein sources have been studied in several laboratories with varying results; neither protein source results in patterns identical to those in human milk fed infants, but the minor differences reported have been judged to be of little or no physiological significance. Debate over which protein source results in serum amino acid patterns and concentrations closest to those in human milk fed infants is difficult to resolve because of so many influencing factors: amount of protein intake, time of blood sampling after feeding, age of the infants studied, laboratory procedures and analytical equipment, type of protein utilized, and the interpretation of the results by the investigator.

Alternate protein sources have been developed to meet the needs of infants who are hypersensitive to cow milk protein. A rich and relatively high quality protein source was found in the soybean and led to the use of soy bean flour in the manufacture of some early milk-free infant formulas. However, indigestible carbohydrate in the soy flour led to undesirably loose and bulky stools. A more satisfactory formula was possible when the soy protein was first isolated from the flour and then processed into a balanced formulation; because of more appropriate heat treatment the protein availability increased substantially. However, the quality still did not quite equal that of casein as measured in the rat assay for protein

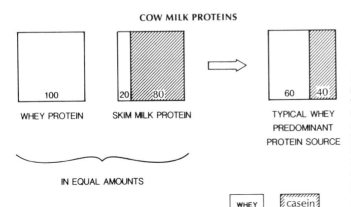

COW MILK PROTEINS

100   WHEY PROTEIN

20 80   SKIM MILK PROTEIN

IN EQUAL AMOUNTS

60 40   TYPICAL WHEY PREDOMINANT PROTEIN SOURCE

WHEY   casein

FIGURE 8. Whey:casein ratios of formulas. The two major milk proteins are whey and casein. Whey is acid soluble, but casein is insoluble and can be a source of curd formation in infants. Human milk protein is whey-predominant (60-70%), whereas cow milk protein has a whey to casein ratio of 20:80. Some manufacturers mix equal parts of whey and skim milk protein to produce a protein source for formula that has a 60:40 whey to casein ratio, more like human milk.

Sidebar 2

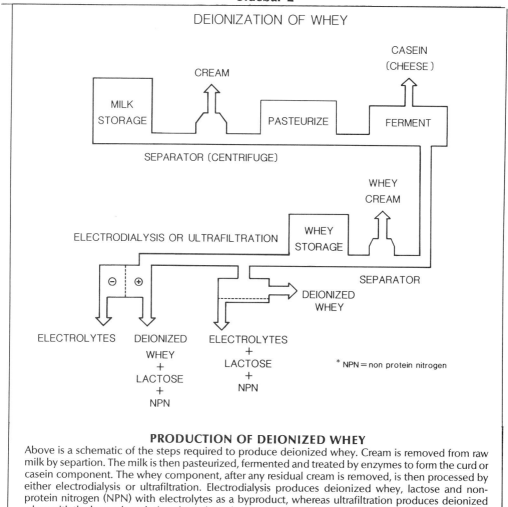

DEIONIZATION OF WHEY

PRODUCTION OF DEIONIZED WHEY

Above is a schematic of the steps required to produce deionized whey. Cream is removed from raw milk by separtion. The milk is then pasteurized, fermented and treated by enzymes to form the curd or casein component. The whey component, after any residual cream is removed, is then processed by either electrodialysis or ultrafiltration. Electrodialysis produces deionized whey, lactose and non-protein nitrogen (NPN) with electrolytes as a byproduct, whereas ultrafiltration produces deionized whey with the byproducts being electrolytes, lactose and NPN. Reducing the mineral level of the whey is essential so that the electrolyte content of the infant formula can be controlled.

equivalency, the protein equivalency ratio (PER). (The PER is more thoroughly discussed in the section on Preclinical Testing of Formulas.) The protein quality of soy protein was improved to nearly equal milk protein by supplementation with a small amount of L-methionine. The rat fed a soy protein diet responds dramatically to supplemental methionine because of its unusually high methionine requirement. Most modern soy formulas are therefore made with soy protein isolate supplemented with methionine. Further studies have shown that the response to supplemental methionine in human infants depends on the dietary protein level.

To meet the needs of infants who are hypersensitive to several intact proteins, who must avoid exposure to intact protein for other reasons, or who have difficulty digesting protein, several infant formula products with the protein component composed of hydrolyzed casein were developed by Mead Johnson & Company, beginning in the 1940s. To manufacture the hydrolysate, casein is incubated with enzyme until very few peptide bonds remain. The average peptide molecular weight is about 200, with less than 1% having molecular weights greater than 500 and none detectable above 1200 daltons. This compares to casein which has a molecular weight of 70,000 daltons and whey which can reach a molecular weight of 150,000 daltons. The crude hydrolysate is purified and tested for antigenicity before being used in the infant formula products. This same hydrolysate was also the first, intravenous, "elemental" nitrogen source for parenteral nutrition. This protein source has not only proven useful in protein sensitive infants, but there are indications it may also be useful in treating that component of infantile colic that is related to intact protein hypersensitivity. The casein hydrolysation process is shown in Figure 9.

Utilizing this protein hydrolysate, Mead Johnson applied special processing techniques to develop a series of special formulas to meet the nutritional needs of those rare individuals who have inborn errors of amino acid metabolism. Lofenalac for dietary management of infants with phenylketonuria (PKU) was made by removing phenylalanine from casein hydrolysate and utilizing this modified hydrolysate to manufacture the product. Similarly, most of the tyrosine and phenylalanine were removed from casein hydrolysate in the manufacture of Low Phe-Tyr Diet Powder for patients with tyrosinemia. Crystalline amino acids were used to make MSUD Diet Powder free of branched-chain amino acids for patients with maple syrup urine disease and to make Phenyl Free for use by older patients with phenylketonuria. For general use, Protein Free Diet Powder was developed so that customized amino acid mixtures can be added to provide an appropriate infant formula for patients with other inborn errors of amino acid metabolism. More recently, several other companies have also developed specialty products for metabolic disorders.

Modular protein sources are available in the U.S. for use in supplementing infant feedings when more protein is desired or if a low fat/low cholesterol or low sodium diet is needed. Calcium caseinate, relatively low in sodium, is provided by Mead Johnson as Casec. Cow milk whey protein is available as ProMod from Ross Laboratories, as is a casein and electrolyte mix, Protein Mineral Module. Two other modular protein sources utilizing cow milk whey are Promix made by Navco and Propac offered by Chesebrough-Pond's.

FAT

Fat provides 40-50% of the energy intake of the breast-fed infant. In spite of the fact that much of the fat is saturated, it is well absorbed and utilized, perhaps due to the predominant location of the saturated fatty acids at the β- or 2 position on the glycerol chain in the triglyceride molecules.[8] On the other hand, un-

modified fat from cow milk and beef tallow is not as well absorbed by the young infant. Accordingly, fat in modern American infant formula is predominantly of vegetable origin.

Corn and soy oil are commonly used in infant formulas and contain abundant essential fatty acids; both are rich in linoleic acid, and soy oil also contains a significant amount of linolenic acid, which may be important for the preterm infant. While such oils are readily absorbed, their high degree of unsaturation makes them dissimilar to human milk fat, and excesses can lead to increased cell membrane fragility and hemolysis, particularly in the preterm infant, if sufficient vitamin E is not present as an antioxidant to protect them. Consequently, a **blend of carefully selected vegetable and occasionally some animal oils is used to make the fatty acid profile more similar to that seen in human milk.** Coconut oil is frequently used in such blends because it is relatively rich in short and medium chain fatty acids that are components of human milk and are easily digested and absorbed by infants. Certain animal fats are occasionally used for the same purpose, although such formulas may not meet the requirements for Kosher certification.

A point of controversy

" . . . the fat blend in SMA is practically exactly the same in composition as that of breast milk; whereas, the all-vegetable fat blends of Enfamil and Similac are completely different from the fatty acid breakdown of human milk."

John Silverio, M.D.
Director of Clinical Nutrition
Wyeth Laboratories, Inc.

By saponifying coconut oil, separating the medium chain fatty acids, and then re-esterifying them, MCT Oil is made. Medium chain triglycerides (MCT) are hydrolyzed by lipases up to 5 times more readily than long chain triglycerides. The resulting fatty acids are absorbed directly into the blood stream without undergoing chylomicron formation for secretion into the lymphatics. Use of MCT also has been associated with increased calcium absorption in preterm infants fed formulas in which MCT replaces a portion of the long chain triglycerides.[9] It is therefore useful as a readily digestible caloric supplement with negligible osmolality and has been used to make formulas (e.g., Portagen, Pregestimil, Mono- and Disaccharide Free Diet Powder) designed for patients who may have fat malabsorption

FIGURE 9. Casein hydrolysis process. Casein is incubated with enzymes to break the peptide linkages and the resultant hyrolysate filtered and tested for its peptide distribution. If the resulting peptide mixture meets the established criteria for non-allergenicity, the hydrolysate is accepted for mixing with other ingredients to provide a non-allergenic formula.

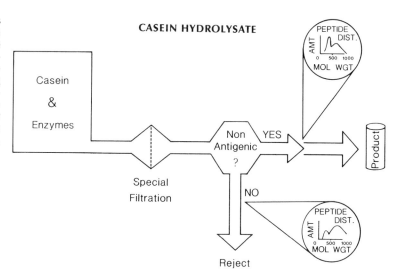

associated with short gut syndrome, cystic fibrosis, severe chronic diarrhea, and monosaccharide intolerance.

Modular fat components include not only MCT Oil, but also the various oils available in food stores such as corn oil, etc. Figure 10 depicts some fat sources and the four main types of fats in each: MC = medium chain, LC Sat = long chain saturated, MONOUNSAT = monounsaturated, and PUFA = polyunsaturated fatty acid. By blending vegetable oil from sources such as corn or soy with coconut oil, a fat blend (e.g., corn + coconut) very similar in fatty acid composition to human milk is achieved.

FAT COMPOSITION AND SOURCES

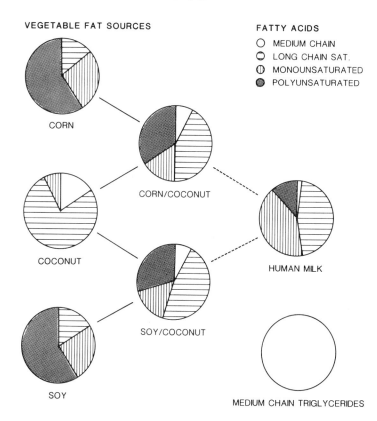

FIGURE 10. Composition of fat sources. Fat sources contain various amounts of medium chain, long chain saturated, monounsaturated and polyunsaturated fatty acids. No one vegetable fat source simulates the fatty acid pattern of human milk. However, by combining vegetable fats, the resultant blend can approximate the pattern found in human milk.

CARBOHYDRATE

The carbohydrate in human milk, as in all animal milks, is primarily lactose; a minor, but significant portion is composed of carbohydrate oligomers. Lactose is a disaccharide and human milk is iso-osmolar; if an equivalent amount of carbohydrate were a monosaccharide (e.g., glucose), the milk would be hypertonic. Milk based formulas also contain lactose, which facilitates calcium absorption. In preterm infants, however, the activity of the intestinal enzyme lactose is not fully developed so lactose may not be completely digested and absorbed. Since energy needs are high in these patients, using glucose polymers (corn syrup solids) to replace some of the lactose allows preparation of a formula with increased caloric density while avoiding excessive osmolality. The reduced lactose load enhances formula tolerance.

Occasionally, infants become intolerant to lactose (e.g., following moderately severe diarrhea which depresses intestinal lactase activity), or are born with a metabolic abnormality in the utilization of galactose resulting in galactosemia. Such patients require **lactose-free diets.** Since soy protein formulas do not contain any lactose or bioavailable galactose, and carbohydrate is easily supplied by sucrose and/or glucose polymers, soy formulas are frequently fed to these infants. **In some infants, diarrhea can lead to a significant reduction in intestinal sucrase activity and consequently to sucrose intolerance;** formulas providing glucose polymers as the only carbohydrate were developed to provide for these infants as well as those with lactose intolerance.

Rarely, diarrhea can be so protracted and severe as to lead not only to disaccharide intolerances, but also to glucose polymer intolerance and even monosaccharide (glucose) malabsorption and intolerance. For such infants, formulations have been developed which are complete *except* for reduction or elimination of the carbohydrate. Mono- and Disaccharide Free Diet Powder contains casein hydrolysate, MCT Oil, and a minimal amount of modified food starch (to enhance mixing and physical stability of formula during storage and feeding) along with a balance of all other essential nutrients. This formulation is useful not only in severe carbohydrate intolerance but also for the protein and fat malabsorption which may accompany it. RCF is an intact soy protein based formula which is complete *except* for the carbohydrate, and Protein Mineral Module contains casein and electrolytes. All of these formulas require that carbohydrate be added as dictated by the needs and tolerance of the patient.

Modular carbohydrate products provided by formula manufacturers are Moducal and Polycose. Both are glucose polymers (corn syrup solids) prepared by partial digestion of corn starch. Their molecular size averages 4 to 6 glucose units. Lactose, glucose, and fructose are also available from pharmacies, and sucrose from either pharmacies or food stores, for use as additional carbohydrate sources in these special formulas.

VITAMINS

Vitamins are included in complete infant formulas in the United States in accordance with the Infant Formula Act of 1980, which came from best available estimates of requirements from the scientific literature or recommendations of the Committee on Nutrition of the American Academy of Pediatrics. In general, water-soluble vitamin needs parallel caloric intake and can therefore be incorporated in the formula according to caloric content. Recommended fat-soluble vitamin intakes, however, tend to be relatively more constant and independent of caloric intake, e.g., 400 units of vitamin D per day regardless of energy consumed. Fortunately, for term infants, total daily formula intake tends to be relatively constant over time and so the daily fat-soluble vitamin requirement can be incorporated in the appropriate amount of formula. On the other hand, **preterm infants present a special challenge. Their formula intake may well double during the first 6 weeks of life, but still be much less than in the term infant.** If the requirement of fat-soluble vitamins is provided in the typical daily formula intake of the 1000-gm infant, then the increased formula intake will supply about twice the requirement at a body weight of 2000 gm. On the other hand, supplying a lower fat-soluble vitamin content in the formula means the small, preterm infant would likely need to be supplemented with liquid vitamin preparations which may be very hyperosmolar. Accordingly, some infant formula manufacturers have increased the vitamin content of feedings intended for these fragile infants in order to provide their estimated vitamin needs without additional supplementation, recognizing that even twice the recommended levels of these

Sidebar 3

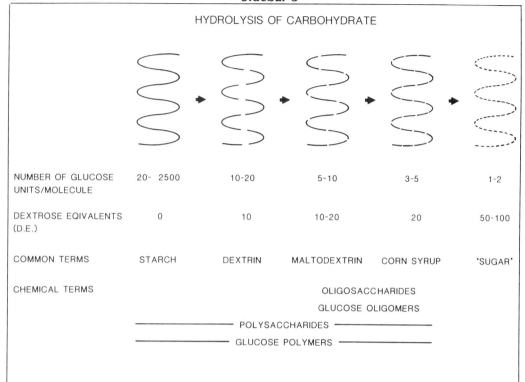

HYDROLYSIS OF CARBOHYDRATE				
NUMBER OF GLUCOSE UNITS/MOLECULE	20- 2500	10-20	5-10	3-5	1-2
DEXTROSE EQIVALENTS (D.E.)	0	10	10-20	20	50-100
COMMON TERMS	STARCH	DEXTRIN	MALTODEXTRIN	CORN SYRUP	"SUGAR"

CHEMICAL TERMS

OLIGOSACCHARIDES

GLUCOSE OLIGOMERS

POLYSACCHARIDES

GLUCOSE POLYMERS

* D.E. reducing sugar content as per cent of d-glucose

HYDROLYSIS OF CARBOHYDRATE

The breakdown of large starch molecules into smaller and smaller glucose polymers is achieved via hydrolysis and is depicted in the figure above. Notice that this process can be interrupted at any point to yield the size of glucose polymer desired. This is important in infant formula manufacture because:

1. It allows the formulation of lactose-free products with small molecular weight carbohydrates that can be readily utilized by infants who cannot digest lactose.
2. By varying the amounts of the various glucose polymers in the formula, i.e., starch, dextrin, corn syrup, "sugar," etc., the osmolality of the finished product can be controlled while still providing the proper total amount of carbohydrate.
3. Starch molecules can be utilized to keep fats in a stabilized emulsion.

fat-soluble vitamins does not approach the toxic range in the more resilient larger preterm infants.

MINERALS

The safe range of sodium intakes for newborn infants is narrow compared to older individuals due to their renal immaturity. While term human milk levels are adequate for term infants, some preterm infants become hyponatremic on these intakes, possibly due in part to their rapid growth rates and limited renal capacity to conserve sodium in the first few weeks of life. On the other hand, excess sodium intake sometimes results in hypernatremia and edema. For this reason, sodium

content of infant formulas is closely monitored to keep it within a safe but adequate range, although levels in formulas for preterm infants are maintained at a higher amount.

Potassium content in formulas is kept within physiologic proportions of the sodium and chloride levels. Adequate chloride necessary for normal metabolism of hydrogen ion is assured by ongoing monitoring of formula production (see quality control discussion below). Molar equivalents of Na:K are generally kept in the range of 0.3:1 to 1:1, whereas (Na + K)/C1 molar ratio is usually between 1.5 and 2.5, consistent with ratios seen in human milk.

The bones of the rapidly growing infant require abundant calcium and phosphorus to assure normal development. However, the relatively low solubility of these minerals creates challenges for incorporating large amounts into infant feedings. While human milk levels are adequate for the term infant, a significant number of preterm infants on these levels will develop hypophosphatemia, hyperphosphatasia, hypocalcemia, rickets and pathological fractures. The hypercalciuria that diminishes with phosphorus supplementation in such patients is evidence that phosphorus is the primary limiting nutrient in this phenomenon. Studies of bone mineral content, mineral balance, and fetal accretion rates also indicate that more calcium and phosphorus are needed than provided in human milk or routine infant formula. Accordingly, the formulas designed for preterm infants all have increased calcium and phosphorus contents. In some instances, a portion of the calcium and phosphorus settles to the bottom of the container and must be resuspended by intermittent agitation for reliable delivery.

The fraction of iron utilized from human milk has been shown to be greater than that from cow milk or most diets containing solid foods; however, iron is present in human milk in very low amounts. **Heat processing of the cow milk used to make infant formulas improves iron availability from formulas;** furthermore, young infants fed a low protein, milk based formula containing a similar amount of iron as human milk had similar iron absorption.[10] The amount of iron in today's non-iron fortified infant formulas is slightly greater than in human milk. For infants at risk for iron deficiency, iron-fortified formula providing 1 to 2 mg of iron/100 kcal is recommended. Typical iron-fortified formulas provide 12 mg of iron per quart. The speculation that iron containing formulas may increase the risk of infection significantly has not been substantiated.

The wide variety of fluoride contents in water across the United States led to uncertainty among some pediatricians regarding appropriate fluoride supplementation schedules for formula-fed infants. At one time, a number of plants at which infant formulas were made used water from municipal supplies which had been supplemented with fluoride. **In 1979, it was decided that manufacturers would use only water that was low in fluoride content to make infant formulas.** Thus, the potential for undesirable intake levels of fluoride resulting from adding local fluoridated water to a fluoride-containing formula was reduced and health care workers could be assured there was no significant amount of fluoride in the formula. They can now make an informed decision regarding the treatment of their patients with fluoride, based on the local water and other relevant considerations.

MISCELLANEOUS INGREDIENTS

As scientific evidence indicates the potential necessity for a new substance in the infant's diet, it is generally incorporated quickly into infant formulas after appropriate testing for safety and tolerance. Such factors that have been added in the past have included choline, inositol, taurine, and carnitine. The desirability of other substances such as cholesterol are still under study and are being debated.

NUTRIENT LEVELS

Over the past few decades, the nutrient profile of human milk and term infant needs have been relatively well defined. The Committee on Nutrition (CON) of the American Academy of Pediatrics (AAP) has published recommendations for the nutrient intake of infants. The Infant Formula Act passed by the U.S. Congress in 1980 codifies the recommendations of this committee and requires that all infant formulas distributed for general use fall within these limits.[11] Investigations comparing growth and development of infants consuming infant formulas to those who are breastfeeding reveal that modern formula performs at least as well as human milk. Nevertheless, research continues to seek further improvement in formulas as knowledge of human milk and infant nutrition expands. See the Appendix for actual nutrient contents in the various formulations, available as of this date.

OTHER CONSIDERATIONS

Osmolality

Figure 11 depicts the contribution to the total osmolality of the formula made by each of the major components of a formula that has 20 kcal/oz, with 12% of the calories provided as protein, 45% of the calories as fat and 43% of the calories as carbohydrate. **Clearly, the saccharides are the major contributors to formula osmolality.** Osmolality can be an important determinant of formula tolerance. If the osmolality is too high, it may draw water from the intestinal cells, in-

COMPONENTS OF OSMOLALITY IN FORMULAS

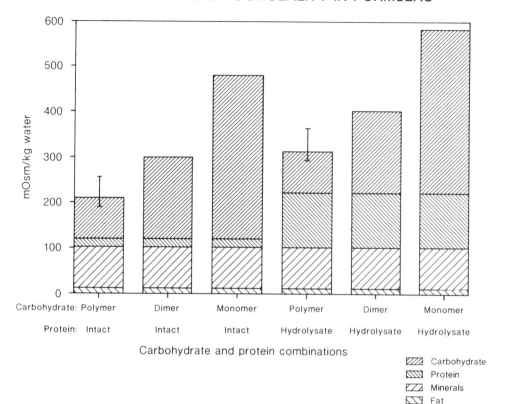

FIGURE 11. Contribution to osmolality. The major contributors to the osmolality of a formula are the minerals, the carbohydrate, and hydrolyzed protein, if used. Glucose polymers with their relatively large molecular size and low dextrose equivalents ratings produce formulas with lower osmolalities than those in which glucose, fructose, or disaccharides are used. Manufacturers control formula osmolalities by choosing the appropriate carbohydrate source(s).

terfere with nutrient and water absorption, and/or cause diarrhea. Thus, selected saccharides can be used to produce a formula that will meet nutrient specifications and have an appropriate osmolality.

Renal Solute Load

The reserve renal capacity of the full term, and particularly the preterm infant, newborn is limited. Hence, renal solute load is an important factor to consider in infant formula design. Two calculations are used to compare renal solute factors of infant formulas.

For preterm infants the potential renal solute load (PRSL, milliosmoles or MOSM) is calculated:

$$PRSL = (gm\ of\ protein)/0.175 + Na + K + Cl + phosphorus$$

where the mineral units are millimoles and all are expressed either per unit volume or per

unit of energy.[12] The first term on the right calculates the potential number of millimoles of urea which could be formed from the protein. The actual renal solute load in the preterm infant is normally somewhat less than the PRSL, since not all of the ingested protein nitrogen and minerals are excreted in the urine. Although there are some urinary constituents not included in the calculation for PRSL, the equation accounts for the major factors and serves as a basis for comparison of potential renal stress to preterm infants. Thus, for a preterm infant ingesting a typical formula designed for him at a rate of 120 kcal/kg/day, PRSL might be 31 mOsm/kg/day.

For term infants, the estimated renal solute load (ERSL) is calculated:

$$ERSL = (gm\ of\ protein)/.25 + Na + K + Cl$$

where the units are as described above for PRSL.[13] In this case, the first term on the right allows for retention of some of the nitrogen and calculates fewer millimoles of urea being excreted from the protein. Also, the phosphorus term is not used to account for retention of some of the minerals. In contrast to calculating the *entire potential renal solute load* described above for preterm infants, this calculation is an attempt to estimate the *actual renal solute load* expected to be experienced by the infant; it serves as a basis for comparison of the load various formulas might put on the kidneys.

Sanitation

One of the major factors leading to the early failures in the use of human milk substitutes was inadequate sanitation practice. Where modern water and sewage facilities are available in the United States and mothers are educated in the appropriate principles of hygiene, the incidence of infection in formula-fed infants does not differ from that in breast-fed infants. All liquid formula products are commercially sterile and powders contain only limited amounts of nonpathogenic bacteria. When these products are used as directed, including dilution with boiled water in clean vessels and storing appropriately, they are bacteriologically as safe as the milk from an appropriately cleaned breast.

Non-Nutritional Factors

Fresh human milk does contain a number of non-nutritional factors and benefits not present in modern formulas. These include such things as living white blood cells, antibodies to organisms in the mother's environment, hormones, as well as factors that encourage the growth of selective types of bacteria in the intestinal tract and inhibit colonization by others. While some future formula may also contain some of these, many scientific and regulatory issues remain to be resolved.

QUALITY CONTROL OF INFANT FEEDINGS

Control over the quality of human milk is provided by natural physiological processes and is limited by the capacity of the mother to adapt to stresses of disease, malnutrition, environmental toxins, state of hydration, and hygiene. While such abilities are remarkable, when superimposed on genetic variability, the composition of human milk varies considerably from mother to mother. These considerable variations, however, are usually within the range to which normal term infants can readily adapt. When human milk is collected in a milk bank, it can be analyzed and quality control measures can be imposed to ensure the safety and nutritional adequacy of the milk that is accepted. No universal standards have yet been established. Some advantageous attributes of human milk may be compromised in the milk banking process.

Modern infant formulas undergo strict quality control procedures in compliance with applicable government regulations to assure product quality; i.e., the proper nutrients are being supplied to the infant in amounts predetermined as acceptable and as specified on the label. As there are over 30 quantitive descriptors of composition in an infant formula, this is a challenging task.

The assurance of a quality product requires the coordinated interaction of many departments within the manufacturing firm. For consistent, high-quality infant formula, it is essential to integrate quality control considerations into all phases of product development and manufacturing including product planning, research testing, product development, pilot plant scale-up and manufacturing. Quality control personnel perform stability studies as well as analytical studies at each step. By being part of the development process, quality control personnel become knowledgeable about the raw materials used, the composition of the product while in process, and the effects of the process itself upon the product. This knowledge is helpful in providing a smooth manufacturing process as quality control personnel can aid in trouble-shooting any problem that arises.

The production process for an infant formula is outlined in Figure 12. Quality control checkpoints have been denoted by double lines. These checkpoints are summarized in Figure 13.

Acceptable limits for nutrient levels are established by (1) Food and Drug Administration regulations and (2) considerations of safety and adequacy in infants and the variability of the nutrient content in the raw ingredients.

Composition

Quality control must start with the acquisition of ingredients. All suppliers must be qualified to assure that they can consistently provide the needed ingredients within rigid tolerance limits of quality and comply with "good

FORMULA MANUFACTURING

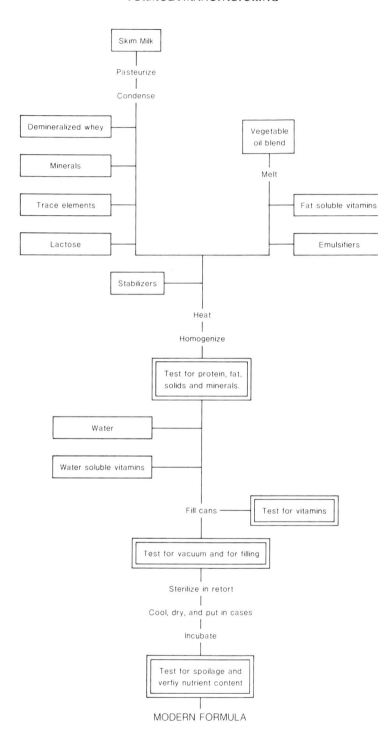

FIGURE 12. Routine infant formula production. Typical liquid infant formula manufacture might start out as skim milk which is pasteurized, condensed, and often combined with demineralized whey. Minerals, trace elements, and lactose are added as needed. This mixture is combined with a blend of vegetable oils, fat-soluble vitamins, and emulsifiers, and stabilizers are added. The resultant mixture is then heated, homogenized and tested for macronutrient contents which are adjusted by dilution and additions as needed. Water-soluble vitamins are added, and cans filled and sealed under vacuum with testing for vitamin content during the process. Each can is checked for vacuum integrity and appropriate filling, and the formula is retort sterilized, cooled, and put into cases. After quality control verifies nutrient contents and an appropriate incubation period has elapsed, the absence of spoilage is confirmed and the product is distributed for use.

Infant Formula Quality Control Checkpoints

Specifications established by unanimous agreement of multidisciplinary panel of experts ✔

Ingredients analyzed for compliance with specifications ✔

Batch instructions compared to master instructions ✔

Certification that each instruction was followed ✔

Witness that each instruction was followed ✔

Analytical confirmation of nutrient composition ✔

Individual batch composition compared with trend analysis ✔

Appropriate container fill verified ✔

Processing temperatures verified by:
  (a) On-line analysis of proper thermal processing ✔
  (b) Incubation test to assure proper thermal processing ✔

Comprehensive review of batch record and analytical ✔

Normal physical condition verified by infant caretaker ✔

Shelf-life assured by statisical sampling & analysis ✔

FIGURE 13. Quality control checkpoints. Multiple checks occur during design, selection of ingredients, manufacturing, testing, and surveillance of infant formulas to assure that infants who depend on them as their sole source of nutrition will be safely and adequately fed.

manufacturing practices." The standards of quality defined by the Food Chemicals Codex, the U.S. Pharmacopeia, the National Formulary or other official references are used with emphasis on properties determined to be critical in the product development steps. Usually multiple suppliers are qualified and used to assure uninterrupted availability of quality ingredients for manufacturing. Each incoming shipment is evaluated upon receipt and must meet applicable compositional and microbiological specifications prior to acceptance for use in the manufacture of infant formula.

The nutrient content of the formula is assured by numerous checks. The exact amount of each ingredient that is incorporated in each batch is recorded by a trained production worker, then confirmed by a second person.

For the final product, multiple nutrients are analyzed on every batch, and **systems are utilized to assure the inclusion of each specified ingredient in every batch of formula.** Long-term trends in nutrient content of formulas and ingredients are closely monitored to assure that seasonal or other supply fluctuations do not affect product quality or consistency.

Multiple quality control checks are also made, recorded and verified during the manufacturing of each batch of formula to assure appropriate processing temperatures, proper container filling, and other aspects of product safety and quality, in compliance with all applicable federal and state regulations.

Microbiology

Microbiological safety is assured by several measures. Only processing procedures that have been shown to be safe and effective are used. Liquids are generally rendered commercially sterile by heat treatment of the finished product. Alternatively, aseptic processing techniques can be used. Liquids are incubated for specified time periods and some samples are subjected to storage at elevated temperatures according to rigorously defined procedures. These samples are then reevaluated for commercial sterility. Powder products are cultured to assure that total bacterial count is less than the limits set by the U.S. Government and that no coliforms or other potential pathogens are present.

The primary containers are subjected to special tests to assure integrity of seals and surfaces that might be potential sites of bacterial entry. The products are stored and shipped under controlled conditions. The ultimate quality assurance check is the evaluation of product appearance, odor, etc. that is done by the nurse, mother, or other infant caretaker before the product is fed to the infant.

Throughout the shelf life of the product, sample packages or cans of product are stored at room and elevated temperatures. Representative packages are opened periodically and evaluated for product quality and nutrient content so that any departure from expectations can be assessed and handled in an appropriate and expeditious manner.

PRECLINICAL AND CLINICAL EVALUATION OF INFANT FORMULAS

An essential part of establishing product safety, tolerance and adequacy is the thorough preclinical and clinical testing that is done commensurate with changes in or development of infant formulas. Animal studies may be useful to verify protein quality and bioavailability of selected nutrients before clinical studies are begun in human infants. A new product is released for general use only after carefully controlled clinical studies wherein performance while on the new formulation is compared to performance while on human milk and/or formulas for which there is a substantial history of successful use in infants. Such clinical studies are designed by rigorous scientific standards and are implemented after scientific review and Institutional Review Board approval.[14]

PRECLINICAL—ANIMAL STUDIES

Protein Quality

The nutritional quality of any protein is related to the balance or distribution of amino acids in the protein, the availability of those amino acids from the diet, and the needs of the test subject. There is no universally accepted test for comparing the quality of protein sources. However, a generally recognized compromise is the protein equivalency ratio (PER) assay.

In this test, young rats are fed a diet containing 10% control or test protein; growth relative to protein intake is measured and the test diet performance is expressed as a percentage of that on the control diet. Casein is the official reference or control protein in the PER test conducted as specified by the Association of Official Analytical Chemists.[14] The American Academy of Pediatrics Committee on Nutrition has recommended and the Food and Drug Administration regulations on infant formula specify that the **PER of proteins used in infant formulas not be less than 70% of casein** and that the equivalent of at least 1.8 gm of protein/100 kcal with a PER 100% of casein be supplied, with total protein content never exceeding 4.5 gm/100 kcal.[14]

Minerals

Animal studies may also provide useful insight about mineral interactions with each other and with other nutrients in infant formulas. In these studies, the amount of intake can be controlled and determined. Likewise, the amounts excreted can be measured as indices of relative bioavailability. Results of such studies must be interpreted with recognition of the limitations of the models used but do provide information that can aid in assessing the suitability of ingredient sources or the effects of processing on bioavailability.

CLINICAL STUDIES

Protein Utilization

Graham et al. have described special studies which compare protein utilization in human infants at 6.4-6.7% protein calories, similar to the level in human milk.[15] New protein sources or new combinations of proteins in infant formula are often tested in a carefully controlled research environment to extend and verify preliminary observations from animal studies. Further clinical evaluations are also performed using classical nitrogen balance methodologies, standard growth, and acceptance and tolerance studies. These clinical studies sometimes include measurement of fasting and/or postprandial plasma amino acid profiles and urea nitrogen levels.

Fat Utilization

Utilization of fat from a new fat source or new blend of fats or oils is determined by careful fat balance studies. These are studied as a component of the formula to be marketed. Information on utilization of fats as appropriate calorie sources is also provided by subsequent growth studies.

Carbohydrate Utilization

The suitability of a carbohydrate for use in infant formulas can be evaluated by breath hydrogen, stool pH, and stool characteristics of infants enrolled in clinical studies. Growth is also an indirect indication of carbohydrate utilization, since the carbohydrate constitutes 40-50% of the calories in many formulas.

Mineral Balance/Availability

Balance studies are performed to determine the absorption of calcium, phosphorus, magnesium, and other key minerals in infants. More recently, stable isotope methods have begun to be used to evaluate mineral absorption in selected cases of critical minerals. Additionally, the bone mineral content achieved while consuming various diets has been measured by photon absorptiometry as another measure of the relative availability of calcium/phosphorus from the feedings.

Measurements of serum concentrations of various minerals have also been used to assure that the form and levels provided by the formulas support normal physiological function in infants. Careful attention is paid to potential excesses as well as to potential deficiencies. A number of indirect parameters such as alkaline phosphatase and parathyroid hormone (calcium/phosphorus/vitamin D and its metabolites), ferritin (iron stores), and ceruloplasmin assays are useful in determining nutrient adequacy of minerals.

Figure 14 depicts a mineral retention study done in preterm infants. In this case, the mineral being observed is calcium, but similar studies are done for other minerals.

In Figure 14, it can be seen that as the preterm infant is thriving (gaining weight), the amount of calcium retained increases. The shaded area is the 95% confidence interval for the infants studied, whereas the solid central curve is the mean fetal accretion rate at the corresponding weight. Calcium retention here is measured as the difference between calcium intake via formula and calcium excretion in the stools and urine.

Vitamins

Vitamins are generally supplied in amounts required by the Infant Formula Act of 1980. Nevertheless, blood concentrations of selected vitamins are often monitored during clinical studies in infants to assure adequacy and safety. Particular attention is directed to this when new vitamin contents are used such as in formulations designed for preterm infants.

Specific Growth Studies

Figure 15 depicts the results of a typical growth study. Infants are observed over an extended period of time and their intake and growth noted. The two outside lines represent the range of normal growth and the middle dark line is the mean growth curve. Plots for individual infants are then made; in this case, all infants grew within the normal range.

Fomon et al. described a 112-day growth study that provides an excellent clinical evaluation of the nutritional adequacy of an infant formula in an integrated way.[16] With very cooperative parents and infants of one sex (males and females have different growth patterns), intake and growth are carefully determined and the results from infants consuming test and control formulas compared to each other as well as to historical data from similar studies.

Acceptance, Tolerance, and Growth

After evaluating a new formula with a relatively small group of infants in metabolic balance studies, and somewhat larger groups in growth studies, large numbers of infants are then enrolled in controlled studies of general acceptance and tolerance in a "real world" setting. Infants in such studies consume the products for several months and mothers or nurses record the volume consumed, the number and character of the stools, any gastrointestinal disturbances, and any other pertinent observations. The infant's pediatrician may record the weight and length of the infant at regular intervals for additional data on growth, and depending on the study, may collect a small blood and/or urine sample for laboratory evaluation. The results from the randomly assigned study groups are statistically analyzed and compared to assure that the new product performs in a manner equal to or better than the control feeding and with no more frequent complications.

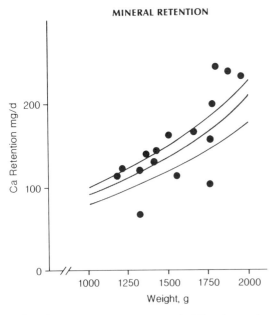

MINERAL RETENTION

FIGURE 14. Mineral retention study. Mineral retention studies done in a clinical environment help assure that the formula is providing appropraite mineral levels to the growing infant. This study depicts the calcium retention observed in preterm infants (points with shaded area showing the composite 95% confidence interval) compared to the known fetal accretion rate for that gestational weight (central dark line).

TERM MALE INFANT GROWTH STUDY

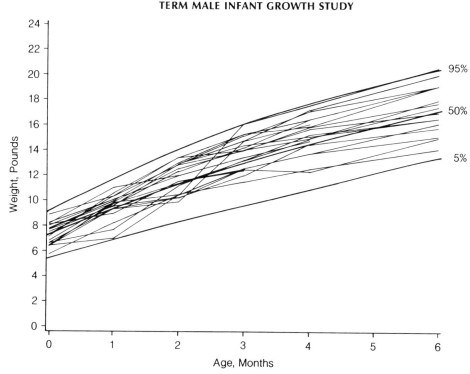

FIGURE 15. Clinical growth studies. Clinical studies are done with new formulas to assure that infants are growing within normal ranges. Growth plots for individual infants in a study are shown here superimposed on the range of normal growth. The heavy line in the middle is the mean growth curve.

SUMMARY

Modern infant formulas meet the needs of infants when breast milk is not available. They are a complete nutritious substitute and, in the case of specific infant conditions, may provide life-giving nutrition that would not otherwise be available.

Infant formulas meet high standards to assure nutrient content and microbiological safety as verified by an intensive quality assurance program. Formulas undergo animal and clinical testing to assure adequate protein quality, adequate nutritional utilization, and safe and acceptable usage before they are marketed.

Infant formula manufacturers will continue to utilize the latest scientific knowledge to provide for the nutritional requirements of all infants and make available to them the best-suited human milk substitute possible.

Acknowledgments. The authors would like to gratefully acknowledge the editorial assistance of Mary Alice Springer of the Medical Communications Staff, Mead Johnson Nutritional Group.

REFERENCES

1. Underwood BA, Van Arsdell H, Blumenstiel E, Scrimshaw NS. Implications of available information on breast-feeding worldwide. In Bond JT, Filer LJ Jr, Leveille GA, et al (eds): Infant and Child Feeding. New York, Academic Press, 1981;77–96.
2. Cone TE Jr. History of infant and child feeding: from the earliest years through the development of scientific concepts. In Bond JT, Filer LJ Jr, Leveille GA, et al (eds): Infant and Child Feeding. New York, Academic Press, 1981;4–34.
3. Greenberg MH. Neonatal feeding. In Smith GF, Vidyasager D (eds): Historical Review and Recent Advances in Neonatal and Perinatal Medicine, Vol 1. Evansville, IN, Mead Johnson Nutritional Division, 1983;55–78.
4. Thomson AM, Hytten FE. Psychophysiological aspects of human lactation. In Bond JT, Filer LJ Jr, Leveille GA, et al (eds): Infant and Child Feeding. New York, Academic Press, 1981;37–46.
5. Koch F. Über die Pioniere der frühen Kinderheilkunde in und aus Giessen. Der Kinderartz 1984;15:1623–1627.
6. Moro E. Ernährungversuche mit Soxhlet's "Nährzucker." Klin Wochenschr 1903;6:4–16.
7. Lifshitz F. Nutrition for special needs in infancy. In Lifshitz F (ed): Nutrition for Special Needs in Infancy: Protein Hydrolysate. New York, Marcel Dekker, Inc., 1985;1–10.
8. Sarett HP. The modern infant formula. In Bond JT, Filer LJ Jr, Leveille GA, et al (eds): Infant and Child Feeding. New York, Academic Press, 1981;99–121.
9. Andrews BF, Lorch V. Improved fat and calcium absorption in LBW infants fed a medium chain triglyceride formula. Pediatr Res 1974;8:378.
10. Gross S. Relationship between the protein and iron content of

cow's milk and hematologic values in infancy. Rep Ross Conf Pediatr Res 1979;62:89–101.

11. Forbes GB, Woodruff CW (eds): Pediatric Nutrition Handbook, 2nd ed. Elk Grove Village, IL, American Academy of Pediatrics, 1985;185–187.

12. Ziegler EE, Fomon SJ. Fluid intake, renal solute load, and water balance in infancy. J Pediatr 1971;78:561–568.

13. Fomon SJ. Infant Nutrition, 2nd ed. Philadelphia, W.B. Saunders Co., 1974;249.

14. Cordano A. Pre-clinical and clinical evaluation of new infant formulas. Nutr Res 1984;4:929–934.

15. Graham GG, Placko RP, Morales E, et al. Dietary protein quality in infants and children. VI. Isolated soy protein milk. Am J Dis Child 1970;120:419–423.

16. Fomon SJ, Thomas LN, Filer LJ, et al. Food consumption and growth of normal infants fed milk-based formulas. Acta Pediatr Scand 1971;Suppl 223.

24

Infant Feeding Practices: Commercially Prepared Baby Foods

GEORGE A. PURVIS, Ph.D.
SANDRA J. BARTHOLMEY, Ph.D.

ABSTRACT

The evolution of infant feeding practice in the United States during the past 200 years has closely paralleled the availability of foods and the development of the food processing industry. The interesting history of baby foods has been well documented.

The original objective for baby foods was to provide normally utilized foods in convenient form for weaning infants. Efficiency of production, food safety, scientific approaches to determining appropriate foods, and documenting nutritional adequacy of infant diets have emerged as equally important objectives.

The most pronounced changes in infant feeding practice have occurred during the last 20 years. These changes are described along with the associated changes in recommendations and nutritional status. The descriptive comments contain categories of infant foods, product descriptions and characteristics. An important part of product description is the use of the foods—intended and real—regulations governing infant foods and nutritional contributions infant foods make to the total diet.

Infant nutrition status is reviewed in detail. The component parts of nutrition status include contribution of baby foods to total nutritional adequacy of the diet and changes in status associated with feeding practice.

Controversial topics in infant feeding including ingredients, salt and other additives are reviewed briefly.

INTRODUCTION

The preparation and feeding of commercially prepared baby foods has been an evolutionary phenomenon during the past 60 years. As late as the 1920s, feeding practice followed recommendations of a number of physicians that weaning should not occur until 10-12 months of age.[1] The diet proposed by Holt in 1899 for infants at 10 months of age included beef juice, followed by thin gruels from oats, wheat, barley, farina, or arrowroot added to each feeding.[2] A number of foods that were primarily derived from malted cereal were offered as baby foods with the assumption they were in addition to bottle feeding.[3]

Another significant factor in the evolution of modern feeding practice was a series of studies conducted by Clara Davis in the 1920s and 1930s. Davis' work focused on identifying foods that infants would, in the absence of adult intervention, select to eat, and determining whether the foods and amounts selected would be adequate to maintain growth and health. The results of her studies have been widely interpreted by health professionals to mean that, given a wide variety of choices, children will instinctively select and eat a well-balanced diet. As pointed out in a recent revisitation of those studies,[4] the self-selection interpretation was not entirely correct, but the impact on food habits was dramatic. An important point made by the studies, and since confirmed by several generations of infants, is that **during the first year infants are capable of digesting foods eaten by adults** (particularly meats) while maintaining normal growth.[4] Sackett published a report in 1956 which inicated that foods could be used "safely" in young infants.[5]

The real basis of commercial foods prepared specifically for infants had its beginning during the 1920s and was primarily associated with the rapid development of the food processing industry.[6] Improvement in food processing technology has made possible appropriate foods for convenient feeding of infants. Not only were purees developed to form an appropriate consistency, but serving size was adjusted to more closely approximate an infant's nutritional needs. Processing trial-and-error and experience have brought us where we are today in infant feeding.

We owe a debt of gratitude to the wars of Napoleon Bonaparte. While thousands of French soldiers were dying gloriously in battle, other thousands were perishing miserably from scurvy and slow starvation. The desperate and impoverished French government offered an award to anyone who could devise a method of ensuring fresh, wholesome food for French armies and navies. Nicolas Appert, genius chef, pickler, preserver, wine maker, brewer and distiller, claimed the prize in 1809. Appert simply sealed fresh or cooked meat, fish, fruits, eggs and vegetables in air-tight bottles, immersed them in boiling water for varying periods, and was able to keep his "processed" foods in edible condition. Although losses from spoilage were frequently heavy, this trial-and-error method set the stage for preserving food by sterilization. Half a century later, Louis Pasteur's discovery of heat treatment as a method for assurance of microbiological safety followed.[7]

Food science has since built on those primitive heating methods to clearly define the techniques to assure microbiological safety, maintain nutritional quality, inactivate undesirable enzyme systems, and provide the cooked flavors that have formed standards for feeding habits of the entire population, including infants. The following discussion begins with a brief history of the three main categories of infant foods followed by an overview of pediatric feeding recommendations, most of which have been based on existing practices in the absence of basic clinical studies. Descriptions of current baby food categories—dry cereals, purees and juices—provide an introduction to the section on changes in feeding patterns and the nutritional contribution of baby foods to the overall nutritional adequacy of the infant diet.

HISTORY OF BABY FOODS

Precooked infant cereal is traditionally fed as the first supplemental food. The heritage of infant cereal has derived from baby foods used during the 1890s which were predominantly malted foods—either malted milk (Horlick's Malted Milk) or Mellin's food, which was malted carbohydrate hydrolyzed to a soluble form.[2]

The modern form of infant cereal, Pablum, was a product developed in 1933 by Dr. Alan Brown at The Hospital for Sick Children in Toronto.[8] For many years, the term Pablum was synonymous with the desirable characteristics of a partially hydrolyzed, precooked, and sterile cereal-based food. The combination has been established as a well-tolerated form of carbohydrate most frequently used as the first supplementary food.

The second category, canned baby foods, in their present form was initiated during the 1920s, with approximately 10 food manufacturers active in the area. Included among these were the current three manufacturers—Gerber, Heinz, and Beech-Nut—but also Clapp's, Armour, Smith, Stokely and Libby, McNeil and Libby were included.[8] Originally, the varieties were limited largely to fruits and vegetables. The process was relatively simple—prepare the fruit or vegetable in the manner customary for canning and further process it through equipment to reduce particle size and remove indigestible materials, fibrous texture, stone cells, and seeds to yield a "pureed" product. Combinations evolved from practices of parents resulting in convenient combinations.

Many of the foods were developed to provide an alternative to practices that were in place. An example: A practice during the 1930s was to cook, grind and strain meat. A natural extension of this practice was to utilize food processing equipment to finely divide (or puree) meat and process it in small, convenient serving size containers. The resulting product is not only more convenient and safer, but the quality is more favorable since juices are not lost, cooking is controlled (adequate for safety but not excessive), flavorings are not added (salt and spices), and the fat content is controlled and uniform.

The containers were small metal cans, usually 4 to 4½ oz. Conversion to glass containers did not occur until 1955–1963.[8] The motivation for use of canned baby foods was then, and remains, convenience, safety and confidence.

Fruit juices are a third category of foods; adaptation of these products has been relatively recent in infant feeding practice. The primary advantages demonstrated by fruit juices for infants are serving size, convenience, availability in glass jars to which a nipple can be attached, assurance of safety and freedom from particulate materials.

FEEDING PRACTICES

The evolution of feeding practices has been closely associated with development of the food supply. Early feeding practice depended entirely on breastfeeding, with conversion to "artificial" foods only when necessary. The poor sanitary quality of foods available at the turn of the century resulted in less than satisfactory results. The infant mortality rate reflected poor sanitation and quality of foods for supplementary feeding. In New York City, for example, 14.3% of children under five years of age died during 1896, 22% from diarrheal diseases. In 1921, the mortality rate had dropped to 9.6% and diarrheal disease claimed only 7% of these deaths.[9]

The history of infant feeding has been well documented, and comprehensive review reveals a fascinating drama. Dr. Thomas Cone wrote a book on the subject in 1976—*200 Years of Feeding Infants in America.*[10] The American Dietetic Association published a set of essays in 1968 related to the history of infant nutrition. The book of essays was appropriately dedicated to Lydia Roberts, a pioneer in child and infant nutrition research from 1930 until her death in 1965.[11] Gerber Products Company published *The Story of an Idea* in 1953,[12] which described the history of baby foods. All these publications are commended to the scholar who wishes to pursue this interesting history.

A major factor in recognition and definition of feeding practice was formation of the Committee on Nutrition of the American Academy of Pediatrics in 1955. The Committee was unique. Members were invited not only from the Academy membership, but liaison and advisory participants came from industry, government agencies and professional societies. Through this forum, infant feeding practices were defined and recommendations were published that focused on the practices most advantageous for pediatricians, and also provided clear guidance for food manufacturers and regulatory agencies. As a result a recommendation for "solid food" was published in 1958[13] and has been updated and expanded to encompass individual nutrients: iron in 1976,[14] vitamin and mineral supplements in 1980,[15] and fluoride in 1972[16] and 1986.[17] These recommendations have substantial value from a practical sense, but more importantly, they recognize the need, value, proper use and potential misuse of supplementary foods.

In the development of infant feeding programs, particularly in support of breastfeeding as the source of basic infant nutrition, it is important to recognize the nutritional contribution of supplementary foods. Satisfactory nutrition in the totally breast-fed infant requires a source of calories in addition to breast milk at 4 to 6 months. For lactating mothers whose nutrition may be marginal, additional calories for the infant may be needed as early as the second month.[18]

Several categories of commercially prepared foods have been developed to fulfill nutritional needs of infants and to satisfy the requirements of caregivers for convenience and safety. In the following section basic supplementary food categories are defined.

BASIC SUPPLEMENTARY FOOD CATEGORIES

Dry Cereals

Dry infant cereals are low moisture, vitamin- and mineral-enriched foods which contain 373-396 calories/100 gm. Their primary purpose is to serve as a concentrated source of calories, vitamins and minerals (particularly iron) to supplement the diet of infants whose needs for these nutrients are not met by human milk, infant formula or other milk. Manufacture of infant cereal involves hydrolysis of cereal flour (rice, barley, oat) with an enzyme source, and heating to precook and gelatinize the starches. The serving size and form of feeding is flexible. The recommended serving is ½ oz (14.2 gm) mixed with 70 ml (2.4 oz) milk, juice, formula or water.

In order to reduce the incidence of allergy arising from an unnecessarily complex diet, single grain cereals—rice, oatmeal and barley—are generally recommended as starting cereals. Mixed cereal based on three or more grains (oat, corn, wheat, rice, soya) provides greater variety to older infants. High protein cereal (based on soya flour, with added oat and wheat flour) offers low cost and high protein in addition to variety. Cereal with fruit appeals to the flavor preferences of older infants and provides a rich source of iron.

Dry cereals are supplemented with iron, thiamin, riboflavin, niacin, calcium and phosphorus to contribute to adequate intakes of these important nutrients.

Purees

Fruits and vegetables are essentially the pureed version of the specific food sterilized in a container that provides an appropriate serving size. The ranges of nutrient values are characteristic of their component ingredient fruits or vegetables. The caloric ranges, for example, are 40-80 calories per container (4.5 oz) for vegetables and 60-100 calories per container (4.5 oz) for fruit.

Numerous combinations of vegetables, meat, cereal and fruit are available, each component of which contributes food value dependent on the characteristics of the individual foods used in the combination (Table 1).

Since there are over 300 infant food combinations and forms in the U.S., each individual product will not be discussed. Manufacturers provide upon request detailed background information for their food products. Nutrient labeling is provided for virtually all foods in the U.S., and ingredients are stated in descending order of concentration. Extensive analytical data, instructions for use, and background preparation information are also available from food manufacturers.

The serving sizes of foods in jars are:

Strained Foods—Fruits and desserts 4¾ oz or 134 gm
　　　　　　　 —other foods　　　　　 4½ oz or 128 gm
　　　　　　　　　　　　　　　　　 2½ oz or　71 gm

Strained foods are defined as having a particle size that can pass through a finishing screen of .033 inches.

Junior Foods—Fruits and desserts 7¾ oz or 220 gm
　　　　　　 —other foods　　　　 7½ oz or 212 gm

Junior foods generally have a coarser texture than strained and incorporate larger particles to provide practice in chewing.

Strained and Junior Meats　 3½ oz or 99 gm
　　　　　　　　　　　　　 2½ oz or 71 gm

Dry versions of strained foods also are available as "instant baby food." Cereals, fruits, vegetables, dinner combinations and desserts are packaged in 1 or 1.5 oz containers supplying 2 to 5 servings. Cereals also are available in 3.5 oz containers. Serving size and consistency of the meal are adjusted by varying the amount of water added to the dry food.

Juices

Strained juices provide a maximum of 4% of the daily caloric intake of infants during the first 12 months. Juice is strained and homogenized, containing no particulate matter such as intact fruit cells, supplemented with vitamin C to a uniform content equivalent to fresh orange juice and placed in a container (4.2 oz or 124 ml) of convenient volume for infant feeding. The vitamin C contribution is sufficient to provide 8-23% of the total vitamin C intake for infants 4 to 9 months of age. Juices are full-strength and prepared without added sugar. Infant juices contain, in addition to added vitamin C, the entire complement of nutrients endogenous to the fruit. **Infant juices are generally good sources of potassium and vitamin B$_6$ and may provide significant quantities of thiamin and folic acid as well.**

NUTRIENT INTAKE

During the 1960s, a new level of consumer consciousness developed in the U.S. population. Consumer activism was the rule, and it at-

TABLE 1.　　Nutrition Information Per Serving of Representative Combination Infant Foods*

			Percent of Calories As			Average Nutrient Values Per Serving Size Percent of U.S. RDA For Infants						
	Serving Size	Calories	Protein	Carbo-hydrates	Fat	Protein	Vit A	Thiamin	Ribo-flavin	Niacin	Iron	Vit B$_6$
Strained Dinner												
Beef Egg Noodle	4.5 oz	90	18	53	30	15	30	6	8	10	2	10
Strained High Meat Dinner												
Ham with Vegetables	4.5 oz	100	32	36	36	45	15	15	15	20	4	20
Strained Cereal w/Fruit												
Oatmeal w/Apple-sauce and							Vit C					
Bananas†	4.5 oz	100	16	84	9	8	45	45	45	45	45	45

†Vitamin- and Mineral-Fortified.
*Nutrient Values 1986. Gerber Products Company, 445 State Street, Freemont, MI 49412.

tained not only acceptance but popularity. A White House Conference on Food, Nutrition and Health in 1969 addressed questions raised by activists but made it clear that substantial voids existed in the knowledge concerning feeding of infants as well as other specific populations.[19]

From the questions raised by the White House Conference came several programs to collect information on infant feeding in the U.S. Gerber Products Company was asked to conduct studies in 1969 which were used as "pilot" evaluations to answer specific questions. More comprehensive nutrition studies were conducted by Gerber Products Company in 1972 and have continued to the most recent studies conducted in 1986. Other studies [the Ten State Survey in 1968-1970 and HANES I and HANES II (Health and Nutrition Evaluation Study)] have evaluated specific population groups in considerable detail and have made extremely valuable contributions to in-depth knowledge of infant nutrition.

Several interacting factors affect an infant's dietary intake: pediatric recommendations, mothers' perceptions of the needs of their babies, and the climate of concern about health issues related to diet. General recommendations are, of course, useful guidelines, but the decision to feed what and when to an individual infant rests primarily on the infant's unique developmental pattern. Wide variation in feeding patterns is, therefore, the rule rather than adherence to a rigid time frame.

The Gerber Nutrition Surveys are presented here in detail because they are compatible with a discussion that emphasizes baby foods, and they represent a statistically valid national sample. The contrast in observed feeding patterns between the first and latest surveys provides insight into changes in nutrient intake and compliance with feeding recommendations.

The most reliable method to determine food intake and, therefore, nutrient intake, is to ask people what, how much and when they eat. Dietary records kept over a period of several days provide useful, accurate information concerning usual patterns of dietary intake.[20] In the Gerber surveys, dietary intake of infants was determined by food records kept by mothers. The data were analyzed to determine usual nutrient intake, as well as portion size, food preferences, and age of introduction of supplemental foods. The following information summarizes data collected from four-day dietary records of infants 2-12 months of age during the earliest (1972, n=377) and latest (1986, n=637) survey years.[21]

ENERGY

Although there were marked changes in the relative amounts of food types provided to infants, the total intake of energy throughout the first year of life did not change significantly from 1972-1986. The average intake of energy calculated for each ranged from 75-122% of the Recommended Dietary Allowance across all ages.[22] The composition of the diet, however, has undergone dramatic change during this period. Breast milk and infant formula provided at least 50% of the total energy intake up to three months of age in 1972, and in excess of one-half of total calories for the first six months in 1986. Cow milk was a significant source of calories much later in age in 1986 than in 1972. As an index for comparison, cow milk provided more calories than infant formula and human milk by five months of age in 1972, but not until 10 months during 1986.

A trend toward later introduction of baby foods parallels the later introduction of cow milk. During 1972, baby foods provided 17% of total calories at two months of age and nearly 30% at three months of age. Corresponding values from 1986 were 2% and 8% respectively. Infant cereal accounted for more than one-half of this amount in 1986. The consumption of commercially prepared baby foods became a significant source of energy at four months of age in 1972, providing 32% of total calories. During 1986 baby foods provided only 14% of total energy at four months of age. **This trend is consistent with contemporary recommendations to delay the introduction of supplemental foods until 4 to 6 months of age.** Overall, baby foods provided 27% of total calories during the first year of life in 1972 and only 19% in 1986.

The time of introduction of table foods was similar in both surveys conducted in 1972 and 1986. Small amounts of table foods were provided to infants during the early months and became a more important source of energy progressively throughout the year. By 12 months of age, table foods provided approximately 50-60% of total calories.

The provision of adequate energy to the active, growing infant is of paramount importance. Unfortunately, the association of calories with obesity often results in a misunderstanding of infant need for calories.

Survey data obtained in 1986 do not support the viewpoint that infants are being overfed. In the 1986 survey fewer than 4% of infants younger than 6 months of age had caloric intake greater than the 90th percentile (145

Legend for All Figures

- ▣ Breast Milk
- 🍼 Formula
- 🥛 Cow's Milk
- 🥄 Baby Foods
- 🍽️ Table Foods
- 💊 Vitamins

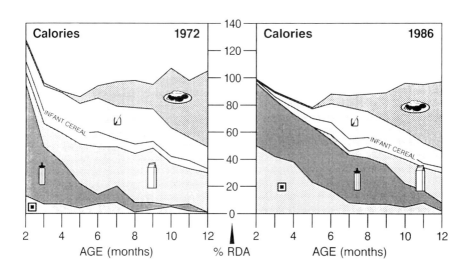

kcal/kg/day). After 6 months of age, the recommended energy allowance decreases from 115 to 105 kcal/kg/day.[22] Only 7% of infants in this age group received intakes greater than the 90th percentile (135 kcal/kg/day).

It is important to emphasize that the energy intake of individual infants is quite variable. Energy allowances for individual children are more appropriately derived from observations of appetite, activity, growth, and weight gain in relation to body fat.[22]

PROTEIN INTAKE

The average protein intake of infants age 2-12 months was above the RDA for each age during 1972 and exceeded 200% after five months. Human milk, infant formula and cow milk together provided the RDA of this nutrient throughout the first year. Baby foods

provided an average 24% of total dietary protein from 3-12 months of age. Table foods become a more significant source of dietary protein towards the end of the first year providing one-third to one-half the total protein between 10 and 12 months.

The protein intake of infants in 1986 decreased somewhat from that in the earlier survey, but average intake in each age range remained near or above the RDA. Infant formula and breast milk were used more frequently and cow milk less frequently in 1986 than in 1972. This change in diet resulted in less protein being contributed by cow milk. To illustrate this point, cow milk provided more than 50% of total dietary protein to infants 5-9 months of age in 1972 and less than 25% for this age group in 1986. Infants 10-12 months of age received 40% of protein from cow milk in 1972 but only 31% in 1986. Baby foods

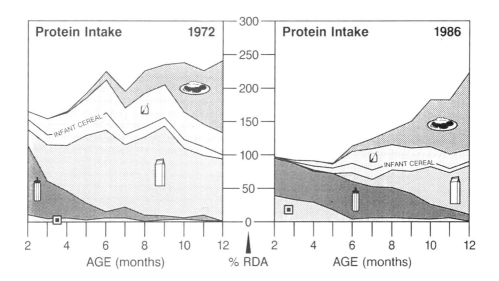

provided substantial amounts of protein after the fifth month in 1986 and supplemented the protein from milk sources to achieve average intakes corresponding to the RDA. Table foods contributed increasing amounts of protein in 1986 and were a significant source after about 8 months of age.

A criticism of diets for U.S. infants has been that they contain excess protein. The 1986 survey data support this. **Starting at 6 months of age, infant diets provided protein in excess of 12% of the RDA and continued to supply progressively greater amounts through the first year to reach more than twice the RDA at 12 months of age.** The amount of protein contributed by commercial baby food peaked at 30% of total protein by 7 months, falling to 11% by one year of age. In 1986 cow milk and table food supplied more than 50% of the dietary protein by 9 months and increased to more than 80% by the end of the first year.

FAT INTAKE

In 1972, fat consistently provided approximately one-third of an infant's calories throughout the first year of life. In 1986, this was true only for the second six months. During the first six months, breast milk or infant formula supplied over 40% of total calories as fat.

Current recommendations do not generally support fat restriction during the first year. The infants in the surveys reported here received from 30-40% of their calories as fat during the second half of their first year, which is suggest-

ed as "sensible for adequate growth and development" by the American Academy of Pediatrics.[23]

The contribution made by baby foods to dietary fat intake in 1972 peaked at 18% at six months of age, then gradually declined as table foods and cow milk became more prominent in the diet. In 1986, baby foods contributed less fat at a later period during the first year—a maximum of only 12% between 7 and 9 months of age—reflecting the trend for later introduction of supplemental foods as well as the decreased usage of baby foods over the 14-year span.

MINERAL INTAKE

Iron

Iron is of particular importance in infant nutrition because requirements are high during infancy, and the number of foods traditionally provided to infants that are rich sources of iron is limited. Although human milk contains a relatively modest amount of iron (approximately 0.5 mg/L), its bioavailability (about 50%) is greater than that of any other food examined.[24] The other important sources of bioavailable iron to the infant are iron-fortified infant formula (average 10-15 mg/L) and iron-fortified infant cereal (average 45 mg/100 gm).

The average iron intake of infants less than 6 months old decreased markedly from 1972 to 1986. This decrease was primarily caused by a reduction of the amount of iron added to infant cereals from 100 mg/100 gm to 45 mg/

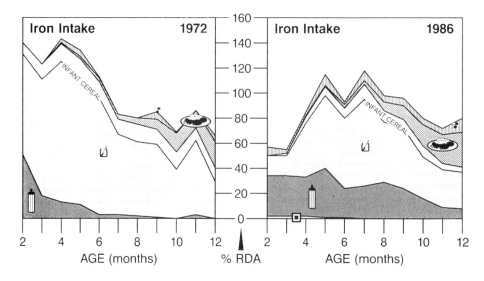

100 gm in 1974. At the same time, the iron fortificant, sodium iron pyrophosphate, was replaced with a small particle size electrolytic iron having a relative bioavailability 2-4 times greater than iron pyrophosphate.[25] Baby foods (primarily dry cereal) provided an average of 80% of an infant's dietary iron in 1972. In 1986, baby foods supplied an average 52% of dietary iron to babies less than one year of age. Table foods provided modest amounts of iron to the diet but were limited to the latter part of the first year. Pharmaceutical vitamin preparations containing iron provided on average less than 7% of total iron during 1986.

In 1972, 58% of the infants surveyed received less than 100% of the RDA for iron. Thirty-seven percent received less than two-thirds of the RDA for iron. These percentages increased slightly during 1986 to 62 and 45%, respectively. Since iron adequacy is recognized as the most critical issue in infant nutrition in the U.S., **assurance of adequate iron intake and recommendation for iron should be strong points in infant nutrition programs.** The American Academy of Pediatrics recommends the use of iron-fortified cereals up to 2 years of age as a means to reduce the risk of iron deficiency in this vulnerable group.[26] This recommendation is particularly important, since the 1986 American Academy of Pediatrics statement sanctioned the use of whole cow milk after 6 months of age if a significant portion of calories are derived from supplemental and, one hopes, iron-rich foods.[27]

Calcium

The milk component of the diet is by far the most important source of calcium, an essential mineral for proper bone growth. Human milk and infant formula provided calcium at or near the RDA until three months of age in 1972 and until five months of age in 1986. After these ages, cow milk gradually replaced formula as the major source of calcium in the diet. The non-milk component of the diet, other than infant cereals, was a relatively unimportant source of this nutrient until table foods became more prominent after 9 months of age.

Although the average intake of calcium was well above the RDA at each age, some infants were not fed adequate quantities of milk. This situation resulted in an increase of infants who did not receive the RDA for calcium—from 9% in 1972 to 42% in 1986. The percentage of infants who received less than two-thirds of the RDA also increased from 2% in 1972 to 10% in 1986. These statistics emphasize the importance of dairy products and calcium-enriched infant cereals in the diet of infants.

Phosphorus

The sources of phosphorus in the diet of infants during 1972 and 1986 closely paralleled those of calcium. Human milk and infant formula provided the major portion of phosphorus intake during the early months of life and, as these sources declined, cow milk provided adequate quantities. Baby foods pro-

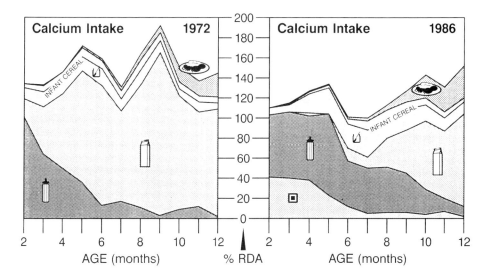

vided a maximum of 25% of dietary phosphorus at 6 months of age in 1972 and 35% in 1986. This contribution by baby foods gradually declined as table foods and cow milk become more prominent in the diet during the latter part of the year.

The average calcium/phosphorus intake ratio of infants in 1986 was 1.5:1 during early infancy and decreased to 0.9:1 at 12 months of age. These ratios closely approximate the calcium/phosphorus ratios recommended by the National Academy of Sciences—National Research Council of 1.5:1 during the early months and 1:1 at the end of the first year.[28]

Magnesium

In 1972, cow milk and baby foods, particularly infant cereals, supplied most of the dietary magnesium throughout the first year. At every age surveyed, infants received on average generous amounts of magnesium above the RDA. For any month surveyed, however, human milk and table foods contributed less than 5% of the RDA for magnesium during the first year.

Magnesium intake in 1986 was near the RDA after 3 months when baby foods supplied at least 25% of the RDA. In contrast to 1972,

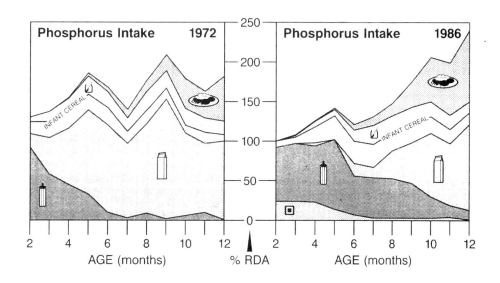

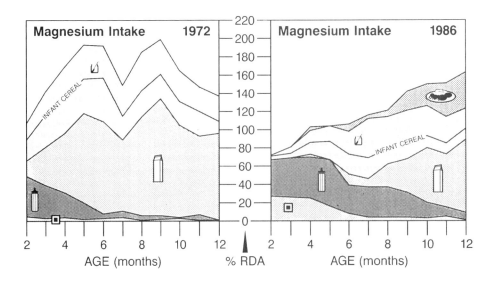

human milk and infant formula provided most of the dietary magnesium through the first 5 months in 1986. After 5 months of age, baby foods continually supplied close to one-third the dietary magnesium until table foods and cow milk became the principal contributors at the end of the first year.

Even though 50% of the infants surveyed in 1986 received over 100% of the RDA for magnesium, 25% received less than two-thirds of the RDA. Although magnesium deficiency is rare and primarily associated with kwashiorkor in infancy, persistent vomiting and diarrhea can also result in the loss of magnesium-rich intestinal secretions.[29]

Trace Minerals

Zinc and iodine are two trace minerals for which adequate evidence exists on which to base recommended dietary allowances. For other trace elements—copper, fluoride, chromium, selenium and molybdenum—ranges of safe intakes are provided by the National Research Council because less information is available on which to base allowances. Of these, only copper has had both a reliable method for analysis and a consistent representation in nutrient data banks since 1972. For these reasons, only zinc, iodine and copper are discussed here.

Zinc. Average zinc intake by infants was near the RDA at all ages in 1972 and in 1986. In both survey years, infant formula was the major source of dietary zinc in the early months. In 1972, however, cow milk and baby food became the primary sources of zinc at 5

months of age and continued to supply substantial amounts until 10 months at which time table foods became a significant source of zinc in the diet.

In 1986, infant formula continued to supply close to one-half the RDA for zinc through the eighth month. Cow milk and table foods gradually became more prominent in the diet after this time, providing 94% of the RDA for zinc by the twelfth month. Baby foods contributed an average of 17% of the RDA for zinc after the first 3 months of age.

Although average zinc intakes were close to the RDA at each month, 27% of infants in the 1986 survey failed to receive two-thirds of the RDA for zinc. These data support suggestions that mild or marginal zinc deficiencies in apparently healthy children[30] and infants[31] in the U.S. may not be uncommon.

Iodine. Iodine intake was 2-4 times the RDA in both 1972 and 1986. In 1972, infant formula or cow milk provided 1.5-3 times the RDA throughout the first year. Baby food contributed an average additional 25% of the RDA from the fifth through the twelfth months. Table foods supplied increasing amounts—up to 1.5 times the RDA for iodine—in the second half of the year.

In 1986, either human milk or infant formula could have provided all the iodine needed by the infants surveyed through the fifth month of age. After 5 months, cow milk and table food supplied increasingly substantial amounts of iodine—up to 3 times the RDA—by 12 months of age. Baby foods provided an average 16% of the RDA for iodine after the sixth month. With average intakes so

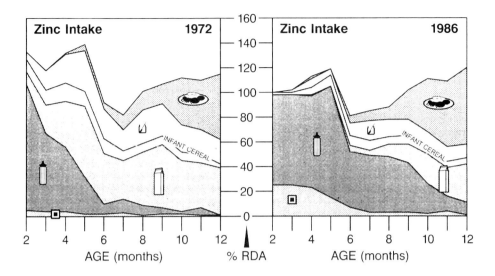

far above the RDA, it was surprising that as many as 5 infants of the 637 surveyed in 1986 received less than two-thirds of the RDA for iodine, a record approached only by vitamins A and C.

During the last 60 years, iodine nutriture has undergone a complete reversal in the U.S. from the problem of endemic goiter to one of excessive iodine intake. Besides the usual dietary sources of iodine, iodophors in cleaning agents used on dairy equipment and as dough-conditioners in breads are rich sources of inadvertent dietary iodine which passes readily into human milk.[32] Although no evidence has been found of adverse effects related to an increased dietary intake of iodine, further increases should be viewed with caution.[33]

Copper. An RDA has not been established for copper, but the National Research Council has established a safe and adequate daily intake of 0.5-0.7 mg for infants up to 6 months of age and 0.7-1.0 mg for infants 6-12 months of age.[34]

In contrast to iodine, copper was more often provided below the range of estimated safe and adequate intake than within or above it. In 1972, infant formula was the major source of dietary copper until the fifth month when baby foods became the primary source. Baby foods continued to provide close to one-half of total dietary copper until 10 months of age when table foods made up a larger share of the diet.

In 1986, infant formula provided at least one-half the total copper intake until 7 months

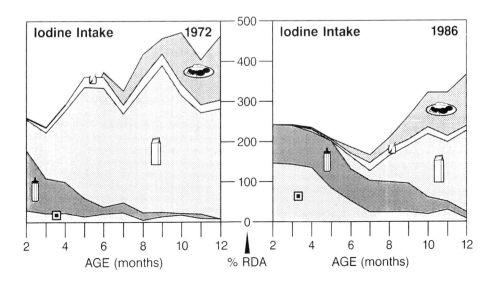

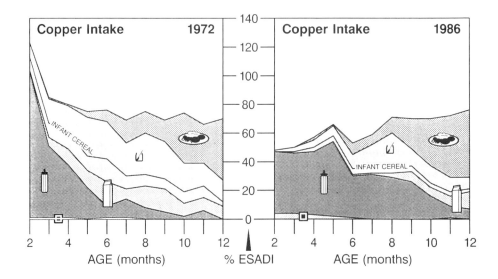

of age. During that time, baby foods were the second largest source of copper in the infant diet. After 8 months, table foods supplied increasing amounts of copper, until by 12 months of age more than one-half the copper intake was from table foods.

Although 56% of the infants surveyed in 1986 received less than two-thirds of the estimated safe intake of copper, healthy infants have maintained positive copper balance with one-half the average estimated safe and adequate amount of copper.[35] A sufficient safety margin apparently is provided by the estimated safe and adequate daily intakes.

Sodium

The National Research Council has established a safe and adequate daily intake for sodium of 115-350 mg (5-15 mEq) for infants up to 6 months of age and 250-750 mg (11-33 mEq) for infants 6 to 12 months of age.[34]

The sodium intake of infants decreased considerably in the period between 1972 and 1986. There are several factors responsible for this change. Increased and prolonged use of human milk and infant formula over the past 15 years has resulted in a decrease in the use of cow milk. Because cow milk is a relatively rich source of sodium compared to formula and breast milk, the net result of these changes has been a decrease in the amount of sodium provided by the milk component of the diet.

The removal of added salt from commercially prepared baby foods also has contributed to the overall reduction in the sodium intake of infants. Also, baby foods of low en-

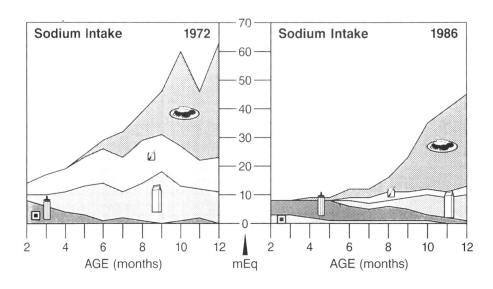

dogenous sodium content such as fruits have tended to replace those of higher sodium concentration. Nevertheless, the small contribution of sodium by baby foods has resulted in a significant change only for infants less than 8 months of age, due to the large contribution of sodium from table foods added to the diet of the older infant.

During both 1972 and 1986, the primary source of sodium in the diet after about 8 months of age was table food. These foods provided more sodium than all other sources combined by 10 months in 1972 and by 9 months in 1986. Infant dietary intake of sodium stayed within the estimated safe and adequate daily intakes through 9 months of age in 1986. After that, sodium intake exceeded suggested levels by 6 to 39%. If the sodium intake of older infants is a concern, prudent selection or delayed introduction of table foods would be the most efficacious dietary change. **Many concealed sodium sources are not recognized in the infant's diet: cow milk and milk products, bread and bakery products, processed meats and canned vegetables and salted, home-prepared foods are some examples.**

Although there is no evidence to suggest that current low intakes of sodium are harmful, an additional source of sodium may be beneficial under certain conditions that increase sodium losses in sweat such as high environmental temperatures.[36]

VITAMIN INTAKES

The remaining nutrients generally are available in adequate amounts. Since individual dietary intakes vary considerably, some individual infants may be at nutritional risk. Infants who were provided with a diet consistent with recommendations, namely human milk, or iron-fortified infant formula supplemented appropriately with a variety of additional foods, received an adequate supply of individual nutrients.

Vitamin A

Vitamin A was available in abundance in the diets of infants during both 1972 and 1986. Human milk, infant formula and cow milk provided at least 100% of the RDA of this nutrient until 2 months of age in 1972 and until 6 months in 1986. Baby foods, particularly vegetable and vegetable-containing foods, provided substantial quantities of vitamin A above the RDA during the remainder of the first year. Contributions from table foods increased with age and provided similar amounts of vitamin A in 1986 and in 1972.

Pharmaceutical vitamin preparations containing vitamin A were provided to infants at all ages. This fact may account for the generous vitamin A supplementation to an already adequate dietary source.

The percentage of infants who received less

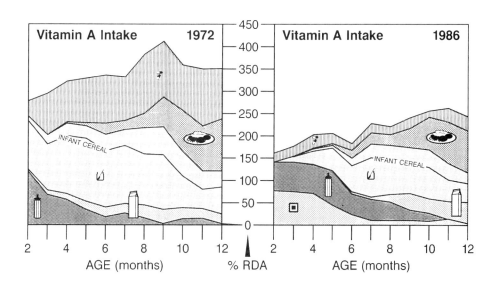

than the RDA for vitamin A decreased from 8% in 1972 to 6% in 1986. One percent of infants received less than two-thirds of the RDA for this nutrient in 1986. That any should not have received the full recommended amount of this essential nutrient is surprising.

Vitamin C

American babies certainly are in no danger of developing scurvy. Vitamin C was a plentiful component of the diet of infants at each age during both 1972 and 1986. Human milk and infant formula provided this nutrient in quantities at or near the RDA during the early months. The contribution by these foods was greater in 1986 than in 1972, but the difference was minimal until about 4 months of age.

Pasteurized cow milk is a poor source of vitamin C, and its contribution to the diet was insignificant during both survey years. It is, therefore, **important to provide an additional source of vitamin C after breastfeeding or formula-feeding is replaced with cow milk.**

Baby foods, particularly vitamin C-fortified fruits and juices, were the largest source of vitamin C in the diet of the infants surveyed. Baby foods complemented the decreasing vitamin C provided by the milk component of the diet to achieve the RDA.

Table foods provided increasing amounts of vitamin C during the latter part of the first year. Pharmaceutical vitamin preparations provided the full RDA for vitamin C in 1972 and about one-third the RDA in 1986 to infants over 6 months old.

Eight percent of the infants in both 1972 and 1986 received less than the RDA of vitamin C, a most surprising finding considering the availability of vitamin C-supplemented infant juices and fruits and vitamin preparations.

Thiamin

The average intake of thiamin by infants during 1972 and 1986 exceeded the RDA at each age examined. Human milk and infant formula supplied quantities of thiamin close to the RDA until 3 months of age during 1972 and 5 months in 1986. The trend for extended usage of infant formula in place of cow milk resulted in a pronounced decrease in thiamin provided by cow milk. Nevertheless, the total contribution of this vitamin by the milk component of the diet did not change dramatically.

Baby foods supplemented the thiamin provided by the milk component of the diet and were a substantial source of this nutrient. Infant cereals are fortified with thiamin (as well as riboflavin, niacin and iron), and are the largest baby food source of this nutrient. Table foods also provided thiamin to the diet of infants, but substantial contributions from this source were limited to the latter part of infancy. The use of pharmaceutical vitamin preparations containing thiamin decreased during the period between 1972 and 1986 but were still provided at each age. The reduction in thiamin supplementation may be the result of fewer pediatric recommendations to supplement with thiamin or other water-soluble vitamins.

Twenty-six percent of the infants surveyed

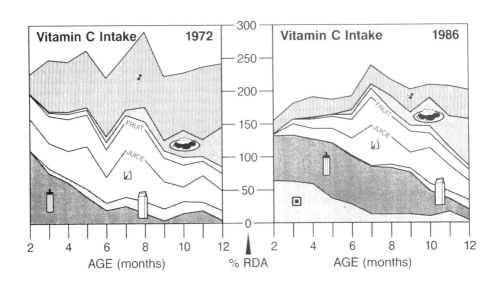

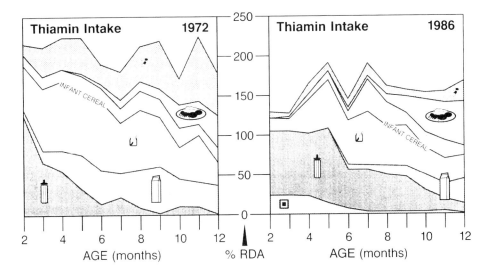

during 1986 received less than the RDA for thiamin. The corresponding value in 1972 was 7%.

Riboflavin

The average intake of riboflavin was well above the RDA for each month of infancy during both 1972 and 1986. Human milk and infant formula provided abundant quantities of riboflavin during the early months of infancy. Cow milk, a rich source of this vitamin, provided large quantities particularly after the fifth month. The milk component of the diet satisfied the RDA for riboflavin throughout the first year of life during both 1972 and 1986.

Additional sources of riboflavin in the infant diet were baby foods, particularly riboflavin-fortified infant cereals, and table foods. Ribo-

flavin also was furnished by vitamin supplements but, as observed for other B vitamins, this source was less important during 1986.

All but one infant of 377 infants surveyed in 1972 received the RDA for riboflavin, but 19% received less than this amount during 1986.

Niacin

The niacin intake of infants during the first year of life was generally similar for 1972 and 1986. Human milk and infant formula, as for most nutrients, made the largest contribution during the early months. As these foods were discontinued, cow milk became a significant source. Although cow milk is a poor source of preformed niacin, it contains substantial quantities of tryptophan, which can be converted to niacin.[37]

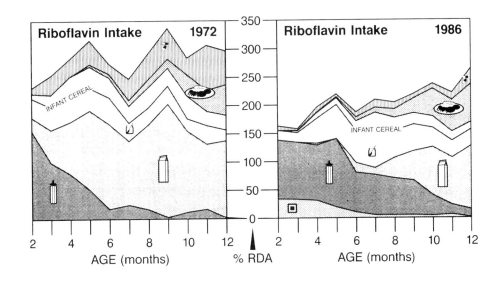

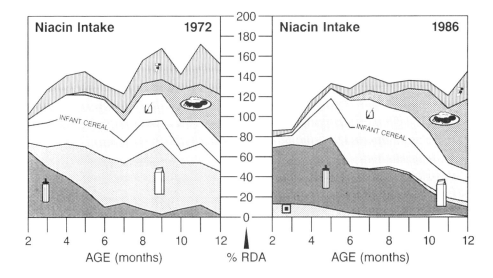

Baby foods are important sources of niacin. Fortified infant cereals provided about one-half of the niacin from baby foods, and meats were another important source. Baby foods were necessary to supplement the niacin in milk to attain average intakes near the RDA in both survey years.

Table foods provided increased quantities of niacin during the latter period of infancy, and vitamin supplements supplied a small but constant amount of niacin during the same period.

Vitamin B₆

Average intakes of vitamin B_6 were higher during 1972 than during 1986, although total average intakes remained close to the RDA. The quantity of vitamin B_6 provided by infant formula and human milk during the first 6 months increased during 1986 but did not totally compensate for the decreased contribution of cow milk. Baby foods are good sources of this nutrient but decreased in usage during this period. **A trend toward providing more fruit-containing baby foods and fewer meat-containing varieties was partially responsible for the decreased contribution of vitamin B_6 from baby foods.**

Table foods contributed increasingly substantial amounts of B_6 during the latter part of the year, and vitamin supplements also provided small amounts of vitamin B_6.

The percentage of infants who received less than the RDA for vitamin B_6 increased from 16.5% in 1972 to 48% in 1986. Similarly, the number of infants who received less than two-thirds of the RDA increased from 3% to 24%

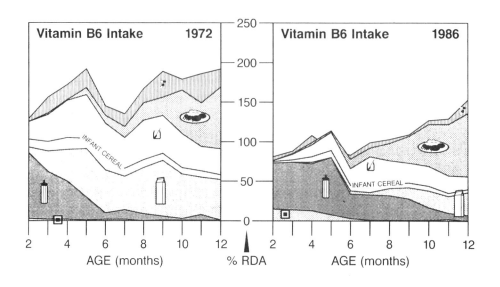

during this period. This decrease in vitamin B_6 intake, especially by very young infants, should alert health professionals to watch for evidence of frank B_6 deficiency—increased irritability and abdominal distention, diarrhea and vomiting.[38]

CONTROVERSIES

The past 15 years have witnessed remarkable changes in infant feeding practices. Breastfeeding is enjoying a dramatic resurgence, and the use of evaporated milk formula has been virtually eliminated. In addition, the nutrition composition of many infant foods has changed significantly. Commercially prepared infant foods are now formulated without added salt. Also, the sugar content of these foods has been significantly reduced.

Several controversial subjects have developed concerning commercially prepared infant foods. Some of the commonly held misconceptions can possibly be dispelled by a series of brief statements.

- **Artificial preservatives are not, and have never been, used in baby foods.** Thermal processing and diligent handling practices eliminate the need for chemical preservatives.
- Artificial colors or flavors are not used in baby foods.
- **Monosodium glutamate (MSG) has not been used in baby foods since November 1969.**
- Salt has not been added to baby foods since October 1977.
- Sugar content was significantly reduced in baby foods during the period 1972-1977. The primary purpose was to reduce caloric density of foods.
- Modified food starch is an acceptable, wholesome ingredient used in some baby food products in amounts ranging from 2-6%.

Some basic questions were raised during the White House Conference in 1969 and were reviewed by a National Academy of Sciences Committee. Each of these topics was reviewed in a separate report.[39–41] Several paragraphs can summarize the somewhat exhaustive conclusions of each.

MSG. Monosodium glutamate was used as a flavor enhancer in some meat-containing baby foods prior to 1969. Safety questions were raised over extremely high concentrations—several times the quantities used in food.[42] As a result of lack of clinical safety information, MSG has not been used as an ingredient in foods for infants since 1969.

Salt. Salt intake in infancy has been of interest and concern to nutrition scientists for approximately 20 years. The controversy around the level of salt intake was precipitated by a hypothesis proposed by Dahl, which suggested that salt in infant food predisposed individuals to hypertension in later life.[43]

The response to this alarming hypothesis was a review conducted by an *ad hoc* National Academy of Sciences Committee which recommended that the amount of salt added to infant foods not exceed 0.25%.[44] A further review of the subject was conducted by the American Academy of Pediatrics in 1978 which confirmed the previous findings.[45]

Eliminating the use of salt in infant foods has not been associated with altered consumption of salt in later life.[46] A reasonable recommendation is that further efforts to reduce the intake of sodium in infancy would be unwise. The infant food manufacturing practice has not included salt as an ingredient in foods for infants since 1977.

Modified Food Starch. The safety and suitability of modifed food starch has been clearly established in three reviews of the topic since 1969.[47,48,49] The *ad hoc* National Academy of Sciences Committee considered the issue in 1970 and concluded that modified food starch is safe and suitable in the amounts and forms used.[47] The evaluation was reviewed in 1979 and the safety and suitability of modified food starch in baby foods was reaffirmed.[48] More recent data have been reviewed on the digestibility of modified starch. The original conclusion stands.[51]

The safety and suitability of modified food starch continue to be questioned by consumer advocacy groups, primarily because the modification process is complex and difficult to define in lay terms. Modification of starches strengthens or stabilizes starch added to foods so that when heated or stored, the foods maintain desirable texture and consistency. Strengthening and stabilization of starches in baby foods are accomplished by inserting trace amounts of chemical cross-links (phosphate or adipate) between hydroxyl groups in starch granules. The safety and digestibility of these modified food starches have been thoroughly evaluated and remain clearly established.

SUMMARY

Commercially prepared foods for infants have developed in a relatively recent period— during the past 60 years. This development offers parents a variety of convenient, safe and quality foods in convenient, waste-free containers. The technology and science for commercial preparation of infant foods as developed in North America are now available worldwide.

Optimal nutrition can be assured with a variety of foods, appropriately introduced and fed according to standard recommendations. The variety and combinations of baby foods available in the United States make it possible to feed infants in this country in a manner to provide excellent nutritional status.

QUESTIONS AND ANSWERS

Questions mothers ask most often about feeding their babies supplemental foods.

1. When?
2. What?
3. How?

1. When does my baby need supplemental foods in addition to breast milk or formula?

Because babies develop at different rates, it is difficult and unwise to set a rigid time schedule for the introduction of supplementary foods. The time to start supplemental foods will depend on the individual infant's rate of growth, level of activity and stage of development. The baby's weight, appetite, activity level and neuromuscular development should, therefore, be considered in deciding when to start supplemental foods. Some signs of the time to start are:

When the baby has doubled in weight since birth, or weighs about 13 pounds, *AND*

When the breast-fed baby frequently demands to be fed more than 8-10 times in a 24-hour period; or

When the baby consistently drinks more than a quart of infant formula per day;

When the baby often seems hungry.

These events usually coincide with developmental signs of readiness to take food from a spoon.

The American Academy of Pediatrics bases its recommendations for the introduction of supplemental foods on developmental criteria that usually appear at approximately 4-6 months of age.[49] By this time, the extrusion reflex of early infancy has disappeared, and the ability to swallow non-liquid foods is established. The intestine is also developing defense mechanisms to protect the infant from foreign proteins; the ability to digest and absorb proteins, fats and carbohydrates is increasing rapidly; and continuing maturation of the kidneys increases their ability to handle osmolar loads with less water.

Nutritional considerations suggest that supplemental iron, vitamin D and fluoride may be necessary especially in exclusively breast-fed infants.

By 5-6 months of age, neuromuscular control is sufficiently developed to allow the infant to sit with support and have good control of head and neck. At this stage of development, the infant "will be able to indicate desire for food by opening the mouth and leaning forward, and to indicate disinterest or satiety by leaning back and turning away."[50]

2. What foods do I offer first?

Because infant requirements for iron are high, the most common recommendation for a baby's first supplemental food is iron-fortified infant cereal. Rice cereal is a popular first choice because of its low allergenic potential. Oatmeal and barley cereals can be introduced after rice cereal is accepted by the baby.

Finely pureed, single-ingredient vegetables and fruits are usually given after the baby is familiar with cereals. Offering a wide variety of plain vegetables and fruits engenders healthy eating habits. Pureed meats may also be offered along with cereal, vegetables and fruits.

After single-ingredient foods are accepted, combination foods are the next step. Iron-fortified, mixed grain cereals can be added to the baby's diet. Mixed vegetables and vegetable-meat combinations offer variety to the vegetable portion of a meal. Mixed fruit juices and pureed mixed fruits widen the selection of vitamin C-fortified fruit choices. Casserole-type combinations of meat, vegetables and cereals, when served with milk, provide main course dishes with an appropriate balance of protein, carbohydrates and fats.

When the baby begins to make chewing motions (lateral movements of the jaw), chewing practice and development can be encouraged with a variety of increasingly more textured foods. The gradual replacement of pureed foods with more adult-type food textures and consistencies continues through the child's first two years. Iron-fortified infant cereals are recommended as a reliable source of dietary iron through two years of age.

3. How do I feed supplemental foods?

New foods should be introduced gradually to allow the baby time to accept them and to help identify foods causing sensitivity or reaction. New foods are, therefore, added one at a time, in small amounts, and continued for three or four days before adding another food.

Two or three small spoonfuls of food give the baby the experience of a new taste and texture. Feeding the new food for three or four days allows the baby to become familiar with the food, and any food sensitivities (rash, diarrhea, vomiting) can be easily identified with the offending food.

Baby food should never be diluted and fed from a bottle. Babies may choke on food or thick liquids sucked through a nipple. Foods should be offered to a baby from a small feeding spoon.

REFERENCES

1. Cone TE Jr. History of American Pediatrics. Boston, Little, Brown, 1979;147.

2. Cone TE Jr. History of American Pediatrics. Boston, Little, Brown, 1979;146.
3. Cone TE Jr. History of American Pediatrics. Boston, Little, Brown, 1979;145.
4. Storey M, Brown JE. Do young children instinctively know what to eat? N Engl J Med 1987;316:103–106.
5. Sackett WW Jr. Use of solid foods early in infancy. GP 1956;14:98–102.
6. May EC. The Canning Clan. New York, Macmillan, 1937;304.
7. May EC. The Canning Clan. New York, Macmillan, 1937;1–2.
8. Gerber Products Company. History of the Fremont Canning Company and Gerber Products Company 1901–1984 prepared by Sidney C. Brooks. Fremont, MI, GPC, 1985.
9. Cone TE Jr. History of American Pediatrics. Boston, Little, Brown, 1979;159.
10. Cone TE Jr. 200 Years of Feeding Infants in America. Columbus, OH, Ross Laboratories, 1976.
11. American Dietetic Association. Lydia J. Roberts Award Essays. Chicago, ADA, 1968.
12. Gerber Products Company. Story of an Idea. Fremont, MI, GPC, 1953.
13. Committee on Nutrition, American Academy of Pediatrics. On the feeding of solid foods to infants. Pediatrics 1958; 21:685–692.
14. Committee on Nutrition, American Academy of Pediatrics. Iron supplementation for infants. Pediatrics 1976;58:765–768.
15. Committee on Nutrition, American Academy of Pediatrics. Vitamin and mineral supplement needs in normal children in the United States. Pediatrics 1980;66:1015–1021.
16. Committee on Nutrition, American Academy of Pediatrics. Fluoride as a nutrient. Pediatrics 1972;49:456–460.
17. Committee on Nutrition, American Academy of Pediatrics. Fluoride supplementation. Pediatrics 1986;77:758,761.
18. World Health Organization. Joint WHO/UNICEF Meeting on Infant and Young Child Feeding, Geneva, WHO, 1979;15.
19. White House Conference on Food, Nutrition and Health, Final Report. Washington, DC, U.S. Government Printing Office, 1969;50.
20. Tremblay A, Sevigny J, Leblanc C, Bouchard C. The reproducibility of a three-day dietary record. Nutr Res 1983;3:819–830.
21. Gerber Products Company. Gerber Infant Nutrition Survey. Fremont, MI, GPC, 1972;1986.
22. Committee on Dietary Allowances, Food and Nutrition Board. Recommended Dietary Allowances, 9th ed. Washington, DC, National Academy of Sciences, 1980;23.
23. Committee on Nutrition, American Academy of Pediatrics. Prudent life-style for children: dietary fat and cholesterol. Pediatrics 1986;78:521–525.
24. Saarinen VM, Siimes MA, Dallman PR. Iron absorption in infants: high bioavailability of breast milk iron as indicated by the entrinsic tag method of iron absorption and by the concentration of serum ferritin. 1977;91:36–39.
25. Rios E, Hunter RE, Cook JD, et al. The absorption of iron as supplements in infant cereal and infant formulas. Pediatrics 1975;55:686–693.
26. Committee on Nutrition, American Academy of Pediatrics. Iron supplementation for infants. Pediatrics 1976;58:765–768.
27. Committee on Nutrition, American Academy of Pediatrics. The use of whole cow's milk in infancy. Pediatrics 1983;72:253–255.
28. Committee on Dietary Allowances, Food and Nutrition Board. Recommended Dietary Allowances, 9th ed. Washington, DC, National Academy of Sciences, 1980;133.
29. Guthrie HA. Introductory Nutrition, 4th ed. St. Louis, C.V. Mosby Co., 1979;154–155.
30. Hambidge KM, Hambidge C, Jacobs M, Baum JD. Low levels of zinc in hair, anorexia, poor growth, and hypogeusia in children. Pediatr Res 1972;6:868–874.
31. Walravens PA, Hambidge KM. Growth of infants fed a zinc

32. Matovinovic J. Iodine. In Olson RE et al (eds): Present Knowledge in Nutrition, 5th ed. Washington, DC, The Nutrition Foundation, Inc., 1984;587–606.
33. Committee on Dietary Allowances, Food and Nutrition Board. Recommended Dietary Allowances, 9th ed. Washington, DC: National Academy of Sciences, 1980;147–150.
34. Committee on Dietary Allowances, Food and Nutrition Board. Recommended Dietary Allowances, 9th ed. Washington, DC: National Academy of Sciences, 1980;178.
35. Alexander FW, Clayton BE, Delves HT. Mineral and trace-metal balances in children receiving normal and synthetic diets. Quart J Med New Series XLIII, 1974;169:89–111.
36. Darrow DC, Cooke RE, Segar WE. Water and electrolyte metabolism in infants fed cow's milk mixtures during heat stress. Pediatrics 1954;14:602–617.
37. Fomon SJ. Infant Nutrition, 2nd ed. Philadelphia, W.B. Saunders, 1974;371.
38. Silver HK, Kempe CH, Bruyn HB. Handbook of Pediatrics, 9th ed. Los Altos, CA, Lange Medical Publications, 1971;53.
39. Filer LJ Jr. Comments on the Safety of MSG. Washington, DC, National Academy of Sciences, 1970.
40. Subcommittee on Safety and Suitability of MSG and Other Substances in Baby Foods, Food Protection Committee, Food and Nutrition Board, National Research Council. Safety and Suitability of Salt for Use in Baby Foods. Washington, DC, National Academy of Sciences, 1970.
41. Subcommittee on Safety and Suitability of MSG and Other Substances in Baby Foods, Food Protection Committee, Food and Nutrition Board, National Research Council. Safety and Suitability of Modified Starches for Use in Baby Foods. Washington, DC, National Academy of Sciences, 1970.
42. Grocery Manufacturers of America. Compendium of Papers Compiled by Members of the GMA Technical Committee for Food Protection and Members of the GMA Legal Committee on the Proposed Panel Recommendations of the White House Conference on Food, Nutrition and Health. Washington, DC, GMA, 1970; part 1, p. 58.
43. Dahl LK, Heine M, Tassinari L. High salt content of Western infant's diet: possible relationship to hypertension in the adult. Nature 1963;199:1204.
44. Subcommittee on Safety and Suitability of MSG and Other Substances in Baby Foods, Food Protection Committee, Food and Nutrition Board, National Research Council. Safety and Suitability of Salt for Use in Baby Foods. Washington, DC, National Academy of Sciences, 1970;11.
45. Committee on Nutrition, American Academy of Pediatrics. Sodium Intake by Infants in the United States, FDA Contract No. 223-76-2091. Chicago, American Academy of Pediatrics, 1979.
46. Whitten CF, Stewart RA. The effect of dietary sodium in infancy on blood pressure and related factors. Acta Paediatr Scand 1980;Suppl. 279.
47. Subcommittee on Safety and Suitability of MSG and Other Substances in Baby Foods, Food Protection Committee, Food and Nutrition Board, National Research Council. Safety and Suitability of Modified Starches for Use in Baby Foods. Washington, DC, National Academy of Sciences, 1970;22.
48. Life Sciences Research Office. Evaluation of the Health Aspects of Starch and Modified Starches as Food Ingredients (SCOGS-115), FDA Contract No. 223-75-2004. Bethesda, MD: Federation of American Societies for Experimental Biology, 1979;64.
49. Committee on Nutrition, American Academy of Pediatrics. On the feeding of supplemental foods to infants. Pediatrics 1980;65:1178–1181.
50. Fomon SJ, Filer LJ Jr, Anderson TA, Ziegler EE. Recommendations for feeding normal infants. Pediatrics 1979;63:52–59.
51. Filer LF Jr: Modified food starch: An update. J Am Dietet Assoc (in press).

Appendix

At the suggestion of several of authors in this book, the following table of current infant formulas available in the United States is provided. Serious consideration was given to including nutritional information on representative formulas manufactured outside of the United States as well. However, it became apparent that choosing fairly such formulas would be an impossible task in view of the hundreds available from different companies compounded by the variations on these imposed by the varying regulations of different countries. This table is meant to include formulas manufactured in the United States and designed for term and preterm infants. Also included are special formulas designed for the management of allergy and carbohydrate intolerance, as well as the additional needs of premature infants being fed mothers' milk. The many special formulas designed for infants with inborn errors of metabolism have not been included in this table.

Every attempt has been made to provide the current (1988) nutrient contents of the formulas listed. However, improvements are constantly under development as new medical knowledge and technology become available. Consult the formula manufacturer directly for the most current nutrient contents of any specific formula.

Abbreviations and conventions used include the following: form = formula, am. acids = amino acids, MCT = medium chain triglycerides, PUFA = polyunsaturated fatty acids, HOSO = high oleic safflower oil, coc = coconut, lact = lactose, gluc = glucose, syr = syrup, sucr = sucrose, tap = tapioca, intol = intolerance, ERSL = estimated renal solute load, PRSL = potential renal solute load, P = powder (in caloric density row labelled kcal/oz), and parentheses indicate a product concentration which is available only in the hospital setting. Where nutrient levels in parenthetical or bracketed product forms deviate from the usual amounts for that product, these levels are shown in corresponding parentheses or brackets. The vitamin E:PUFA ratio is calculated as the number of IU of vitamin E per gram of total polyunsaturated fatty acids. The estimated renal solute load is calculated as the grams of protein $\times 4$ + the mmoles of sodium + potassium + chloride in 100 kcal of formula. The potential renal solute load (which applies to premature infants) is calculated as the grams of protein/0.175 + mmoles of sodium + potassium + chloride + phosphorus in each 100 kcal of formula. The osmolarity is expressed as the mosmoles present in 100 kcal formula prepared at standard dilutions. For complex modular formula, the values given are the nutrients provided by the product in each 100 calories of final formula when made to the recommended caloric density with the appropriate additive as directed.

NUTRIENT CONTENT OF INFANT FORMULAS (units per 100 kcal)

		——————— Routine Cow Milk Based Formulas ———————			
Manufacturer	Mother	Mead Johnson	Ross	Wyeth	Ross
Product	Human milk	Enfamil	PM 60/40	S.M.A.	Similac
kcal/oz	21.3	[P],(13),20,(24),40	P,(20)	P,(13),20,(24,27),40	[P],(13),20,(24,27),40
Protein,gm	1.46	2.20	2.22,(2.34)	2.20	2.22,(2.71)
whey:casein	70:30	60:40	60:40	60:40	18:82
source	human milk	cow whey + milk	cow whey + caseinate	cow whey + milk	cow milk
Fat,gm	5.42	5.60	5.59,(5.56)	5.30	5.37,(5.27)
linoleic acid,mg	540.00	1460.00	1300.00	500.00	1300.00
E:PUFA, IU/gm	0.49	1.90	1.47,(1.6)	2.00	[1.56],1.60
polyunsat:saturated	0.32	0.63	0.62,(0.76)	0.32	[0.61],0.82
MCT added,% fat					
source	human milk	coconut + [corn] soy	corn(soy) + coconut	oleo + coconut + HOSO + soy	[corn]soy + coconut
Carbohydrate,gm	10.00	10.30	10.20	10.60	10.70
source	lactose	lactose	lactose	lactose	lactose
Vitamin A,IU	310.00	310.00	300.00	300.00	300.00
Vitamin D,IU	3.05	62.00	60.00	60.00	60.00
Vitamin E,IU	0.32	3.10	2.5,(3.0)	1.40	[2.5],3.00
Vitamin K,µg	0.29	8.60	8.00	8.00	8.00
Thiamin,µg	29.17	78.00	100.00	100.00	100.00
Riboflavin,µg	48.61	156.00	150.00	150.00	150.00
Pyridoxine,µg	28.50	62.00	60.00	62.50	60.00
Cyanocobalamin,µg	0.07	0.23	0.25	0.20	0.25
Niacin,µg	208.00	1250.00	1050.00	750.00	1050.00
Folic acid,µg	6.94	15.60	15.00	7.50	15.00
Pantothenic acid,µg	250.00	470.00	450.00	315.00	450.00
Biotin,µg	0.56	2.30	4.50	2.20	4.40
Vitamin C,mg	5.56	8.60	9.00	8.50	9.00
Choline,mg	12.50	15.60	12.00	15.00	16.00
Inositol,mg		4.70	24.00	4.70	4.70
Taurine,mg	5.56	5.90	6.70	5.90	6.70
Calcium,mg	38.89	69.00	56.00	63.00	75.00,(90.00)
Phosphorus,mg	19.44	47.00	28.00	42.00	58.00,(70.00)
calcium:phosphorus	2:1	1.5:1	2:1	1.5:1	1.3:1
Magnesium,mg	4.86	7.80	6.00	7.00	6.00,(7.00)
Iron,mg	0.04	0.16,1.88	0.22	0.2,1.8	0.22,1.8
Zinc,mg	0.17	0.78	0.75	0.80	0.75
Manganese,µg	0.08	15.60	5.00	22.00	5.00
Copper,µg	35.00	94.00	90.00	70.00	90.00
Iodine,µg	15.28	10.20	6.00	9.00	15.00
Sodium,mg	25.00	27.00	24.00	22.00	32.00
Potassium,mg	73.00	108.00	86.00	83.00	120.00
Chloride,mg	58.00	62.00	59.00	55.50	75.00
ERSL,mOsm	10.43	14.49	13.79,(14.27)	13.45	15.46,(17.42)
Osmolarity,mOsm	40.00	40.00	38.50	40.00	abt. 38.00
Primary indication	term infants	term infants	infants needing low minerals	term infants	term infants

NUTRIENT CONTENT OF INFANT FORMULAS (units per 100 kcal)

	Premature Infant Formulations			
Manufacturer	Mead Johnson	Ross	Wyeth	Ross
Product	Enfamil Premature Form	Similac Special Care	S.M.A. Preemie	Similac LBW
kcal/oz	20,(24)	(20),(24)	(24)	(24)
Protein,gm	3.00	2.71	2.40	2.71
whey:casein	60:40	60:40	60:40	18:82
source	cow whey + milk	cow whey + caseinate	cow whey + milk	cow milk
Fat,gm	5.10	5.43	5.40	5.53
linoleic acid,mg	1070.00	700.00	500.00	720.00
E:PUFA, IU/gm	3.93	4.00	2.38	3.33
polyunsat:saturated	0.35	0.32	0.32	0.24
MCT added,% fat	40.00	50.00	10.00	
source	coconut + soy + MCT	coconut + soy + MCT	oleo + coc + HOSO + soy + MCT	soy + coconut + MCT
Carbohydrate,gm	11.00	10.60	10.50	10.50
source	lact + gluc oligomers	lact + gluc oligomers	lact + gluc oligomers	lact + gluc oligomers
Vitamin A,IU	1200.00	680.00	300.00	300.00
Vitamin D,IU	330.00	150.00	60.00	60.00
Vitamin E,IU	4.60	4.00	1.90	3.00
Vitamin K,μg	13.00	12.00	8.60	8.00
Thiamin,μg	250.00	250.00	100.00	125.00
Riboflavin,μg	350.00	620.00	160.00	150.00
Pyridoxine,μg	250.00	250.00	60.00	60.00
Cyanocobalamin,μg	0.30	0.55	0.30	0.25
Niacin,μg	4000.00	5000.00	750.00	1050.00
Folic acid,μg	35.00	37.00	12.50	15.00
Pantothenic acid,μg	1200.00	1900.00	450.00	450.00
Biotin,μg	2.30	37.00	2.20	4.40
Vitamin C,mg	35.00	37.00	8.60	12.00
Choline,mg	15.60	10.00	16.00	16.00
Inositol,mg	4.70	5.50	4.00	4.70
Taurine,mg	6.00	6.70	6.00	6.70
Calcium,mg	117.00	180.00	90.00	90.00
Phosphorus,mg	59.00	90.00	50.00	70.00
calcium:phosphorus	2:1	2:1	1.8:1	1.3:1
Magnesium,mg	4.90	12.00	8.60	10.00
Iron,mg	0.25	0.37	0.38	0.37
Zinc,mg	1.00	1.50	1.00	1.00
Manganese,μg	13.00	12.00	25.00	5.00
Copper,μg	160.00	250.00	86.00	100.00
Iodine,μg	7.90	6.00	10.00	15.00
Sodium,mg	39.00	50.00	40.00	44.00
Potassium,mg	111.00	140.00	90.00	150.00
Chloride, mg	85.00	90.00	66.00	110.00
PRSL,mOsm	26.49	27.14	21.10	27.06
Osmolarity,mOsm	32.00	32.00	30.20	32.00
Primary indication	preterm infants	preterm infants	preterm infants	preterm infants

NUTRIENT CONTENT OF INFANT FORMULAS (units per 100 kcal)

	Soy Protein Formulations					
Manufacturer	Mead Johnson	Ross	Ross	Wyeth	Loma Linda	Loma Linda
Product	ProSobee	Isomil	Isomil SF	Nursoy	Soyalac	i-Soyalac
kcal/oz	P,20,40	P,20,40	20,40	20,40	20,40	20,40
Protein,gm	3.00	2.66	2.66	3.10	3.10	3.10
whey:casein						
source	soy isolate	soy isolate	soy isolate	soy isolate	soy solids	soy isolate
Fat,gm	soy	soy	soy	soy	soy	soy
	5.30	5.46	5.46	5.30	5.50	5.50
linoleic acid,mg	1000.00	1300.00	1300.00	500.00	2810.00	2810.00
E:PUFA, IU/gm	2.07	1.58	1.58	2.00	0.70	0.70
polyunsat:saturated	0.52	0.82	0.82	0.32	3.67	3.67
MCT added,% fat						
source	coconut + soy	soy + coconut	soy + coconut	oleo + coc + HOSO + soy	soy	soy
Carbohydrate,gm	10.00	10.10	10.10	10.20	10.00	10.00
source	gluc oligomers	corn syrup + sucrose	gluc oligomers	sucrose	corn syr + sucr + soy	sucr + tap dextrin
Vitamin A,IU	310.00	300.00	300.00	300.00	312.00	312.00
Vitamin D,IU	62.00	60.00	60.00	60.00	62.00	62.00
Vitamin E,IU	3.10	3.00	3.00	1.40	2.30	2.40
Vitamin K,µg	15.60	15.00	15.00	15.00	7.80	7.80
Thiamin,µg	78.00	60.00	60.00	100.00	78.00	78.00
Riboflavin,µg	94.00	90.00	90.00	150.00	94.00	95.00
Pyridoxine,µg	62.00	60.00	60.00	62.50	70.00	71.00

(Continued)

NUTRIENT CONTENT OF INFANT FORMULAS (units per 100 kcal) (Continued)

	Mead Johnson ProSobee P,20,40	Ross Isomil P,20,40	Soy Protein Formulations Ross Isomil SF 20,40	Wyeth Nursoy 20,40	Loma Linda Soyalac 20,40	Loma Linda i-Soyalac 20,40
Manufacturer Product kcal/oz						
Cyanocobalamin,μg	0.31	0.45	0.45	0.30	0.31	0.31
Niacin,μg	1250.00	1350.00	1350.00	750.00	1250.00	1240.00
Folic acid,μg	15.60	15.00	15.00	7.50	23.00	24.00
Pantothenic acid,μg	470.00	750.00	750.00	450.00	469.00	473.00
Biotin,μg	7.80	4.50	4.50	5.50	9.40	9.60
Vitamin C,mg	8.10	9.00	9.00	8.50	12.00	12.00
Choline,mg	7.80	8.00	8.00	13.00	16.00	19.00
Inositol,mg	4.70	5.00	5.00	4.06	16.00	18.00
Taurine,mg	5.90	6.70	6.70	5.90	6.10	6.10
Calcium,mg	94.00	105.00	105.00	90.00	94.00	102.00
Phosphorus,mg	74.00	75.00	75.00	63.00	55.00	71.00
calcium:phosphorus	1.3:1	1.4:1	1.4:1	1.4:1	1.7:1	1.4:1
Magnesium,mg	10.90	7.50	7.50	10.00	12.00	11.00
Iron,mg	1.88	1.8	1.8	1.7	1.9	1.9
Zinc,mg	0.78	0.75	0.75	0.80	0.78	0.78
Manganese,μg	31.00	30.00	30.00	30.00	156.00	47.00
Copper,μg	94.00	75.00	75.00	70.00	78.00	117.00
Iodine,μg	10.20	15.00	15.00	9.00	7.80	7.80
Sodium,mg	43.00	47.00	47.00	30.00	42.00	42.00
Potassium,mg	116.00	140.00	140.00	105.00	117.00	117.00
Chloride,mg	81.00	65.00	65.00	56.00	65.00	78.00
ERSL,mOsm	19.13	18.10	18.10	17.97	19.00	19.40
Osmolarity,mOsm	26.50	34.00	20.71	39.10	32.00	36.20
Primary indication	term infants cow milk intol lactose intol sucrose intol	term infants cow milk intol lactose intol	term infants cow milk intol lactose intol sucrose intol	term infants cow milk intol lactose intol	term infants cow milk intol lactose intol	term infants cow milk intol lactose intol corn sensitivity

NUTRIENT CONTENT OF INFANT FORMULAS (units per 100 kcal)

	Complete Special Formulas			Complex Modular Formulas: Nutrients Provided by Product per 100 Cal*				
Manufacturer	Mead Johnson Portagen	Mead Johnson Nutramigen	Mead Johnson Pregestimil	Mead Johnson Mono-/Di-Saccharide Free Diet Powder	Ross RCF	Mead Johnson Protein Free Diet Powder	Mead Johnson Enfamil Human Milk Fortifier,(P)	Ross Similac Natural Care (24)
Product kcal/oz	P	P,20	P		24		1 pkg/25 ml human milk	1:1 with human milk
Protein,gm	3.50	2.80	2.80	2.80	2.96	0.00	1.03	1.35
whey:casein	0:100	hydrolysate	hydrolysate	hydrolysate + am. acids	soy isolate		60:40	60:40
source	sodium caseinate	casein hydrolysate	casein hydrolysate	casein hyd. + am. acids	soy		cow whey + milk	cow whey + milk
Fat,gm	4.80	3.90	4.10	4.20	5.33	3.90	trace	2.72
linoleic acid,mg	390.00	2000.00	1360.00	391.00	2170.00	2300.00	350.00	350.00
E:PUFA, IU/gm	8.00	1.35	1.60	9.60	1.56	0.67	4.00	4.00
polyunsat:saturated	2.8	4.5	4	3.7	0.91	4.5		0.32
MCT added,% fat	86.00		42.00	85.00				
source	corn + MCT	corn	corn + MCT	corn + MCT	soy + coconut	corn	milk	corn + soy + MCT
Carbohydrate,gm	11.50	13.40	13.50	4.20	0.00	12.50	4.00	5.30
source	gluc oligomers + sucr	gluc olig + mod tapioc	gluc olig + mod tapioc	modified tapioca		gluc olig + mod tapioc	lact + gluc oligomers	lact + gluc oligomers
Vitamin A,IU	780.00	310.00	310.00	375.00	300.00	250.00	1150.00	340.00
Vitamin D,IU	78.00	62.00	62.00	75.00	60.00	62.00	380.00	75.00
Vitamin E,IU	3.10	3.10	2.30	3.75	3.00	1.60	5.00	2.00
Vitamin K,µg	15.60	15.60	15.60	18.80	15.00	15.60	13.40	6.00
Thiamin,µg	160.00	78.00	78.00	78.00	60.00	78.00	275.00	125.00
Riboflavin,µg	190.00	94.00	94.00	94.00	90.00	94.00	368.00	310.00
Pyridoxine,µg	200.00	62.00	62.00	63.00	60.00	63.00	284.00	125.00

(Continued)

NUTRIENT CONTENT OF INFANT FORMULAS (units per 100 kcal) (Continued)

	Complete Special Formulations			Complex Modular Formulas: Nutrients Provided by Product per 100 Cal*				
Manufacturer Product	Mead Johnson Portagen	Mead Johnson Nutramigen	Mead Johnson Pregestimil	Mead Johnson Mono-/Di-Saccharide Free Diet Powder	Ross RCF	Mead Johnson Protein Free Diet Powder	Mead Johnson Enfamil Human Milk Fortifier,(P)	Ross Similac Natural Care (24)
kcal/oz	P	P,20	P		24		1 pkg/25 ml human milk	1:1 with human milk
Cyanocobalamin,µg	0.62	0.31	0.31	0.31	0.45	0.31	0.31	0.28
Niacin,µg	2000.00	1250.00	1250.00	1250.00	1350.00	1250.00	4560.00	2500.00
Folic acid,µg	15.60	15.60	15.60	15.60	15.00	15.60	34.00	18.50
Pantothenic acid,µg	1040.00	470.00	470.00	470.00	750.00	470.00	1160.00	950.00
Biotin,µg	7.80	7.80	7.80	7.80	4.50	7.80	1.20	
Vitamin C,mg	8.10	8.10	8.10	11.70	9.00	7.80	35.00	18.50
Choline,mg	13.00	13.30	13.30	13.30	8.00	13.10		
Inositol,mg		4.70	4.70	4.70	5.00	4.70		
Taurine,mg		5.90	5.90	7.80	6.70			3.35
Calcium,mg	94.00	94.00	94.00	94.00	105.00	94.00	88.00	105.00
Phosphorus,mg	70.00	62.00	62.00	62.00	75.00	52.00	49.00	52.50
calcium:phosphorus	1.3:1	1.5:1	1.5:1	1.5:1	1.4:1	1.8:1	1.8:1	2:1
Magnesium,mg	20.00	10.90	10.90	10.90	7.50	10.90		6.00
Iron,mg	1.88	1.88	1.88	1.88	0.25	1.88		0.185
Zinc,mg	0.94	0.78	0.62	0.63	0.75	0.62	0.46	0.75
Manganese,µg	120.00	31.00	31.00	31.00	30.00	16.00	13.20	6.00
Copper,µg	160.00	94.00	94.00	94.00	75.00	94.00	118.00	125.00
Iodine,µg	7.00	7.00	7.00	7.00	15.00	7.00		10.00
Sodium,mg	47.00	47.00	47.00	43.00	48.00	13.00	10.30	25.00
Potassium,mg	125.00	109.00	109.00	109.00	115.00	59.00	23.00	70.00
Chloride,mg	86.00	86.00	86.00	86.00	88.00	23.00	26.00	45.00
ERSL,mOsm	21.67	18.46	18.46	18.29	19.35	2.73	9.41	13.78
Osmolarity,mOsm	22.00	42.60	45.60	36.30	14.80	37.60	8.00	17.50
Primary indication	fat malabsorption	any protein intol disaccharide intol	moderate malabsorb any protein intol disaccharide intol	severe malabsorption (protein, fat and/or carbohydrate) (add carbohydrate)	carboydrate malabs. (add carbohydrate)	amino acid intol (add amino acids or protein)	preterm infants	preterm infants

*When made to recommended caloric density with appropriate additive as directed.

Index